THE CLINICAL SCIENCE OF NEUROLOGIC REHABILITATION

SECOND EDITION

CONTEMPORARY NEUROLOGY SERIES

THE CLINICAL SCIENCE OF NEUROLOGIC REHABILITATION

SECOND EDITION

BRUCE H. DOBKIN, M.D.
Professor of Neurology
Medical Director
Neurologic Rehabilitation and Research Program
University of California Los Angeles, School of Medicine
UCLA Medical Center

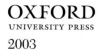
UNIVERSITY PRESS
2003

OXFORD
UNIVERSITY PRESS

Oxford   New York
Auckland   Bangkok   Buenos Aires   Cape Town   Chennai
Dar es Salaam   Delhi   Hong Kong   Istanbul   Karachi   Kolkata
Kuala Lumpur   Madrid   Melbourne   Mexico City   Mumbai
Nairobi   São Paulo   Shanghai   Taipei   Tokyo   Toronto

Copyright © 2003 by Oxford University Press, Inc.

Published by Oxford University Press, Inc.
198 Madison Avenue, New York, New York, 10016
http://www.oup-usa.org

Oxford is a registered trademark of Oxford University Press

Library of Congress Cataloging-in-Publication Data
Dobkin, Bruce H.
The clinical science of neurologic rehabilitation /
Bruce H. Dobkin.—2nd ed.
p. ; cm. — (Contemporary neurology series ; 67)
Rev. ed. of: Neurologic rehabilitation /
Bruce H. Dobkin, c1996.
Includes bibliographical references and index.
ISBN 0-19-515064-3
1. Nervous system—Diseases—Patients—Rehabilitation.
I. Dobkin, Bruce H.
Neurologic rehabilitation. II. Title. III. Series.
[DNLM: 1. Nervous System Disease—rehabilitation.
2. Brain Injuries—rehabilitation.
3. Spinal Cord Injuries—rehabilitation.
WL 140 D633c 2003]   RC350.4 .D63 2003   616.8'043—dc21   2002070037

The science of medicine is a rapidly changing field. As new research and clinical experience broaden our knowledge, changes in treatment and drug therapy do occur. The author and publisher of this work have checked with sources believed to be reliable in their efforts to provide information that is accurate and complete, and in accordance with the standards accepted at the time of publication. However, in light of the possibility of human error or changes in the practice of medicine, neither the author, nor the publisher, nor any other party who has been involved in the preparation or publication of this work warrants that the information contained herein is in every respect accurate or copmlete. Readers are encouraged to confirm the information contained herein with other reliable sources, and are strongly advised to check the product information sheet provided by the pharmaceutical company for each drug they plan to administer.

9 8 7 6 5 4 3 2 1
Printed in the United States of America
on acid-free paper

We shall not cease from exploration
And the end of all our exploring
Will be to arrive where we started
And know the place for the first time.
    T.S. Elliot, "Little Gidding" in *Four Quartets*

"Do we ever have enough information to be pessimistic?"
    In the days and years following his traumatic spinal cord injury.
    Craig H. Dobkin, experiential educator

"What's the purpose of life? We are the audience of the universe. Our job is
    to enjoy it, do what we do best, and leave it a better place."
    In the months following his stroke.
    Ray Bradbury, storyteller, playwright, futurist

Preface

The first generation of rehabilitation interventions for patients disabled by neurologic diseases has passed. It was kicked off by the need to manage victims of polio and war injuries in the middle of the last century. The surge in disabled survivors led to the disciplines of physical, occupational, and speech therapy, to physicians with expertise in acute and chronic care, to dedicated rehabilitation units, and to government funding for these activities. The second generation of rehabilitation interventions started in the mid-1980s, when both medicine and healthcare insurers asked for evidence-based practices. Clinicians began to look for the scientific bases of their interventions, developed reliable and valid assessment and outcome measures, and best of all, became less defensive about their practices. The rehabilitation community appropriated the same theme song: "How do we know what we do is better than something else?"

We are on the brink of embracing the third generation of rehabilitation interventions. This generation of thinkers and doers will draw upon the data from neuroscience and engineering to harness the physiology of the nervous system and to modulate its function after injury. This new generation may implant neurons, regrow axons, and use the brain to control prostheses. The potential utility of these interventions will still depend on the ability of rehabilitationists to engage and train cerebral and spinal networks to lessen impairments and disability.

Some cacophony accompanies my attempt to draw together a text that blends what has been done, what is being done, and what could be done to best manage our patients. Themes of neurologic disability provide the bass line, sometimes subordinated to the melodies of cerebral geography and neuroscientific notes. The literature is silent, ambivalent, or at odds too often. So I take the prerogative of the composer to play fortissimo when struck by excellence or by mediocrity. If we do not stop playing the easiest rhythms to manage patients, if we do not better prepare ourselves for the chords of the near future, then those who practice neurologic rehabilitation will be heard pianissimo.

The name of this second edition of my book, *Neurologic Rehabilitation*, has been changed to *The Clinical Science of Neurologic Rehabilitation*. The title reflects my sense that fundamental research now drives the field of neurologic rehabilitation even more than it could in 1996. The need for a second edition has arisen from the fine work of creative researchers around the world. Theorists and experimentalists have designed and carried out more insightful studies in the past 6 years than at any time in the history of neurologic rehabilitation.

The text continues to cover the basics about what we do and what we ought to attempt to do to limit the disabilities of our patients. The book continues to challenge the reader's imagination by emphasizing neuroscientific information that can be wedded to the themes that run through the practices of neurologic rehabilitation. This book does not talk down. It calls for readers to compose a piece that will merge the scientist's biologic approaches with the clinician's experienced hands.

As I wrote in the preface to the first edition, I have marked arbitrary borders in this survey of the concerns, practices, and scientific grounding of the rehabilitation specialists who care for people with diseases and injuries of the nervous system. The boundaries are Imaginot Lines. The book encompasses sites from clinical and basic science research that underpin present and future efforts in neurorestoration. I especially emphasize studies about how we learn skills and gather knowledge, which are the essences of rehabilitation practices. The growing body of neuroscientific knowledge regarding motor control, motor learning, sensorimotor integration, and cognitive processing challenges us to consider how we may provide patients with the best of all possible interventions. I emphasize the good clinical trials that have tested interventions. I place special emphasis on neuroimaging. Functional imaging, done properly, offers an especially robust physiologic marker to assess mechanisms of gains after brain injury. By revealing network and representational plasticity, imaging helps us understand how physical, cognitive, pharmacologic, and biologic interventions affect the functional anatomy of the brain and spinal cord.

The book appropriates some of the property of disciplines such as neuroanatomy and neurophysiology, developmental neurobiology, neuropharmacology, kinesiology and biomechanics, muscle physiology, cognitive psychology, the physics of neuroimaging, and bioengineering. These mutable boundaries of knowledge are expanding at a dizzying rate, especially in the neurosciences relevant to recovery.

Only one surveyor writes over this landscape. I have been influenced and intrigued over the last 20 years by my own experiences in research and practice related to neurologic rehabilitation at the University of California Los Angeles, by the researchers referenced in these chapters, and by many others who cannot be acknowledged in a short volume. So personal biases and space restrictions will set the final Imaginot Line for this book. That should not limit the reader's imagination about the rich future of neurologic rehabilitation. This text aims to encourage physicians, therapists, and clinical scientists to push their personal boundaries toward sound interventions that merge basic and clinical research with the practical arts of therapy.

Los Angeles, California   B.D.
bdobkin@mednet.ucla.edu

Contents

PART **I**

NEUROSCIENTIFIC FOUNDATIONS FOR REHABILITATION

Chapter 1

Organizational Plasticity in Sensorimotor and Cognitive Networks

Function follows structure. The central (CNS) and peripheral (PNS) nervous system matrix is a rich resource for learning and for retraining. This chapter begins with the structural framework of interconnected neural components that contribute to motor control for walking, reaching, and grasping, and to cognition and mood. I then review what we know about cellular mechanisms that may be manipulated by physical, cognitive, and pharmacologic therapies to lessen impairments and disabilities. These discussions of functional neuroanatomy provide a map for mechanisms relevant to neural repair, functional neuroimaging, and theory-based practices for neurologic rehabilitation.

Injuries and diseases of the brain and spinal cord damage clusters of neurons and disconnect their feedforward and feedback projections. The victims of neurologic disorders often improve, however. Mechanisms of activity-dependent learning within spared modules of like-acting neurons are a fundamental property of the neurobiology of functional gains. Rehabilitation strategies can aim to manipulate the molecules, cells, and synapses of networks that learn to represent some of what has been lost. This plasticity may be no different than what occurs during early development, when a new physiologic organization emerges from intrinsic drives on the properties of neurons and their synapses. Similar mechanisms drive how living creatures learn new skills and abilities.

3

Activity-dependent plasticity after a CNS or PNS lesion, however, may produce mutability that aids patients or mutagenic physiology that impedes functional gains.

Our understanding of functional neuroanatomy is a humbling work in progress. Although neuroanatomy and neuropathology may seem like old arts, studies of nonhuman primates and of man continue to reveal the connections and interactions of neurons. The brain's macrostructure is better understood than the microstructure of the connections between neurons. It is just possible to imagine that we will grasp the design principles of the 100,000 neurons and their glial supports within 1 mm^3 of cortex, but almost impossible to look forward to explaining the activities of the 10 billion cortical neurons that make some 60 trillion synapses.[1] Aside from the glia that play an important role in synaptic function, each cubic millimeter of gray matter contains 3 km of axon and each cubic millimeter of white matter includes 9 meters of axon. The tedious work of understanding the dynamic interplay of this matrix is driven by new histochemical approaches that can label cells and their projections, by electrical microstimulation of small ensembles of neurons, by physiological recordings from single cells and small groups of neurons, by molecular analyses that localize and quantify neurotransmitters, receptors and gene products, and by comparisons with the architecture of human and nonhuman cortical neurons and fiber arrangements.

Functional neuroimaging techniques, such as positron emission tomography (PET), functional magnetic resonance imaging (fMRI), and transcranial magnetic stimulation (TMS) allow comparisons between the findings from animal research and the functional neuroanatomy of people with and without CNS lesions. These computerized techniques offer insights into where the coactive assemblies of neurons lie as they simultaneously, in parallel and in series, process information that allows thought and behavior. Neuroimaging has both promise and limitations (see Chapter 3).

What neuroscientists have established about the molecular and morphologic bases for learning motor and cognitive skills has become more critical for rehabilitationists to understand. Neuroscientific insights relevant to the restitution of function can be appreciated at all the main levels of organization of the nervous system, from behavioral systems to interregional and local circuits, to neurons and their dendritic trees and spines, to microcircuits on axons and dendrites, and most importantly, to synapses and their molecules and ions. Experience and practice lead to adaptations at all levels. Knowledge of mechanisms of this activity-dependent plasticity may lead to the design of better sensorimotor, cognitive, pharmacologic, and biologic interventions to enhance gains after stroke, traumatic brain and spinal cord injury, multiple sclerosis, and other diseases.

SENSORIMOTOR NETWORKS

Motor control is tied, especially in the rehabilitation setting, to learning skills. Motor skills are gained primarily through the cerebral organization for procedural memory. The other large classification of memory, declarative knowledge, depends upon hippocampal activity. The first is about how to, the latter is the what of facts and events. Procedural knowledge, compared to learning facts, usually takes considerable practice over time. Skills learning is also associated with experience-specific organizational changes within the sensorimotor network for motor control. A model of motor control, then, needs to account for skills learning. To successfully manipulate the controllers of movement, the clinician needs a multilevel, 3-dimensional point of view. The vista includes a reductionist analysis, examining the properties of motor patterns generated by networks, neurons, synapses, and molecules. Our sightline also includes a synthesis that takes a systems approach to the relationships between networks and behaviors, including how motor patterns generate movements modulated by action-related sensory feedback and by cognition. The following theories, all of which bear some truth, focus on elements of motor control.

Overview of Motor Control

Mountcastle wrote, "The brain is a complex of widely and reciprocally interconnected systems," and "The dynamic interplay of neural activity within and between these systems is the very *essence* of brain function." He proposed: "The remarkable capacity for improvement of function after partial brain lesions is viewed as evidence for the adaptive capacity of such distributed systems to achieve a goal, albeit slowly and with error, with the remaining neural apparatus."[2]

A distributed system represents a collection of separate dynamic assemblies of neurons with anatomical connections and similar functional properties.[3] The operations of these assemblies are linked by their afferent and efferent messages. Signals may flow along a variety of pathways within the network. Any locus connected within the network may initiate activity, as both externally generated and internally generated signals may reenter the system. Partial lesions within the system may degrade signaling, but will not eliminate functional communication so long as dynamic reorganization is possible.

What are some of the "essences" of brain and spinal cord interplay relevant to understanding how patients reacquire the ability to move with purpose and skill?

No single theory explains the details of the controls for normal motor behavior, let alone the abnormal patterns and synergies that emerge after a lesion at any level of the neuraxis. Many models successfully predict aspects of motor performance. Some models offer both biologically plausible and behaviorally relevant handles on sensorimotor integration and motor learning. Among the difficulties faced by theorists and experimentalists is that no simple ordinary movement has only one motor control solution. Every step over ground and every reach for an item can be accomplished by many different combinations of muscle activations, joint angles, limb trajectories, velocities, accelerations, and forces. Thus, many kinematically redundant biological scripts are written into the networks for motor control. The nervous system computes within a tremendous number of degrees of freedom for any successful movement. In addition, every movement changes features of our physical relationship to our surrounds. Change requires operations in other neural networks, such as frontal lobe connections for divided attention, planning, and working memory.

Models of motor behavior have explored the properties of neurons and their connections to explain how a network of neurons generates persistent activity in response to an input of brief duration, such as seeing a baseball hit out of the batter's box, and how networks respond to changes in input to update a view of the environment for goal-directed behaviors, such as catching the baseball 400 feet away while on the run.[4] A wiring diagram for hauling in a fly ball, especially with rapidly changing weights and directions of synaptic activity, seems impossibly complex. Researchers have begun, however, to describe some clever solutions for rapid and accurate responses that evolve within interacting, dynamic systems such as the CNS.[5] Each theory contains elements that describe, physiologically or metaphorically, some of the processes of motor control. These theories lead to experimentally backed notions that help explain why rehabilitative therapies help patients.

GENERAL THEORIES OF MOTOR CONTROL

Sherrington proposed one of the first physiologically based models of motor control. Sensory information about the position and velocity of a limb moving in space rapidly feeds back information into the spinal cord about the current position and desired position, until all computed errors are corrected. Until the past decade or two, much of what physical and occupational therapists practiced was described in terms of chains of reflexes. Later, the theory expanded to include reflexes nested within Hughling Jackson's hierarchic higher, middle, and lower levels of control. Some schools of physical therapy took this model to mean that motor control derives in steps from voluntary cortical, intermediate brain stem, and reflexive spinal levels.[6] Abnormal postures and tone evolve, in the schools of Bobath and Brunnstrom (see Chapter 5), from the release of control by higher centers. These theories for physical and for occupational therapy imply that the nervous system is an elegantly wired machine that performs stereotyped computations on sensory inputs. Lower levels are subsumed under higher ones. This notion, however, is too simple. All levels of the CNS are highly integrated with feedforward and feedback interactions. Sensory inputs are critical, however.

Another theory of motor control suggests that stored central motor programs allow sensory stimuli or central commands to generate movements. Examples of stored programs include the lumbar spinal cord's central pattern generators for stepping and the cortical "rules" that allow cursive writing to be carried out equally well by one's hand, shoulder, or foot. This approach, however, needs some elaboration to explain how contingencies raised by the environment and the biomechanical characteristics of the limbs interact with stored programs or with chains of reflexes. A more elegant theory of motor control, perhaps first suggested by Bernstein in the 1960s, tried to account for how the nervous system manages the many degrees of freedom of movement at each joint.[7] He hypothesized that lower levels of the CNS control the synergistic movements of muscles. Higher levels of the brain activate these synergies in combinations for specific actions. Other theorists added a dynamical systems model to this approach. Preferred patterns of movement emerge in part from the interaction of many elements, such as the physical properties of muscles, joints, and neural connections. These elements self-organize according to their dynamic properties. This model says little about other aspects of actions, including how the environment, the properties of objects such as their shape and weight, and the demands of the task all interact with movement, perception, and experience.

Most experimental studies support the observations of Mountcastle and others that the sensorimotor system learns and performs with the overriding objective of achieving movement goals. All but the simplest motor activities are managed by neuronal clusters distributed in networks throughout the brain. The regions that contribute are not so much functionally localized as they are functionally specialized. Higher cortical levels integrate subcomponents like spinal reflexes and oscillating brain stem and spinal neural networks called pattern generators. The interaction of a dynamic cortical architecture with more automatic oscillators allows the cortex to run sensorimotor functions without directly needing to designate the moment-to-moment details of parameters such as the timing, intensity, and duration of the sequences of muscle activity among synergist, antagonist, and stabilizing muscle groups.

For certain motor acts, the motor cortex needs only to set a goal. Preset neural routines in the brain stem and spinal cord carry out the details of movements. This system accounts for how an equivalent motor act can be accomplished by differing movements, depending on the demands of the environment, prior learning, and rewarded experience. Having achieved a behavioral goal, the reinforced sensory and movement experience is learned by the motor network. Learning results from increased synaptic activity that assembles neurons into functional groups with preferred lines of communication.[8] Thus, goal-oriented learning, as opposed to mass practice of a simple and repetitive behavior, ought to find an essential place in rehabilitation strategies.

Several experimentally based models suggest how the brain may construct movements. Target-directed movements can be generated by motor commands that modulate an equilibrium point for the agonist and antagonist muscles of a joint.[9] During reaching movements, for example, the brain constructs motor commands based on its prediction of the forces the arm will experience. Some forces are external loads and need to be learned. Other forces depend on the physical properties of muscle, such as its elasticity. The computations used by neurons to compose the motor command may be broadly tuned to the velocity of movements.[10]

Using microstimulation of closely related regions of the lumbar spinal cord, Bizzi and colleagues have also defined fields of neurons in the anterior horns that store and represent specific movements within the usual workspace of a limb, called primitives.[11] Combinations of these simple flexor and extensor actions may be fashioned by supraspinal inputs into the vast variety of movements needed for reaching and walking. The motor cortex, then, determines which spinal modules to activate, along with the necessary coefficient of activation, presumably working off an internal, previously learned model of the desired movement. The representations for the movement, described later, are stored in sensorimotor and association cortex. Thus, some simplifying rules generate good approximations to the goal of the reaching or stepping movement. Systems for error detection, especially within connections to the cerebellum, simultaneously make fine adjustments to reach the object.

A variety of related concepts about neural network modeling for the generation of a reaching movement have been offered.[12,13] Much work has gone into what small groups of cortical cells in the primary motor cortex (M1) encode. The activity of these neurons may encode the direction or velocity of the hand as it moves toward a target[14] or the forces at joints or the control of mechanical properties of muscles and joints.[15] Other theories suggest how ever larger groups of neurons may interact to carry out a learned or novel action.[16,17]

Motor programs can also be conceptualized as cortical cell assemblies stored in the form of strengthened synaptic connections between pyramidal neurons and their targets, such as the basal ganglia and spinal cord for the preparation and ordered sequence of movements.[18] Indeed, multiple representations of aspects of movement are found among the primary and secondary sensorimotor cortices. The neurons of each region have interconnections and cell properties that promote some common responses, such as being tuned in a graded and preferred fashion to the direction or velocity of a reaching movement, to perceived load, and to other visual and proprioceptive information, including external stimuli such as food.[19] Many other frames of reference, such as shoulder

torques, the equilibrium points of muscle movements mentioned above, and the position of the eyes and head also elicit neuronal discharges when a hand reaches into space. As a motor skill is trained, cells in M1 adapt to the tuning properties and firing patterns of other neurons involved in the action.[20] Learning-dependent neuronal activity, in fact, has been found in experiments with monkeys with single cell recordings of neurons in all of the motor cortices. Each distributed neighborhood of neurons is responsible for a specific role in aspects of planning and directing movements. The matrix of cortical, subcortical, and spinal nodes in this network model of motor control are described later, along with some of the attributes that they represent.

Figure 1–1 diagrams anatomical nodes of the sensorimotor system, emphasizing the map for locomotor control with some of its most prominent feedforward and feedback connections. These reverberating circuits calibrate motor

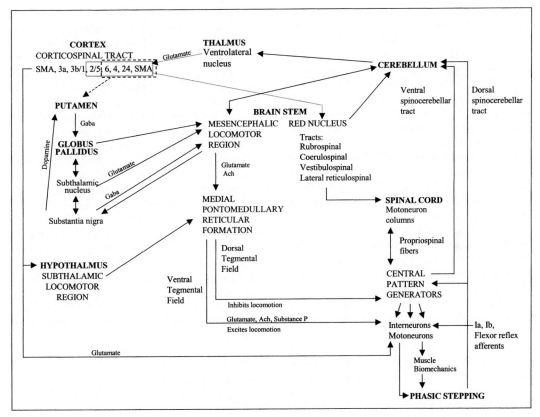

Figure 1–1. Prominent cortical, subcortical, and spinal modules and their connections within the sensorimotor networks for locomotor control.

control. Each anatomic region has its own diverse neuronal clusters with highly specified inputs and outputs. These regions reflect the distributed and parallel computations needed for movement, posture, coordination, orientation to the environment, perceptual information, drives, and goals that formulate a particular action via a large variety of movement strategies. The distributed and modular organization of the sensorimotor neurons of the brain and spinal cord provide neural substrates that arrange or represent particular patterns of movement and are highly adaptable to training.

No single unifying principle for all aspects of motor control is likely. The one certain fact that must be accounted for in theories about motor control for rehabilitation is that the nervous system, above all, learns by experience. The rehabilitation team must determine how a person best learns after a brain injury. At a cellular level, activity-dependent changes in synaptic strength are closely associated with motor learning and memory. Later in the chapter, we will examine molecular mechanisms for learning such as long-term potentiation (LTP), which may be boosted by neuropharmacologic interventions during rehabilitation. After a neurologic injury, these forms of adaptability or neural plasticity, superimposed upon the remaining intact circuits that can carry out task subroutines, can be manipulated to lessen impairments and allow functional gains.

To consider the neural adaptations needed to gain a motor skill or manage a cognitive task, I selectively review some of the anatomy, neurotransmitters, and physiology of the switches and rheostats drawn in Figure 1–1. Most of the regions emphasized can be activated by tasks performed during functional neuroimaging procedures, so rehabilitationists may be able to weigh the level of engagement of these network nodes after a brain or spinal injury and in response to specific therapies. The cartoon map of Figure 1–1 is a general road atlas. It allows the reader to scan major highways for their connections and spheres of influence. Over the time of man's evolution, these roads have changed. Over the scale of a human lifetime, built along epochs of time from milliseconds to minutes, days, months, and years, the maps of neuronal assemblies, synapses, and molecular cascades that are embedded within the cartoon map evolve, devolve, strengthen and weaken. After a CNS or PNS injury or disease, the map represents what was, but not all that is. If some of the infrastructure persists, a patient may solve motor problems by practice and by relearning.

The following discussion of structure and function takes a top-down anatomic approach, given that diseases and injuries tend to involve particular levels of the neuraxis. Within each level, but with an eye on the potential for interactive reorganization throughout the distributed controllers of the neuraxis, I select especially interesting aspects of biological adaptability within the neuronal assemblies and distributed pathways that may be called upon to improve walking in hemiparetic and paraparetic patients and to enhance the use of a paretic arm.

Cortical Motor Networks

PRIMARY MOTOR CORTEX

Neurophysiologic and functional imaging studies point to intercoordinated, functional assemblies of cells distributed throughout the neuraxis that initiate and carry out complex movements. These neuronal sensorimotor assemblies show considerable plasticity as maps of the dermatomes, muscles, and movements that they represent. In addition, they form multiple parallel systems that cooperate to manage the diverse information necessary for the rapid, precise, and yet highly flexible control of multijoint movements. This organization subsumes many of the neural adaptations that contribute to the normal learning of skills and to partial recovery after a neural injury.

The primary motor cortex (M1) in Brodmann's area (BA) 4 (Fig. 1–2), lies in the central sulcus and on the precentral gyrus. It receives direct or indirect input from the adjacent primary somatosensory cortex (S1) and receives and reciprocates direct projections to the secondary somatosensory cortex (SII), to nonprimary motor cortices including BA 24, the supplementary motor area (SMA) in BA 6, and to BA 5 and 7 in the parietal region. These links integrate the primary and nonprimary sensorimotor cortices.

Organization of the Primary Motor Cortex

The primary motor cortex has an overall somatotopic organization for the major parts of the

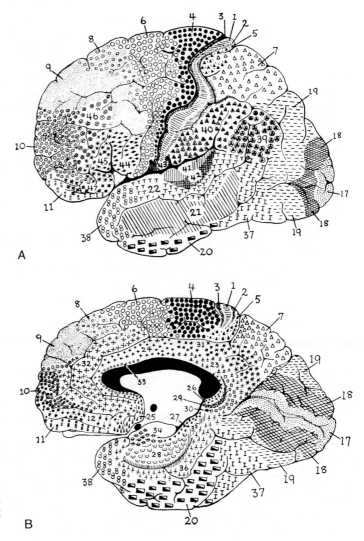

Figure 1–2. Brodmann's areas cytoarchitectural map over the (A) lateral and (B) medial surfaces of the cortex.

body, not unlike what Penfield and Rasmussen found in their cortical stimulation studies in the 1940s.[21] In addition, separable islands of cortical motoneurons intermingle to create a more complex map for movement than the neatly portrayed traditional cartoons of a human homunculus.[22] For example, M1 has separate clusters of output neurons that facilitate the activity of a single spinal motoneuron. Cortical electrostimulation mapping studies in macaques reveal a central core of wrist, digit, and intrinsic hand muscle representations surrounded by a horseshoe-shaped zone that represents the shoulder and elbow muscles. The core zones representing the distal and proximal arm are bridged by a distinct region that represents combinations of both distal and proximal muscle groups. These bridging neurons may specify multijoint synergistic movements needed for reaching and grasping.[23] This arrangement also is a structural source for modifications in the strength and distribution of connections among neurons that work together as a skill is learned. Some individual neurons overlap in their control of muscles of the wrist, elbow, and shoulder.[24,25] In addition, representations for movements of each finger overlap with other fingers and with patches of neurons for wrist actions.[26,27] They, too, are mutable controllers and a mechanism for neuroplasticity.

A single corticospinal neuron from M1 may project to the spinal motoneurons for different muscles to precisely adjust the amount of muscle coactivation.[28] Branching M1 projections, however, rarely innervate both cervical and lumbar cord motor pools. Strick and colleagues found that only 0.2% of neurons in M1 were double-labeled retrogradely in macaques from both lower cervical and lower lumbar segments, compared to 4% that were double-labeled from the upper and lower cervical segments.[29] The individual and integrated actions of multiple cortical representations to multiple spinal motoneurons reflect important aspects of motor control, as well as another anatomic basis for representational neuroplasticity.

Functional neuroimaging studies in humans performed as they make individual flexor–extensor finger movements point to overlapping somatotopic gradients in the distributed representation of each finger.[30,31] A 2–3 mm anatomical separation was found between the little finger (more medial) and the second digit (more lateral). A reasonable interpretation of the data is that the cortical territory activated by even a simple movement of any joint of the upper extremity constitutes a relatively large fraction of the representation of the total limb because representations overlap considerably.[25] This overlap is consistent with the consequences of a small stroke in clinical practice. A stroke confined to the hand region of M1 tends to affect distal joints more than proximal ones and tends to involve all fingers approximately equally (see Color Fig. 3–5 in separate color insert).

The M1 encodes specific movements and acts as an arranger that pulls movements together. The relationships of the motoneurons for representations of movements are dynamically maintained by ongoing use. Horizontal and vertical intracortical and corticocortical connections modulate the use-dependent integrations of these ensembles.[32] Intermingled functional connections among these small ensembles of neurons offer a distributed organization that provides a lot of flexibility and storage capacity for aspects of movement. These assemblies manage the coordination of multijoint actions, the velocity and direction of movements, and process the order of stimuli on which a motor response will be elicited to carry out a task.[16] The assemblies also make rapid and slow synaptic adaptations during learning.

Thus, a cortical motoneuron can activate a small field of target muscles; and an assembly of interacting motoneurons within M1 can represent the selective activation of one or more complex movements. The allocation of cortical representational space in M1 and adjacent somatosensory areas depends on the synaptic efficacy associated with prior experience among neuronal assemblies that represent a movement or skin surface. Temporally coincident inputs to the assemblies of the sensorimotor cortex during practice produce skilled synergistic, multijoint movements.[33] This arrangement is a basis for neuronal representational plasticity, which involves practice-induced fluxes in the strength of neural liaisons. This view of cortical maps, as opposed to the more rigid cartoon of the homunculus, especially makes sense when one considers that a reaching and grasping movement can incur rotations at the shoulder, elbow, wrists, and fingers with 27° of freedom using at least 50 different muscles. Many of these muscles have multijoint actions and provide postural stability for a range of different movements.[34]

Primary Motor Cortex and Hand Function

What aspects of hand movement are encoded by M1? The M1 has been described as a computational map for sensorimotor transformations, rather than a map of muscles or of particular movement patterns.[19] Its overlapping organization contributes to the control of the complex muscle synergies needed for fine coordination and forceful contractions.[35] After lesioning M1 in a monkey, the upper extremity is initially quite impaired. The hand can be retrained, however, to perform simple movements and activate single muscles. This rehabilitation leads to flexion and extension of the wrist, but the monkey cannot learn to make smooth diagonal wrist movements using muscles for flexion and radial deviation.[28] The animal accomplishes this motion only in a stepwise sequence. The M1, then, activates and inactivates muscles in a precise spatial and temporal pattern, including the controllers for fractionated finger movements. Using some clever hand posture tasks to dissociate muscle activity, direction of movement at the wrist, and the direction of movement in space, Kakei and colleagues showed that substantial numbers of neurons in M1 represent both muscles and directional movements.[36]

The primary motor cortex motoneurons have highly selective and powerful effects on the spinal motor pools to the hand, especially for the intrinsic hand muscles of primates, which includes humans, with good manipulative skills.[37] This cortical input lessens the spinal reflex and synergistic activity that better serves postural and proximal limb movements. The coding of movement patterns and forces during voluntary use of the hand relates to the coactivation of assemblies of neurons acting in parallel, not to the rate of firing of single neurons.[38] In single cortical cell recordings in M1, the burst frequency codes movement velocity and the burst duration codes the duration of the movement. Velocity correlates with the amount of muscle activation. The force exerted by muscles is a summed average of the ouput of single cells that fire at variable rates and the synchronization of assemblies of M1 neurons during specific phases of a motor task.[39] Single cell activity in the motor cortex is most intense for reaching at a particular magnitude and direction of force.[14] The direction of an upper extremity movement may be coded by the sum of the vectors of the single cell activities in motor cortex in the direction of the movement.[40]

The activity of a single corticomotoneuron can differ from the activity of an assembly of neighboring motoneurons. When a small assembly of cells becomes active, the discharge pattern of a neuron within that population may change with the task. As the active population evolves to include cells that had not previously participated or to exclude some of the cells that had been active, the assembly becomes a unique representation of different information about movement.

Thus, M1 is involved in many stages of guiding complex actions that require the coordination of at least several muscle groups. The M1 computes the location of a target, the hand trajectory, joint kinematics, and torques to reach and hold an object—the patterns of muscle activation needed to grasp the item—and relates a particular movement to other movements of the limb and body. These parameters may be manipulated by therapists during retraining functional skills. The degree to which discharges from M1 represent the extrinsic attributes of movements versus joint and muscle-centered intrinsic variables is still unclear. A remarkable study in monkeys sheds additional light.

Brief electrical microstimulation reveals a homunculus-like organization of muscle twitch representations. Longer trains lasting 500 ms, which approximates the time scale of neuronal activity during reaching and grasping, at sites in the primary motor and premotor cortex of monkeys evokes a map of complex postures featuring hand positions near the face and body. Indeed, out of over 300 stimulation sites, 85% evoked a distinct posture. The map from cortex to muscles also depends on arm position in a way that specifies a final posture. For example, when the elbow started in flexion, stimulation at one site caused it to extend to its final posture. When starting in extension, the elbow flexed to place the hand at the same position. Spontaneous movements of the hand to the mouth followed the same pattern of motion and EMG activity as stimulation-evoked movements. Thus, within the larger arm and hand representation, stimulation-evoked postures were organized across the cortex as a map of multijoint movements that positioned the hand in peripersonal space. Primary motor cortex represented particularly the space in front of the monkey's chest. Premotor cortex stimulation always included a gripping posture of the fingers when the hand-to-mouth pattern was evoked, presumably related to the action of feeding. All the evoked postures suggested typical behaviors such as feeding, a defensive movement, reaching, flinching, and others. Evoked postures were also found for the leg, in which stimulation elicited movements that converged the foot from different starting positions to a single final location within its ordinary workspace, much like what has been found with lumbar spinal cord microstimulation (see section, Spinal Sensorimotor Activity).

Functional imaging studies reveal a small activation in ipsilateral motor cortex during simple finger tapping. A study by Cramer and colleagues found a site of ipsilateral activation when the right finger taps to be shifted approximately 1 cm anterior, ventral, and lateral to the site in M1 activated by tapping the left finger.[41] This bilateral activity may be related to the uncrossed corticospinal projection, to an aspect of motor control related to bimanual actions, or to sensory feedback. The M1 in monkeys contains a subregion located between the neuronal representations for the digits and face in which approximately 8% of cells are active during ipsilateral and bilateral forelimb movements.[42] Ipsilateral activations by PET and fMRI may actually include BA 6 rather than M1, since the separation of M1 from SMA and from BA 6 is difficult enough in postmortem brains and far more unreliable in functional imaging studies.[43] Many nonprimary motor areas are also activated by simple finger movements,[44] suggesting that the same regions of the brain participate in simple and complex actions, but that the degree of activation increases with the demands of the task.

Since motoneurons in M1 participate in, or represent particular movements and contribute to unrelated movements, cells may functionally shift to take over some aspects of an impaired movement in the event a cortical or subcortical injury disconnects the primary cortical activators of spinal motoneurons. As described later in this chapter and in Chapters 2 and 3, these motor and neighboring sensory neurons adapt their synaptic relationships in remarkably flexible ways during behavioral training. Future experimental studies of the details of these computations, of the neural correlates for features of upper extremity function, and of the relationships between neuronal assemblies in distributed regions during a movement will have practical implications for neurorehabilitation training and pharmacologic interventions.

The Primary Motor Cortex and Locomotion

Supraspinal motor regions are quite active in humans during locomotion.[45,46] In electrophysiologic studies of the cat, motoneurons in M1 discharge modestly during locomotion over a flat surface under constant sensory conditions. The cells increase their discharges when a task requires more accurate foot placement, e.g., for walking along a horizontally positioned ladder, compared to overground or treadmill locomotion. Changing the trajectory of the limbs to step over obstacles also increases cortical output.[47] As expected, then, M1 is needed for precise, integrated movements.

Some pyramidal neurons of M1 reveal rhythmical activity during stepping. The cells fire especially during a visually induced perturbation

from steady walking, during either the stance or swing phase of gait as needed. These neurons may be especially important for flexor control of the leg. A pyramidal tract lesion or lesion within the leg representation after an anterior cerebral artery distribution infarct almost always affects foot dorsiflexion and, as a consequence, the gait pattern. Transcranial magnetic stimulation studies in man show greater activation of corticospinal input to the tibialis anterior muscle compared to the gastrocnemius.[48] The tibialis anterior muscle was more excitable than the gastrocnemius during the stance phase of the gait cycle in normal subjects who walked on a treadmill. This phase requires ankle dorsiflexion at heel strike (see Chapter 6). For functional neuroimaging studies of the leg, the large M1 contribution to dorsiflexion of the ankle makes ankle movements a good way to activate M1 (see Color Fig. 3–8 in separate color insert). The considerable interest in this movement within M1 also suggests that a cognitive, voluntary cueing strategy during locomotor retraining is necessary to best get foot clearance during the swing phase of gait and to practice heel strike in the initial phase of stance. The alternative strategy to flex the leg enough to clear the foot, when cortical influences have been lost, is to evoke a flexor reflex withdrawal response.

For voluntary tasks that require attention to the amount of motor activity of the ankle movers, M1 motoneurons appear equally linked to the segmental spinal motor pools of the flexors and extensors.[49] This finding suggests that the activation of M1 is coupled to the timing of spinal locomotor activity in a task-dependent fashion, but may not be an essential component of the timing aspects of walking, at least not while walking on a treadmill belt. Spinal segmental sensory inputs, described later in this chapter, may be more critical to the temporal features of leg movements during walking. The extensor muscles of the leg, such as the gastrocnemius, especially depend on polysynaptic reflexes during walking modulated by sensory feedback for their antigravity function.[50] Primary motor cortex neurons also represent the contralateral paraspinal muscles and may innervate the spinal motor pools for the bilateral abdominal muscles.[51] Potential overlapping representations between paraspinal and proximal leg muscle representations may serve as a mechanism for plasticity with gait retraining.[52]

Primary motor cortex also contains the giant pyramidal cells of Betz. These unusual cells reside exclusively in cortical layer 5. They account for no more than approximately 50,000 of the several million pyramidal neurons in each precentral gyrus. Approximately 75% supply the leg and 18% project to motor pools for the arm,[53] but Betz cells constitute only 4% of the neurons of the leg representation that are found in the corticospinal tract.[54] The Betz cells appear to be important innervators of the large, antigravity muscles for the back and legs. They phasically inhibit extension and facilitate flexion, which may be especially important for triggering motor activity for walking. Consistent with this tendency, pyramidal tract lesions tend to allow an increase in extension over flexion in the leg.

Ankle dorsiflexion and plantar flexion activate the contralateral M1, S1, and SMA in human subjects, although the degree of activity in functional imaging studies tends to be smaller than what is found with finger tapping (see Fig. 3–7). With an isometric contraction of the tibialis anterior or gastocnemius muscles, the bilateral superior parietal (BA 7) and premotor BA 6 become active during PET scanning, probably as a result of an increase in cortical control of initiation and maintenance of the contraction.[55] Greater exertion of force and speed of movement give higher activations, similar to what occurs in M1 when finger and wrist movements are made faster or with greater force. When walking on uneven surfaces and when confronted by obstacles, BA6 and 7, S1, SMA, and the cerebellum participate even more for visuomotor control, balance, and selective movements of the legs. An increase in cortical activity in moving from rather stereotyped to more skilled lower extremity movements also evolves as a hemiparetic or paraparetic person relearns to walk with a reciprocal gait (see Fig. 3–8).

NONPRIMARY MOTOR CORTICES

The premotor cortex and SMA exert what Hughlings Jackson called "the least automatic" control over voluntary motor commands. These cortical areas account for approximately 50% of the total frontal lobe motoneuron con-tribution to the corticospinal tract and have specialized functions. Each of the six cortical motor areas that interact with M1 has a separate and independent set of inputs from adjacent and remote regions, as well as parallel, separate outputs to the brain stem and spinal cord.[56] Table 1–1 gives an overview of their relative contributions to the corticospinal tract and their functional roles. These motor areas also interact with cortex that does not have direct spinal motoneuron connections. For example, although motorically silent prefrontal areas do not directly control a muscle contraction, they play a role in the initiation, selection, inhibition, and guidance of behavior by representational knowledge. They do this via somatotopically arranged prefrontal to premotor, corticostriatal, corticotectal, and thalamocortical connections.[57]

Functional imaging has revealed a somatotopic distribution of activation during upper extremity tasks in SMA, dorsal lateral premotor, and cingulate motor cortices.[58] Somatotopy in the secondary sensorimotor cortices, at least for the upper extremity, may be based on a functional, rather than an anatomical representation.[59] For example, the toe and foot have access to the motor program for the hand for cursive writing, even though the foot may never have practiced writing. An fMRI study that compared writing one's signature with the dominant index finger and ipsilateral big toe revealed that both actions activated the intraparietal sulcus and premotor cortices over the convexity in the hand representation.[59] The finding that one limb can manage a previously learned task from another limb may have implications for compensatory and retraining strategies after a focal brain injury.

Premotor Cortex

Whereas M1 mediates the more elementary aspects of the control of movements, the premotor networks encode motor acts and program defined goals by their connections with the frontal cortical representations for goal-directed, prospective, and remembered actions. BA 6 has been divided into a dorsal area, in and adjacent to the precentral and superior frontal sulcus, and a ventral area in and adjacent to the caudal bank of the arcuate sulcus at its inferior limb. In the dorsal premotor area,

Table 1–1. Some Relative Differences Between the Motor Cortices and Corticospinal Motoneurons Based on Studies of Macaques

| | | | CORTICAL AREA | | | | |
	M1	SMA	Cingulate Dorsal	Cingulate Ventral	Cingulate Rostral	Premotor Dorsal	Premotor Ventral
Total number of CS neurons:							
Forelimb (low cervical)	15,900	5200	4600	2600	2200	6100	300
Forelimb (high cervical)	10,400	5000	1900	2300	2500	7200	2300
Hindlimb (L-6–S-1)	23,900	5800	3700	2500	400	5200	6
Total frontal lobe CS projections (%)	46	15	9	7	4	17	2
Functional movement roles	Execute action	Self-initiated selection; learned sequence; Bimanual action	Movement sequence from memory		Reward-based motor selection	Visually guided reaching	Grasp by visual guidance

M1, primary motor cortex; SMA, supplementary motor area; CS, corticospinal.
Source: Adapted from data from Cheney et al., 2000.[396]

separate arm and leg representations are found along with both distal and proximal upper extremity representations.[29] In humans, the dorsal premotor region is activated by motor tasks of any complexity. The ventral premotor region, near the frontal operculum, activates with complex tasks such as motor imagery, observing another person grasping an item, and preshaping the hand to grasp an object. The ventral region has connections with the frontal eye fields and visual cortex, putting it in the middle of an action observation and eye–hand network that appears to help compensate for M1 lesions of the hand. Lesions of the ventral premotor and dorsal precentral motor areas over the lateral convexity cause proximal weakness and apraxia (see Chapter 9).

Supplementary Motor Area

Based upon PET studies in humans, the SMA includes a pre-SMA, which is anterior to a line drawn from the anterior commissure vertically up through BA 6, and the SMA proper, just caudal to this.[60] Tasks that require higher order motor control such as a new motor plan activate the pre-SMA, whereas simple motor tasks activate the caudal SMA. After an M1 lesion in the monkey, these premotor areas contribute to upper extremity movements, short of coordinated cocontractions and fractionated wrist and finger actions.[28] Lesions of the SMA cause akinesia and impaired control of bimanual and sequential movements, especially of the digits, consistent with its role in motor planning.[61]

The SMA plays a particularly intriguing role within the mosaic of anatomically connected cortical areas involved in the execution of movements. Electrical stimulation of the SMA produces complex and sequential multijoint, synergistic movements of the distal and proximal limbs. Surface electrode stimulation over the mesial surface of the cerebral cortex in humans prior to the surgical excision of an epileptic focus has revealed the somatotopy within SMA and suggests that it is involved not only in controlling sequential movements, but also in the intention to perform a motor act.

As an example of hemispheric asymmetry, stimulation of the right SMA produced both contralateral and ipsilateral movements, whereas left-sided stimulation led mostly to contralateral activity.[62] In humans, the SMA is involved in initiating movements triggered by sensory cues. The SMA is also highly involved in coordinating bimanual actions and simultaneous movements of the upper and lower extremities on one side of the body.[63] The practice of bimanual tasks is sometimes recommended after a brain injury to visuospatially and motorically drive the paretic hand's actions with patterns more easily accomplished by the normal hand (see Chapter 9). The success of this strategy may depend upon the intactness of secondary sensorimotor cortical areas.

Cingulate Cortex

At least 3 nonprimary motor areas also contribute to motor control from their locations in BA 23 and 24 along the ventral bank of the cingulate cortex, at a vertical to the anterior commissure and immediately rostral to the more dorsal SMA.[64] The representation for the hand is just below the junction of BA 4 and the posterior part of BA 6 on the medial wall of the hemisphere. In BA 24, a rostral cingulate zone is activated by complex tasks, whereas a smaller caudal cingulate zone is activated by simple actions.[60] The posterior portion of BA 24 in cingulate cortex sends dense projections to the spinal cord, to M1, and to the caudal part of SMA.[65] This BA 24 subregion also interacts with BA 6. The rostral portion targets the SMA. Functional imaging studies usually reveal activation of the mesial cortex during motor learning and planning, bimanual coordination of movements, and aspects of the execution of movements, more for the hand than the foot. Limited evidence from imaging in normal subjects suggests that all the nonprimary motor regions are activated, often bilaterally to a modest degree, by even simple movements such as finger tapping.[44] The activations increase as behavioral complexity increases. As noted, after a CNS injury, greater activity may evolve in M1 and nonprimary motor cortices when simple movements become more difficult to produce.

The portion of the corticospinal tract from the anterior cingulate projects to the intermediate zone of the spinal cord. The anterior cingulate cortex also has reciprocal projections with the dorsolateral prefrontal cortex, discussed later in this chapter in relation to working memory and cognition. The anterior cingulate receives afferents from the anterior and midline thalamus and from brain stem nuclei that send fibers with the neuromodulators dopamine, serotonin, noradrenaline, and a variety of neuropeptides, pointing to a role in arousal and drives. The difficulty in spontaneous initiation of movement and vocalization associated with akinetic mutism that follows a lesion disconnecting inputs to the cingulate cortex can sometimes improve after treatment with a dopamine receptor agonist. On the other hand, the dopamine blocker haloperidol decreases the resting metabolic rate of the anterior cingulate.[66] The anterior cingulate, in line with its drive-related actions, participates in translating intentions into actions.[66] For example, area 24 is activated in PET studies mainly when a subject is forced to choose from a set of competing oculomotor, manual, or speech responses.[65] The anterior cingulate presumably participates in motor control by facilitating an appropriate response or by suppressing the execution of an inappropriate one when behavior has to be modified in a novel or challenging situation. The region may be especially important for enabling new strategies for motor control in patients during rehabilitation.

SPECIAL FEATURES OF MOTOR CORTICES

Rehabilitationists can begin to consider the contribution of the cortical nodes in the motor system to motor control, to anticipate how the activity of clusters of neurons may vary in relation to different tasks, to test for their dysfunction, and to adapt appropriate interventions. For example, patients with lesions that interrupt the corticocortical projections from somatosensory cortex to the primary motor cortex might have difficulty learning new motor skills, but they may be able to execute existing motor skills.[67] The lateral premotor areas, especially BA 46 and 9, receive converging visual, auditory, and other sensory inputs that integrate planned motor acts. As discussed later in the section on working memory (see Working Memory and Executive Function Network, these regions have an important role in the temporal organization of behaviors, including motor sets and motor sequences.[68] In the presence of a lesion that destroys or disconnects some motor areas, a portion of the distributed functional network for relearning a movement or learning a new compensatory skill may be activated best by a strategy that engages non-

primary and associative sensorimotor regions. Therapists may work around the disconnection of a stroke or traumatic brain injury with a strategy that is cued by vision or sound, self-paced or externally paced, proximal limb-directed, goal-based, mentally planned or practiced, or based on sequenced or unsequenced movements. Task-specific practice that utilizes diverse strategies may improve motor skills in part by engaging residual cortical, subcortical, and spinal networks involved in carrying out the desired motor function.[69,70] Strategies that engage neuronal assemblies dedicated to imagery and hand functions are of immediate interest as rehabilitation approaches.

Observation and Imitation

Functional activation studies reveal that many of the same nodes of the motor system produce movement, observe the movements of other people, imagine actions, understand the actions of others, and recognize tools as objects of action.[71] Motor imagery activates approximately 30% of the M1 neurons that would execute the imagined action. Observation and imitation of a simple finger movement by the right hand preferentially activated two motor-associated regions during an fMRI study by Iacoboni and colleagues: (1) Broca's ventral premotor area that encodes the observed action in terms of its motor goal, i.e., lift the finger, and (2) the right anterior superior parietal cortex that encodes the precise kinesthetic aspects of the movement formed during observation of the movement, i.e., how much the finger should be raised.[72] *Mirror neurons* are a subset of the neurons activated by both the observation of a goal-directed movement, e.g., another person's hand reaching for food, and by the subject's action in reaching for an item.

Mirror neurons represent action goals more than movements. They may be critical for the earliest learning of movements from parents. Thus, the brain's representation of a movement includes the mental content that relates to the goal or consequences of an action, as well as the neural operations that take place before the action starts (see Experimental Case Study 1–1). In a sense, the cognitive systems of the brain can be thought of as an outgrowth of the increasing complexity of sensory manipulations for action over the course of man's evolution. Indeed, one of the remarkable changes in how

EXPERIMENTAL CASE STUDY 1–1:
Mirror Mapping, Mental Imagery and the Dance

I have watched my wife learn a new dance—the movements of a ballet, a modern dance, a center piece tango for the Los Angeles production of *Evita* back in 1980. How is she able to observe the choreographer's actions and immediately reproduce what seem to me like an infinite number of head, torso, arm and leg movements that flow and rapidly evolve with practice? What she sees resonates with her sensorimotor system. She knows a vocabulary of movement from 20 years of studio classes and stage performance. She understands the choreographer's movements by mapping what she observes onto a sensorimotor representation of each phrase of what she observes. Her ability to imitate is almost automatic. As the choreographer sweeps into action, she watches intently. Her body winks abbreviated gestures that start to replicate the fuller movement she observes. She is making a direct match[81] between the observation and the execution of a vocabulary of motion. This imitation calls upon mirror neurons that are active with observation of goal-oriented movement. Indeed, the choreographer learns from her. He observes and imitates some of the movement variations that she injects into the dance. He almost unconsciously imitates those added movements, she imitates his. Back and forth they go, building the dance.

Her image of the dance gains an internal representation, engaging the same neural structures for action that were engaged during perception. Standing in a line at the supermarket, stirring a sauce, sitting at the edge of the studio, standing in the wings of the theatre just before a performance, her imagery rerepresents the vision and affective components of the dance. Mental practice multiplies the number of repetitions of dance movements, extending her physical practice. Cerebral reiteration may prime and facilitate her performance, perhaps not as efficiently as the full movements with their kinaesthetic feedback, but good enough for her to be aware that she possesses explicit knowledge of the dance.

She practices during sleep. I know this. I am kicked abruptly in our bed several times a night whenever she is learning a dance or dreams of dance. Stages of sleep may reactivate and consolidate the representation of her movements. Whether asleep or in the moments before she glides onto the stage, she engages her systems of imagery and imitation to practice, soundly building associations among auditory, visual, visuospatial, and sensorimotor nodes of inferior frontal, right anterior parietal, and parietal opercular cortices, linked to the amygdala and orbitofrontal cortices. These networks integrate and command her complex range of tightly bound actions as when she physically performs. The mental steps of the dance gradually disappear from consciousness, replaced by implicit memory, a striatal sequence of breathing and releasing with movement phrases of the dance tied to the bars of the music, like an athlete in the zone, like the singer whose lyrics meld into melody, or like the actor expressing words without thinking about the lines of the play.

The choreographer's actions, the dancer's focused observation, understanding by mapping an internal representation, imitation, sensorimotor binding, mental and physical practice reactivating neuronal assemblies for phrases of movements, combinations of movements infused with emotion, the performance, the reward of an audience taken by the power struggle and passion of the tango dancers, *brava, bravo!*

Observation and imagery may serve as no less a prescription for bringing about relearned movements during neurorehabilitation.

---

neuroscience understands brain function has been the realization that the same cortical networks that allow us to perceive and move also serve the memory of perception and movement.[68] The mirror properties of some of the neurons in Broca's area (BA 44) during imitation suggest that language may have evolved from a mirror system that recognizes and generates actions.[73] On closer inspection with functional imaging, the action recognition system that is engaged by observing a person grasping a cup is just posterior and below the portion of Broca's area that is activated by internally speaking an action verb.[74]

The posterior superior temporal sulcus also responds to the sight of movements such as reaching. Some mirror neurons here respond to the direction of the observed upper limb's movement and others respond to cues about the other person's directed attention to the target based on the face, eye gaze, and body posture.[75] The ability to understand the behavior of other people may have evolved from the interaction of superior temporal sulcus neurons with neurons along the border between the rostral anterior cingulate and medial prefrontal cortices.[76] The medial prefrontal region is involved in the explicit representation of states of the self. Along with the temporal region's representation of the intentional actions of others, the two regions interact to understand and manipulate the social behavior of others in keeping with a person's own mental state. Thus, many aspects of higher cognitive, language, and social functions may have evolved from a system that represents actions.[77] The links between the actions of others and oneself may serve as a neural basis of the golden rule—do to others what you have observed and imagined them doing to you. It is a short leap to imagine how a problem in detecting the goal-directed actions of others in relation to oneself can create some of the behaviors of patients with traumatic brain injuries and the thought disorders associated with illnesses like schizophrenia.

Action observation, imitation of a movement, and imagining a movement are carried out within a mirror system of the motor network. For neurologic rehabilitation, these findings suggest that the practice required to relearn skills may be augmented by engaging networks dedicated to the observation of another person's actions and by mental rehearsal.[78,79]

Shaping the Hand

The ventral premotor area includes *canonical neurons* that respond to the visual presentation of 3-dimensional objects, especially graspable items, as well as when a subject grasps the item.[80] These neurons connect to the anterior intraparietal area, which contains motor-dominant neurons that respond to grasping and manipulation, visual-dominant neurons, and visuomotor neurons activated by bimanual actions and object presentations. These neurons interact with M1 and subcortical areas to encode the shape of the hand—grasping, precision grip, finger prehension, and whole hand prehension—as the fingers reach for an object.

In a study of monkeys, reversible inactivation of mirror neurons led to motor slowing, but no difficulty in shaping the hand.[80,81] Inactivation of canonical neurons caused clear impairment of hand shaping in relation to the visualized characteristics of objects, although the monkeys could still grasp and manipulate objects a bit clumsily and improve their grasp by using tactile information. Inactivation of a larger expanse of the ventral premotor area caused bilateral deficits and signs of peripersonal neglect for contralateral hemispace. Inactivation of the anterior intraparietal region produced a similar deficit and slowness in hand shaping as occurs after a small premotor lesion. In contrast, inactivation of the hand region of M1 in the same monkeys caused a flaccid paresis, loss of individualized finger movements, and the inability to use the hand. Similar regions have been activated by tasks during functional neuroimaging in human subjects and similar deficits may be called an apraxia after focal strokes in these regions.[82,83]

Patients with hemiparesis may improve their ability to reach and grasp by drawing upon this canonical system. Practice must involve reaching for usable items of different sizes that are smaller than the hand, visual attention to the item and to the affected wrist and fingers, and attempts to preform the fingers to the shape of each object.

Precision Grip

The ability to grasp and manipulate small, easily crushed items requires fine motor control and is often lost in patients who need neurologic rehabilitation. Cortical regions that participate include those for hand shaping. A precision grip, compared to a palmar grip, recruits exclusively or augments the activation of the bilateral ventral premotor cortex (BA 44), rostral cingulate motor area, and the bilateral ventral lateral prefrontal, supramarginal, and right intraparietal cortices.[84] Of course, the contralateral M1, S1, and SMA are activated in all conditions. The sensorimotor control necessary to generate small fingertip forces requires greater activation of the bilateral ventral premotor area, the rostral cingulate motor area, and the right intraparietal cortex compared to the cortical response when subjects apply large forces.[84] The M1 and S1 do, up to a point, show greater activation as the force or speed of finger movements increase. Thus, these distributed regions, which include mirror and canonical neurons, are involved in controlling the small fingertip forces typically needed for manipulation. The greater level of activation points to greater somatosensory processing, a richer neural representation for this learned difference in force exertion, or a greater need for inhibition of a cortical node in the motor network to dampen the force. If M1 or BA 6 are partially spared after a brain injury, extensive practice of precision grip tasks that takes advantage of sensory feedback may increase the synaptic efficacy of this network and improve fine motor control.

Somatosensory Cortical Networks

A key design of the cerebral cortex is the substrate to permit flexible associations between sensory inputs and motor behaviors. Neuronal assemblies in primary and nonprimary motor cortex and in prefrontal and parietal regions become active during specific movements and with sensory cues that trigger the movements. The modulation of motor output by sensory inputs appears to be important at every level of the neuraxis,[85] starting from segmental spinal cord inputs that help drive locomotion. For example, ascending sensory afferent information reaches the thalamus and primary and secondary somatosensory cortex partly to help adjust the gain of M1 neurons according to their output requirements. The pyramidal projections, in turn, provide dorsal horn inputs that modulate sensory inputs from the periphery. *The manipulation of sensory experience by therapists and patients may be the most formidable tool for the rehabilitation of motor skills.*

PRIMARY SENSORY CORTEX

The primary sensory cortex SI, which includes BA 3a, 3b, 1, and 2, receives thalamically relayed cutaneous and proprioceptive inputs. The divisions of these regions are not always outlined quite the way Brodmann mapped them.[86] Other anatomic and functional neuroimaging studies find additional subregions and somewhat different borders, which may acount for variations in the localization of activations between subjects during functional imaging studies. For example, although BA 2 is regularly located on the anterior wall of the postcentral gyrus, the border between BA 4 and BA 3 in the fundus of the central gyrus can be indistinct. A high density of cholinergic

muscarinic M2 receptors in the primary sensory areas does, however, distinguish the sensory from more anterior motor areas.[86] Indeed, the density of different neurotransmitter receptors in the cortical layers of each Brodmann area seems to be distinct, especially between the motor and sensory areas, reflecting differences in their activity for sensing and action. The central sulcus divides the agranular (lacking layer IV neurons) motor cortex from the caudal 6-layered granular somatosensory cortex. The two regions are also distinguishable by the relatively low density of glutaminergic, muscarinic, GABAergic, and serotonergic receptors in agranular, compared to granular cortices.[87] Knowledge of these neurotransmitter receptor differences may prove valuable for the design of pharmacologic interventions to augment motor learning.

Area 3b projects to 3a, 2, 1, and SII, but not to M1. Areas 3a, 2, and SII project to M1. BA 3b does project to the anterior and ventral parietal cortical fields that in turn project topographically to M1, as well as to SMA, BA 6, and the putamen. As a general rule, projections from one area receive reciprocal inputs.

The primary somatosensory cortex responds in a time-locked fashion to stimuli, permitting temporally and spatially accurate information. The secondary somatosensory cortex, which generally corresponds to BA 43 at the upper bank of the Sylvian fissure just posterior to the central sulcus, integrates sensory inputs for a longer time, "smearing" single tactile inputs from a train of stimuli, perhaps for processes related to sensorimotor integration.[88] The SII is also linked to the ventral premotor area, to BA 7, and to connections of the insula with the limbic system. In an fMRI study that required object discrimination, tactile input from SII to BA 44 appeared necessary to control and direct finger movements during object exploration in the absence of vision.[83] Ablation of SII in monkeys severely impairs tactile learning, but tactile sensation is normal. BA 43 is often activated bilaterally by a unilateral movement during a PET or fMRI task. The absence of this activation may serve as a physiologic marker for the loss of the sensorimotor network necessary for skills learning during rehabilitation.

The smallest sensory receptive fields, the lips and fingertips, have the highest density of inputs. The receptive fields in BA 2 for the finger pads are large, extending over several fingers.[89] BA 3a cells respond primarily to muscle and tendon mechanoreceptors. Area 3b contains a somatotopic representation of the body with small, sharply defined receptor fields provided by afferents from low threshold, slowly adapting Merkel afferents and rapidly adapting Meissner afferents. The slowly adapting receptor afferents allow the discrimination of separate points on the skin and detect roughness. The rapidly adapting receptors permit awareness of motion across the skin and the feedback to prevent items from slipping from grasp. Microstimulation of mechanoreceptors during functional neuroimaging may give further insights into sensory neurophysiology and adaptability in humans.[90] Thus, stretch and kinematic information from muscle and joint receptors reach the cerebellum and thalamus, then ascend to BA 3a, M1, and SII to initiate sensorimotor integration. These links are critical for motor skills learning driven by interventions that optimize typical sensory inputs during skilled movements.

Sensory experience that bears behavioral importance leaves a lasting memory.[91,92] The size of cortical representations from the skin varies with tactile and motor experience during the acquisition of a skill.[93] Thus, musicians may have larger representations for their digital finger pads and joint proprioceptors than people who do not carry out fine sensorimotor tasks. As a digit participates in a task, its sensory receptive fields become smaller and more succint, more neurons are excited, the synapses between neurons that receive coincident skin inputs strengthen, and, as described later in this chapter, dendritic spines increase among these neurons. By similar mechanisms, highly repetitive and stereotyped inputs to the digits can degrade somatosensory representation and motor performance, perhaps leading to a focal hand dystonia in some patients.[94]

Primary somatosensory cortex has a key role in both the storage and retrieval of representations of sensory information.[95] When subjects train to make sensory discriminations of vibratory stimuli on one fingertip, learning the vibration frequency stimulus does not transfer to other digits.[96] The learned discriminations for punctate pressure and roughness will, however, transfer to the finger that neighbors the trained one and to the same digit of the other hand. Each area of S1 that processes specialized stimuli, then, contains information stored in stimulus-specific cortical fields, each with it own receptive field, feature selectivity, and callosal connectivity. The SII is also essential for learning about roughness and pressure.[97]

The profound effects of sensory inputs on motor function and the dual functions of S1 for information processing, storage, and retrieval suggest that rehabilitation strategies should include methods to optimize sensory inputs during the retraining of a sensorimotor skill. Chapters 5 and 9 include studies of these methods. Functional neuroimaging studies of the brain during the acquisition of a skill involving the upper or lower extremity reveal the effects of these sensory inputs on neural activity and on remodeling sensorimotor maps (see Chapter 3).

PARIETAL SENSORY CORTEX

BA 5 and 7, separated by the intraparietal sulcus from BA 39 (corresponding broadly to the angular gyrus), and BA 40 (approximately the supramarginal gyrus) complete the parietal sensory region. The cell types and neurotransmitter receptor densities of the cortical layers vary within areas of the parietal cortex. BA 5 and 7 can be conceived as parasensory association areas. Along with the visual and auditory cortices, these two areas process sensory information and, with their hippocampal connections, store perceptual memories. BA 5 and 7 represent higher order processing than occurs in the computations of the primary sensorimotor cortices. For example, when a monkey reaches for an object of interest or manipulates it, neurons in BA 5 are more active than those in BA 2 as the finger joints move and as the surface of the object moves across the skin.[89] BA 5 interacts with the primary sensorimotor and dorsal premotor cortices to encode the intrinsic kinematics of a moving limb to guide an action. For example, neurons in the superior parietal lobe of monkeys distinguish between the presentation of a right or left arm, whether the arm is real or a fake replica, and encode the arm's position in relationship to the monkey's body.[98] Thus, neurons in BA 5 are concerned with both the location and identity of a visual stimulus. Their properties may help incorporate external objects into the body's schema when tools or prosthetic limbs are used. Hemineglect syndromes after a parietal stroke often involve this region.

Neurons in BA 7 have large visual receptive fields, encode a multimodal, abstract representation of space, and play a role in visual guidance of movements, especially actions retrieved from memory.[99] The region integrates sensory information to plan actions. As discussed previously, neurons in BA 7 become preferentially activated for preshaping a hand to match the shape of the object before the hand grasps it.[100] Patients with a hemiparetic hand or proprioceptive loss require greater use of the visually guided and tactile components of reaching and grasping to retrain preshaping.

Neurons in the posterior parietal cortex and intraparietal sulcus become active when a person prepares to move a hand. Localizing the distributed network for motor intention leads further away from primary and secondary sensorimotor regions. In this case, the posterior temporal cortex is also activated during the extraction of contextual and intentional sensory cues for a goal-driven behavior.[101] Patients with an apraxia from a left parietal lesion may not be able to mimic the use of objects because of a disturbance in the ability to evoke actions from stored motor representations or because patients no longer understand the goals of ac-

tions.[102] Thus, the left parietal parasensory cortex represents actions in terms of knowledge about the upper extremity. A lesion here impairs following meaningless actions on command or by imitation. The right parietal parasensory region participates in the visuospatial analysis of gestures. Approaches to rehabilitation may differ, depending on the mechanism of the apraxia (see Chapter 9).

Pyramidal Tract Projections

Estimates of the contribution of M1 in man to the corticospinal tract that enters each medullary pyramid range from 40% to 60% of the 1 million fibers within the white matter tract.[103] Approximately 70% of the corticospinal tract arises from the primary and nonprimary motor cortices and approximately 30% arises from the primary somatosensory cortices (Table 1–2). From 70% to 90% of pyramidal fibers decussate into the lateral corticospinal tract in the cord and 10% to 30% remain uncrossed and form the ventral corticospinal tract.[104] Figure 1–3 shows the distribution of decussated and undecussated fibers from pri-

Table 1–2. Approximate Contributions to the Contralateral Pyramidal Tract at the C-6 Level from Cortical Sensorimotor Regions in the Macaque

Brodmann's Equivalent Cortical Area	Crossed (%)	Ipsilateral in Lateral or Ventral Column
MOTOR		
4	36	Yes
24	6	
23	4	
6	7	
SMA	15	Yes
SOMATOSENSORY		
3a	2	
3b/1	10	
2/5	13	Yes
7	2	
SII	2	
Insula	1	

SMA, supplementary motor area; SII, secondary somatosensory cortex.
Source: Adapted from Darian-Smith et al., 1996.[89]

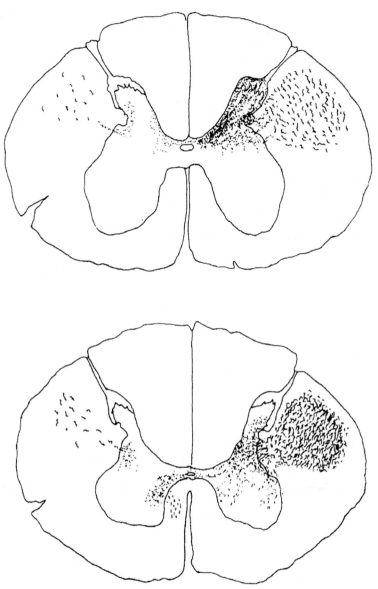

Figure 1–3. The drawing reconstructs the corticospinal pathways derived from antegrade labeling of primary sensori-motor cortex in the macaque and other nonhuman primates. The *top* figure shows the mostly decussated inputs to the dorsal horn (right) after injection of WGA-horseradish peroxidase into the cortical lamina of BA 3b, 1, and 2 on the left. Note that some fibers cross dorsal to the central canal of the spinal cord to return to the side of origin and a modest number of fibers descend uncrossed in the ipsilateral lateral corticospinal tract. The *bottom* figure shows the crossed and uncrossed projections revealed after injection of BA 4 on the left with WGA-horseradish peroxidase. Although most descending fibers (right) have decussated, a moderate number recross under the central canal and two separate tracts in the lateral and ventral funiculi contain undecussated fibers. These ipsilateral inputs may be important for bilateral proximal movements and bimanual movements. The uncrossed and recrossed fibers are a resource of spared pathways for motor gains after a unilateral cerebral injury. Source: adapted from Ralston and Ralston, 1985[54] and Tuszynski, M (in press).

mary sensory cortex in BA 3b, 2, and 1 and from M1. In addition, some sensory and motor fibers of the pyramidal projections into the spinal cord recross within the cord. Their function is uncertain, perhaps related to the coordi-nation of bilateral motor activities, but both un-crossed and recrossing axons may contribute to some recovery of function after a unilateral cere-bral or spinal injury. The asymmetry in the cor-ticospinal tracts, in which the ventral and lateral tracts are larger in about 75% of spinal cords on the right side,[105] may offer another source of spared fibers after a cerebral injury to enable substitution of pathways that ordinarily play a more modest role in motor control.

The dorsal and ventral horn targets of the descending corticospinal fibers have perhaps been underappreciated (Fig. 1–3).[54,89,106] Each projection from BA 4, SMA, cingulate, parietal, and insular sensorimotor cortices extends to all spinal segments. Each has a rather distinctive distribution of excitatory axon branches. All projections target some terminals in the spinal intermediate zone (Rexed laminae V–VII), where they end on intrinsic interneurons and propriospinal neurons. Propriospinal neurons, in turn, have broad segmental and rostrocaudal connections, further distributing commands from the cortex.

Some of the projections from motor areas, especially from BA 4 and SMA, synapse directly on motoneurons in the central and dorsolateral ventral horn (lamina IX), which innervate distal limb muscles. Other frontal and cingulate axons terminate in the neck of the dorsal horn (laminae IV and V), but not in the pure sensory input regions of the substantia gelatinosa (laminae I and II). A modest number of fibers from areas 3a, 3b, 1, 2, and 5 and insular cortex do terminate in laminae I and II, but most end in the intermediate zone, medially in the neck of dorsal laminae III–VI. The descending inputs from M1 and SMA appear to be more diffuse in their axodendritic and cell body terminations within Rexed laminae II/IV to IX in the ventral horn compared to the terminations from somatosensory cortex in laminae I to VI/VII of the dorsal horn. Thus, the descending motor inputs have powerful depolarizing and rather widespread influences on the motor pools that need to be coordinated for stabilizing and multijoint movements. The somatosensory cortical projections terminate mostly on distal regions of the dendritic tree of dorsal horn neurons. A more distal synapse tends to modulate, rather than depolarize a neuron.

A general somatotopy exists in the terminations of the corticospinal projections, but morphologic data point to a convergence of inputs to each segment of the cord from a fraction of most cortical regions. This broad input is most notable within the cervical and lumbar enlargements for the arm and leg. The axons and terminals of the pyramidal projections are also heterogeneous, supporting direct as well as indirect excitatory and inhibitory responses in spinal neurons.[54]

UNCROSSED AND RECROSSING AXONS

The somatosensory projection includes a modest number of decussated fibers that reach the cord in the dorsolateral white matter column and recross through the isthmus above the central canal back to the side of cerebral origin (Fig. 1–3). It also includes a small undecussated projection to laminae V/VI. Some M1 axons from the lateral funiculus also cross the isthmus under the central canal to medial and ventral regions of the ventral horn on the side of their cortical origins. An uncrossed projection from ipsilateral area 4 in the lateral column's corticospinal pathway terminates in lamina VIII and more sparsely in laminae V/VI. The fibers of the medioventral ipsilateral corticospinal tract synapse especially with motoneurons for axial and girdle muscles. They are said to minimally, if at all, reach the lumbar cord. Several spinal cord regeneration studies described in Chapter 2 suggest, however, that the ventromedial uncrossed tract is robust enough to play a role in the recovery of lower extremity function. Some of the ventral funiculus pyramidal fibers also cross the anterior commissure below the isthmus to connect to motoneurons of the opposite ventral horn.[103]

Ipsilateral corticomotoneuronal projections are readily stimulated by TMS in neonates. These projections ordinarily decline by 18 months to 3 years old,[107] most likely as part of a developmental, activity-dependent pruning of descending axons. The uncrossed axons may persist in children who experience a perinatal brain injury that causes hemiplegic cerebral palsy. Residual ipsilateral corticospinal pathways may help control distal, as well as proximal upper limb movements in these children.[42] Both ipsilateral and double-crossing fibers within the spinal gray may also serve as a source of spared pyramidal inputs that sprout dendrites after a cerebral or spinal cord injury in adults.

Thus, information from sensorimotor regions of the cortex reaches spinal motoneurons via multiple parallel pathways, taking a contralateral and a less robust ipsilateral path. The behavioral parameters for a motor task are distributed among the coactive descending sensorimotor pathways. Particular information about any parameter is weighted more strongly in one or several of the parallel inputs to the spinal motor pools. Parallel and distributed processing acts at both a cellular and systems level and provides the fabric for use-dependent plasticity, a major focus of rehabilitation interventions.

INDIRECT CORTICOSPINAL PROJECTIONS

Corticorubrospinal, corticoreticulospinal, and corticovestibulospinal projections contribute to limb and trunk muscle contractions, especially for sustained contractions. Such contractions of muscle are important for stabilizing the trunk and proximal muscles during actions. The reticular and vestibular descending pathways project bilaterally in the ventral and ventrolateral funiculi of the spinal cord, reaching the ventromedial zone of the anterior horns to contribute to postural and orienting movements of the head and body and synergistic movements of the trunk and limbs. Kuypers suggested that the interneurons of the ventromedial intermediate zone of spinal gray matter represent a system of widespread connections among a variety of motor neurons, whereas the dorsal and lateral zones, which receive direct corticospinal inputs, are a focused system with a limited number of connections.[106]

Other corticomotoneurons project directly and by collaterals to the upper medullary medial reticular formation. Their spinal projections overlap the descending reticulospinal pathway to the same spinal cord gray matter in the intermediate zone. Some reticulospinal fibers run from the ventrolateral pons and accompany the corticospinal pathway in the dorsolateral column. Within these pathways, then, potential redundancy exists that could, after an injury, allow partial sparing or reorganization, especially for axial and proximal movements. Indeed, a patient with severe hemiparesis who cajoles minimal voluntary flexion in the affected leg or extension of the elbow, wrist, and fingers may rely on corticorubrospinal and corticoreticulospinal pathways for functional hip and knee flexion during walking or extension for reaching to an object and on corticovestibulospinal projections for leg extension and postural control.

Corticospinal fibers from M1, SMA, and BA 24 and 2/5 project to the parvicellular nucleus of the red nucleus, which sends most of its output to the olivary nucleus. This half of the red nucleus apparently has only modest connections to its lower half, the somatotopically arranged magnocellular nucleus. The magnocellular division of the red nucleus also receives cortical sensory inputs. Magnocellular neurons create the rubrospinal tract, which crosses and intermingles with corticospinal fibers. The rubrospinal fibers terminate on interneurons and directly on some motoneurons in the dorsolateral intermediate zone of the ventral horn, where they contribute to motor control of the limbs. Similar movement-related cell discharges occur in M1 and in magnocellular cells, as well as in the basal ganglia and cerebellum, which points to their close functional relationship.[108] The neurons are tuned to particular directions of movement, best worked out for hand reaching. These cells respond to skin touch and joint movements. The red nuclei help control the extremities and digits for skilled steering and fractionated movements. These midbrain neurons, which also receive cerebellar projections, may independently subserve some aspects of the motor control for the distal arm after a hemispheric injury.[109]

Subcortical Systems

THE BASAL GANGLIA

Distributed, parallel loops characterize the subcortical volitional movement circuits that involve the basal ganglia and cerebellum. These circuits are critical for the procedural learning of motor skills and for cognition.

Basal ganglia outputs, primarily from the internal segment of the globus pallidus and pars reticulata region of the substantia nigra, project to motor and prefrontal areas and to brain stem motor sites. The input nuclei include the caudate, putamen, and ventral striatum. The subthalamic nucleus, globus pallidus externa, and pars compacta of the substantia nigra modulate activity primarily within the basal ganglia circuits. Many anatomical and physiological studies demonstrate the parallel and segregated arrangement, rather than convergent integration, of the motor pathways in the circuit M1-putamen-globus pallidus-thalamic ventrolateral nucleus-M1.

The frontal lobe–basal ganglia–thalamocortical circuits include (*1*) a skeletomotor circuit from the precentral motor fields, (*2*) the oculomotor circuit from the frontal and supplementary eye fields, (*3*) the prefrontal circuit from the dorsolateral prefrontal and lateral orbitofrontal cortex, (*4*) the limbic circuit from the anterior cingulate and medial orbitofrontal cortex, and (*5*) a circuit with inferotemporal and posterior parietal cortex.[110,111] Many of the cortical regions that input the basal ganglia are also targets of basal ganglia output. For rehabilitation, the possibility holds that circuits for a particular domain of function or for a limited region of the body may reorganize and substitute for a damaged network.

Within the topographically organized, closed loops of the skeletomotor pallidothalamocortical system, localized regions of the globus pallidus organize into discrete channels. For the primate's arm, separable channels project to particular locations in M1, SMA, and the ventral premotor area via the ventrolateral thalamus.[112] The face and leg representations in M1 are targets of globus pallidus interna output. In addition to the SMA and ventral premotor area, at least 4 other premotor regions connect to both the spinal cord and the basal ganglia, including the dorsal premotor and the rostral cingulate in BA 24. Discrete regions of the ventrolateral thalamus modulate these loops. These channels presumably process different variables for movement. Corticostriatal pyramidal neurons in M1 are anatomically and functionally distinct from corticospinal neurons. The former respond more to sensory inputs and perimovement activities that are directionally specific, whereas corticospinal neurons fire more in relation to muscle activity.[113] The basal ganglia path to M1 affects parameters such as the direction and force of movement. The premotor path carries out higher-order programming, such as the internal guidance and sequence of a movement.

The input and output architecture of the sensorimotor striatum has a modular design that remaps cortical inputs onto distributed local modules of striatal projection neurons.[114] One type of striatal interneuron, *tonically active neurons*, bind these modular networks temporally during behavioral learning. These neurons are sensitive to signals associated with motivation and reward from adjacent parallel circuits, such as those from the limbic channel.

Dopamine and possibly cholinergic influences mediate the response properties of these tonically active interneurons. This organization allows the basal ganglia to participate in concurrently ongoing skeletomotor, oculomotor, cognitive, and limbic drive activities. Together, the circuits internally generate a movement, execute an automatic motor plan, and acquire and retain a motor skill. They are closely allied to the frontal-subcortical circuits that participate in a range of human behaviors. In considering rehabilitation strategies, activities of significance to a patient that motivate practice with rewards of success are most likely to activate these circuits. This strategy is one of the bases for task-oriented therapy, reviewed in Chapter 5. In addition, pharmacologic agents that affect the neurotransmitters of the striatum, including dopamine, glutamate, acetylcholine, and γ-aminobutyric acid (GABA), may alter the net excitatory and inhibitory activities of these systems after a CNS injury and, when combined with training, enhance motor learning.

CEREBELLUM

The cerebellum plays an important role in creating and selecting the internal models necessary for movements.[115] Internal models are computationally efficient ways to generate an appropriate sensorimotor behavior under different circumstances. These experience-based models can either predict the sensory consequences of motor plans or control the motor plans that produce a desired sensory outcome.[116] Thus, instead of reinventing the wheel of neural strategy for every motor act, especially for tasks that require eye–hand coordination, the cerebellum draws on its real world experience and employs a test hypothesis, its internal model, to plan and detect errors as the hand reaches for an object.[117]

The cerebellar cortex is a 50,000 cm^2 continuous sheet. The large Purkinje cells represent the sole output system to the cerebellar nuclei and they receive two main inputs. Climbing fibers project from the olive and mossy fibers project from cortex, brain stem, and spinal cord and terminate on the granule cell-Purkinje cell complex. When learning a new task, the climbing fiber, which detects movement, alters the effectiveness of the synapses between the granule cell's parallel fibers and Purkinje cells. A Purkinje cell's dendrites form 200,000 synapses with mossy fiber afferents, but each Purkinje cell receives only one climbing fiber. Granule cells release glutamate. Purkinje cells release GABA.

Relating these structural features to function has led to competing hypotheses.[118] The parallel fibers may wire different muscles together for coordinated movements. The strength of synaptic efficacy between parallel fibers and Purkinje cells may set the force and timing of muscle contractions. Learning a new, complex sensorimotor skill in the rat leads to an increase in the number of synapses between parallel fibers and Purkinje cells, and these changes last for 4 months after training stops.[119] On the other hand, the olive's climbing fibers that wrap Purkinje cells may act like a timer that determines which muscles contract or relax in 100 ms ticks. These actions may contribute more to modifying performance than to learning the motor skill.[119a]

Like the loops through the basal ganglia, parallel arrangements also hold for the cerebellar projections to the ventrolateral nucleus of the thalamus. One loop connects M1-pons-dorsal dentate nucleus-cerebellar cortex-thalamic ventrolateral nucleus-M1. Another goes from the motor cortices to the red nucleus as noted earlier, where a rubrocerebellar loop includes the olive, lateral reticular nucleus, and cerebellar nucleus interpositus. These loops, like those of the basal ganglia, help sort out valid and invalid cues for initiating and planning movements, which is mostly a dentate nucleus and frontal lobe circuit function.

The detection and correction of any mismatch between intended and actual movements are functions of the interpositus nucleus and spinocerebellar circuit. Postural control is managed by the fastigial nucleus with its vestibular and reticular inputs. The olivocerebellar system functions as an oscillatory circuit that can generate timing sequences for coordinated movements as well as cause tremors. The mossy fibers, with input and output connections to spinal and brain stem motor regions, inform the cerebellar cortex of the place and rate of movement of the limbs. These fibers put the motor intention generated by the cerebral cortex into the context of the status of the body at the time the movement is executed.[120] Purkinje cells may encode some of the experience-dependent computations, such as position, velocity, acceleration, and inherent viscous forces of a moving

limb, that aid experience-dependent learning within the cerebellum's cortical and subcortical connections.[10] Remarkably, the output of the cerebellums's elaborate cortical network produces only inhibition of the cerebellar nuclei.

Motor Functions

The cerebellum participates in the seamless synthesis of complex, multijoint movements from simpler component actions. Pure cerebellar lesions, for example, cause upper extremity ataxia that decompose the coordination for reaching between the elbow and shoulder. Functional imaging with PET during coordinated forearm and finger movements, compared to isolated forearm or finger movements during reaching and pointing, reveals greater activity in the contralateral anterior and bilateral paramedian cerebellar lobules.[121] This region receives upper extremity spinocerebellar and corticocerebellar inputs. The posterior parietal cortex, a multimodal integrating region that receives projections from the dentate nucleus,[122] is also more active, perhaps as it processes visual data about the target and proprioceptive information about limb position. These interactions are critical for activating internal models for eye–hand coordination.

Although most studies of the cerebellum relate to postural control and upper extremity actions, the cerebellum also plays a major role in locomotion. Damage to its medial structures, including the fastigium, disturbs standing and walking, but not voluntary limb movements. Lateral lesions that include the dentate alter voluntary multijoint movements. Balance deficits vary with the location of the lesion. Damage to the anterior vermis affects anteroposterior sway. Posterior vermis and flocculonodular lobe damage causes sway in all directions and poor tandem walking.[123]

Purkinje cells are rhythmically active throughout the step cycle.[124] The information they receive must be important. Neurons of the fastigial and interpositus nuclei burst primarily during the flexor phase of stepping. The cerebellum receives inputs from alpha and gamma motor neurons and Ia interneurons, as well as from segmental dorsal root afferents. This input is copied not only to the cerebellum, but also to corticomotoneurons and to the locomotor regions of the dorsolateral midbrain and pons (Fig. 1–1).[125,126] During locomotion, and even with passive ankle movements, the neurons of the dorsal spinocerebellar tract in the dorsolateral funiculus of the lumbar cord fire in relation to both Ia and Ib afferent activity.[124] This activity provides the cerebellum with detailed information about the performance of leg movements. Ventral spinocerebellar neurons project to the cerebellar cortex from the contralateral lateral funiculus and burst during locomotion, reflecting activity in spinal central pattern generators, discussed later in this chapter. Spinoreticulocerebellar pathways also carry bilateral information predominantly from the spinal circuits for stepping.

Thus the cerebellum receives and modulates locomotor cycle-related signals. The neocerebellum monitors the outcome of every movement and optimizes movements using proprioceptive feedback. Given the great computational interest the cerebellum has in the details of afferent information from joints and muscles, *rehabilitation therapies for walking and for upper extremity actions should aim to provide this key motor pathway with the sensory feedback that the spinal cord and cerebellum recognize as typical of normal walking and of typical reaching-related inputs.* The sorts of motor functions that the cerebellar inputs and outputs attend to, such as timing and error correction for accuracy as the hand approaches an object, are especially important for patients to practice when a lesion undermines motor control.

Cognitive Functions

The cerebellum is also a node in the distributed neural circuits that subserve aspects of cognition relevant to movement. The cerebellum influences at least a few prefrontal regions via thalamic projections and through the dentate nucleus.[127] Corticopontine projections arise from the dorsolateral, dorsomedial, and frontopolar prefrontal cortex and project, in a highly ordered fashion, to paramedian and peripeduncular nuclei of the ventral pons to form part of the pontocerebellar pathway.[128] These frontal lobe areas, discussed later in the chapter (cognitive network), participate in the planning, initiation, and execution of movements, and the verification of willed actions and thoughts. The rostral cingulate, septal nuclei, hippocampus, and amygdala provide limbic connections to the cerebellum.

These nodes may provide visual and spatial attributes of objects, such as their location and direction of motion, and assist recall of this information.[128] Thus, regional activations of the cerebellum can be expected across a range of motor and cognitive tasks during functional neuroimaging. An fMRI study, for example, demonstrated independent activation of separate cerebellar regions during a task of visual attention and during motor performance.[129] Initiation of even a simple motor task activated the hot spot for attention, but a sustained motor task did not. The cerebellum, then, influences sensory, motor, attentional, planning, working memory, and rule-based learning systems as it acquires new information and builds internal models based on previous experience for the analysis and smooth control of actions. A careful neuropsychologic evaluation often reveals aspects of frontal lobe-like dysfunction in patients who have lesions within the cerebellar network.

THALAMUS

The thalamus receives all sensory information from the internal and external world as well as all processed sensorimotor information from the spinal cord, cerebellum, basal ganglia, and substantia nigra. The thalamic nuclei are not passive relays. They almost certainly perform distributed, parallel processing of sensory information and filter the flow of information to the cortex. Filtering may depend on a subject's level of alertness or consciousness. All thalamic relay nuclei respond to excitatory inputs with either tonic or burst firing. The burst pattern may play a role in attending to a stimulus.[130] Separate channels are maintained within the somatic sensory and motor thalamus for cutaneous sensation, for slowly adapting and rapidly adapting inputs, for each of the cerebellar nuclei, and for the vestibular and spinothalamic systems.[131] Somatotopic relations are maintained in much of this sensory space. Anatomic studies reveal almost no convergence of lemniscal, cerebellar, pallidal, or substantia nigral afferents in the thalamus. Each is independent. Thus, individual channels of the thalamocortical projections control separate functional units of motor cortex which, in turn, independently influence the basal ganglia, cerebellum, and other subcortical motor nuclei. These parallel systems may include a partially reiterative capacity to allow some sparing or compensation after a sensorimotor network injury.

Each thalamic nucleus projects widely to up to seven primary and nonprimary sensorimotor areas. This divergence of projections produces convergence of a variety of thalamic inputs to targets. Why would so many thalamic cells with similar receptive fields converge onto the same assemblies of cortical neurons? One thought is that information about a cutaneous stimulus requires cells only in a single receptive field to respond, but a moving stimulus must be coded for recognition by a population of responding cells. When learning a motor skill, coding across a population leads to temporally convergent inputs that strengthen synapses between neighboring representations for the stimulated skin. This thalamic mediated activity-dependent plasticity induces rapid cortical reorganization (see Experimental Case Studies 1–4).

Brain Stem Pathways

The pontine nuclei receive projections from the prefrontal and limbic areas noted in the discussion of the cerebellum, as well as from other association cortices such as the posterior parietal, superior temporal, occipitotemporal, and parahippocampal cortices. Each cortical area projects to a specific lateral basis pontis region. As a general organizing principle, interconnected cortical areas like these share common subcortical projections.

Vestibulospinal and rubrospinal neurons are rhythmically modulated by cerebellar inputs, primarily for extensor and flexor movements, respectively. In addition, chains of polysynaptically interacting propriospinal neurons have been identified in the lateral tegmentum of the pons and medulla and reach the upper cervical cord. Reticulospinal and propriospinal fibers intermingle on the periphery of the ventral and lateral spinal tracts, where reticulospinal paths may come to be replaced by propriospinal ones.[132] The shortest propriospinal fibers are closest to the gray matter. These fibers connect motor neurons to axial, girdle, and thigh muscles. Short propriospinal fibers descend for one or two segments. In a sense, the axial and proximal leg motor pools are wired to interact together. The brain stem pro-

jections and propriospinal fibers may participate in the hemiplegic patient's recovery of enough use of truncal and antigravity muscles on the paralyzed side to aid walking and proximal arm function.

HAND FUNCTIONS

Rudimentary synergistic movements such as opening and closing the hand persist after a pyramidectomy, probably through the activity of the descending rubrospinal, vestibulospinal, and reticulospinal systems.[133] These descending pathways mediate skilled forelimb movements, especially movements related to feeding.[134] The rubrospinal tract provides a potential path for independent, flexion-biased movements of the elbow and hand.[109] The more individuated a movement, the greater the amount of corticomotoneuronal activity needed to superimpose control on subcortical centers and directly upon spinal motoneurons to multiple muscles. Substitution of a brain stem pathway for a cortical one by retraining after a brain injury may reorganize subcortical controllers and increase motor recovery.

LOCOMOTOR FUNCTIONS

The brain stem, particularly the reticular formation, includes important structures for automatic and volitional control of posture and movement. Interacting with the cortex, deep cerebellar nuclei, substantia nigra, and globus pallidus, the brain stem has convergent areas involved in locomotion (Fig. 1–1). Reticulospinal and propriospinal projections from the mesencephalic locomotor region (MLR) and pedunculopontine region synapse with lumbar spinal neurons and carry the descending message for the initiation of locomotion.[135] In animal experiments, electrical and pharmacologic stimulation of these two regions, as well as stimulation of the cerebellar fastigial nucleus and the subthalamic nucleus that project to reticulospinal neurons, produce hindlimb locomotor activity. The step rate is modulated by the intensity of stimulation.[136] The locomotor regions modulate spinal pattern generators for stepping in animal models and, presumably, in humans.

A hemisection of the upper lumbar spinal cord is followed by considerable recovery of locomotion in monkeys and cats, mediated at least in part by descending ventrolateral retic-ulospinal fibers on the intact side that cross at a segmental level below the transection.[137] In rats, the initiation of hindlimb locomotion is not compromised after a thoracic spinal cord injury (SCI) until almost all of the ventral white matter of the cord is destroyed. Fibers from the pontomedullary medial reticular formation descend in a diffuse fashion in the ventral and ventrolateral funiculi,[138] so a partial lesion of this white matter spares some of the brain stem projections and preserves locomotion. The regions that participate in the initiation of stepping also participate in the control of body orientation, equilibrium, and postural tone.

Cholinergic agonists, excitatory amino acids, and substance P elicit or facilitate locomotion when injected into the medial pontine reticular formation. Cholinergic antagonists and GABA abolish MLR-evoked locomotion. Dopamine and amphetamine also initiate locomotion by modulating amygdala and hippocampal inputs to the nucleus accumbens, which projects to the MLR via the ventral pallidal area.[139] The lateral reticulospinal tract contains glutaminergic fibers and noradrenergic fibers that descend from the locus coeruleus. The use of systemic drugs that increase or block the neurotransmitters of this network may enhance or inhibit the automatic patterns of stepping in patients.

These brain stem locomotor regions are affected by a variety of neurologic diseases. Patients with Parkinson's disease and progressive supranuclear palsy lose neurons in the pedunculopontine nucleus. Their gait deviations include difficulty in the initiation and rhythmicity of walking. In a case report, a patient who suffered a small hemorrhagic stroke in the dorsal pontomesencephalic region on the right abruptly lost the ability to stand and generate anything but irregular, shuffling steps while supported, despite the absence of paresis and ataxia.[140] Patients with infarcts in this locomotor region can be retrained to walk on a treadmill, which engrains the initiation and maintenance of stepping.

Locomotor activity also requires constant processing of information from the environment. Brain stem circuits help mediate this information. Visual control of walking includes an egocentric mechanism. A person perceives the visual direction of the destination with respect to the body and walks in that direction.

Steering is based on optic flow, the pattern of visual motion as the person's focus expands in the direction of the walk. The observer adjusts direction so as to cancel the error between the heading perceived from optic flow and the goal.[141] Less accurate steering can also be accomplished in the absence of vision, using vestibular or auditory signals.

Cells of the superior colliculus that project to the motor and premotor cortex are an example of a system that manages the task of coordinating the sensory cues for orientation behaviors during ambulation and other activities. Physiological studies of the superior colliculus reveal a sensory convergence system in which motor responses are not irrevocably linked to a particular stimulus, but vary with visual, auditory, somatosensory, and other stimuli.[142] The output message from what are mostly multimodal cells is a synthesis of the spatial and temporal characteristics of the stimuli. This synthesis allows a remarkably simple neural mechanism for a very flexible range of motor responses in the face of a changing environment. In clinical practice, visual input may compensate for proprioceptive impairments during gait retraining, but may impede stepping and postural adjustments when associated with perceptual deficits.

Spinal Sensorimotor Activity

The pools of spinal interneurons and motoneurons translate the internal commands of the brain into simple (reflexes), rhythmic (walking, breathing, swallowing), and complex (speaking, reaching for a cup) movements. These motor pools integrate descending commands with immediate access to sensory feedback about limb position, muscle length and tension, tactile knowledge about objects, and other segmental inputs. The sensory and motor pools of the cord conduct simple and polysynaptic movement patterns, recruit motor units for movements, and participate in rhythmic activity called pattern generation. Most importantly, the spinal motor pools are an integral part of motor learning. Indeed, the spinal cord reveals a considerable degree of experience-dependent plasticity that is induced, adjusted, and maintained by descending and segmental sensory influences.[143,144] Another form of spinal plasticity results in pain after a peripheral nerve injury. This central sensitization of dorsal horn nociceptive neurons produces hyperalgesia and allodynia by a molecular learning mechanism akin to LTP.

MOTONEURON COLUMNS

The motoneurons of the spinal cord are arranged in 11 rostrocaudal columns, shown in Figure 1–4. These columns originate and terminate at several levels of the cord. Continuous columns are found medially in the ventral gray horns from C-1 to L-3 (column 1), and more laterally from C-8 to S-3 (column 2), L-

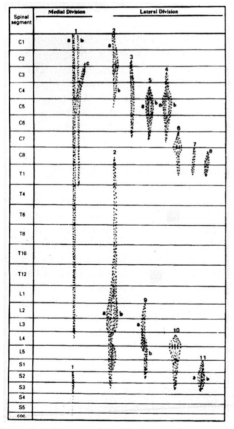

Figure 1–4. Drawing of the 11 columns of motoneurons of the spinal cord. The motor pools of each column are interconnected by propriospinal connections and the columns themselves interact for axial, limb girdle, and distal motor functions. Source: Routal and Pal, 1999[145] with permission.

1 to S-2, and L-4 to S-3.[145] Of interest for locomotor control, column 2 innervates the erector spinae and hip muscles. Short propriospinal connections across these spinal segments also link and coordinate multiple muscles and multijoint movements under the influence of supraspinal controllers. As described later under Spinal Primitives, the caudal thoracic and the lumbar motor pools are also linked to the circuitry for locomotor rhythm generators and for stereotyped movements called primitives. This rostrocaudal organization allows considerable computational flexibility. The columnar organization becomes a source for plasticity when descending activity is diminished by a CNS injury. Any descending or segmental afferent activity becomes a weightier input that may help drive activity in all the cells of the column and between columns, but this plasticity requires practice of motor skills. These columns are potentially important targets for biologic interventions that reinstate some supraspinal input after a spinal cord injury (see Chapter 2).

VENTRAL HORNS

Within a ventral horn, motoneurons can be mapped in three dimensions.[146] The more rostral a muscle's origin, the more rostral its cells are found in the cord. The hip flexor motoneurons are more rostral than the extensors. The muscles of the most distal joints have their motoneurons situated most dorsally in the ventral horn. Mediolaterally, the hip adductor and abductor pools are most medial, the flexors of the hip and knee are more lateral, and the extensors of the hip and knee are most lateral. The motoneurons for the axial muscles are always medial to those for more distal muscles.

The anatomical organization of the spinal pools and their passive and active membrane properties, fatigue characteristics, and responses to various neurotransmitters permit considerable adaptability. The muscles innervated at the other end of the motor unit are also quite adaptable, as discussed in Chapter 2. Modulatory inputs from amines and peptides alter motor pool excitability over a variety of time scales to assist the timing and magnitude of muscle contractions.[147] Sensory inputs and descending synaptic inputs create different orders of recruitment of motoneurons, including by order of size in keeping with Henneman's principle, by synchronous activation of all motor pools, and by selective recruitment of otherwise high-threshold units for rapid and forceful movements.[148]

SPINAL REFLEXES

Many theories of physical therapy focus on the use of brain stem and spinal reflexes as a way to retrain voluntary movement and affect hypotonicity and hypertonicity. Tonic and phasic stimuli can modify the excitability of spinal motor pools, postural reflexes, and muscle cocontractions.

The response to muscle stretch during passive movement, postural adjustment, and voluntary movement is not inflexible. Moment to moment adjustments in reflexes have been partly accounted for by a variety of mechanisms.[149,150] They include:

1. The mechanical, viscoelastic properties of muscle that vary in part with changes in actinomysin cross-bridges and alterations in connective tissues

2. Peripheral sensory receptors that respond to a perturbation from primary and secondary muscle spindles and Golgi tendon organs, but are regulated over a wide range of responsiveness by central commands

3. The convergence of segmental and descending inputs on Renshaw cells and motoneurons and interneurons that can summate in many ways, so that excitation of one peripheral receptor will not always produce the same stereotyped reflex response

4. Joint and cutaneous flexor reflex afferents that are activated during limb movements and vary in the degree to which they set the excitability of interneurons

5. Presynaptic inhibition of afferent proprioceptive inputs to the cord that are constantly affected by the types of afferents stimulated, as well as by descending influences

6. Long-latency responses to muscle contraction that supplement the short-latency, segmental monosynaptic component of the stretch reflex to compensate especially for a large change in mechanical load

7. The variety of sources of synaptic contacts on alpha-motoneurons, along with the intrinsic membrane properties that affect their excitability and pattern of recruitment of muscle fibers

Wolpaw and colleagues demonstrated activity-driven plasticity within the spinal stretch reflex, revealing that even the neurons of a seemingly simple reflex can learn when trained. The investigators operantly conditioned the H-reflex in monkeys to increase or decrease in amplitude.[151] An 8% change began within 6 hours of conditioning and then gradually changed by 1% to 2% per day. This modulation of the amplitude of the H-reflex required 3000 trials daily. The alteration persisted for several days after a low thoracic spinal transection, which suggests that the spinal circuitry for the H-reflex below the transection had learned and held a memory trace. A long-term change in presynaptic inhibition mediated by the Ia terminal presumably mediated this learning. Subsequent studies revealed that operant conditioning depends on corticospinal input, but not on other descending tracts.[152] In addition, cerebellar output to the cortex contributes to the corticospinal influence.

Using electromyographic biofeedback, the stretch reflex of the human biceps brachii muscle was successfully conditioned to increase or decrease in amplitude, but also required considerable training, approximately 400 trials per session.[153] Evidence for the effects of physical activity and training on the strength of spinal reflexes has also been found in active compared to sedentary people. The H-reflex and disynaptic reciprocal inhibition responses were small in sedentary subjects, larger in moderately active subjects, and largest in very active ones.[154] The reflexes were lowest, however, in professional ballerinas. The greater need for corticospinal input to the cord to stand en pointe and the sustained cocontractions involving the gastrocnemius and soleus complex probably lead to a decrease in synaptic transmission at Ia synapses, reducing the reflex amplitude. Thus, activity-dependent plasticity in the spinal motor pools contributes to the long-term acquisition of motor skills. Short-term, task-specific modulation of the gain of the H-reflex also occurs. The stretch reflex in leg extensor muscles is high during standing, low during walking, and lower during running.[155] A higher gain with standing provides greater postural stability. The gain also changes with the phases of the step cycle.

Thus, coupled spinal input and output activity can be trained, although training takes considerable and specific forms of practice. This adaptive plasticity may be of value in developing therapies to reduce spasticity and abnormal spinal reflex activity and, more importantly, to modulate the recovery of standing and walking in hemiparetic and paraparetic patients. Sensory inputs drive this plasticity.

CENTRAL PATTERN GENERATION

All mammals that have been studied, including a nonhuman primate,[156] possess a lumbar rhythm–generating network that can conduct reciprocal stepping movements.[124] This self-oscillating interneuronal network is found in a section of the lumbar spinal cord after it is severed from all descending and dorsal root inputs, leaving only the isolated cord segment and its ventral roots (Fig. 1–5B). The isolated lumbar spinal cord, after stimulation by drugs such as clonidine or dihydroxyphenylalanine, produces cyclical outputs in the ventral roots called *fictive locomotion*.[157,158] This primitive locomotor circuit, whose premotor and interneurons are imbedded within the motor pools, is called a *central pattern generator* (CPG). The CPGs of an intact spinal cord can excite and inhibit interneurons in reflex pathways using Ia and cutaneous inputs (Fig. 1–6).

Glutamate from the corticospinal tract, GABA, and glycine are the primary neurotransmitters from premotor inputs to the CPG. Serotonin, norepinephrine, thyrotrophin releasing hormone, substance P, and other peptides project to the CPG from brain stem nuclei. The effects of neurotransmitters and neuromodulators are complex. The lumbar stepping motoneurons are especially influenced by descending serotonergic and noradrenergic brain stem pathways, which are especially found in reticulospinal projections. These messengers set the gain for sensory and motor output and modulate the oscillatory behavior of spinal neurons and specific aspects of the locomotor pattern.[159] The serotonin pathway accounts for nearly all serotonin in the cord. Multiple serotonin receptor subtypes are distributed rostrocaudally. They interact with other receptors, including the glutamate NMDA receptor, and modulate reflexes and aspects of locomotion.[160] Amine and peptide neuromodulators tonically facilitate or depress ongoing motor acts, initiate and prime the circuits to respond more effectively to inputs, and alter the cellular and synaptic properties of neurons within a network, enabling the same CPG or group of CPGs to generate different motor patterns for different behaviors.[161] After a spinal or supraspinal injury, the distribution and availability of these neurotransmitters

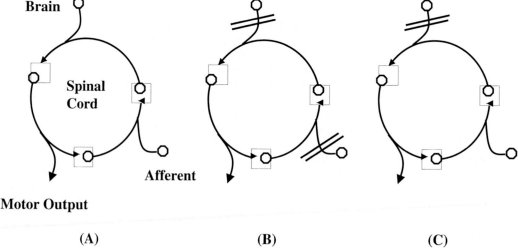

Figure 1–5. (*A*) The cartoon shows the descending supraspinal inputs and segmental afferent inputs that modulate the oscillating central pattern generators (CPGs) of the spinal cord. Motor outputs go to the flexor and extensor muscles of the legs. (*B*) Diagram of the isolated spinal cord. Flexor and extensor motor outputs are elicited by direct stimulation of the lumbar CPGs. (*C*) When isolated from supraspinal influences, segmental proprioceptive, cutaneous and other inputs drive flexor and extensor outputs for stepping.

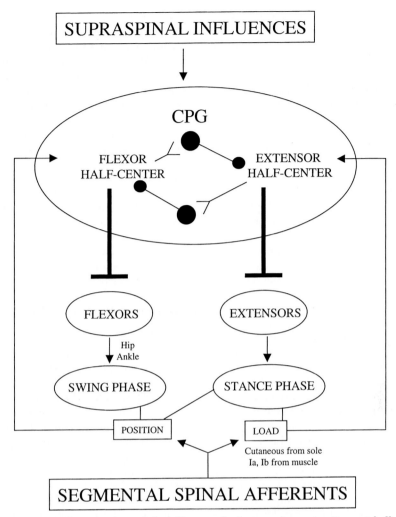

Figure 1–6. The central pattern generator includes half-centers for flexion and extension. Segmental afferents esepcially related to limb load and limb position during stance and swing phases of walking alter the level of inhibition and excitation in a state-dependent fashion.

change. One notion for a clinical intervention is to supplement by oral or intrathecal administration one or more neurotransmitter agonists to affect the initiation or automaticity of flexor and extensor alternating leg movements for walking that are managed by CPGs.

The precise distribution of the spinal CPGs is the subject of many studies. Experiments in rats suggest that the origin of patterned motor output extends over the entire lumbar region and into caudal thoracic segments.[162] Motoneurons at the L-1 and L-2 levels seem especially important to the CPG in animal studies.[163,164] This level is a potential cephalad target for biologic interventions such as axonal

regeneration aimed at restoring walking after a spinal cord injury.

Elementary CPGs probably control different muscles around a joint. For example, when one group of interacting neurons fires, a withdrawal reflex results. A different pattern that allows stepping emerges when another partially overlapping combination of neurons becomes activated. Many types of neural circuits that produce rhythmically recurring motor patterns have been described.[165–167] The recurrent burst patterns arise by networking common cellular mechanisms such as reciprocal inhibition, mutual excitation, spike frequency adaptation, and pacemaker-like or plateau properties.[165]

The CPGs must alter their output in response to even simple changes in conditions, such as variations in the characteristics of the surface walked. For effective stepping, as for upper limb movements, the motor output has to be timed precisely to changing positions, forces, and movements of the limbs. Descending and afferent sensory input timed to the gait cycle transform a group of oscillatory networks into coordinated activity (Fig. 1–5A). Sensory inputs from the hips, knees, and the dorsum and soles of the feet interact with the rhythm generators of the cord (Fig. 1–6).[168–171] These stretch, load, positional, and other inputs contribute to the timing of leg movements during the stance and swing phases of the gait cycle.

In studies of animals, small movements at the hip influence the rhythm-generating network, especially the transition as the hip is extended at the end of the stance phase to initiate the swing phase (see Gait Analysis in Chapter 6). During locomotion at ordinary speeds, the mechanism for swinging the leg forward is not triggered until a particular degree of posterior positioning of the limb is reached.[172] Flexor activity does not occur for swing in one leg until the extensors are loaded in the stance limb. Also, the magnitude of activity in knee and ankle extensor muscles and the duration of extensor muscle bursts during stance help generate a normal motor pattern for walking in both animal and human studies.[173,174] Sensory inputs have task-specific effects as well. The same sensory input from the foot that increases hip and knee flexion if applied during the swing phase of the gait cycle will increase activation of the extensor muscles if applied during the stance phase. *To best retrain walking in patients, strategies must incorporate optimal step-related sensory drives.*

Computer simulations of locomotion that model neural oscillators for each leg joint (Fig. 1–6), along with inputs from proprioceptors, the senses, and rhythmic movements of the musculoskeletal system, show the relative simplicity of a locomotor system designed around centrally generated patterns.[175] This organization allows flexibility and stability in an unpredictable environment and permits a change in a single parameter, such as a cortical or brain stem signal, to switch walking to running. Indeed, the mechanics of walking can be modeled as a simple inverse pendulum that moves forward by gravitational and inertial forces.

The evolution of the mechanics of walking has simplified the level of neural control needed for automatic stepping. The CNS controllers for walking may only have to issue suggestions to the spinal oscillators, rather than commands, which are reconciled with the physics of the body's muscles, joints, and bones and with the task.

The spinal cord, then, is not a passive node in the sensorimotor network. These sensorimotor pools are not a mere slave to supraspinal commands and simple segmental reflexes. The locomotor region of the spinal cord plays an important role in processing sensory information and in making decisions (see, Experimental Case Studies 1–2). In addition, sensorimotor tasks that involve practice lead to experience-dependent learning within the spinal cord's smartly organized circuits.

Evidence For A Central Pattern Generator in Humans

The definitive experiment to show the presence of a CPG would require isolation of the lumbar cord from supraspinal and segmental afferent inputs. Thus, only indirect evidence is possible. Striking similarities between humans and other animals weigh in favor of pattern generation in both.[176] Clinical studies of people with SCI have described spontaneous alternating flexion and extension movements of the legs. In a remarkably detailed evaluation of patients with operative verification of complete versus incomplete transection after traumatic SCI, Riddoch could not elicit rhythmic flexion-extension movements below complete thoracic lesions. He found almost exclusively a flexor response to cutaneous stimulation.[177] Reflexive extension followed by flexion was found in patients with partial preservation of anatomical continuity. In another study, however, subjects with operative verification of complete transection after traumatic SCI reported spontaneous slow, irregular alternating stepping or bicycling-like movements when supine that lasted up to 10 minutes.[178] We have observed slow, spontaneous alternating flexor and extensor leg movements in supine patients with severe or complete spinal injuries above T-8 following sessions of treadmill training for stepping that incorporates partial body weight support.[179] Involuntary lower extremity stepping-like movements were recorded from a subject with a chronic incomplete cervical

EXPERIMENTAL CASE STUDIES 1–2:
Plasticity in Spinal Locomotor Circuits

The cat's deafferented spinal cord below a low thoracic transection can generate alternating flexor and extensor muscle activity a few hours after surgery when DOPA or clonidine are administered intravenously or when the dorsal columns or dorsal roots are continuously stimulated. This is called *fictive locomotion*. Several weeks after a complete lower thoracic spinal cord transection without deafferentation, adult cats and other mammals have been trained on a treadmill so that their paralyzed hindlimbs fully support their weight, rhythmically step, and adjust their walking speed to that of the treadmill belt in a manner that is similar to normal locomotion.[375,376] Postural support alone is detrimental to subsequent locomotion, whereas rhythmic alternating movements of the limbs with joint loading seems critical to the recovery of locomotor output.[377] Serotonergic and noradrenergic drugs enhance the stepping pattern[378] and strychnine, through a glycinergic path, quickly induces it in spinalized animals who have trained only been to stand.[379]

The transected animal also transiently learns locomotor-related tasks such as stepping over an object.[186] The cat retains its learned, stereotyped locomotor patterns for at least 6 weeks after treadmill training and rapidly relearns to walk on the treadmill after another period of training.[380] Step training in the spinal transected cat and rat also affects the firing thresholds of motoneurons in the cord below the lesion. Changes in excitability are related to an increase in the GABA-synthesizing enzyme, GAD67, in the cord after spinal transection and glycine-mediated inhibition.[381] The trained spinalized cat's lumbar cord can make other adaptations. After the nerve to the lateral gastrocnemius and soleus was cut, the lumbar locomotor circuits compensated for the induced gait deficit, a yield at the ankle during stance that produced a more forward placement of the foot and shortened the stance phase, by 8 days postneurectomy.[382] The data show that compensatory changes can be attributed to spinal rather than to supraspinal pathways and that some combination of inputs from cutaneous and group I afferents led to the change in gait pattern.

Sensory feedback from cutaneous and proprioceptor inputs during stepping has a powerful affect on locomotor rhythm and muscle activation. The step phase transitions from stance to swing are triggered by afferent feedback related to extension at the hip and the unloading of leg extensor muscles.[161] One possible explanation is that group Ib Golgi tendon input during early stance inhibits the generation of flexor activity. As this input wanes near the end of stance, it releases the flexor burst generating system and enables the initiation of the swing phase.

SCI.[180] The movements were evoked when the subject was supine with the hips and knees in extension and when the subject was suspended over a treadmill belt. Noxious input from one hip appeared to initiate the rhythmical locomotor activity. In parallel to this human example, cats after a low thoracic spinal transection perform hindlimb stepping on a treadmill that is enabled by noxious stimulation below the lesion and hip extension caused passively by the posterior movement of the treadmill belt (see Experimental Case Studies 1–2).

Other evidence for a CPG in humans includes the occurrence of rhythmic myoclonic activity generated by a patient's transected spinal cord. Peripheral stimulation of flexor reflex afferents induced, slowed, or interrupted a subject's symmetrical 0.3–0.6 Hz rhythmic activity in extensor muscles.[181] Dimitrijevic and colleagues induced step-like locomotor activity in subjects with chronic complete spinal

cord injuries by epidural electrical stimulation of the posterior spinal cord below the level of the lesion.[182] They placed quadripolar electrodes at vertebral levels T-11 through L-1 and measured surface EMG activity in five muscles of each leg. Nonpatterned stimulation with 6–9 volts at 25–50 Hz at the L-2 level of the spinal cord produced the most rhythmic unilateral, but occasionally bilateral, alternating flexor-extensor muscle activity. Bilateral activity was found only when the electrodes happened to be placed in the midline. The L-2 level is especially important for hip flexion and, as noted above, has also been a key level for activation of CPGs in mammals. Stimulation at T-10 produced rhythmic irregular flexor withdrawal movements. Stimulation at 100 Hz at L-2 changed locomotor-like activity to tonic muscle firing. The current probably stimulated dorsal root fibers and, perhaps, dorsal column fibers. Neuromodulation by spinal electrical stimulation is being evaluated as a potential neuro-prosthesis for locomotion (see Chapter 4).

A parallel can be drawn between the the results of step training in the cat and in humans after a complete SCI. After a low thoracic spinal cord transection, the segmental sensory inputs discussed above have been used to train cats[183–186] and rats[187] to step independently on a moving treadmill belt over a range of speeds. In people with a complete thoracic SCI who are suspended with body weight support over a moving treadmill belt while therapists move their legs reciprocally through the step cycle, sensory inputs such as levels of loading on the stance leg and the degree of hip extension prior to the swing phase lead to step-like, alternating EMG activity.[174,179,188–191] Some subjects swing their legs without physical assistance and take a few steps that require only placement of the foot at the end of swing.[174,179]

Figure 1–7A shows the rhythmical EMG activity elicited from a subject with a clinically complete thoracic SCI. If considered in parallel to the spinal transected cat experiments in Experimental Case Studies 1–2, this rhythmic activity suggests the possiblity that spinal automaticity in humans can be driven by locomotor-related sensory inputs that are recognized by CPGs. Repetitive step training of a subject with a complete SCI may lead to greater amplitude of the elicited EMG bursts and improved organization, as shown in Figure 1–7B. This training-induced change supports the potential for activity-dependent plasticity in the motor pools and their motor units and functional stepping despite partial disconnection from supraspinal influences.

Thus, the lumbosacral spinal cord in humans recognizes patterned afferent input related to the step cycle and produces basic locomotor

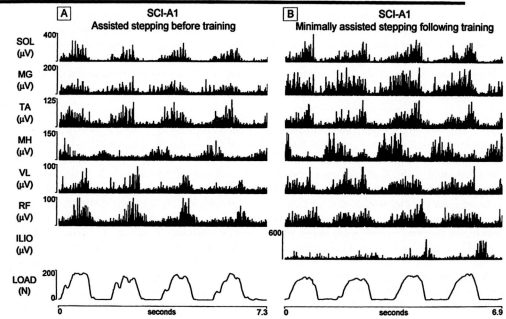

Figure 1–7. Electromyographic (EMG) activity from the flexor and extensor muscles of the legs in a subject with a complete thoracic spinal cord injury obtained during fully assisted treadmill stepping with 40% body weight support early (A) and late (B) after training. The level of weightbearing is shown at the bottom, highest during the phase of single and double-limb stance. The EMG about the ankle and knee muscles increased in amplitude, including the medial hamstrings (MH) and vastus lateralis (VL) at the knee and the soleus (SOL) and medial gastrocnemius (MG) at the ankle over the time of training, which suggests the recruitment of more motor units. The double burst that evolved in the tibialis anterior (TA) is typical of its normal pattern of firing. The rectus femoris (RF) came on only during stance and the iliopsoas (IL) fired at onset of swing (see Chapter 6 for details about normal firing patterns). Source: UCLA Locomotor Laboratory. S. Harkema, V.R. Edgerton, B. Dobkin.

synergies. The spinal cord, then, can learn.[192] This training approach has been operationalized using body weight–supported treadmill training BWSTT) in people with incomplete SCI and hemiplegic stroke (see Chapter 6).[179,193–196] Although a network of CPGs may be less useful in humans than for quadripeds who need coupling between the step cycles of the forelimbs and hindlimbs, it seems unlikely that evolution would dismiss the computational flexibility offered by the interaction of spinal reflexes, CPGs, and, as discussed in the next section, motor primitives.

SPINAL PRIMITIVES

The motoneurons and interneurons of the lumbar cord also participate in another type of organization that appears to simplify the problem of motor contol. Bizzi and colleagues combined a spinal cord transection with electrical or chemical microstimulation of the ventral gray matter of frogs, rats, and nonhuman primates.[9] The investigators found that rostral-caudal stimulation of separate volumes of gray matter produced movements that the investigators quantified as force vectors. Within each volume or module, a discrete set of synergistic limb muscle contractions was elicited that directed the limb toward an equilibrium point. In the frog, for example, they modeled the synergistic coactivation of muscles that stabilized the leg in four positions within its usual workspace.[197] As few as 23 out of over 65,000 possible combinations of activations of 16 limb muscles reproducibly stabilized the hindlimb within the flexion and extension synergies associated with its range of functional movements, in spite of wide variations in the force output of the muscles. By superimposing the vectors of the force fields that were elicited across all the spinal modules, the investigators calculated that the set of modules, which they call "primitives," stored the movements that carry out typical motor tasks within the leg's workspace. This intrinsic spinal organization, which is likely to be present in man, permits great dynamic stability and simplifies the computational work of supraspinal controllers for reaching and for locomotion. The primitives presumably act together under the control of supraspinal commands to create a rich repertoire of movement behaviors. When M1 or other regional motoneurons fire in a direc-

tionally tuned way, for example, they may be selecting spinal primitives. Corticoreticulospinal and corticovestibulospinal pathways are good candidates for leveraging the spinal primitives. By superimposing supraspinal and segmental sensory inputs, a vast number of movements and postures can be computed for the motor control of important synergies.

The spinal organization of force field modules may provide a basis for computational flexibility even when a stroke or SCI interrupts descending influences on the cord. In this circumstance, segmental afferent activity may become a more dominant input for resculpting locomotor or reaching activity. For walking, the details of experiential practice in cats and rats[198] and in humans[174,179,195,199] are critical for improving reciprocal stepping. As noted earlier, important sensory inputs relate to the rate and degree of hip extension, the level of limb weight bearing, the timing of interlimb movements and of shifts in bearing weight at the transition between stance and swing, and the speed of walking. Such inputs, provided repetitively, may activate any conserved organization of primitives and CPG circuitry of the cord and provide a clinical benefit (see Chapters 6 and 9). This sensory information also activates and reorganizes spared cortical and subcortical assemblies of motoneurons that may contribute to the recovery of better motor control. Functional neuroimaging studies reveal the details of the networks involved.

FUNCTIONAL IMAGING OF THE SENSORIMOTOR NETWORK

Details about how functional imaging studies are performed, as well as how they contribute to our knowledge of neuroplasticity after brain and spinal cord lesions, are provided in Chapter 3. Functional neuroimaging studies also reveal the physiologic anatomy of the sensorimotor network. For example, PET and fMRI show the somatotopic organization of movement representations in the primary sensorimotor cortex in remarkable detail.[200] Positron emission tomography and fMRI also map the secondary sensorimotor cortices for modality-specific activities such as preparation for a movement, internal generation of the movement, and visualizing or imagining an action. Association cortex and regions that represent cognitive functions become more active as the task grows in complexity. Of great interest for rehabilitation, PET, fMRI, TMS, and other techniques described in Chapter 3, reveal the networks engaged as motor tasks are learned.[201,202] For example, a high level of synaptic activity in primary and secondary sensorimotor cortices accompanies the early stages of learning a motor skill.[203] Studies of patients as they do therapy to acquire a skill could be used to monitor this gain in cerebral activity and its relationship to the success of the rehabilitation strategy.

Physiologic imaging techniques also reveal how the nature of a task, such as its difficulty, whether it is internally or externally cued, and how it is learned, alters the probability that a cerebral region will come into play.[204] A PET study, for example, performed as subjects learned a new sequence of eight finger movements by trial and error, revealed that the right-handed task activated the left dorsolateral prefrontal cortex (DLPFC) that includes BA 9 and 46 and the right anterior cingulate cortex (BA 24 and 32).[205] These areas were not involved in carrying out an overlearned sequence of finger movements. During new learning, then, subjects must monitor their movements and maintain successful responses in their working memories. Once subjects perform a skilled task automatically, they may be able to direct their attention elsewhere. When the subjects were asked to pay attention to their overlearned movements, the anterior cerebral regions again became active, though less intensely. The primary sensory area was more active as attention returned to the fingers. The bilateral cerebellar nuclei and the vermis and caudate were also activated significantly during new learning and novel problem-solving, compared to the other conditions.[206]

Functional imaging of the sensorimotor areas during the rehabilitative training of an important task may be used to determine whether critical tissue for learning is activated by the training strategy. For example, the recovery of prelearned finger movements is associated with activation of the same primary sensorimotor and SMA cortices as learning a novel, difficult task.[207] Despite some potential limitations,[208] PET, fMRI, and TMS allow the generation and testing of hypotheses about motor and cognitive processes and, as discussed in Chapter 3, about adaptive functional changes

after a cerebral, spinal, or peripheral nerve injury.

HAND AND FOOT ACTIVATIONS

Regional cerebral blood flow (rCBF) studies of normal subjects by PET reveal cortical areas most activated during simple upper extremity motor tasks. Activity increases in the contralateral M1 and the premotor, SMA, ventral premotor, and parietal cortical areas that are linked to it during proximal and distal arm, finger, and whole-hand movements.[209] Color Figure 1–8 (in separate color insert) is a fine example of the association of cortical and subcortical activations during self-paced, flexion and extension of the fingers or toes.[210] In half of the subjects, the ipsilateral putamen was activated. The toe activated the dorsal putamen and the fingers localized more ventral and medial. When a subject decides which fingers to move or learns a finger tapping sequence, the caudate and putamen become active rostral to the anterior commissure, consistent with a separate cortico-basal ganglia-thalamo-cortical loop. Passive movements of the hand and foot also activate sensorimotor cortices (see Chapter 3), which is useful for studying plasticity-related motor recovery over time when subjects start with paralysis of a limb.

In a PET experiment that helps define the distributed motor system, subjects were studied under four conditions. They moved a joystick (1) after a tonal cue according to a previously trained sequence, (2) in random directions, (3) when the correct movement was specified by one of the four tones they heard, and (4) when the correct movement was the opposite of what had been specified by the tones on the previous task.[209] The rCBF during these tasks was compared to simply moving the joystick forward at the same rate as the other tasks after a sound cue. The SMA had greater metabolic activity in the first two conditions. These tasks required internal generation of a movement, whereas the second two were directed by external cues. Activity within the left superior parietal cortex increased in all four conditions, suggesting that the process by which movement is selected is coded here. The bilateral premotor cortices, which are synaptically linked to the parietal region, were activated in all conditions as well. In the random condition, several frontal areas and the cingulate sulcus were activated, pointing to the contribution of these areas for self-initiated acts.

Control of Muscle Strength

Another experiment points to the contribution of parallel, cortical networks in a distributed motor system. Muscle strength increased by having individuals practice at imagining they were contracting a particular muscle.[211] Indeed, when the abductor digiti quinti was exercised to increase its strength and when subjects only imagined that they practiced abduction against resistance, the abductor of the untrained hand also increased in strength. This neural, as opposed to muscular, origin for strengthening also seems to occur during physical exercise before any muscle hypertrophy is evident. Mental exercise that improves muscle strength is associated with an increase in electroencephalographic-derived cortical potentials.[212] Positron emission tomography and other techniques suggest that this strengthening derives from the activation of central motor planning areas outside of M1. These areas increase the coordination and strength of outputs to spinal motoneurons.[213] The transfer of the motor program to the nonexercised digit may have been via the corpus callosum or by bilateral activation of the SMA. It appears, from limited studies, that BA 4 makes callosal connections, but not in the hand and foot areas. The bilateral SMAs, however, are highly interconnected with each other and with contralateral BA 4.[131] Increased strength, as opposed to an increase in skill, is probably not associated with a need for reorganization of movement representations for the active muscles.[214]

LOCOMOTOR NETWORKS

Positron emission tomography,[45] SPECT,[215] and near-infrared spectroscopy[46] can be carried out in association with walking on a treadmill. Supine rest was compared to 30 minutes of treadmill walking after injection with a fluorodeoxyglucose tracer and placing the subject back into the scanner. Cerebral activity for glucose increased bilaterally in the cerebellar vermis and the bilateral occipital cortex and paramedian BA 3, 4, 6 (including the SMA), 40 and 43. This activity presumably reflects the inte-

gration of visual and somatosensory information with motor activity in the leg region for motor control during rather rhythmic stepping. In some studies, the anterior cingulate and prefrontal cortices are active, perhaps especially in relation to the rhythmic movement and attention needed for treadmill locomotion. When normal subjects imagine doing locomotive leg movements while supine, functional imaging reveals significant increases in activation in the SMA and leg region of the primary sensorimotor cortex bilaterally and in the cingulate gyrus and cerebellar vermis.[46,216] A PET study of postural standing revealed significant activation of the vermis.[217] Rehabilitation specialists will be able to apply PET, fMRI, and other functional imaging techniques to detect and promote the reorganization of cortical networks for walking.

STUDIES OF REPRESENTATIONAL PLASTICITY

Cortical sensory and motor neurons are not permanently fixed in the way they subserve sensing and movement. On the contrary, these neurons quickly adapt to changing demands as new sensory and motor associations are experienced. In the adult and developing animal (see Experimental Case Studies 1–3 and 1–4) and in humans (see Chapter 3), the topographical maps of sensory and motor neuronal representations are capable of rapid and long-term physiologic and structural reorganization.[33,218,219] Electrophysiologic and metabolic imaging experiments reveal changes in the cortical maps for sensorimotor,[220] visual retinotopic,[221] auditory tonotopic,[222] and other representations induced by experience. This mutability is a ubiquitous property of adult cortical output and receptive fields.

Table 1–3 summarizes the sequence of important steps that lead to a memory trace for a skill. Consideration of these steps may give clinicians insight into the training and other input conditions that optimize remodeling and, in turn, improve motor control and higher cognitive activities during rehabilitation. How these modifications of functional pathways are modulated and how they may be manipulated to enhance and not to inhibit functional recovery is one of the most impor-

Table 1–3. **General Steps for Learning Motor Skills**

1. Goal-oriented, skilled movement task
2. Behavior reinforced by a learning paradigm
3. Repetitive practice under varying conditions
4. Sensory feedforward drive of motor cortex
5. Sensorimotor feedback
6. Neuronal representational map for movement expands by unmasking latent synapses
7. Increased synaptic efficacy of connections with related sensorimotor cortices and spinal motor pools
8. Dendritic branching and growth of spines
9. Lasting cortical and subcortical representational map for the skilled movement

tant applications of basic neuroscience to neurorestoration.

Motor Maps

Representational plasticity in M1 has been induced in a variety of animal models. Much of this work reconstructs movements of the forelimb digits and wrist evoked by cortical electrical microstimulation of small neuronal assemblies to produce representational maps of movements. Studies of changing neuronal assembly representations have been combined with a search for the molecular, physiologic, and morphologic changes that accompany reorganization.[27,223–226] Experimental Case Studies 1–3 describes motor map plasticity in uninjured animals. Representational and morphologic changes that arise after a CNS injury are reviewed in Chapter 2.

Activity-dependent representational changes in human subjects parallel those in animal models. Motor learning induces adaptations in the cortical maps that represent movements during the training of skilled hand movements.[227,228] A sequential finger opposition task practiced for a few minutes a day improves the speed and precision of performance, accompanied by a more extensive representation in M1 for the involved digits that evolves in stages. The cerebral activation by PET or fMRI is specific to the practiced fine motor coordination task and does not evolve with an untrained finger movement sequence. A different skilled finger sequence may overlap with elements of the same representation. Imaging also reveals fast and slow learning. An initial habituation-like decrease in M1 activation occurs during a session of practice. Several weeks

of practice and the acquisition of a skilled series of movements leads to the emergence of an enlarged representation for the digits. More remarkable, the practice of just 120 synchronous movements of the thumb and foot induces representational changes in which TMS reveals a short-term change in which the cortical locus for stimulation of the thumb moves toward the foot region.[229] This representational plasticity is consistent with the latent connnections of cortical motoneurons in M1 and the rather wide distribution of pyramidal projections to spinal motoneurons discussed earlier.

In normal subjects, TMS over M1, which selectively activates the corticospinal projections, has revealed representational plasticity during simple movements and with the acquisition of more complex skills. In a study of rapidly induced representational plasticity, TMS evoked either a flexor or extensor thumb movement in each subject at baseline. The subjects then practiced making repetitive thumb movements in the opposite direction. Within 5 to 30 minutes, thumb movements evoked by TMS changed to the direction of the practiced movement and this kinematic change persisted for up to 15 minutes.[230] In another study, subjects practiced a five-finger piano exercise for 2 hours a day for 5 days. Transcranial magnetic stimulation-evoked movements showed an enlarging motor cortical area targeting the long finger flexors and extensors and a decreased threshold for activation as subjects learned the skill.[231] In another experiment, cortical output maps to the muscles involved in a serial reaction time task, in which subjects had to learn from ongoing experience which buttons to push, enlarged as subjects learned the task.[232] Up to that point, the subjects had implicit or

EXPERIMENTAL CASE STUDIES 1–3:
Motor Map Plasticity

Motor maps also show functional reorganization. Merzenich and colleagues mapped the motor cortical zones that represent the digital, hand, wrist, elbow, and shoulder movements of monkeys before and after 11 hours of behavioral training.[383] Training involved having the primates retrieve food pellets from small food wells without using their thumbs. The M1 territories evoked by digital movements required for the task increased significantly (Fig. 1–9). New movement relationships emerged in the map between digit and wrist extensor activity that were inherent to success at the task. The cortical surface over which this increased coupling of neurons evolved corresponded to a network as great or greater than the spread of the axonal arbors of intracortical pyramidal cells.

Other experiments by this group support long held notions about the plasticity of the movement maps of the primary motor cortex.[384] The results also extend the work of others who found that the cortex of primates is composed of multiple representations of distal forelimb movements. For example, Merzenich and colleagues studied each hand's representation for movement in M1 as squirrel monkeys performed an unpracticed task that required skilled use of the arm and digits. In the hemisphere contralateral to the preferred hand, they found representations, especially for digit flexion, wrist extension, and forearm supination, to be greater in number, cover a larger area, and show greater spatial complexity compared to the nondominant hand's cortical representations for the same task.[385] The investigators concluded that the number of rerepresentations and the type of movements that overlap are quite variable between individuals and between the hemispheres of an individual. These differences derive in part from ontogenetic development and from experience, such as coactivating muscles or using them in a particular sequence in everyday activities.

Several neurotransmitters may participate in the changes in representational maps with experience and activity. A reduction in intracortical inhibitory pathways mediated by GABA permits the expression of new receptive fields.[282] Cholinergic and N-methyl-D-aspartate (NMDA) receptor modulation is also required.[386] These messengers apparently unmask preexisting synapses that had been functionally ineffective. For example, following deafferentation, tonic inhibition was diminished in rat and cat somatosensory cortex and the responsiveness of neurons to acetylcholine increased. This uncovered new receptive fields and strengthened existing ones.[387] Drugs used in clinical practice may alter these transmitters and receptors and affect plasticity.

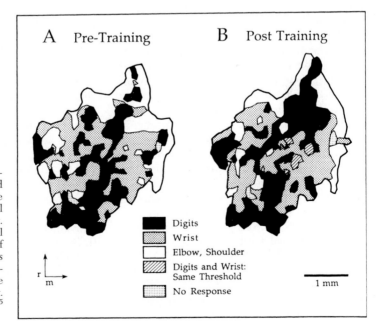

Figure 1–9. Movement maps derived by recording from a grid placed over Brodmann area 4 of the macaque before and after the animal was trained in a food-retrieval task. The upper cortex shows territorial gains for the neuronal assemblies of the digits (black) and new evocations by combined digit and wrist movements (parallel lines) that were needed to learn the motor task. Source: Merzenich et al., 1990,[395] with permission.

unconscious knowledge of the task. When they achieved explicit or verbalizable knowledge of how to do the task, the map of cortical output returned to baseline. These examples of rapid motor learning with enlarging maps suggest that synaptic connections are rapidly unmasked and the motoneurons form new movement associations. Once the procedure is overlearned and automatic, the same level of synaptic excitation for learning is no longer needed. Indeed, the internal knowledge about automatic performance may be stored elsewhere, perhaps in the basal ganglia and cerebellar networks.[203]

Cortical and subcortical networks, of course, also reveal adaptations with motor learning. For example, subjects moved a robotic manipulandum against a changing force field to targets on a screen. Within 6 hours of completion of practice on this novel task, in which performance skills were unchanged, a PET study revealed that the brain had come to engage new areas to consolidate learning the skill.[233] The internal model for the new skill shifted from an increase in activation of the visuomotor association cortex in BA 46, prior to practice, to an increase in rCBF in the contralateral posterior parietal and ipsilateral anterior cerebellar cortices. A reduction in activation was found in the bilateral middle frontal gyri in BA 46. These results and other studies reveal that the prefrontal cortex temporarily maintains arbitrary sensorimotor information, followed by long-term storage of an internal model for the skill.

The properties of neurons and their synapses are continuously shaped by use-dependent experience as a motor skill is learned. Bizzi and colleagues recorded from M1 neurons in monkeys as they performed the same reaching movements with a manipulandum in a force field to assess for plasticity during learning.[234] Loads on the arm strongly modulated the activity of M1 neurons. Both muscle and movement representations were found in M1. The investigators showed that both motor performance during the task and motor learning involved the same neuronal population. Apparently, single neurons change their activity as a new internal model for motor learning evolves. In parallel, the entire neuronal population reorganizes in relation to the direction of movements and to activation of muscles to transmit signals appropriate for the behavioral goal and motor performance. Thus, plasticity

induced by practice supports both motor performance and motor learning. This association is critical to theories about how to enhance motor skills after a CNS or PNS injury.

Sensory Maps

Experimental studies in rodents and monkeys also provide insights into somatosensory representational plasticity induced by changing sensory inputs and by learning. In a series of primate studies (Experimental Case Studies 1–4), Merzenich and colleagues found that cortical representational changes are especially likely to arise during training paradigms that involve learning and the acquisition of specific skills. The more a set of neurons is activated by a sensory stimulus, as when a primate learns to perform a task with repeated use of the same skin surface, the more widespread the cortical sensory representation becomes for the most stimulated area of skin. The investigators do not, however, always correlate an enlargement of the map with an increase in the primate's skill in the sensory discrimination task. The improvements the investigators observed as a result of training may be better associated with enhancement in the neural representation of the stimulus at another cortical or subcortical area that the investigators did not map. It is also possible that a physiologic variable more closely associated with greater skill was coded by a property of the neurons other than the spatial and temporal responses that were measured.[92]

In another clever experiment, monkeys practiced for a month to make fine sensory discriminations between two narrow bars gripped against the skin of three fingers for approximately 50 ms.[235] One bar crossed the digits proximally, the other pressed the same digits distally. Each bar pressed the skin of the three digits simultaneously, but the bars pressed at slightly different times. Evoked neuronal spikes from BA 3b revealed a dramatic change in the organization of the sensory fields for the digits. Instead of the usual separate zones for individual fingers, multiple-digit receptive fields evolved. Two large, continuous zones partially replaced the normally segregated representation for the skin of adjacent digits. The change occurred only in the cortex, not in the ventroposterior nucleus of the thalamus. This experiment demonstrates that Hebbian synap-

EXPERIMENTAL CASE STUDIES 1–4:
Sensory Map Plasticity

Using a mapping technique with an array of microelectrodes over the cortical surface of monkeys, Merzenich and colleagues conducted a series of experiments that demonstrate the mutability of somatosensory representations.[388] Following the amputation of a digit in adult monkeys, the sensory representation of adjacent digits in cortical areas 3b and 1 enlarged topographically by approximately 1 mm to occupy the territory that had been filled by the sensory neurons associated with the lost digit.[389] The change evolved over several weeks. Also, the details of the animal's touch maps improved in neighboring fingers.

In another experiment, monkeys were rewarded for touching a rotating disk that had an uneven surface with the tip of a digit for approximately 1.5 hours a day.[388] Compared to controls and to touching a static disk, reorganization of receptive fields in BA 3a and 3b evolved rapidly. The cortical representation of the stimulated phalanx enlarged immediately after stimulation and returned to the prestimulation size within 30 days. In other paradigms, stimulation of a small skin surface during a behavioral task leads to the emergence of a greatly expanded cortical zone of a coherent response that correlates with the improvement in the animal's ability to make relevant discriminations about the applied stimuli.[91]

A focal brain lesion model in the monkey is of special interest to rehabilitationists. A cortical lesion in area 3b was made where stimulation of one of the fingers had produced neuronal activation. The investigators induced the primate to use the same skin area of the hand in a reinforcing behavioral task by having it manipulate food pellets to eat. By the time the monkey was able to do so efficiently, the cortical region that represented the lesioned finger had shrunk, the map of surrounding finger areas enlarged, and a separate representation of the lesioned finger's skin arose in area 3a.[390] The investigators suggested that behaviorally important stimulation at a constant skin location led to an increase in the synaptic effectiveness for the related thalamocortical inputs, which produced a larger thalamic receptive field. In addition, changes in synaptic effectiveness within the local intracortical somatosensory neural network seemed to account for some of the variations in representations they observed. Horizontal connections that link cortical neurons over 6 to 8 mm have been found in the visual system. Axons of primary sensorimotor cortex pyramidal cells have as many as five intracortical collateral axons that form synapses over distances of 6 mm.[391] This increase in synaptic efficacy is equivalent to the neuroplasticity mechanism of unmasking synaptic connections after an injury.

Subcortical representational maps are also mutable. Local anesthetic injected into dorsal column nuclei resulted in the emergence of a new receptive field for each affected neuron within minutes, which suggests that new fields arise from unmasking previously ineffective inputs.[392] In another model of tactile learning, neurons of different cortical layers responded rapidly to changes in sensory experience within the whisker's receptive fields in rats.[269] Unmasking of latent synapses appeared less important than strengthening specific synapses in the thalamus and cortex. These two mechanisms are related and account for much of the modulation of sensory representational plasticity in humans.

tic plasticity, discussed shortly, can act across individual digits within BA 3b in relation to the timing of sensory input and practice.

In human subjects, studies of sensory representational plasticity and the effects of sensory inputs on motor cortex point to the influences that sensory inputs have on sensorimotor plasticity. For example, brief anesthesia of the median or radial sensory nerves immediately reduces the size of the representation of the first dorsal interosseus muscle elicited by TMS over the M1 representation. The effect is related to the loss of the muscle's cutaneous sensory input, since ulnar-innervated motor function was unaffected by the nerve block.[236] Thus, tonic sensory input from cutaneous and digital joint receptors affects the excitability of M1. With practice, task-dependent somatosensory maps are acquired rapidly and are later activated when that task is performed.[237] The somatosensory cortex switches between different preexisting maps, as does M1, depending on the requirements of the task. For rehabilitation, these studies provide more evidence of the impact of sensory inputs that are appropriate to a task on activity-dependent plasticity.

Another experiment found that repetitive stimulation of the ulnar nerve for 2 hours increased the excitability of M1 and increased the representation for ulnar, but not median-innervated hand muscles during testing with TMS.[238] In another paradigm, TMS that stimulated the abductor pollicus brevis, paired with low frequency stimulation of the median nerve to that muscle, induced greater excitability to the muscle within 30 minutes and the effect lasted up to 1 hour.[239] The anatomic localization for this plasticity, such as M1 alone, S1, or the spinal cord, is uncertain. This example of artificially driving sensorimotor integration likely involves a thalamocortical interaction. For clinical rehabilitation, these two TMS studies suggest the need to test a strategy of a synchronous combination of peripheral nerve stimulation of weaker muscles or stimulate with TMS during the retraining of a motor skill that incorporates those muscles. Direct cortical stimulation of S1 or M1 in monkeys with small surface electrodes at 50 Hz or less, combined with training, would be of great interest to see if such drive alters the rate or level of skills learning and sensorimotor representational plasticity.

Whether a specific frequency or magnitude of cortical stimulation can raise the excitability of M1S1 or of a nonprimary motor region to enhance relearning after a brain or spinal injury is far from certain. In a more general sense, however, the synaptic efficacy of motor representations are enabled by repetitive activation of somatosensory afferents, driven by spinal segmental sensory information associated with the kinematics, kinetics, and temporal features of movements during skills practice.

As discussed in Chapter 3, peripheral nerve, brain, and spinal cord injury may lead to new somatosensory maps appreciated by fMRI, PET, and other neuroimaging and stimulation techniques.[220,240–243]

BASIC MECHANISMS OF SYNAPTIC PLASTICITY

Having reviewed some of the anatomy and representational plasticity that accompanies motor control and sensorimotor learning, I selectively explore some of the burgeoning data at the level of neurons and molecules that help explain remodeling of sensorimotor representations by experience and by CNS and PNS lesions. Many important issues have yet to be explained at the level of cell connections, cell properties, and the molecules of neuron-to-neuron interactions at synapses. Nearly every step in the mechanisms by which experience modifies the properties of neuronal assemblies and networks reveals activity-dependent plasticity. I emphasize information that may trigger ideas relevant to rehabilitation training and neuropharmacologic interventions.

The level of activity of a network is modulated by the strength of excitatory and inhibitory connections and the intrinsic excitability of the neurons of an assembly and network. The best regarded mechanism for cortical representational remodeling is the induction of synaptic plasticity by LTP, guided by Hebb's rules.[33]

Hebbian Plasticity

In the 1940s, Hebb described an increase in synaptic strength between neurons that fire together. Hebbian learning arises when neurons detect temporally correlated inputs, meaning behaviorally important stimuli that cause them to respond in a temporally coherent fashion. The synaptic strengthening is called *associative*, because it associates the firing of a postsynaptic neuron with the firing of a presynaptic one. Subsequently, when a presynaptic neuron bursts, the postsynaptic one is more likely to fire. Whereas the active synapse strengthens, other unrelated synapses on the postsynaptic neuron do not. Either *homosynaptic facilitation or depression* results. The Hebbian learning rule, then, states that connection weights will be increased or decreased depending on whether presynaptic and postsynaptic activity is correlated or uncorrelated, respectively. Studies suggest that this relationship maintains the capacity of a circuit to store new information and prevents the saturation of connections.[244] Correlation-based Hebbian mechanisms that modify the properties of connections over time may seem to work against the homeostatic mechanisms that stabilize networks and learning. On the other hand, *homeostatic plasticity* may operate over longer time scales and by altering postsynaptic receptor numbers, but still closely linked to the mechanisms of Hebbian plasticity.[245]

Kandel and colleagues proposed another rule for learning-related synaptic plasticity. A third neuron can mediate the firing of the presynaptic neuron to facilitate or inhibit the synaptic strength between a presynaptic and postsynaptic neuron.[246] This modulatory interneuron allows for *heterosynaptic plasticity*. The homosyaptic Hebbian response produces a relatively short-term memory. The heterosynaptic synapse ensures that the memory persists.

Widely projecting neurotransmitter systems, such as norepinephrine, dopamine, serotonin, and acetylcholine may be especially important in modulating Hebbian synaptic strengthening to save an association. Whereas LTP may be critical for short-term homosynaptic Hebbian plasticity, repeated heterosynaptic activity may recruit the signalling pathways and gene expression that grow new synapses.[247] The combination of homosynaptic and heterosynaptic plasticity can create new combinations of synaptic excitation and inhibition for the complex encoding of cortical development, memory, and synaptic remodeling throughout life.

Cortical Ensemble Activity

Many experiments have shown that the selective response properties of single neurons can change by associating inputs from other neurons across a narrow window in time or by manipulating a neuron's membrane potential by external stimuli so it is more or less excitable.[33] These cell-conditioning experiments support the relationship between Hebbian synaptic plasticity and changes in selective neuronal responses.[248] Experimental Case Studies 1–5 describe several insightful experiments in active rats. These studies support the neuroimaging data in humans of time-dependent plasticity within a neuronal network.[233] In general, the neuronal ensembles in M1, for example, increasingly encode sensorimotor contingencies as a new task is learned. A subgroup of M1 neurons come to represent new and behaviorally relevant information by subtle changes in their temporal patterns of firing, by more correlated firing, and by their firing rates.

Long-Term Potentiation and Depression

Long-term potentiation and long-term depression (LTD) appear to be fundamental cellular mechanisms for learning and memory. They are the most robust forms of a persistent modification of synaptic transmission in response to a brief stimulus. The cascade for synaptic plasticity involves the modulation of neuronal excitability by N-methyl-D-aspartate (NMDA) receptor activation, induction by triggering mechanisms for plasticity after NMDA recep-

EXPERIMENTAL CASE STUDIES 1–5:
Listening to Neuronal Ensembles

Cortical ensemble activity can be studied during a motor learning task by listening to the activity of small groups of neurons, usually from 20 to 60 randomly chosen cells located near the tip of the intracerebral recording electrodes. For example, electrode recordings were made from sensorimotor striatal neurons of rats as they learned to correctly move through a maze by making turns when they heard a tone.[393] As the rats improved in learning this skill or procedural task, marked changes occurred in the recruitment and firing patterns of the recorded neurons. These changes were found when the starting gate opened and locomotion began, at the onset of auditory cues, upon making turns to the left or right, and at the end of the maze when a reward was given. The changes in ensemble activity could also have occurred among midbrain dopaminergic neurons that will shift their responses toward the earliest indicator of a reward in a procedural learning task and to other primary and secondary sensorimotor regions.

Other investigators recorded from neuronal assemblies in rat motor cortex as the animals learned a task in which they had to hold down a lever for variable times with a forepaw and release it in response to an auditory or tactile stimulus.[394] Correct trials occurred when the rodents sustained the press until being cued and released the lever with a short reaction time. Three measures of neuronal ensemble activity—the average firing rate, temporal patterns of firing, and correlated firing among neurons—changed as the learned skill improved and the reaction time shortened. The investigators were able to predict the outcome of single trials based upon these modifications in ensemble activity.

tor activation, and maintenance of the potentiated or depressed state. The cascade occurs both presynaptically and especially postsynaptically. In experimental protocols, LTP is induced by brief, high-frequency stimulation of afferent paths, whereas LTD requires more prolonged, low-frequency stimulation that leads to a reduction in synaptic drive.

Although best studied in the hippocampus, LTP and LTD have also been demonstrated in normal somatosensory, motor, and visual cortices.[249–251] In the cerebellum, LTP, LTD, and a probable nonsynaptic type of memory storage have been demonstrated.[252] For the nonsynaptic mechanism, activity-dependent changes in the intrinsic excitability of granule cells creates a more global change in signal integration. Cerebellar LTD is a fundamental mediator of aspects of motor learning.[253] Long-term potentiation has also been demonstrated in activity-dependent corticostriatal synaptic plasticity, which would favor the initiation of a learned movement.[254] Mechanisms for spinal cord learning also include repeated sensory inputs during practice that produce LTP and LTD.[255,256] LTP may also contribute to learning-induced synaptic plasticity and representational changes after a supraspinal injury.[69]

The link between learning-induced synaptic plasticity and LTP in motor cortex is firming up. The strengthening of connections in the M1 representation for the contralateral forelimb in the rat as it learns a skilled motor task is achieved by LTP in excitatory synaptic transmission in the horizontal cortico-cortical connections in layers II/III.[32,257,258] In keeping with the general hypothesis that stimuli that increase the NMDA current or decrease inhibition (see Molecular Mechanisms in this chapter) will produce more robust LTP, cortical layers II, III, and IV show robust associative synaptic plasticity. In the rat model, motor learning compared to motor activity also led to a significant increase in the number of synapses per neuron in layers II/III.[259] In addition, induction of LTP by daily electrical stimulation of the corpus callosum in rats with chronically implanted electrodes increased the density of dendritic spines, the same change that occurs in rats housed in visually and physically stimulating environments that induce activity-dependent plasticity.[260]

Ascending inputs to M1 also induce LTP. Asanuma and colleagues showed that the stimulus parameters in sensory cortex for producing LTP in the motor cortex were within the range of the discharges of sensory cortical neurons that respond to ordinary peripheral afferent stimulation.[261] The investigators also showed that repetitive activity of pyramidal neurons produces LTP in spinal interneurons. Although tetanic stimulation of the ventrolateral nucleus of the thalamus (VL) alone did not induce LTP, the researchers produced associative LTP in the VL when they combined VL and sensory cortex stimulation. They proposed that repeated practice of a particular movement increased the excitability of a selected group of VL terminals by associative LTP, so that the VL's untrained, diffuse input became able, with training, to excite selected cortical efferent zones without further input from the sensory cortex. They hypothesized that thalamocortical circuits are initially diffuse, leading to excessive muscle contractions during a new movement. The circuits become more specific as practice induces LTP and greater sensorimotor integration.

The synaptic strengthening in M1 by LTP during the learning of a new motor skill may shift the population of involved synapses close to their maximum range of operation.[257] If LTP were saturated by the task, interference with further learning could theoretically arise. This susceptibility to saturation tends to happen when a motor memory is in its short-term fragile form, before it has progressed to a long-term, consolidated internal model for an action. In one experiment, subjects reached with a robotic arm within a changing force field. They learned and retained two conflicting motor skills a day later only if the training sessions were separated by at least 5 hours.[262] Presumably, mechanisms such as ongoing neuronal firing and synaptic changes that continue for some hours after learning one task can disrupt the initial learning of a second task that reuses a similar internal model for an action. Practice for the second task also degraded what was learned in the first task.

In the rehabilitation setting, where therapists coax the relearning of motor skills by a nervous system that has been depleted of some of its learning and storage capacity, practice paradigms may need to consider the potential for saturation. At the molecular level, a small residual of LTP capacity or striking a new balance with LTD may be sufficient to support additional learning. In addition, procedural and declarative learning both appear to have an initial, time-limited stage that involves regions of the brain that maintain the procedural or declarative memory. Other regions store the memory. This shifting process may also reduce the likelihood of saturation.

Molecular Mechanisms

The details of the cellular and molecular bases for LTP and LTD are still evolving. Kandel and colleagues have demonstrated the conservation of mechanisms from the Aplysia snail's gill-withdrawal reflex to the mammalian hippocampus.[247] A general model for induction of LTP starts with the release of glutamate from presynaptic boutons. The neurotransmitter acts upon both α-amino-3-hydroxy-5-methyl-4-isoxazoleproprionic (AMPA) receptors and NMDA receptors. Sodium then flows through the AMPA receptor. Calcium cannot flow through the NMDA receptor because magnesium blocks its receptor channel. Upon depolarization of the postsynaptic neuron, the magnesium block is overcome and sodium and calcium flow into the dendritic spine of the synapse via the NMDA receptor. The neurotrophin BDNF contributes to depolaring the postsynaptic neuron. The rise in calcium within the spine initiates a cascade that triggers LTP at that synapse. Metabotropic glutamate receptors, particularly the ones in the family of G protein–coupled receptors, may also need to be activated for the generation of LTP in some types of synapses.

Subsequent biochemical pathways translate the calcium signal in a dendritic spine into an increase in synaptic strength. This cascade of events continues to be explored.[251] Several of the steps may be important to a future neuropharmacology for neurorehabilitation. One of the apparently mandatory steps for signal transduction occurs when calcium binds to calmodulin to activate α-calcium-calmodulin-dependent protein kinase II (CaMKII). Once this molecule autophosphorylates, it is no longer dependent on a continued rise in calcium. A key molecular switch in cortical experience-dependent plasticity,[263] CaMKII phosphorylates AMPA receptors at the postsynaptic membrane and increases the number of delivered AMPA receptors. This step expresses

LTP. Thus, protein synthesis of AMPA receptors appears necessary for LTP. The local calcium increase also activates other protein kinases that may aid LTP, particularly protein kinase C (PKC), cyclic adenosine 3′,5′-monophosphate (cAMP)-dependent protein kinase A (PKA), a tyrosine kinase, and mitogen-activated protein kinase (MAPK). These kinases help lock a synapse or cell into a set of specific and enduring synaptic weights. The kinases also participate in many other signal transduction processes relevant to plasticity. Thus, the ability to manipulate them pharmacologically would give clinicians a potential tool to enhance the learning of skills and retain new information after a CNS lesion.

In the hippocampus, for example, PKC moves from the cytoplasm to the nucleus where it activates a regulatory protein for transcription named cAMP response element-binding protein (CREB). A cascade of genes that make new proteins to enhance synaptic strength and generate new dendritic synapses for learning and memory is then turned on by CREB. A gene mutation in CREB or PKA pathways would reduce the persistence of declarative memory, but initial learning, which is dependent on NMDA-dependent plasticity, would be normal. Long-term potentiation induction does not require new protein synthesis, but synthesis is necessary if memory storage in the hippocampus CA1 field is to persist for 24 hours. Kinases move from protein to protein within a dendritic spine or presynaptic terminal to phosphorylate proteins and alter their function. Phosphatases, which dephosphorylate proteins, also have an important role in synaptic plasticity.[264] The serine/threonine phosphatases include calcineurin, which plays a key role in limiting the induction and maintenance of LTP and in triggering the induction of LTD.

Long-term depression is a common cerebellar learning mechanism. It occurs at the parallel fiber–Purkinje cell synapse and at the climbing fiber synapse.[252] The climbing fiber increases calcium influx and the parallel fiber releases glutamate onto metabotropic and AMPA receptors. In many respects, LTD is a reversal of the processes that lead to LTP, although the total effects of the two can be additive. In LTD, the AMPA and NMDA receptor–mediated excitatory postsynaptic current decreases along with a postsynaptic decrease in responsiveness to glutamate.

Any manipulation that increases calcium influx at the dendritic spine or leads to a subsequent increase in a strategic protein kinase may induce LTP and aid learning in the rehabilitation setting. Finding drugs that act as memory molecules is a major pursuit of pharmaceutical companies.

Growth of Dendritic Spines

Motor learning induces genes that modify cell structures and functions, such as increasing the number of synaptic spines.[259] Indeed, dendritic spines increase with the induction of LTP.[265] Growing evidence points to the relationship between morphologic remodeling of the postsynaptic membrane as a late response to LTP and functional changes in synaptic strength.[266] In one proposal for this remodeling process, the induction of LTP increases the number of AMPA receptors in a postsynaptic dendritic spine. The postsynaptic membrane enlarges, then splits into several spines.[267] The new spines send a retrograde message to the presynaptic membrane to trigger structural changes there. The number of synapses related to the initial activity-induced signal then increases. Long-term depression may involve the inverse of this process. A decrease in AMPA receptors and membrane material leads to a decrease in the size of the postsynaptic membrane, and finally to the loss of the dendritic spine.

The expression of synaptic plasticity may be influenced by the properties of dendrites.[268] Dendrites reveal a great variety of forms of excitability that arise, in part, from their diverse morphology and differences in the types and distribution of their voltage-gated and nonvoltage-dependent membrane channels. This flexibility adds to the computational power of synaptic plasticity.

Synapse duplication by LTP induction and weaning by LTD maintain the specificity of information processing between activated neuronal terminals and target cells and increases storage capacity for new learning. This morphologic mechanism also helps explain how the effects of an enriched environment and learning paradigms may increase synapse number and dendritic arborization.[269–271] For example, an enriched environment for rats, meaning lots of mates, tunnels, and toys to climb, increases the number of new dendritic boutons with postsynaptic contacts, presumably by synaptic mechanisms for activity-dependent learning.[272]

Kleim and colleagues used cortical microstimulation and morphologic techniques to reveal parallel changes between learning-dependent functional reorganization and synaptogenesis. The region of M1 that represents wrist and digit movements enlarged its representation as rats trained in a skilled reaching task for food pellets. This representational map expansion and synaptogenesis colocalized to the wrist and digit region of M1 in layer V of rats trained in the skilled reaching task compared to rats that carried out unskilled reaching.[273] The number of afferent synapses per neuron increased by approximately 30%, presumably strengthening intracortical connections and consolidating skills learning. Thus, an initial unmasking of latent synapses for the neuronal assemblies representing the digits led to an increase in the number of synapses through task-specific training for just a $1/2$ hour/day for 10 days.

Neurotrophins

Neurotrophins are also important effectors of morphologic changes with activity-dependent plasticity. Several of the neurotrophins, discussed further in Chapter 2 (see Table 2–5), are induced by LTP and by activity-dependent plasticity. In the most studied model of LTP memory processing in the hippocampus, the genes expressed during the establishment of LTP include brain-derived neurotrophic factor (BDNF) whose protein increases in the CA1 region during hippocampus-dependent learning.[274] Neural activity associated with physical activity in rodents helps regulate neurotrophins such as BDNF and fibroblast growth factor (FGF-2).[275] The combination of a motor activity in a learning situation, such as swimming in a water maze, increases activity-induced expression of the neurotrophins during the learning phase. This expression likely affects the molecular and cellular events that influence cortical plasticity, motor learning, and memory, including greater synaptic efficacy and dendritic sprouting.

The neurotrophins and their tyrosine receptor kinase (trk) receptors, modulate the development and maintenance of synapses and the rapid modifications of synaptic structure and function.[276] Neurotrophins such as BDNF were thought to be produced by target neurons and to pass from postsynaptic to presynaptic neurons. Their production and movement is more complex. For example, fluorescent-labeled BDNF was shown in a set of experiments to move antegrade down presynaptic axons in an activity-dependent fashion, although some moved retrograde from the postsynaptic neuron in association with a learning task.[277]

For hippocampal learning, BDNF rapidly modulates presynaptic transmission over seconds to minutes. In addition, the neurotrophin modulates postsynaptic hippocampal transmission and plasticity. By activating postsynaptic trkB receptors, BDNF depolarizes the postsynaptic neuron, probably by opening sodium channels and calcium channels, leading to the cascade for LTP.

The rise in calcium at a dendritic spine that induces LTP also induces the postsynaptic secretion of morphogenic levels of neurotrophins at the membrane. As functional modulators of LTP, secreted neurotrophins prolong the effects of presynaptic neurotransmitters and postsynaptic responsiveness. For example, when BDNF binds to its receptor on a presynaptic neuron, it activates many signaling steps. One of these cascades leads to the production of synapsin, which tethers tiny vesicles of neurotransmitters such as glutamate and GABA and helps control their availability and release.[278] As morphogenic modulators, certain neurotrophins structurally modify existing synapses by low-level secretion. The neurotrophins also trigger sprouting of terminal arbors and dendritic spines with activity-dependent secretion of larger amounts to induce new synaptic contacts.

Given that most of the identified neurotrophins are available for pharmacologic testing, they offer a potential means for enhancing synaptic efficacy during the relearning of skills or cognitive functions that were compromised by a neurologic disease. Neurotrophins and drugs that mimic them, as well as other potential "memory-related molecules" such as neuropeptides, cytokines, and neurotransmitters that act as neuromodulators rather than for synapse-specific transmission, offer great promise. They all have complex actions, however, so flooding the brain with one could also have adverse clinical effects.

Neuromodulators

Chemical neurotransmission across synapses permits the computational flexibility and regulation that contribute to synaptic plasticity. Many proteins are involved in the biosynthesis, storage, reuptake after release, and degradation of neurotransmitters. Other proteins participate in bringing the vesicles that are filled with neurotransmitters to the nerve terminal where the packets dock, fuse, and undergo endocytosis, then recycle. The processes that mediate neurotransmitter release are essential for information processing and the goal of learning and memory.[279] The growing number of known details about the molecular mechanisms of neurotransmitter synthesis and release may lead to better pharmacologic means to selectively increase and decrease the activity of chemical messengers to augment activity-dependent plasticity. Further studies may reveal genetic differences between people in, for example, their dopaminergic tone, which may correlate with neuropsychiatric disorders and differences in the ability to learn.

The release of a neurotransmitter across the synaptic cleft transduces a physiologic signal after the messenger binds to the postsynaptic receptor. Table 1–4 lists the primary actions of neurotransmitters at a synapse.[247] Fast synaptic transmission occurs when neurotransmitters such as acetylcholine (Ach), GABA, glycine, and glutamate activate ion channels. On a longer time scale, monamines such as norepinephrine and dopamine, peptides, and the classic neurotransmitters such as Ach activate G protein–coupled receptors, which then activate a cascade of secondary messengers. Glial cells can also modulate synaptic transmission by releasing or taking up most neurotransmitters.[280] At least five of the major neurotransmitters are known to modulate the distributed, parallel networks for sensorimotor and cognitive processes.[281] Histamine is perhaps the least studied. Projections from the hypothalamus may affect attention, mood, motivation, learning, and vigilance. Four other neuromodulators project widely, especially to the frontal lobes.

Table 1–4. Synaptic Actions Mediated by Neurotransmitters

1. Activate ligand-gated ion channel for rapid synaptic action for milliseconds
2. Activate a receptor and a second messenger kinase to produce a synaptic action lasting minutes
3. Activate second-messenger kinases that go to the nucleus to initiate gene-regulated neuronal growth and persistent synaptic change
4. Mark the specific synapses that regulate local protein synthesis for long-term stability of synapse-specific facilitation
5. Mediate attention and signal-to-noise processes needed for memory and recall

ACETYLCHOLINE

Acetylcholine from the nucleus basalis projects to the cortex and amygdala. Pedunculopontine cholinergic neurons modulate thalamocortical input and the striatum. Muscarinic receptors are most involved in cortical neuromodulation.

Among their activities, Ach projections gate behaviorally relevant sensory information. With greater output of Ach, the response to a sensory input is greater. With less neurotransmitter neuromodulation of the sensory input, the responsiveness of target neurons decreases. For example, the cortical sensory representational expansion that usually follows the partial loss of input from the skin after a peripheral nerve injury will not occur if the lesion is made after unilateral destruction of the basal forebrain's cholinergic input.[282]

Acetylcholine produces a long-lasting slow depolarization of pyramidal cells, which facilitates their firing.[283] By modulating incoming action potentials, Ach fine tunes cortical responses, lends focus, and enhances the appreciation of sensory inputs. The effects of Ach on cortical neurons are generally excitatory, but Ach can cause inhibition by its secondary effect of stimulating GABA-releasing neurons. The activation of inhibitory interneurons may also sharpen the impact of a sensory input.

Acetylcholine has other modulatory effects over longer time scales. It influences second-messenger activities that raise protein kinase C levels and intracellular calcium stores, both of which contibute to dendritic growth and plasticity. It also enhances glutaminergic activity to contribute to LTP. Thus, cholinergic or cholinomimetic drugs, which are widely available to physicians, may have practical value in augmenting synaptic plasticity, whereas cholinergic antagonists may be harmful to the recovering brain.

Merzenich and colleagues carried out a series of elegant experiments to assess a cholinergic neuromodulating mechanism for plasticity in primary auditory cortex of rats.[222] The investigators mapped the auditory cortex with microelectrodes to sample frequency-intensity responses from 45 pure tone frequencies at 15 sound intensities. With this tonotopic map, they then paired a particular tone with electrical stimulation of the nucleus basalis. The representation of that tone enlarged progressively by 1 to 3 weeks later. The amount of remodeling was considerably larger after nucleus basalis stimulation compared to operant conditioning with a behavioral training paradigm. Acetylcholine is released from one-third of the neurons of the nucleus. Most of the other neurons release GABA. The responses in the auditory cortex were ascribed to cholinergic neuromodulatory effects. Thus, paired auditory and cholinergic stimulation enhanced the behavioral relevance of the tone, consistent with the connections of the nucleus basalis to limbic and paralimbic structures.

DOPAMINE

Dopaminergic projections from the ventral tegmental tract relate a reward to the cognitive effort, which reinforces associative learning. The reward is associated with a preceding event or stimulus. During initial learning, when rewards happen unpredictably, dopamine neurons are activated by rewards. They lose this response when rewards become predictable. Neuronal learning in relation to dopamine depends more on reward prediction errors than a stimulus–reward association.[284] This teaching signal is found in the actions of dopaminergic neurons in the ventral tegmental tract in relation to sensory and cognitive functions and in the substantia nigra in relation to sensorimotor and procedural learning. Microdialysis of the human amygdala during tasks that require working memory, during reading, and with word-pair learning reveal an increase in the release of dopamine during performance of the cognitive task.[285] The ventral tegmental tract, once considered only a mediator of pleasure, is involved especially in learning given that it rewards attention to what is significant or surprising.

Dopamine also modulates LTP. Dopamine agonists sharpen or focus NMDA-mediated and other depolarizing synaptic signals, especially on apical dendrites in frontal cortex.[286] In addition, dopamine, like norepinephrine, decreases background firing rates and increases the signal-to-noise ratio for focused attention. The neurotransmitter enhances the salience of a task. In addition to pharmacologically available dopamine, inhibitors of dopamine breakdown, dopamine receptor agonists, and d-amphetamine and methylphenidate,[287] all increase the availability of the dopaminergic signal. Amphetamine may enhance the phasic release of dopamine and thereby participate in a more typical neural processing of reward than what direct supplementation of dopamine allows.[288] In addition, amphetamine combined with a novel environment or task has a greater action than the drug alone.[289] It would not be surprising, then, to find instances in which patients during their rehabilitation benefit from drugs that drive dopaminergic receptors to enhance task-specific signaling.

Merzenich and colleagues, again using the paradigm of electrical stimulation paired with pulsed tones of different frequencies, demonstrated how the dopamine system may shape both primary and secondary auditory cortex.[290] As with nucleus basalis stimulation, the cortical representation of a particular tonal frequency expanded when a 4 kHz tone preceded ventral tegmental area (VTA) stimulation. An adjacent representation for 9 kHz diminished if VTA stimulation was preceded by the 4 kHz pulse and followed the 9 kHz pulse. Stimulation of the VTA, then, increased the saliency of the tones to reorganize tonal representations. As noted earlier, the functional properties of cortical neurons can be defined both by their selective responsiveness to certain input parameters as well as by their interactions with other neurons of a cooperative neuronal assembly. The combination of VTA stimulation paired with auditory stimulation induced the synchronization of neuronal activity over a large area of primary and secondary auditory cortices. Thus, large-scale experience-related reorganization included association cortex, which itself has widespread connections to limbic and sensory regions. This interaction associates neuromodulatory dopamine activity to emotion, to auditory or other sensory stimuli, and to learning.

NOREPINEPHRINE

The noradrenergic (NA) fibers from the locus ceruleus (LC) project to much of the cortex. These projections suppress spontaneous background neural activity, which may increase the signal-to-noise ratio and modulate resistance to distraction. This system helps mediate arousal and selective attention.[291] The firing rate of NA cells has been suggested as a control on attentional selectivity.[292] A moderate rate of coupled firing of LC neurons in monkeys facilitated a state of selective responding during a task that required visual discrimination of a target stimulus. High tonic activity impaired performance. The investigators suggested that heightened selectivity would be a disadvantage in an uncertain or stressful environment in which an ongoing behavior has to be jettisoned for a more adaptive one, such as interrupting the feeding of offspring when a predator appears. The acquisition of a new skill also depends less on the speed with which the most correct behavior is discovered and more on a fuller exploration of alternatives until the skill is learned. Locus ceruleus activity may both increase and decrease attentional selectivity to increase behavioral responsiveness to a novel stimulus. Pharmacologic doses of norepinephrine-like drugs may not, then, have the same effect as natural tonic firing that pulses, rather than floods target neurons.

Neurotransmitter modulators may interact. In sensory cortices, for example, Ach acting on a muscarinic receptor and norepinephrine acting on an α-1 receptor facilitated NMDA receptor-dependent LTD at the same synapse.[293] This combination modulates the plasticity of receptive fields in visual cortex in an experience-dependent fashion. In the studies from Merzenich and colleagues described above, some interaction between dopamine and Ach seems likely in their dual modulation of aspects of auditory cortex plasticity.

SEROTONIN

Serotonergic (5-hydroxytryptamine) [5-HT]) projections from the brain stem dorsal and median raphe nuclei play roles in sensory, motor, and cognitive arousal.[294] Projections from the pontomesencephalic nuclei go to the cortex, including the hippocampus, amygdala, and sensorimotor areas, as well as to the cerebellum, thalamus, and hypothalamus. Serotonergic projections from the caudal medulla go to the spinal cord where they act upon the proximal and axial muscle motoneurons, the locomotor CPG, and sympathetic neurons. Serotonin colocalizes with neuropeptides at ventral horn synapses, so their modulatory effects can be complex. Serotonergic activity changes markedly with the sleep–wake cycle. One general theory of the action of serotonergic cells is that they facilitate motor output while suppressing sensory information processing. With a decrease in activation, sensory processing is disinhibited and automatic motor activity disfacilitated, which permits more focused information processing.[295] Serotonin may improve reaction times without increasing errors made in performing a task.[296]

The selective serotonin-reuptake inhibitors (SSRI antidepressants), some tricyclics, and MDMA (*Ecstasy*) are indirect serotonin agonists. Pindolol is a weak antagonist. Serotonergic receptor subtypes are numerous, so different drugs that increase serotonin may act differently.[297]

EFFECTS ON LEARNING-INDUCED REORGANIZATION

Pharmacologic agents may act on multiple neurotransmitters. D-amphetamine, for example, affects the presynaptic release of dopamine, noradrenaline, and serotonin and inhibits their reuptake from the synaptic cleft. The drug facilitates LTP and affects the consolidation and storage of memory. This makes pharmacologic manipulation of neuromodulators somewhat unpredictable. Motor and cognitive training under the positive influence of neuromodulating drugs is, nonetheless, a highly visible target for clinical trials aimed at enhancing plasticity and recovery. Short-term plasticity in somatosensory cortex produced by the coactivation of associative pairing of tactile stimuli is enhanced by amphetamine and blocked by memantine, an NMDA antagonist, and by lorazepam, a GABA agonist.[298] These drug classes had similar enhancing and blocking effects on short-term motor cortex plasticity.[220,299] The challenge for rehabilitation is to design protocols that will test the efficacy of the combination of behavioral interventions and drugs that augment long-term representational and synaptic plasticity.

COGNITIVE NETWORKS

Between the sensory inputs and the motor outputs that control the execution of motor acts sit the challenging black boxes of attention, motivation, perception, forms of memory, recognition, information storage, language, task management and other executive functions, and mood and behavior. Central nervous system lesions often degrade cognition in clinically obvious and in much more subtle ways. Rehabilitation approaches to these interlocked processes are underdeveloped. Studies of neural structure and function may enable rehabilitationists to readdress the way they conceptualize complex functions. Successful interventions depend on going well beyond simple black-box notions. This section examines concepts about structure and function relevant to the interventions discussed in subsequent chapters.

Overview of the Organization of Cognition

Different views about the functional organization of cognition are not unexpected. Neuroscience has much less evidence about how we think than about how we move. Investigators employ probes that tease out bits of information that are then incorporated into a more intricate model. Controversy flourishes with each new cleverly designed probe. For example, are regions of the brain divided according to the content of the information they process, such as perceiving visual motion? Or, is the brain organized around the sorts of processes it computes, such as judging and categorizing? This argument has been played out especially by researchers who believe that the perception of faces is a function of domain-specific modules, one of which is in the fusiform gyrus. Other researchers find weightier evidence for the handling of faces by domain-general mechanisms that can also appreciate certain nonface visual stimuli.[300] These two hypotheses are not mutually exclusive. Separable cognitive functions may be organized in distinct modules that carry out specific tasks, as highly distributed processes, by both.

Cognition presumably evolved out of the Darwinian need to augment increasingly complex sensorimotor functions. The smallest neural network may be a circumscribed group or module of neurons that represents a basic sensory or motor interaction between humans and their environment. Each module processes particular types of information, such as certain visual characteristics of a face. Other modules in a distributed network contribute to the identification of the face. Simple representations sprawl out into prefrontal, parietal, and frontal cortex with experience, adding associations with other modules and larger numbers of networks. From the sensory and motor areas that support specific functions, regions of later phylogenetic and ontogenetic development support more integrative functions with the prefrontal cortex at the top of the hierarchy that represents and executes actions.[301]

Although the functional organization of cognition involves the role of microcircuits of neurons, an underappreciated role is played by individual neurons specialized to contribute to the structure of cognition.[302] Such neurons probably exist in language and facial recognition cortex. Although most studies assess networks and the learning properties of synapses, microelectrode studies in humans point to neurons in the medial temporal lobe that respond only to particular stimuli, such as specific words, faces, categories of objects, and the encoding and retrieval of paired stimuli such as the words in a word association task.[303] The presence of highly specialized neurons may be genetically determined, so other neurons and assemblies may not be able to substitute for them.[302]

Functional brain imaging has boosted the evaluation of the neural correlates—both shared and unique—in the activation patterns of different cognitive processes. At least three ways to view cognitive brain maps are suggested by functional imaging and electrophysiologic recordings performed during cognitive tasks. First, the role of a specific Brodmann area or a smaller subdivision can be related to a process that participates within a cognitive domain, such as the activation of the ventral prefrontal cortex in the maintenance of a recent memory. Second, a more general approach associates the role of each region engaged by a task to operations that can be recruited by various tasks, such as involvement of BA 10 during verbal or nonverbal retrieval of a remembered event. Third, in a network approach, the role of each region is interpreted within its relationship to the other regions activated by a task. Large-scale networks for learning and memory, for example, include the prefrontal cortex (PFC) and parietal regions for working memory and the left PFC and temporal regions for semantic memory. In addition, local, general and interactive network mapping approaches can be interpolated for a dynamic, multidimensional interpretation of the nodes involved in cognitive processing. Overall, the cerebral regions that process aspects of cognition act more like areas of functional specialization, rather than of functional localization.

Functional neuroimaging maps reveal locations for processing, but may not reveal the upstream and downstream serial and parallel flow of information. Fuster[68] and Mesulam[304] emphasize how cognition arises from the elaboration of information from the senses with increasing associations and modulation by attention, until the sensory input is incorporated into the matter of thought and behavior. Fundamentally encoded visual information, such as color, form, and motion, converges on neurons that receive additional inputs to encode, for example, faces, objects, points in space, and the symbols of words. Motivation, attention, and emotion modulate this encoding as information gets integrated into more complex networks. At the highest synaptic levels imaged by PET or fMRI, perception becomes something recognized, letter symbols have meaning, and events become incorporated into experiences. These highest nodes of large-scale cognitive networks also interact among themselves. Mesulam points to at least five anatomically distinct networks modulated by each other, as well as by systems for attention, motivation, novelty-seeking, imagery, reward-seeking, and emotional impact.[304,305] Sensory information is further manipulated and elaborated by these epicenters. The cognitive networks most often affected by CNS lesions include the following:

1. Explicit memory network centered in the hippocampus and a closely related emotion network centered in the amygdala
2. Working memory and executive function network in lateral prefrontal cortex
3. Spatial awareness network centered in the posterior parietal cortex and frontal eye fields
4. Language network centered in Broca's and Wernicke's areas
5. Face and object recognition network with centers in the midtemporal and temporopolar cortices[300,306]

The neural mechanisms that select and coordinate distributed brain activity for the rapid adaptations needed for learning and thought probably include electrical synchronization of neuronal assemblies in a network.[307] Synchronous networks recorded by electrodes over wide regions of the brain emerge and disappear in waves that last 100–300 ms, which is within the temporal scale of the working brain. Phase-locking of the electrical and metabolic activity of regions of a network are mediated by reciprocal corticocortical and thalamocortical pathways.

Potential rehabilitative interventions for the cognitive effects of disruption of a network derive from the finding that multiple associational, sensory, and motor areas of the brain contain features of what was learned in the past, although a particular modality may carry the highest weight and be especially important.[308] Many cognitive rehabilitation strategies have been developed around the notion that impairments may be ameliorated by tapping into one or more of the distributed grids that remain connected. On the other hand, since cognitive domains appear to be mapped at multiple interconnected sites, a single lesion at any of many sites may degrade network function.

The *transfer effect* is an example of a CNS mechanism that depends on a distributed system. Relearning a few forgotten words of a foreign language or of a poem often triggers the recall of many other words or phrases. This spontaneous recovery is a generic characteristic of the CNS, in which associations are distributed over many processing units, such as

neurons and functionally specialized assemblies. Because an association depends on its connections, relearning a subset of these associations pushes all connections toward the strength they had when initially learned. This change in efficacy, then, improves performance on associations that were not relearned.[309] The transfer effect may serve as one of the bases for rehabilitation retraining.

Explicit and Implicit Memory Network

Declarative or *explicit* memory refers to what can be recalled consciously and reported. This form of memory includes *episodic* memories, which are personal experiences, images and everyday events with their rich contexts and recreation over time, and *semantic* memories, which refer to the recall of factual knowledge about the world and general information about our surrounds. Declarative memory stands in contrast to *implicit* or *procedural* memory, which cannot be overtly reported, such as how one types on a keyboard after training. With nondeclarative memory, past experience influences current behavior, even though we do not consciously recollect the details of what was learned. Procedural memory for skills, as discussed earlier, as well as habits and biases, depends especially upon the cerebellum and neostriatum. Knowledge about the qualities of items that place them in the same category can also be acquired implicitly, so that even an amnesic patient can learn the pattern that classifies items.[310]

Declarative learning depends upon limbic and diencephalic structures. These networks, especially the parahippocampal regions and hippocampus, receive new sensory information regarding facts and events and sketch a memory trace until it is bound onto the remote cortical modules that consolidate the memory.[311] Then, with effortful recollection or inferences drawn from personal experience, a person can tap into large-scale networks of memories. For example, episodic memory mediates a synthesis of all the auto trips a person takes around a city. Even without looking at a paper map, one can make navigational inferences while driving that are built upon past spatial (streets that run east to west) and visual memories (relationships to a previously passed supermarket and theater) and other personal experiences (a conversation with a friend about the intended target) to arrive at a new location. The heart of declarative memory, then, is the process of making associations and the ability to retain relational information over time.

The hippocampal region is not required for immediate recall. The prefrontal cortex manages *working* memory and neighboring areas are involved in the maintenance and manipulation of ongoing working memory. The amygdala is a center that mediates *emotional* memory and modulates the strength and persistence of memories in other memory systems. *Prospective* memory has a declarative component (what needs to be recalled) and a temporal or contextual component (when or where the intention or action is to be carried out). Prospective recall involves a frontal lobe network that enables a person to carry out an intention after a delay. Cerebral trauma often impairs this function. Other specialized areas of the brain allow for rich and stable new associations. Memories of faces and complex visual patterns, for example, are encoded in the inferotemporal cortex, those for words in the midtemporal cortex, memory tasks related to spatial relationships in the superior parietal cortex, and multimodal memory tasks in the posterior parietal and prefrontal cortices.

Priming, an implicit learning strategy, facilitates recognition by using a cue, such as the first letters of a word. The cue biases a subsequent response in the correct direction toward recall. For example, a whole word is recalled after a subject is given only the first syllable of the word. Priming is not sensitive to associations with other knowledge. Priming systems handle information about physical form and structure, rather than about the meanings and associative properties of objects and words.[312] Priming strategies rely on perceptual representations stored by modality-specific memory subsystems, such as those that process word forms and visual objects. Each hemisphere, in fact, may store different representations. For example, changing the font of letters did not affect word-stem priming when fragments of a word were presented to the left hemisphere, but it did impair recognition when presented only to the right hemisphere.[313] Priming is a valuable strategy for working with amnestic subjects following a traumatic brain injury, herpes encephalitis, and posterior cerebral artery infarcts that damage the hippocampus. The medial temporal lobe is not needed for successful priming or for sequence learning.[314]

PATHWAYS AND NEURONAL MECHANISMS OF EXPLICIT MEMORY

The hippocampal region of the medial temporal lobe, a jelly roll of interleaved neuronal fields, projects from the subiculum through the fornix to the cortex. The parahippocampal region includes the parahippocampal and perirhinal cortices, which provide the major inputs to the hippocampus. Damage to the hippocampal formation causes profound amnesia for recently acquired declarative memories, but generally spares remotely acquired memories. Damage to diencephalic structures may also produce an amnestic syndrome by disrupting communication to and from the hippocampus. Color Figure 3–3 (in separate color insert) reveals some of this interacting circuitry by showing the distribution of hypometabolism after a stroke in the dorsal and anterior thalamus. The interconnected regions affected may include the hippocampus-fornix-mammillary body-mammillothalamic tract-anterior thalamic nuclei-posterior cingulate-hippocampus pathway and the perirhinal cortex-dorsomedial thalamus pathway that includes a projection from the amygdala. These connections are especially vulnerable to trauma and to ischemia and hypoxia.

As noted, the medial temporal lobe and striatum are differentially engaged by declarative and procedural learning tasks, respectively. These systems may compete, however, depending upon the demands of learning.[315] The need for flexibly accessible information is supported by the hippocampus and the need to quickly learn automatic stimulus–response associations for a specific situation is supported by the striatum. Poldrack and colleagues found that subjects may rely on the medial temporal lobe early in training, but dependence changes if procedural learning is needed. Activations by fMRI between the hippocampus and caudate correlate negatively as learning proceeds.

The amygdala's collection of nuclei in the anterior medial temporal lobe encodes the implicit and the explicit emotional correlates of experiential memory. A lesion in the amygdala may leave declarative memory intact, but could abolish the autonomic responses that had been associated with the recall of events and biographical information, as well as reduce the ability to recognize emotion in faces.[304,316] The amygdala also provides events with a high emotional valence to enhance attention to them. It helps separate what is mundane from what is important by modulating the salience of events. After a lesion of the left amygdala, for example, a subject loses the usual enhanced perception of aversive words.[317] Input from the amygdala during stressful learning may reduce LTP in the hippocampus.[318] An acute brain injury that produces sudden disability serves as a potential LTP-reducing stressor during rehabilitation.

The neurons of the hippocampus have properties that allow them to rapidly encode the events that make up an episodic memory, retrieve that memory by reexperiencing some facet of prior events, and link the continuing experience to other stored representations of episodic and semantic knowledge. For example, rats have been electrophysiologically studied as they reach the junction of a T-maze, where they must learn whether to turn left or right for a reward.[319] Some neurons in the hippocampus fire as the rat passes each sequence of locations in the maze. The firing pattern of many cells depends upon whether the rat is in the midst of a left or right turn. Other cells fire as the rat moves along the stem of the T regardless of whether the rat has to turn left or right based on prior experiences. The hippocampus, then, has encoded both left-turn and right-turn experiences and has cells that link both experiences.

Microelectrode recordings in humans also reveal neuronal firing patterns that reflect the encoding process of memories.[320] A possible substrate of visual recall was studied, for example, in patients with epilepsy who needed invasive monitoring in preparation for possible surgery to remove a seizure locus.[321] Single neurons were found in the hippocampus, amygdala, entorhinal cortex, and parahippocampal gyrus that selectively altered their rate of firing when subjects viewed a particular category of items or imagined the items. Indeed, the neurons that processed what was viewed, say an object but not faces, animals, or visual patterns, were usually the same cells engaged when the person recalled in the mind's eye what had been viewed. The firing of the same neurons may correlate with some percept common to vision

and imagery. The activation may also represent the actual storage of an image and later activation during retrieval of the image from memory.

Memory Storage

The hippocampus is not the final storage site of declarative memories. Rather, repetitive interactions between the cortex and hippocampus temporarily coactivate widely spread cortical representations until cortical memories are consolidated. The parahippocampal regions receive convergent information from cortical association areas and send back projections to these areas to mediate the persistence of the cortical representations. In prefrontal and temporal regions that are modulated by novelty during an encoding task of words or pictures, the magnitude of activation predicts whether the events will be remembered.[322] Multiple prefrontal-temporal circuits that each depend on the content of the task support the encoding of events to create a flexible, long-term memory trace. These circuits may contribute individually to encoding attributes of visuospatial, phonologic, lexical, and semantic stimuli.[322] Memory retrieval may come about from a top-down frontotemporal signal for voluntary recall, from a medial temporal-to-neocortical backward signal for automatic recall, or from both in relation to the need.[323] Phase-locked synchronization of electrical waves lasting a few hundred ms within the hippocampal-cortical loops may correlate with the acquisition and retrieval of memories.[307] Most importantly, consolidation of a new memory takes time, from hours to days, which accounts for the temporal gradient of retrograde amnesia after an acute traumatic brain injury.

Memory consolidation may require repeated rounds of site-specific synaptic modifications to reinforce experienced-induced plasticity. New memories, then, are initially labile and disruptable before neuronal protein synthesis consolidates long-term memories. When a stimulus associated with a consolidated memory reactivates that memory, some of the cellular events that occurred during the intiial consolidation are reenacted.[324] Evidence from fruitflies to humans suggests that the reactivation of memory during retrieval, whether implicit or explicit knowledge, may return a consolidated memory to a labile state, which can reinforce or degrade knowledge of the old experience. A high degree of attention at the time of retrieval may increase reconsolidation, in part by noradrenergic neuromodulation. This potential for degradation may have a highly negative impact on the patient with deficits in attention and recall after a stroke or traumatic brain injury. In such patients, the retrieval of past knowledge could be contaminated by new stimuli.

Studies of mice with mutations in α-CaMKII, which is required for hippocampal LTP and learning, show that recurrent activation of cortical networks for memory consolidation depends on repetitive LTP-like events.[325] Of interest, NMDA receptor-dependent neurons in the hippocampus reactivate spontaneously in the immediate period after learning. This reentry reinforcement may be one of the drives that consolidates memory in the cortex.[326] Some of this hippocampal replay may occur during sleep, just as REM sleep may serve to reinforce procedural learning.[327,328] Thus, initial encoding and long-term storage through the hippocampus share some of the same mechanisms. Encoding and storage may respond in a similar way to neuropharmacologic interventions with "memory" molecules that will be available in the near future, such as drugs or genetic modulations that increase nuclear calcium levels to activate CREB-mediated transcription and learning.[329]

Neurogenesis

Hippocampal-dependent memory requires synaptogenesis by mechanisms described in the section on LTP. Memory traces may also involve neurogenesis. Neurogenesis in the hippocampus has been found in all adult mammals including humans (see Chapter 2). By experimentally reducing the number of new neurons entering the dentate gyrus of the hippocampus from their source in the subventricular zone, new learning by rats was impeded.[330] Cell proliferation also increases during running, an act in rodents probably associated with learning and recall in the wild, as well as by a home cage enriched by objects for exploration and climbing.[331,332]

Neurogenesis may be modulated by an increase in neurotrophins such as BDNF and FGF. These trophins also increase in the hippocampus with learning and with physical activity in rodents.[275,333] Indeed, blocking the effects of BDNF in the brain by infusing an antisense protein impaired the learning of a spatial task and recall from spatial memory, which are medial temporal lobe functions.[334] Neurogenesis may be necessary to provide additional substrate for the enormous number of hippocampal computations made over the life of an animal. Running on wheels for exercise also increases gene expression in the hippocampus for messenger RNA associated with synaptic structures and neuronal plasticity.[335]

FUNCTIONAL IMAGING OF DECLARATIVE MEMORY

Positron emission tomography and fMRI can assess network and within-region activations for a variety of memory processes. Maps have been made of episodic memory encoding for verbal, spatial, and object information and of episodic retrieval for verbal and nonverbal items, as well as for the success, effort, and mode of retrieval. Encoding and retrieval engage prefrontal cortex, the medial temporal lobe, and parieto-occipital regions, but considerable within-region differences arise across tasks. Semantic retrieval of knowledge about categories, such as animals versus tools or the color of objects based on knowledge of the world, usually engages the left prefrontal cortex (BA 45) and the temporal region. Although fairly reproducible patterns emerge across investigations, the fine details of each study's cognitive activation paradigm and statistical methods leave room for ongoing controversy.[336]

Functional magnetic resonance imaging studies of subjects during declarative memory tasks have revealed two separately localizable memory processes in the medial temporal lobe. The subiculum is more active during retrieval, whereas the parahippocampal cortex is especially activated by encoding new inputs.[337] As a memory task, such as looking at pictures of scenes, becomes more familiar, parahippocampal activation decreases. This area is more responsive to novel or infrequently encountered stimuli.[338] Indeed, the parahippocampal region may act as a novelty detector. The hippocampus is most active in an fMRI paradigm when retrieval is accompanied by conscious recollection of a learning episode,[339] both in making associations and recalling recent facts and events.[340] Medial temporal lobe activity lateralizes depending on the stimulus used during functional imaging. For example, during the encoding of a list of words, activity is mostly on the left. During the learning of pictures and objects, bilateral activation occurs.

Functional imaging may allow clinicians to study whether patients have the ability to learn and retain new information, to determine if they are able to participate in a rehabilitation setting. Studies using fMRI demonstrate that the amount of neural activity in specific brain regions, including the prefrontal and parahippocampal cortices, correlates with how well subjects subsequently remember the pictures or words to which they had been exposed.[341,342] Aspects of the subcomponent processes of memory, such as attending to an experience, rehearsing, encoding, elaborating, and retrieving have also been visualized with increasing specificity using fMRI activation paradigms.[343,344]

Functional imaging during prospective memory tasks and after repetition priming may be of special value in understanding the capacity for learning in patients undergoing cognitive rehabilitation after a traumatic brain injury. Prospective memory allows a person to carry out an intended future action without continuous rehearsal, until the appropriate time or context arises. This form of recall is not simply a special case of pulling an intention from retrograde memory. A PET study mapped the maintenance of an intention to bilateral BA 10 and the right lateral prefrontal (BA 45/46) and inferior parietal areas.[345] Priming for either a perceptual or conceptual task was accompanied by a reduction in the level of activation compared to the naïve or unprimed performance of a task.[346]

Thus, the fMRI pattern of activation or deactivation in regions of interest may be of value in the assessment of the functioning of specific memory processes in patients, in the evaluation of their brain's readiness for the learning that is necessary for successful rehabilitation, and to determine whether particular drugs or cognitive training strategies engage key components of the explicit or implicit memory network.

Working Memory and Executive Function Network

A critical cognitive process during rehabilitation requires patients to bring information to mind, hold it, and process these mental representations. The prefrontal cortex includes the machinery for online information processing for thought, for comprehension, and for carrying out intentions. Remembering often requires planning and a strategy. Tests of strategic memory, such as the free recall of words, the temporal order of a list of items, and judgments about how often an item has been seen, rely on the dorsolateral prefrontal cortex (DLPFC) for processing and on the right frontal pole for monitoring the results of retrieval.[347] Ordinary memory performance is guided by a variety of subjective organizing strategies. The working memory cognitive system in the DLPFC supports these strategies with temporary storage, online manipulations, and transformations of the information needed for an ongoing cognitive task. Short-term memory is a component of working memory and can be thought of and localized (Table 1–5) as a buffer and rehearsal system.[208] Neuroimag-

Table 1–5. Processes of Short-Term Memory Localized by Functional Imaging

Cognitive Process	Cortical Regions Activated
VERBAL SHORT-TERM MEMORY	
Phonological buffer storage	Left ventral parietal
Rehearsal/inner speech scratchpad	Left ventral posterolateral frontal
VISUOSPATIAL SHORT-TERM MEMORY	
Visuospatial buffer	Right ventral parietal
Visuospatial sketchpad	Right prefrontal, parietal, dorsolateral occipital

ing studies show that spatial, visuospatial, and verbal working memory tasks produce an overlapping and distributed pattern of activations, with a fractionation of working memory processes between dorsolateral and ventrolateral frontal regions, depending upon the executive demands of a task.[348] Working memory can handle a limited number of channels of related information, which is the clinical basis for digit span and delayed matching-to-sample tests.

Executive processes, which often operate on the contents of short-term working memory, are also managed in the frontal lobes, primarily in prefrontal cortex. Executive cognition (*1*) focuses attention on relevant information and inhibits irrelevant stimuli; (*2*) manages tasks, which may require switching or dividing attention from one task or stimulus to another; (*3*) plans the sequence of subtasks that may accomplish a goal; and (*4*) codes time and place and monitors the steps of a working memory task.[349] Prefrontal cortex extracts information about the regularities across experiences, integrates relationships among inputs, and then imparts rules that guide subsequent thoughts and actions. These processes are especially vulnerable to a traumatic brain injury. Normal prefrontal cortex and its connections create much of what is most human, from an imaginative hypothesis of a neuroscientist to the skewed beliefs of a terrorist.

PATHWAYS AND NEURONAL MECHANISMS

Working Memory

The anatomical area involved in working memory has been described in both macaque and human studies.[350] BA 46 and 9/46 in mid-DLPFC and a strip just caudal to BA 9 within either BA 6 or 8, monitor information within working memory for spatial, nonspatial, and verbal material. The dorsolateral portion of DLPFC receives large projections from the dorsal posterior parietal region to support working memory for spatial tasks. The oculomotor system also connects here to assist the coding of visuospatial 'where' data. The ventrolateral aspect of the DLPFC receives a large projection from the inferotemporal cortex for tasks that encode 'what' data about objects. Other inputs arise from the superior temporal

and cingulate cortices. The anterior cingulate (BA 24 and 32) is often activated in functional imaging studies along with the DLPFC. Whereas the DLPFC provides top-down management for behaviors appropriate to a task, the cingulate may be more involved in monitoring performance. It signals when control needs to be more strongly engaged.[351] Subregions of the anterior cingulate receive affective and nociceptive inputs, in addition to motor and cognitive influences. The posterior cingulate in BA 23, 30, and 31 also participates in memory and visuospatial processing. These areas are highly connected to both the parahippocampal and DLPFC regions and may serve as a link between them. The cingulate region also provides an emotional and motivational influence on memory.[316] This input is important. Lesions in the retrosplenial cingulate cause amnesia, especially for episodic memories.

Working memory in circuits has parallels at the cellular level. Prefrontal neurons delay their firing in a selective fashion for specific objects and spatial locations, as well as for faces. The delay presumably maintains the internal representation of a cue for what is to be remembered.[348] Some neurons are attuned to one or more attributes, such as spatial location, color, and the sensory stimuli associated with a motor act.[352] The DLPFC neurons also integrate sensory stimuli from different modalities, such as sight and sound, and across time.[85] Experiments with single cell recordings from monkey DLPFC by Fuster and colleagues revealed audio and visual cross-modal association neurons. Different cells, to differing degrees, were activated by a sensory input, sustained a low level of activity in working memory for the association, and were reactivated before and during presentation of a reminder cue.

Executive Prefrontal Cortex

The hippocampus binds stimuli into long-term memories of specific episodes, whereas the prefrontal cortex represents not specific episodes, but the rules for using sensory inputs and declarative knowledge. The dorsal prefrontal cortex in BA 9 and 46 and the ventral prefrontal cortex in BA 12/47 and 45 exert executive control over the storehouses of cortical memory representations.[353] For example, a top-down signal from prefrontal neurons activates single neurons in the inferior temporal lobe after monkeys learn a visual task that came to be represented in the temporal cortex.[354] Along with other data, this points to the influence of prefrontal neurons in focusing attention on task-relevant information that can be drawn from past memory stores. Prefrontal connections to the association cortices serve as an important orchestrator of voluntary recall. The region may also bias brain systems toward a common task, controlling the selection of particular sensory inputs, memories, or motor outputs.[355]

Most fundamentally, the executive prefrontal cortex flexibly selects cortically stored information of many sorts to construct associations and choose actions that are appropriate to both the sensory information at hand and the circumstances in which it is encountered.[356] Patients with frontal injuries often cannot acquire and implement a behavior in the context of a particular task or a changing task. These patients act as if they cannot find the mental rules to guide their behavior. The prefrontal cortex may be the only brain region that can represent cues for behaviors, repertoires of responses, and anticipate the outcomes of actions taken by a subject.[357]

During learning, neural signals akin to rewards strengthen the synaptic connections among the prefrontal neurons that process information that achieves a goal. The reward-related signals, most likely provided by dopamine released from the ventral tegmental tract, produce an activity pattern of stronger associations between the information that is relevant to the goal and the desired outcome.[353]

The neurons of the ventral tegmental area are ideal for guiding goal-relevant behavior. As noted earlier, they initially fire in response to unpredicted rewards. With experience, these dopaminergic neurons are activated by cues that predict rewards and not by the rewards themselves. Their firing is inhibited when a reward does not occur. Dopamine is released to prefrontal neurons more rapidly over the time of learning, which may help link more information into an increasingly complex set of representations for goal-related behaviors. Later, with additional training, the cues that fired the dopamine neurons are transferred to neurons that monitor behaviors more rapidly. The dopamine influx, then, allows for experience-dependent plasticity. The precise molecular mechanism is uncertain, but may work through augmentation of NMDA-receptor mediated glutaminergic transmission by dopamine, leading to LTP. Of interest, dopamine agonists improve executive and working memory aspects of cognition in patients with Parkinson's disease and for some patients with frontal traumatic injuries.[358–360]

FUNCTIONAL IMAGING

Research on working memory, as well as all other aspects of cognitive processing, is a work in progress. Data from functional imaging and TMS studies continue to create and partially settle controversies about how specific regions process mneumonic and executive functions. Since focal and global brain injuries often degrade some of these processes, the clinician needs to consolidate a few of the major anatomical and physiological hypotheses.

Most studies support the finding that the mid-dorsolateral and mid-ventrolateral prefrontal regions play different roles, regardless of whether the task involves spatial, visual, or verbal working memory.[348] The ventrolateral area, including BA 47, is involved in the active retrieval of one or a few pieces of information and the sequencing of responses based upon what information is being stored. For example, right mid-ventral BA 47 was activated primarily when subjects held five verbally given numbers in mind and were asked to repeat them. Thus, this region may carry out active, low-level encoding strategies, such as rehearsal and intentional retrieval. If asked to listen to five numbers and repeat them in reverse order, the left dorsolateral area and BA 47 are activated. A more dorsal activation also occurs in BA 46 and 9 when the task requires a person to monitor or manipulate, for example, a set of spatial locations held in working memory and make comparisons with new stimuli. This spatial memory task activates BA 9 and 46/9 on the right. Activation studies also suggest that prefrontal cortex is organized by fairly separable storage and executive processes.[349] The attention and inhibition requirements of a task, for example, especially activate the anterior cingulate.

One controversy is whether the DLPFC is primarily involved in the maintenance and monitoring of items in working memory or in maintaining a record of the selection of responses. An fMRI study dissected out the finding that during a spatial working memory task, maintenance was associated with bilateral activation of prefrontal area 8 and the intraparietal cortex.[361] Selection of a target location from memory was more associated with activation of BA 46 on the right, area 9/46 or 8, and the right orbitofrontal cortex, along with parietal activations that were more posterior and medial to those identified during maintenance. BA 46 may participate more in the attentional than the mnemonic component of a complex working memory task.[362] These findings help explain why the DLFPC is activated both when subjects select between items on tasks that use working memory and when they self-select between movements on tasks that require a willed action.

Metabolic imaging at rest to assess network activity and functional neuroimaging of tasks that require working memory and executive processing may help clinicians determine the readiness, capacity, and best strategies for cognitive remediation in patients. Therapists must keep the types of definable processes subsumed under working memory and executive functioning in mind as they delineate impairments, assess the causes of disability, and treat components of these cognitive processes (see Chapter 11).

Emotional Regulatory Network

Prefrontal and orbitofrontal cortex often bear the brunt of damage in traumatic brain injuries. Also, the system may degrade in patients with stroke, multiple sclerosis, the cortical and subcortical dementias, and other cerebral disorders. Behavioral and mood syndromes caused by frontal lobe injury are recapitulated by lesions in subcortical structures of the circuits.

The primary structures in the circuitry for emotional regulation include the orbital and ventromedial prefrontal cortex (BA 12), regions of the DLPFC, and the amygdala, hippocampus, and anterior cingulate. Other interconnected structures implicated in aspects of emotion, affective style, and the maintenance, amplification, and attenuation of an emotion include the hypothalamus, insular cortex, and ventral striatum. This system also suppresses negative emotions such as anger and impulsive aggression, partly through serotonergic neuromodulation.[363] Antidepressant and antianxiety medications act on the system through such modulation.

Three distinct neurobehavioral syndromes have been described that involve frontal-subcortical circuits.[364] Mixed behavioral features suggest the involvement of more than one circuit.

1. The *prefrontal syndrome* includes deficits in motor programming, especially evident in alternating, reciprocal, and sequential motor tasks. Executive function impairments include the inability to generate hypotheses and show flexibility in maintaining or shifting sets required by changes in the demands of a task. Patients also exhibit poor organizational strategies for learning tasks and copying complex designs, as well as diminished verbal and drawing fluency. Lesions span the circuit from BA 9 and 10 to the dorsolateral caudate nucleus, to the globus pallidus, and to the ventral anterior and dorsomedian thalamus and back to DLPFC. This circuit is shown to be hypometabolic in Figure 3–3 after an anterior thalamic stroke. Indirect pathways extend from globus pallidus externa to lateral subthalamic nucleus, then to globus pallidus interna and substantia nigra.

2. The *orbitofrontal syndrome* especially affects personality. The range of characteristics include a change in interests, initiative, and conscientiousness, as well as disinhibition, tactless words, irritability, lability, and euphoria. Patients tend to be enslaved by environmental cues. They may automatically imitate the gestures and actions of others. Lesions span the same structures as the dorsolateral syndrome, but in different sectors. Impulsivity and aggression may accompany lesions that affect this area and adjacent prefrontal cortex. Orbitofrontal cortex provides a social context for perceptual information and, through its connections with the prefrontal cortex and amygdala, plays a key role in constraining impulsive outbursts.[363] The frontal-subcortical circuit includes the lateral orbitofrontal cortex (BA 10, 11, and 47) to ventromedial caudate to globus pallidus to ventral anterior and dorsomedian thalamus and back to the orbitofrontal region. Figure 3–4 shows the resting hypometabolic activity that may result from interruption of elements of this circuit after a stroke in-

duced by an anterior communicating aneurysm.

3. The *anterior cingulate syndrome* includes profound apathy, even akinetic mutism. The circuit includes the anterior cingulate (BA 24) to nucleus accumbens to globus pallidus to dorsomedian thalamus and back to BA 24. Other striatal loops are involved as well. Both DLPFC and orbitofrontal subcortical circuits may be part of the substrate of depression.

Spatial Awareness Network

A variety of spatial impairments affect patients undergoing neurorehabilitation. These range from right posterior parietal lesions that cause a hemineglect to the left parietal lesions of the Gerstmann syndrome that includes left/right confusion, finger agnosia, and the inability to report which finger is touched. Poor spatial localization by vision or touch may be detected on the patient's body, within the patient's peripersonal space, or beyond the patient's reach. Short-term or long-term spatial memory may be impaired. The neural network for these distributed functions includes the posterior parietal cortex, especially BA 7, which transforms visual, touch, and proprioceptive stimuli, the frontal eye fields and adjacent prefrontal cortex, and the cingulate region.[99] Figure 9–6 shows the network effects of a thalamic infarction that deafferented the parietal region to produce contralateral spatial hemi-inattention.

Spatial information is represented by the patterns of firing of neuronal groups, which are sensitive, for example, to where a visual image falls on the retina, the angle of the head, and the location of the eyes in their orbits.[365] The parietal regions project to the premotor cortex and putamen as an arm-centered and head-centered spatial coordinate system. Parietal projections also go to the frontal eye fields, superior colliculi, and other areas to control saccadic eye movements to locate objects in space, and send information to the entorhinal cortex, hippocampus, and DLFPC to hold memories about the location of items in space.

The sum of these functions allows the perception and recall of space. The posterior parietal regions seem to provide a holistic impression of space.[99] They assist in planning and carrying out the visual and body-centered guidance for reaching and other visually guided behaviors. The multiple coordinate systems for visuomotor tasks, divided among at least a few bilateral brain regions, offer the potential for therapists to design interventions that work around a focal disruption of one pathway of spatial architecture. Strategies for treating hemi-inattention and related phenomena are discussed in Chapter 9.

Language Network

As discussed under cortical motor networks, language may have evolved from the action observation system, perhaps as primates increased their social interactions for survival in hostile environments. Social isolation may follow the loss of language function in aphasic patients. The traditional aphasia syndromes correlate in a general way with damage to specific sites, but many aphasiologists have questioned the extent to which the traditional aphasia subtype classification (see Table 5–5) relates to localization.[366] Wernicke's region in BA 37, 39, and 40 and Broca's region in BA 44 and 45 and their surrounds are tissues of relative specialization. These areas cannot simply be dichotomized as receptive and expressive language zones. Indeed, the left posterior ventral frontal area that is called Broca's and the left posterior superior temporal gyrus that is called Wernicke's have at least several functional subdivisions with variations in their connectivity.[367]

Language requires at least two mental capacities. The dual elements, which may or may not be separable, include memorized word-specific lexical information that conveys meaning and rules of grammar that constrain words and sentences. These domains have been modeled in many ways to explain the acquisition, processing, computation, and neural bases of lexicon and grammar. One approach of special interest for rehabilitation posits the mental lexicon within the declarative memory system and mental grammar within the procedural memory system.[368] Other systems may be involved. In support of this approach, functional imaging studies of lexical and semantic learning and retrieval show activation in the explicit memory system of the medial temporal and temporoparietal regions and anterior prefrontal cortex. Tasks that probe syntactic processes preferentially activate Broca's area, the SMA, and the left basal ganglia of the implicit system. This conceptualization may be tested in patients with aphasia. The declarative system permits memorization to rebuild a lexicon and the procedural system can be used to retrain grammar through priming and iconic language (see Chapter 5). In addition, neuropharmacologic approaches for enhancing declarative and procedural memory may be effective for word-finding and fluency (see Chapter 9).

In the terms of a neurocognitive network for language, Mesulam has described Wernicke's area as a nodal bottleneck for accessing a distributed grid of connections that hold information about sound-word-meaning relationships.[281] Broca's area is conceived as the bottleneck for transforming neural word representations from Wernicke's and other areas into their corresponding articulatory sequences. The pathway to Broca's area was mapped by magnetoencephalography during the generation of words to visually presented word stems.[369] This study also offers a sense of the time scale required for processing words. With presentation of a novel word stem for completion, the subject's first activation occurred in posterior occipital cortex (at 110 ms after presentation), spread into the ventral anterior occipital cortex (at 120 ms), marched forward and lateralized to the left hemisphere (at 180 ms), spread to posteroventral and lateral temporal areas (at 220 ms), progressively involved the anterior temporal lobe (at approximately 300 ms) and the ventral prefrontal cortex (at approximately 450 ms), and then faded after 500 ms.

Studies that map the brain during elementary tasks offer valuable information regarding processing, but may not reflect the neural architecture of ordinary discourse. A PET study of extemporaneous speech, in which subjects told a story about themselves, found broad activations.[370] Anterior regions included the frontal operculum, anterior insula, SMA, and lateral premotor and medial prefrontal cortices primarily in the left hemisphere. Posterior regions included mostly bilateral perisylvian temporal cortex and inferior portions of the angular gyrus, along with extrasylvian lateral occipital, medial and basal temporal, and paramedian cortices. This wide swath of anatomical substrate for discourse suggests early stages for forming concepts and accessing the lexicon and later stages for phonological encoding and articulation. The pattern progresses from bilateral activation to left-lateralized representation of natural language.

The study of elementary features of language provides key insights regarding specific language functions. Damasio and colleagues proposed that the systems that support concepts, language, and the two-way access between them are anatomically separate.[371,372] A mediational set of neural structures uses convergence zones and feedforward–feedback connections to link separate regions. To support this, they found patients who had impaired verb retrieval and normal noun retrieval associated with a left frontal cortical injury. In contrast, they described other patients who had impaired retrieval of proper nouns and certain classes of common nouns, but normal verb retrieval after a lesion in the left anterior and middle temporal lobe.[371] Naming actions and spatial relations activated frontal and parietal regions of the left hemisphere. The investigators also found segregated systems for different categories of nouns. Backed up by neuroimaging studies, they suggested that systems that mediate access to concrete nouns are in the neighborhood of systems that support concepts for concrete entities. Systems that access verbs are elsewhere, close to the neural entities that support concepts of movement and relationships in time and space. For example, the bilateral posterior temporoparietal region called MT, which is activated by the perception of motion, is also engaged when subjects name an action, such as the word "stirring" when shown a static drawing of a spoon in a bowl. Within these distributed systems, parallel and interlocking streams of corticocortical projections build up the levels of complexity of our knowledge of words.

How ensembles of neurons encode language representations is far from clear. Microelectrode recordings of the brain in people who undergo a craniotomy for epilepsy or tumor surgery suggest that individual cortical neurons in the temporal lobe language region tend to respond to only one aspect of language, such as either when a subject listens to a word or speaks that word.[320] Most neurons, within the limitations of testing human subjects, appear to have a narrow behavioral repertoire. They may respond solely to one word from a list, only second syllables, or only particular linguistic characteristics of language. This narrow band of behavioral response seems to apply to most individual neurons within the cognitive association cortices.[320]

From the point of view of plasticity and treatment of aphasia, these findings support the approach that word forms can be reactivated from their highly distributed fragments in auditory, kinesthetic, and motor cortices.[371] Thus, small differences in the amount and location of damage to the inputs and outputs of the distributed network for language will produce differences in neurolinguistic impairments or aphasia subtypes and affect the degree of eventual recovery.[373,374] Detailed knowledge about these systems should lead to more theory-based aphasia therapy. The plasticity associated with gains in patients who are aphasic, appreciated using functional neuroimaging, is discussed in Chapter 3.

SUMMARY

The anatomic and functional structure of assemblies of neurons, their axonal projections, and their synapses are increasingly informing us about mechanisms of movement and cognition. To understand the basis for the symptoms and signs of patients who need neurologic rehabilitation and to develop neuroscientifically based interventions for treatment, clinicians must understand the details of how information shuttles through the CNS.

Neuronal assemblies with their local circuitry, receptive fields, and stimulus-response characteristics are connected to other functional assemblies in the brain stem and spinal cord by top-down commands and bottom-up sensory inputs. Movement-associated sensory experience and perceptual goals organize voluntary movements and skills learning. The assemblies that participate in the performance of a task are highly distributed and project information in parallel pathways. Goal-oriented behaviors, along with paradigms that optimize implicit and explicit learning, induce plasticity and increase the beneficial output from the anatomical networks that participate in a behavior.

Many signaling pathways contribute to the storage of sensorimotor and cognitive information and to the mechanisms for learning procedural and declarative knowledge. Thus,

many points of entry into these cascades may be available for a neuropharmacology of rehabilitation. For example, activation of NMDA receptors at the membranes of synapses increases the probability of release of glutamate from the presynaptic neuron terminal, increases the number of AMPA receptors needed to produce LTP, fires off neurotrophins for cell health and LTP, changes the excitability of the dendritic membrane, leads to cytoskeletal proteins that bud a new spine and, in the end, adds the infrastructure needed to compute and manifest a memory or skill. Electrical signals carrying information among the nodes of networks and across networks come to be interlocked as stable records for long-term recall. Problem solving, practice, reward, and optimizing sensory inputs relevant to a motor task may be essential for successful adaptation of molecules, cells, circuits, and behaviors.

Functional neuroimaging studies provide a sense of which cortical networks are special contributors to movement and cognition under various conditions. By understanding the task-related conditions that modulate brain regions, rehabilitationists may be able to design physical, cognitive, pharmacologic, and biologic repair interventions that enhance the engagement of the nodes in a network.

Patients who suffer acute injuries and diseases of the brain and spinal cord often evolve a lessening of their impairments and disabilities. Recovery of neuronal and axonal transmission, experience-dependent learning within partially spared tissue, activity-dependent representational plasticity, and compensation by new behavioral strategies may account for much of this improvement. The potential plasticity of residual assemblies and networks is remarkable. Retraining paradigms, pharmacologic interventions, and the biological interventions discussed in Chapter 2 offer exciting new options to lessen the impairments and disabilities of patients. These approaches to augment gains after a CNS or PNS injury rest upon basic scientific knowledge of structure and function.

REFERENCES

1. Shepherd G. The Synaptic Organization of the Brain. New York: Oxford University Press, 1998.
2. Mountcastle V. An organizing principle for cerebral

function: The unit module and the distributed system. In: Schmitt F, Worden F, eds. The Neurosciences Fourth Study Program. Cambridge: MIT Press, 1977:8–21.

3. Mountcastle V. The columnar organization of the neocortex. Brain 1997; 120:701–722.

4. McCormick D. Brain calculus: neural integration and persistent activity. Nat Neurosci 2001; 4:113–114.

5. Strogatz S. Exploring complex networks. Nature 2001; 410:268–276.

6. Horak F. Assumptions underlying motor control for neurologic rehabilitation. In: Lister M, ed. Contemporary Management of Motor Control Problems: Proceedings of the II Step Conference. Alexandria, VA: Foundation for Physical Therapy, 1991:11–27.

7. Bernstein N. The coordination and regulation of movment. London: Pergamon, 1967.

8. Edelman G, Finkel L. Neuronal group selection in the cerebral cortex. In: Edelman G, Gall W, Cowan W, eds. Dynamic Aspects of Neocortical Function. New York: John Wiley, 1984:653–696.

9. Bizzi E, Mussa-Ivaldi F. Neural basis of motor control and its cognitive implications. Trends Cogn Sci 1998; 2:97–102.

10. Thoroughman K, Shadmehr R. Learning of action through adaptive combination of motor primitives. Nature 2000; 407:742–747.

11. Bizzi E, Tresch M, Saltiel P, d'Avella A. New perspectives on spinal motor systems. Nat Rev/Neurosci 2000; 1:101–108.

12. Pouget A, Dayan P, Zemel R. Information processing with population codes. Nat Rev/Neurosci 2000; 1:125–132.

13. Todorov E. Direct cortical control of muscle activation in voluntary arm movements: a model. Nat Neuroscience 2000; 3:391–398.

14. Georgopoulos A, Ashe J, Smyrnis N, Taira M. The motor cortex and the coding of force. Science 1992; 256:1692–1695.

15. Scott S, Gribble P, Graham K, Cabel D. Dissociation between hand motion and population vectors from neural activity in motor cortex. Nature 2001; 413: 161–165.

16. Carpenter A, Georgopoulos A, Pellizzer G. Motor cortical encoding of serial order in a context-recall task. Science 1999; 283:1619–1752.

17. Georgopoulos A, Taira M, Lukashin A. Cognitive neurophysiology of the motor cortex. Science 1993; 260:47–52.

18. Wickens J, Hyland B, Anson G. Cortical cell assemblies: A possible mechanism for motor programs. J Mot Behav 1994; 26:66–82.

19. Kalaska J, Crammond D. Cerebral cortical mechanisms of reaching movements. Science 1992; 255: 1517–1523.

20. Gandolfo F, Li C, Benda B, Schioppa C, Bizzi E. Cortical correlates of learning in monkeys adapting to an new dynamical environment. Neurobiology 2000; 97:2259–2263.

21. Penfield W, Rasmussen T. The Cerebral Cortex of Man: A Clinical Study of Localization of Function. New York: Macmillan, 1950.

22. Schott G. Penfield's homunculus: A note on cerebral cartography. J Neurol Neurosurg Psychiatry 1993; 56:329–333.

23. Park M, Belhaj-Saif A, Gordon M, Cheney P. Consistent features in the forelimb reperesentation of primary motor cortex in rhesus macaques. J Neurosci 2001; 21:2784–2792.

24. Sanes J, Donoghue J, Thangaraj V, Edelman R, Warach S. Shared neural substrates controlling hand movements in human motor cortex. Science 1995; 268:1775–1777.

25. Sanes J. The relation between human brain activity and hand movements. NeuroImage 2000; 11:370–374.

26. Schieber M, Hibbard L. How somatotopic is the motor cortex hand area? Science 1993; 261:489–492.

27. Nudo R, Milliken G, Jenkins W, Merzenich M. Use-dependent alterations of movement representations in primary motor cortex of adult squirrel monkeys. J Neurosci 1996; 16:785–807.

28. Hoffman D, Strick P. Effects of a primary motor cortex lesion on step-tracking movements of the wrist. J Neurophysiol 1995; 73:891–895.

29. He S-Q, Dum R, Strick P. Topographic organization of corticospinal projections from the frontal lobe: Motor areas on the lateral surface of the hemisphere. J Neurosci 1993; 13:952–980.

30. Beisteiner R, Windischberger C, Lanzenberger R, Edward V, Cunnington R, Erdler M, Gartus A, Streibl B, Moser E, Deecke L. Finger somatotopy in human motor cortex. NeuroImage 2001; 13:1016–1026.

31. Indovina I, Sanes J. On somatotopic representation centers for finger movements in human primary motor cortex and supplementary motor area. NeuroImage 2001; 13:1027–1034.

32. Donoghue J. Limits of reorganization in cortical circuits. Cereb Cortex 1997; 7:97–99.

33. Buonomano D, Merzenich M. Cortical plasticity: From synapses to maps. Annu Rev Neurosci 1998; 21:149–186.

34. Sanes J, Schieber M. Orderly somatotopy in primary motor cortex: Does it exist? NeuroImage 2001; 13: 968–974.

35. Lemon R. The output map of the primate cortex. Trends Neurosci 1988; 11:501–506.

36. Kakei S, Hoffman D, Strick P. Muscle and movement representations in the primary motor cortex. Science 1999; 285:2136–2139.

37. Lemon R. Mechanisms of cortical control of hand function. Neuroscientist 1997; 3:389–398.

38. Fetz E. Temporal coding in neural populations? Science 1997; 278:1901–1902.

39. Baker S, Spinks R, Jackson A, Lemon R. Synchronization in monkey motor cortex during a precision grip task. J Neurophysiol 2001; 85:869–885.

40. Schwartz A, Kettner R, Georgopoulus A. Primate motor cortex and free arm movements to visual targets in three-dimensional space. J Neurosci 1988; 8: 2913–2927.

40a. Graziano M, Taylor C, Moore T. Complex movements evoked by microstimulation of precentral cortex. Neuron 2002;34:841–851.

41. Cramer S, Finklestein S, Schaechter J, Bush G, Rosen B. Activation of distinct motor cortex regions during ipsilateral and contralateral finger movements. J Neurophysiol 1999; 981:383–387.

42. Aizawa H, Mushiake H, Inase M, Tanji J. An out-

put zone of the monkey primary motor cortex specialized for bilateral hand movement. Exp Brain Res 1990; 82:219–221.

43. Rademacher J, Burgel U, Geyer S, Schormann T, Freund H-J, Zilles K. Variability and asymmetry in the human precentral motor system: a cytoarchitectonic and myeloarchitectonic brain mapping study. Brain 2001; 124:2232–2258.

44. Kollias S, Alkadhi H, Jaermann T, Crelier G, Hepp-Raymond M-C. Identification of multiple nonprimary motor cortical areas with simple movements. Brain Res Rev 2001; 36:185–195.

45. Dobkin B. Recovery of locomotor control. The Neurologist 1996; 2:239–249.

46. Miyai I, Tanabe H, Sase I, Eda H, Oda I, Konishi I, Tsunazawa Y, Suzuki T, Yanagida T, Kubota K. Cortical mapping of gait in humans: A near-infrared spectroscopic topography study. NeuroImage 2001; 14:1186–1192.

47. Drew T. The role of the motor cortex in the control of gait modification in the cat. In: Shimamura M, Grillner S, Edgerton V, eds. Neurobiological Basis of Human Locomotion. Tokyo: Japan Scientific Societies Press, 1991:201–212.

48. Brouwer B, Ashby P. Corticospinal projections to lower limb motoneurons in man. Exp Brain Res 1992; 89:649–654.

49. Capaday C, Lavoie B, Barbeau H, Schneider C, Bonnard M. Studies on the corticospinal control of human walking. I. Responses to focal transcranial magnetic stimulation of the motor cortex. J Neurophysiol 1999; 81:129–139.

50. Schubert M, Curt A, Dietz V. Corticospinal input in human gait: Modulation of magnetically evoked motor responses. Exp Brain Res 1997; 115:234–246.

51. Murayama N, Lin Y-Y, Salenius S, Hari R. Oscillatory interaction between human motor cortex and trunk muscles during isometric contraction. NeuroImage 2001; 14:1206–1213.

52. Dobkin B. Spinal and supraspinal plasticity after incomplete spinal cord injury: Correlations between functional magnetic resonance imaging and engaged locomotor networks. In: Seil F, ed. Progress in Brain Research. Vol. 128. Amsterdam: Elsevier, 2000:99–111.

53. Schiebel M, Tomiyasu U, Scheibel A. The aging human Betz cell. Exp Neurol 1977; 56:598–609.

54. Ralston D, Ralston H. The terminations of corticospinal tract axons in the macaque monkey. J Comp Neurol 1985; 242:325–337.

55. Johannsen P, Christensen L, Sinkjaer T, Nielsen J. Cerebral functional anatomy of voluntary contractions of ankle muscles in man. J Physiol 2001; 535.2:397–406.

56. Strick P. Anatomical organization of multiple motor areas in the frontal lobe. In: Waxman S, ed. Functional Recovery in Neurological Disease. Vol. 47. New York: Raven Press, 1988:293–312.

57. Goldman-Rakic P. Motor control function of prefrontal cortex. In: Porter R, ed. Motor Areas of the Cerebral Cortex. Vol. 132. New York: John Wiley, 1987:187–197.

58. Grafton S, Woods R, Mazziotta J. Within-arm somatotopy in human motor areas determined by PET imaging of cerebral blood flow. Exp Brain Res 1993; 95:172–176.

59. Rijntjes M, Dettmers C, Buchel C. A blueprint for movement: Functional and anatomical representations in the human motor system. J Neurosci 1999; 19:8043–8048.

60. Picard N, Strick P. Motor areas of the medial wall: A review of their location and functional activation. Cere Cortex 1996; 6:342–353.

61. Grafton S. Cortical control of movement. Ann Neurol 1994; 36:3–4.

62. Fried I, Katz A, McCarthy G, etal. Functional organization of human supplementary motor cortex studied by electrical stimulation. J Neurosci 1991; 11:3856–3866.

63. Debaere F, Swinnen S, Beatse E, Sunaert S, Van Hecke P, Duysens J. Brain areas involved in interlimb coordination: A distributed network. NeuroImage 2001; 14:947–958.

64. Kurata K. Somatotopy in the supplementary motor area. Trends Neurosci 1992; 15:159–160.

65. Paus T, Petrides M, Evans A, Meyer E. Role of the human cingulate cortex in the control of oculomotor, manual, and speech responses: A PET study. J Neurophysiol 1993; 70:453–468.

66. Paus T. Primate anterior cingulate cortex: where motor control, drive and cognition interface. Nat Rev/Neurosci 2001; 2:417–424.

67. Pavlides C, Miyashita E, Asanuma H. Projection from the sensory to the motor cortex is important in learning motor skills in the monkey. J Neurophysiol 1993; 70:733–741.

68. Fuster J. Network memory. Trends Neurosci 1997; 20:451–459.

69. Dobkin B. Activity-dependent learning contributes to motor recovery. Ann Neurol 1998; 44:158–160.

70. Kwakkel G, Wagenaar R, Twisk J, Lankhorst G, Koetsier J. Intensity of leg and arm training after primary middle cerebral artery stroke: A randomised trial. Lancet 1999; 354:191–196.

71. Jeannerod M, Frak V. Mental imaging of motor activity in humans. Curr Opin Neurobiol 1999; 9:735–739.

72. Iacoboni M, Woods R, Brass M, Bekkering H, Mazziotta J, Rizzolatti G. Cortical mechanisms of human imitation. Science 1999; 286:2526–2528.

73. Arbib MA, Billard A, Iacoboni M, Oztop E. Synthetic brain imaging: Grasping, mirror neurons and imitation. Neural Networks 2000; 13:975–997.

74. Hamzei F, Buchel C, Dettmers C, Rijntnes M, Weiller C. The human action recognition system and its relationship to Broca's area: An fMRI study. Neurology 2001; 56(suppl 3):A246.

75. Jellema T, Baker C, Wicker B, Perrett D. Neural representation for the perception of the intentionality of actions. Brain Cogn 2000; 44:280–302.

76. Frith C, Frith U. Interacting minds-a biological basis. Science 1999; 286:1692–1695.

77. Castelli F, Happe F, Frith U, Frith C. Movement and mind: A functional imaging study of perception and interpretation of complex intentional movement patterns. NeuroImage 2000; 12:314–325.

78. Rossini P, Rossi S, Pasqualetti P. Corticospinal excitability modulation to hand muscles during movement imagery. Cereb Cortex 1999; 9:161–167.

79. Decety J. Can motor imagery be used as a form of therapy? J NIH Res 1995; 7:47–48.

80. Fogassi L, Gallese V, Buccino G, Craighero L,

Fadiga L, Rizzolatti G. Cortical mechanism for the visual guidance of hand grasping movements in the monkey. Brain 2001; 124:571–586.

81. Rizzolatti G, Fogassi L, Gallese V. Neurophysiological mechanisms underlying the understanding and imitation of action. Nat Rev/Neurosci 2001; 2:661–670.

82. Binkofski F. Human anterior intraparietal area subserves prehension: A combined lesion and functional MRI activation study. Neurology 1998; 50:1253–1259.

83. Binkofski F, Buccino G, Posse S, Seitz R, Rizzolatti G, Freund H-J. A fronto-parietal circuit for object manipulation in man: Evidence from an fMRI study. Eur J Neurosci 1999; 11:3276–3286.

84. Ehrsson H, Fagergren A, Forssberg H. Differential fronto-parietal activation depending on force used in a precision grip task: An fMRI study. J Neurophysiol 2001; 85:2613–2623.

85. Fuster J, Bodner M, Kroger J. Cross-modal and cross-temporal association in neurons of frontal cortex. Nature 2000; 405:347–351.

86. Zilles K, Palomero-Gallagher N. Cyto-, myelo-, and receptor architectonics of the human parietal cortex. NeuroImage 2001; 14:8–20.

87. Zilles K, Schlaug G, Matelli M. Mapping of human and macaque sensorimotor areas by integrating architectonic, transmitter receptor, MRI and PET data. J Anat 1995; 187:515–537.

88. Forss N, Narici L, Hari R. Sustained activation of the human SII cortices by stimulus trains. NeuroImage 2001; 13:497–501.

89. Darian-Smith I, Galea M, Darian-Smith C, Sugitani M, Tan A, Burman K. The Anatomy of Manual Dexterity. Berlin: Springer-Verlag, 1996.

90. Trulsson M, Francis S, Kelly E, Westling G, Bowtell R, McGlone F. Cortical responses to single mechanoreceptive afferent microstimulation revealed with fMRI. NeuroImage 2001; 13:613–622.

91. Recanzone G, Merzenich M, Schreiner C. Changes in the distributed temporal response properties of SI cortical neurons reflect improvements in performance on a temporally based tactile discrimination task. J Neurophysiol 1992; 5:1071–1091.

92. Recanzone G, Merzenich M, Jenkins W, Grajski K, Dinse H. Topographic reorganization of the hand representation in cortical area 3b of owl monkeys trained in a frequency-discrimination task. J Neurophysiol 1992; 67:1031–1056.

93. Xerri C, Merzenich M, Jenkins W, Santucci S. Representational plasticity in cortical area 3b paralleling tactual-motor skill acquisition in adult monkeys. Cereb Cortex 1999; 9:264–276.

94. Byl N, Merzenich M, Jenkins W. A primate genesis model of focal dystonia and repetitive strain injury: I. Learning-induced dedifferentiation of the representation of the hand in the primary somatosensory cortex in adult monkeys. Neurology 1996; 47:508–520.

95. Harris J, Petersen R, Diamond M. The cortical distribution of sensory memories. Neuron 2001; 30:315–318.

96. Harris J, Harris I, Diamond M. The topography of tactile learning in humans. J Neurosci 2001; 21:1056–1061.

97. Roland P, O'Sullivan B, Kawashima R. Shape and roughness activate different somatosensory areas in the human brain. Proc Natl Acad Sci USA 1998; 95:3295–3300.

98. Graziano M, Cooke D, Taylor C. Coding the location of the arm by sight. Science 2000; 290:1782–1786.

99. Andersen R, Snyder L, Bradley D, Xing J. Multimodal representation of space in the posterior parietal cortex and its use in planning movements. Annu Rev Neurosci 1997; 20:303–330.

100. Taira M, Mine S, Georgopoulos A, Sakata H. Parietal cortex neurones of the monkey related to the visual guidance of hand movement. Exp Brain Res 1990; 80:351–364.

101. Toni I, Thoenissen D, Zilles K. Movement preparation and motor intention. NeuroImage 2001; 14: S110–S117.

102. Freund H-J. The parietal lobe as a sensorimotor interface: A perspective from clinical and neuroimaging data. NeuroImage 2001; 14:S142–S146.

103. Davidoff R. The pyramidal tract. Neurology 1990; 40:332–339.

104. Nathan P, Smith M. Effects of two unilateral cordotomies on the mobility of the lower limbs. Brain 1973; 96:471–494.

105. Nathan P, Smith M, Deacon P. The corticospinal tracts in man. Brain 1990; 113:303–324.

106. Kuypers H. Some aspects of the organization of the output of the motor cortex. In: Porter R, ed. Motor Areas of the Cerebral Cortex. Chichester: John Wiley, 1987:63–82.

107. Eyre J, Tayulor J, Villagra F, Smith M, Miller S. Evidence of activity-dependent withdrawal of corticospinal projections during human development. Neurology 2001; 57:1543–1554.

108. Houk J. Neurophysiology of frontal-subcortical loops. In: Lichter D, Cummings J, eds. Frontal-subcortical circuits in psychiatric and neurological disorders. New York: Guilford Press, 2001:92–113.

109. Kennedy P. Corticospinal, rubrospinal and rubro-olivary projections: A unifying hypothesis. Trends Neurosci 1990; 13:474–479.

110. Alexander G, Crutcher M. Functional architecture of basal ganglia circuits: Neural substrates of parallel processing. TINS 1990; 13:266–271.

111. Middleton F, Strick P. A revised neuroanatomy of frontal-subcortical circuits. In: Lichter D, Cummings J, eds. Frontal-subcortical circuits in psychiatric and neurological disorders. New York: Guilford Press, 2001:44–58.

112. Hoover J, Strick P. Multiple output channels in the basal ganglia. Science 1993; 259:819–821.

113. Turner r, DeLong M. Corticostriatal activity in primary motor cortex of the macaque. J Neurosci 2000; 20:7096–7108.

114. Graybiel A, Aosaki T, Flaherty A, Kimura M. The basal ganglia and adaptive motor control. Science 1994; 265:1826–1831.

115. Houk J, Wise S. Distributed modular architectures linking basal ganglia, cerebellum, and cerebral cortex: Their role in planning and controlling action. Cereb Cortex 1995; 5:95–110.

116. Iacoboni M. Playing tennis with the cerebellum. Nat Neurosci 2001; 4:555–556.

117. Miall R, Reckess G, Imamizu H. The cerebellum coordinates eye and hand tracking movements. Nat Neurosci 2001; 4:638–644.

118. Wickelgren I. The cerebellum: the brain's engine of agility. Science 1998; 281:1588–1590.

119. Kleim J, Swain R, Armstrong K, Napper R, Jones T, Greenough W. Selective synaptic plasticity with the cerebellar cortex following complex motor skill learning. Neurobiol Learn Mem 1998; 69:278–289.

119a. Seidler R, Purushotham A, Kim S-G, Ugurbil K, Willingham D, Ashe J. Cerebellum activation associated with performance change but not motor learning. Science 2002; 296:2043–2046.

120. Llinas R, Walton K. Cerebellum. In: Shepherd G, ed. The Synaptic Organization of the Brain. New York: Oxford University Press, 1998:255–288.

121. Ramnani N, Toni I, Passingham R, Haggard P. The cerebellum and parietal cortex play a specific role in coordination: A PET study. NeuroImage 2001; 14:899–911.

122. Clower D, Dum R, Strick P. Area 7B of parietal cortex is the target of topographical output from the dentate nucleus of the cerebellum. Soc Neurosci Abstr 2001; 27:65.9.

123. Bastian A, Mink J, Kaufman B, Thach W. Posterior vermal split syndrome. Ann Neurol 1998; 44:601–610.

124. Orlovsky G, Deliagina T, Grillner S. Neuronal Control of Locomotion: From Mollusc to Man. Oxford: Oxford University Press, 1999.

125. Jueptner M, Weiller C. A review of differences between basal ganglia and cerebellar control of movements as revealed by functional imaging studies. Brain 1998; 121:1437–1449.

126. Muir G, Steeves J. Sensorimotor stimulation to improve locomotor recovery after spinal cord injury. Trends Neurosci 1997; 20:72–77.

127. Middleton F, Strick P. Cerebellar projections to the prefrontal cortex of the primate. J Neurosci 2001; 21:700–712.

128. Schmahmann J, Pandya D. Anatomic organization of the basilar pontine projections from prefrontal cortices in rhesus monkey. J Neurosci 1997; 17:438–458.

129. Allen G, Buxton R, Wong E, Courchesne E. Attentional activation of the cerebellum independent of motor involvement. Science 1997; 275:1940–1943.

130. Sherman S. Tonic and burst firing: dual modes of thalamocortical relay. Trends Neurosci 1997; 24:122–126.

131. Jones E. Ascending inputs to, and internal organization of, cortical motor areas. In: Porter R, ed. Motor Areas of the Motor Cortex. Chichester: John Wiley, 1987:21–39.

132. Nathan P, Smith M, Deacon P. Vestibulospinal, reticulospinal and descending propriospinal nerve fibres in man. Brain 1996; 119:1809–1833.

133. Schieber M. How might the cortex individuate movements? Trends Neurosci 1990; 13:440–445.

134. Iwaniuk A, Whishaw I. On the origin of skilled forelimb movements. Trends Neurosci 2000; 23:372–376.

135. Jordan L. Brain stem and spinal cord mechanisms for the initiation of locomotion. In: Shimamura M, Grillner S, Edgerton V, eds. Neurobiological Basis of Human Locomotion. Tokyo: Japan Scientific Societies Press, 1991:3–20.

136. Garcia-Rill E, Skinner R. Modulation of rhythmic function the posterior midbrain. Neuroscience 1988; 27:639–654.

137. Eidelberg E, Nguyen L, Deza L. Recovery of locomotor function after hemisection of the spinal cord in cats. Brain Res Bull 1986; 16:507–515.

138. Loy D, Magnuson D, Zhang Y, Onifer S, Mills M, Cao Q, Darnall J, Fajardo L, Burke D, Whittemore S. Functional redundancy of ventral spinal locomotor pathways. J Neurosci 2002; 22:315–323.

139. Morgenson G. Limbic-motor integration. Prog Psychobiol Physiol Psychol 1987; 12:117–170.

140. Masdeu J, Alampur U, Cavaliere R, Tavoulareas G. Astasia and gait failure with damage of the pontomesencephalic locomotor region. Ann Neurol 1994; 35:619–621.

141. Warren W, Kay B, Zosh W, Duchon A, Sahuc S. Optic flow is used to control human walking. Nat Neurosci 2001; 4:213–216.

142. Meredith M, Stein B. Descending efferents from the superior colliculus relay integrated multisensory information. Science 1985; 227:657–659.

143. Edgerton V, Roy R, de Leon R. Neural Darwinism in the mammalian spinal cord. In: Patterson M, Grau J, eds. Spinal Cord Plasticity: Alterations in Reflex Function. Norwell, MA: Kluwer Academic Publishing, 2001:186–206.

144. Wolpaw J, Tennissen A. Activity-dependent spinal cord plasticity in health and disease. Annu Rev Neurosci 2001; 24:807–843.

145. Routal R, Pal G. A study of motoneuron groups and motor columns of the human spinal cord. J Anat 1999; 195:211–224.

146. Vanderhorst V, Holstege G. Organization of lumbosacral motoneuronal cell groups innervating hindlimb, pelvic floor, and axial muscles in the cat. J Comp Neurol 1997; 382:46–76.

147. Rekling J, Funk G, Bayliss D, Dong X-W, Feldman J. Synaptic control of motoneuronal excitability. Physiol Rev 2000; 80:767–852.

148. Burke R. Spinal cord: Ventral horn. In: Shepherd G, ed. Synaptic Organization of the Brain. New York: Oxford University Press, 1998:77–120.

149. Mendell L. Modifiability of spinal synapses. Physiol Rev 1984; 64:260–324.

150. Davidoff R. Skeletal muscle tone and the misunderstood stretch reflex. Neurology 1992; 42:951–963.

151. Wolpaw J, Carp J. Memory traces in spinal cord. Trends Neurosci 1990; 13:137–142.

152. Chen X, Carp J, Chen L, Wolpaw J. Corticospinal tract transection prevents operantly conditioned H-reflex increase in rats. Exp Brain Res 2002; 144:88–94.

153. Evatt M, Wolf S, Segal R. Modification of human spinal stretch reflexes. Neurosci Lett 1989; 105:350–355.

154. Nielsen J, Crone C, Hultborn H. H-reflexes are smaller in dancers from the Royal Danish Ballet than in well-trained athletes. Eur J Appl Physiol 1993; 66:116–121.

155. Stein R, Yang J, Edamura M, Capaday C. Reflex modulation during normal and pathological human locomotion. In: Shimamura M, Grillner S, Edgerton V, eds. Neurobiological Basis of Human Locomotion. Tokyo: Japan Scientific Societies Press, 1991:335–346.

156. Fedirchuk B, Nielson J, Petersen N, Hultborn H. Pharmacologically evoked fictive motor patterns in the acutely spinalized marmoset monkey. Exp Brain Res 1998; 122:351–361.

157. Grillner S. Neurobiological bases for rhythmic motor acts in vertebrates. Science 1985; 228:143–149.

158. Hultborn H, Petersen N, Brownstone R, Nielsen J. Evidence of fictive spinal locomotion in the marmoset. Proceedings of the Annual Meeting of the Society For Neuroscience, Washington, D.C., 1993. Vol. 19.

159. Stein R. Reflex modulation during locomotion: Functional significance. In: Patla A, ed. Adaptability of Human Gait. North Holland: Elsevier, 1991:21–36.

160. Schmidt B, Jordan L. The role of serotonin in reflex modulation and locomotor rhythm production in the mammalian spinal cord. Brain Res Bull 2001; 53: 689–710.

161. Pearson K. Common principles of motor control in vertebrates and invertebrates. Annu Rev Neurosci 1993; 16:265–297.

162. Kjaerulff O, Kiehn O. Distribution of networks generating and coordinating locomotor activity in the neonatal rat spinal cord in vitro: A lesion study. J Neurosci 1996; 16:5777–5794.

163. Hadi B, Zhang P, Burke D, Shields C, Magnuson D. Lasting paraplegia caused by loss of lumbar spinal cord interneurons in rats: No direct correlation with motor neuron loss. J Neurosurg 2000; 93:266–275.

164. Magnuson D, Green D, Sengoku T. Lumbar spinoreticular neurons in the rat: Part of the central pattern generator for locomotion? Ann NY Acad Sci 1998:436–440.

165. Grillner S, Matsushima T. The neuronal network underlying locomotion in lamprey—Synaptic and cellular mechanisms. Neuron 1991; 7:1–15.

166. Smith J, Greer J, Liu G, Feldman J. Neural mechanisms generating respiratory pattern in mammalian brain stem-spinal cord in vitro. J Neurophysiol 1990; 64:1149–1169.

167. Weimann J, Meyrand P, Marder E. Neurons that form multiple pattern generators. J Neurophysiol 1991; 65:111–122.

168. Pearson K. Proprioceptive regulation of locomotion. Curr Opin Neurobiol 1995; 5:786–791.

169. Pearson K, Misiaszek J, Fouad K. Enhancement and resetting of locomotor activity by muscle afferents. Ann NY Acad Sci 1998; 860:203–215.

170. Van Wezel B, Ottenhoff F, Duysens J. Dynamic control of location-specific information in tactile cutaneous reflexes from the foot during human walking. J Neurosci 1997; 17:3804–3814.

171. Nielsen J, Petersen N, Fedirchuk B. Evidence suggesting a transcortical pathway from cutaneous foot afferents to tibialis anterior motoneurones in man. J Physiol 1997; 501:473–484.

172. Duysens J, Pearson K. From cat to man: basic aspects of locomotion relevant to motor rehabilitation of SCI. NeuroRehab 1998; 10:107–118.

173. Dietz V, Duysens J. Significance of load receptor input during locomotion: A review. Posture Gait 2000; 11:102–110.

174. Harkema S, Hurley S, Patel U, Dobkin B, Edgerton V. Human lumbosacral spinal cord interprets loading during stepping. J Neurophysiol 1997; 77:797–811.

175. Taga G, Yamaguchi Y, Shimizu H. Self-organized control of bipedal locomotion by neural oscillators in unpredictable environment. Biol Cybern 1991; 65: 147–159.

176. Duysens J, Van de Crommert H. Neural control of locomotion: The central pattern generator from cats to humans. Gait Posture 1998; 7:131–141.

177. Riddoch G. The reflex functions of the completely divided spinal cord in man, compared with those associated with less severe lesions. Brain 1917; 40: 264–402.

178. Kuhn R. Functional capacity of the isolated human spinal cord. Brain 1950; 73:1–51.

179. Dobkin B, Harkema S, Requejo P, Edgerton V. Modulation of locomotor-like EMG activity in subjects with complete and incomplete chronic spinal cord injury. J Neurol Rehab 1995; 9:183–190.

180. Calancie B, Needham-Shropshire B, Green B, Jacobs P, Willer K, Zych G. Involuntary stepping after chronic spinal cord injury. Brain 1994; 117:1143–1159.

181. Bussel B, Roby-Brami A, Biraben A, Held J. Myoclonus in a patient with spinal cord transection. Brain 1988; 111:1235–1245.

182. Dimitrijevic M, Gerasimenko Y, Pinter M. Evidence for a spinal central pattern generator in humans. Ann NY Acad Sci 1998; 860:360–376.

183. Lovely R, Gregor R, Roy R, Edgerton V. Effects of training on the recovery of full-weight-bearing stepping in the adult spinal cat. Exp Neurol 1986; 92: 421–435.

184. Barbeau H, Rossignol S. Recovery of locomotion after chronic spinalization in the adult cat. Brain Res 1987; 412:84–95.

185. Hodgson J, Roy R, Dobkin B, Edgerton V. Can the mammalian spinal cord learn a motor task? Med Sci Sports Exerc 1994; 26:1491–1497.

186. de Leon R, Hodgson J, Roy R, Edgerton V. Locomotor capacity attributable to step training versus spontaneous recovery after spinalization in adult cats. J Neurophysiol 1998; 79:1329–1340.

187. Giszter SF, Kargo WJ, Davies M, Shibayama M. Fetal transplants rescue axial muscle representations in M1 cortex of neonatally transected rats that develop weight support. J Neurophysiol 1998; 80:3021–3030.

188. Dobkin B, Edgerton V, Fowler E, Hodgson J. Training induces rhythmic locomotor EMG patterns in subjects with complete SCI. Neurology 1992; 42 (Suppl 3):207–208.

189. Dobkin B, Edgerton V, Fowler E. Sensory input during treadmill training alters rhythmic locomotor EMG output in subjects with complete spinal cord injury. Soc Neurosci Abstr 1992; 18:1043.

190. Dietz V, Colombo D, Jensen L, Baumgartner L. Locomotor capacity of spinal cord paraplegic patients. Ann Neurol 1995; 37:574–582.

191. Harkema S, Requejo P, Dobkin B, Edgerton V. Load and phase dependent modulation of motor pool output by the human lumbar spinal cord during manually assisted stepping. Proceedings of the International Symposium on Neurons, Networks, and Motor Behavior, The University of Arizona, Tucson, 1995.

192. Edgerton V, Roy R, DeLeon R, Tillakaratne N, Hodgson J. Does motor learning occur in the spinal cord. The Neuroscientist 1997; 3:287–294.

193. Wernig A, Nanassy A, Miller S. Maintenance of locomotor abilities following Laufband (treadmill) therapy in para- and tetraplegic persons: Follow-up studies. Spinal Cord 1998; 36:744–749.

194. Barbeau H, Pepin A, Norman K. Walking after spinal cord injury: Control and recovery. The Neuroscientist 1998; 4:14–24.

195. Dietz V, Wirz M, Curt A, Colombo G. Locomotor patterns in paraplegic patients: Training effects and recovery of spinal cord function. Spinal Cord 1998; 36:380–390.

196. Dobkin B. Overview of treadmill locomotor training with partial body weight support: A neurophysiologically sound approach whose time has come for randomized clinical trials. Neurorehabil Neural Repair 1999; 13:157–165.

197. Loeb E, Giszter S, Saltiel P, Bizzi E, Mussa-Ivaldi F. Output units of motor behavior: An experimental and modeling study. J Cogn Neurosci 2000; 12:78–97.

198. Edgerton V, de Leon R, Harkema S, Hodgson J, London N, Reinkensmeyer D, Roy R, Talmadge R, Tillakaratne N, Tomiszyk W, Tobin A. Retraining the injured spinal cord. J Physiol 2001; 533:15–22.

199. Barbeau H, Ladouceur M, Norman K, Pepin A, Leroux A. Walking after spinal cord injury: Evaluation, treatment and functional recovery. Arch Phys Med Rehabil 1999; 80:225–235.

200. Lotze M, Erb M, Flor H, Huelsmann E, Godde B, Grodd W. fMRI evaluation of somatotopic representation in human primary motor cortex. NeuroImage 2000; 11:473–481.

201. Kawashima R, Roland P, O'Sullivan B. Fields in human motor areas involved in preparation for reaching, actual reaching, and visuomotor learning: A PET study. J Neurosci 1994; 14:3462–3474.

202. Jenkins I, Brooks J, Frackowiak R, Nixon P, Passingham R. Motor sequence learning: A study with positron emission tomography. J Neurosci 1994; 14:3775–3790.

203. Grafton S, Mazziotta J, Presty S, Friston K, Frackowiak R, Phelps M. Functional anatomy of human procedural learning determined with regional cerebral blood flow and PET. J Neurosci 1992; 12:2542–2548.

204. Rao S, Binder J, Bandettini P. Functional magnetic resonance imaging of complex human movements. Neurology 1993; 43:2311–2318.

205. Jueptner M, Stephan K, Frith C, Brooks D, Frackowiak R, Passingham R. Anatomy of motor learning. I Frontal cortex and attention to action. J Neurophysiol 1997; 77:1313–1324.

206. Jueptner M, Frith C, Brooks D, Frackowiak R, Passingham R. Anatomy of motor learning. II. Subcortical structures and learning by trial and error. J Neurophysiol 1997; 77:1325–1337.

207. Remy P, Zilbovicius M, Leroy-Willig A, Syrota A, Samson Y. Movement- and task-related activations of motor cortical areas: A positron emission tomographic study. Ann Neurol 1994; 36:19–26.

208. Frackowiak R. Functional mapping of verbal memory and language. Trends Neurosci 1994; 17:109–115.

209. Deiber M, Passingham R, Colebatch J, Frackowiak R. Cortical areas and the selection of movement: A study with positron emission tomography. Exp Brain Res 1991; 84:393–402.

210. Lehericy S, van de Moortele P-F, Lobel E, Paradis A, Vidailhet M, Frouin V, Neveu P, Agid Y, Marsault C, Le Bihan D. Somatotopical organization of striatal activation during finger and toe movement: A 3-T functional magnetic resonance imaging study. Ann Neurol 1998; 44:398–404.

211. Yue G, Cole K. Strength increases from the motor program: Comparison of training with maximal voluntary and imagined muscle contractions. J Neurophysiol 1992; 67:1114–1123.

212. Rahnganathan V, Siemionow V, Sahgal V, Yue G. Increasing muscle strength by training the central nervous system without physical exercise. Soc Neurosci Abstr 2001; 27:168.17.

213. Roland P. Cortical organization of voluntary behavior in man. Hum Neurobiol 1985; 4:155–167.

214. Remple M, Bruneau R, VandenBerg P, Kleim J. Sensitivity of cortical movement representations to motor experience: Evidence that skill learning but not strength training induces cortical reorganization. Behav Brain Res 2001; 123:133–141.

215. Fukuyama H, Ouchi Y, Matsuzaki S, Nagahama Y, Yamauchi H, Ogawa M, Kimura J, Shibasaki H. Brain functional activity during gait in normal subjects: A SPECT study. Neurosci Lett 1997; 228:183–186.

216. Honda M, Freund H-J, Shibasaki H. Cerebral activation by locomotive movement with the imagination of natural walking. Human Brain Mapping 1995; 2(Suppl 1):318.

217. Ouchi Y, Okada Y, Yoshikawa E, Nobezawa S, Futatsubashi M. Brain activation during maintenance of standing postures in humans. Brain 1999; 122:329–338.

218. Asanuma C. Mapping movements within a moving motor map. Trends Neurosci 1991; 14:217–218.

219. Florence S, Jain N, Kaas J. Plasticity of somatosensory cortex in primates. Neuroscience 1997; 9:3–12.

220. Boroojerdi B, Ziemann U, Chen R, Butefisch C, Cohen L. Mechanisms underlying human motor system plasticity. Muscle Nerve 2001; 24:602–613.

221. Sabel B. Unrecognized potential of surviving neurons: Within-systems plasticity, recovery of function, and the hypothesis of minimal residual structure. Neuroscientist 1997; 3:366–370.

222. Kilgard M, Merzenich M. Cortical map reorganization enabled by nucleus basalis activity. Science 1998; 279:1714–1718.

223. Nudo R, Jenkins W, Merzenich M. Repetitive microstimulation alters the cortical representation of movements in adult rats. Somatosens Mot Res 1990; 7:463–483.

224. Nudo R, Plautz E, Milliken G. Adaptive plasticity in primate motor cortex as a consequence of behavioral experience and neuronal injury. Semin Neurosci 1997; 9:13–23.

225. Schallert T, Fleming S, Leasure J. CNS plasticity and assessment of forelimb sensorimotor outcome in unilateral rat models of stroke, cortical ablation, parkinsonism and spinal cord injury. Neuropharmacol 2000; 39:777–787.

226. Tillerson JL, Cohen AD, Philhower J, Miller GW, Zigmond MJ, Schallert T. Forced limb-use effects on the behavioral and neurochemical effects of 6-hydroxydopamine. J Neurosci 2001; 21:4427–4435.

227. Karni A, Meyer G, Jezzard P, Adams M, Turner R, Ungerleider S. Functional MRI evidence for adult motor cortex plasticity during motor skill learning. Nature 1995; 377:155–158.

228. Karni A, Meyer G, HipolÄito C, Jezzard P, Adams M. The acquisition of skilled motor performance: Fast and slow experience-driven changes in primary motor cortex. Proc Natl Acad Sci USA 1998; 95:861–868.

229. Liepert J, Terborg C, Weiller C. Motor plasticity induced by synchronized thumb and foot movements. Exp Brain Res 1999; 125:435–439.

230. Classen J, Liepert J, Wise S, Hallett M, Cohen L. Rapid plasticity of human cortical movement representation induced by practice. J Neurophysiol 1998; 79:1117–1123.

231. Pascual-Leone A, Cohen L, Dang N, Hallet M. Acquisition of fine motor skills in humans is associated with the modulation of cortical motor outputs. Neurology 1993; 43(suppl):A157.

232. Pascual-Leone A, Grafman J, Hallett M. Modulation of cortical output maps during development of implicit and explicit knowledge. Science 1994; 263: 1287–1289.

233. Shadmehr R, Holcomb H. Neural correlates of motor memory consolidation. Science 1997; 277:821–825.

234. Li C-S, Padoa-Schioppa C, Bizzi E. Neuronal correlates of motor performance and motor learning in the promary motor cortex of monkeys adapting to an external force field. Neuron 2001; 30:593–607.

235. Wang X, Merzenich M, Sameshima K, Jenkins W. Remodelling of hand representation inadult cortex determined by timing of tactile stimulation. Nature 1995; 378:71–75.

236. Rossini P, Rossi S, Tecchio F, Pasqualetti P, Sabato A, Finazzi-Agrò A. Focal brain stimulation in healthy humans: motor maps changes following partial hand sensory deprivation. Neurosci Lett 1996; 214: 191–195.

237. Braun C, Heinz U, Schweizer R, Wiech K, Bribaumer N, Topka H. Dynamic organization of the somatosensory cortex induced by motor activity. Brain 2001; 124:2259–2267.

238. Ridding M, Brouwer B, Miles T, Pitcher J, Thompson P. Changes in muscle responses to stimulation of the motor cortex induced by peripheral nerve stimulation in human subjects. Exp Brain Res 2000; 131:135–143.

239. Stefan K, Kunesch E, Csohen L, Benecke R, Classen J. Induction of plasticity in the human motor cortex by paired associative stimulation. Brain 2000; 123: 572–584.

240. Nudo R, Friel K, Delia S. Role of sensory deficits in motor impairments after injury to primary motor cortex. Neuropharmacol 2000; 39:733–742.

241. Florence S, Taub H, Kaas J. Large-scale sprouting of cortical connections after peripheral injury in adult macaque monkeys. Science 1998; 282:1117–1120.

242. Ebner F, Rema V, Sachdev R, Syhmons F. Activity-dependent plasticity in adult somatic sensory cortex. Neuroscience 1997; 9:47–58.

243. Jones E, Pons T. Thalamic and brain stem contributions to large-scale plasticity of primate somatosensory cortex. Science 1998; 282:1121–1125.

244. Froc D, Chapman C, Trepel C. Long-term depression and potentiation in the sensorimotor cortex of the freely moving rat. J Neurosci 2000; 20:438–445.

245. Turrigiano G, Nelson S. Hebb and homeostasis in neuronal plasticity. Curr Opin Neurobiol 2000; 10: 358–364.

246. Bailey C, Giustetto M, Huang Y-Y, Hawkins R, Kandel E. Is heterosynaptic modulation essential for stabilizing Hebbian plasticity and memory? Nat Rev/Neurosci 2000; 1:11–20.

247. Kandel E. The molecular biology of memory storage: A dialogue betweeen genes and synapses. Science 2001; 294:1030–1038.

248. Wessberg J, Stambaugh C, Kralik J, Beck P, Laubach M, Chapin J, Kim J, Biggs SJ, Srinivasan M, Nicholelis M. Real-time prediction of hand trajectory by ensembles of cortical neurons in primates. Nature 2000; 408:361–365.

249. Castro-Alamancos M, Donoghue J, Connors B. Different forms of synaptic plasticity in somatosensory and motor areas of the neocortex. J Neurosci 1995; 15:5324–5333.

250. Wang J-H, Ko G, Kelly P. Cellular and molecular bases of memory: Synaptic and neuronal plasticity. J Clin Neurophysiol 1997; 14:264–293.

251. Malenka R, Nicoll R. Long-term potentiation—A decade of progress? Science 1999; 285:1870–1874.

252. Hansel C, Linden D, D'Angelo E. Beyond parallel fiber LTD: The diversity of synaptic and nonsynaptic plasticity in the cerebellum. Nat Neurosci 2001; 4:467–475.

253. Malenka R. Mucking up movements. Nature 1994; 372:218–219.

254. Charpier S, Deniau J. In vivo activity-dependent plasticity at cortico-striatal connections: evidence for physiological long-term potentiation. Proc Natl Acad Sci USA 1997; 94:7036–7040.

255. Randic M, Jiang C, Cerne R. Long-term potentiation and long-term depression of primary afferent neurotransmission in the rat spinal cord. J Neurosci 1993; 13:5228–5241.

256. Grillner S. Ion channels and locomotion. Science 1997; 278:1087–1088.

257. Rioult-Pedotti M, Friedman D, Donoghue J. Learning-induced LTP in neocortex. Science 2000; 290: 533–536.

258. Hess G, Aizenman C, Donoghue J. Conditions for the induction of long-term potentiation in layer II/III horizontal connections of the rat cortex. J Neurophysiol 1996; 75:1765–1778.

259. Kleim J, Lussnig E, Schwarz E, Comery T, Greenough W. Synaptogenesis and FOS expression in the motor cortex of the adult rat after motor skill learning. J Neurosci 1996; 16:4529–4535.

260. Ivanco T, Racine R, Kolb B. Morphology of layer III pyramidal neurons is altered following induction of LTP in sensorimotor cortex of the freely moving rat. Synapse 2000; 37:16–22.

261. Asanuma H, Pavlides C. Neurobiological basis of motor learning in mammals. NeuroReport 1997; 8:I–VI.

262. Shadmehr R, Brashers-King T. Functional stages in the formation of human long-term motor memory. J Neurosci 1997; 17:409–419.

263. Glazewski S, Giese K, Silva A, Fox K. The role of alpha-CaMKII autophosphorylation in neocortical experience-dependent plasticity. Nat Neurosci 2000; 3:911–917.

264. Winder D, Sweatt J. Roles of serine/threonine phosphatases in hippocampal synaptic plasticity. Nat Rev/Neurosci 2001; 2:461–474.

265. Engert F, Bonhoeffer T. Dendritic spine changes associated with hippocampal long-term synaptic plasticity. Nature 1999; 399:66–70.

266. Toni H, Buchs P, Nikonenko I, Bron C, Muller D. LTP promotes formation of multiple spine synapses

between a single axon terminal and a dendrite. Nature 1999; 402:421–425.

267. Luscher C, Nicoll R, Malenka R, Muller D. Synaptic plasticity and dynamic modulation of the postsynaptic membrane. Neuroscience 2000; 3:545–550.

268. Hausser M, Spruston N, Stuart G. Diversity and dynamics of dendritic signaling. Science 2000; 290:739–744.

269. Diamond M, Huang W, Ebner F. Laminar comparison of somatosensory cortical plasticity. Science 1994; 265:1885–1888.

270. Jones T, Kleim J, Greenough W. Synaptogenesis and dendritic growth in the cortex opposite unilateral sensorimotor cortex damage in adult rats: A quantitative electron microscopic examination. Brain Res 1996; 733:142–148.

271. Kleim J, Vij K, Ballard D, Greenough W. Learning-dependent synaptic modifications in the cerebellar cortex of the adult rat persist for at least four weeks. J Neurosci 1997; 17:717–721.

272. Klintsova A, Greenough W. Synaptic plasticity in cortical systems. Curr Opin Neurobiol 1999; 9:203–208.

273. Kleim J, Barbay S, Cooper N, Hogg T, Reidel C, Remple M, Nudo R. Motor learning-dependent synaptogenesis is localized to functionally reorganized motor cortex. Neurobiol Learn Mem 2002; 77: 63–77.

274. Hall J, Thomas K, Everitt B. Rapid and selective induction of BDNF expression in the hippocampus during contextual learning. Nat Neurosci 2000; 3:533–535.

275. Neeper S, Gomez-Pinella F, Choi J, Cotman C. Physical activity increases mRNA for brain-derived neurotrophic factor and nerve growth factor in rat brain. Brain Res 1996; 726:49–56.

276. Poo M. Neurotrophins as synaptic modulators. Nat Rev Neurosci 2001; 2:24–32.

277. Kohara K, Kitamura A, Morishima M, Tsumoto T. Activity-dependent transfer of brain-derived neurotrophic factor to postsynaptic neurons. Science 2001; 291:2419–2422.

278. Jovanovic J, Czernik A, Fienberg A, Greengard P, Sihra T. Synapsins as mediators of BDNF-enhanced neurotransmitter release. Nat Neurosci 2000; 3:323–329.

279. Fon EA, Edwards RH. Molecular mechanisms of neurotransmitter release. Muscle Nerve 2001; 24: 581–601.

280. Smit A, Syed N, Schaap D, van Minnen J, Klumperman J, Kits K, Lodder H, Van Der Schors R, Van Elk R, Sorgedrager B, Brejc K, Sixma T, Geraerts W. A glia-derived acetylcholine-binding protein that modulates synaptic transmission. Nature 2001; 411:261–268.

281. Gu Q. Neuromodulatory transmitter systems in the cortex and their role in cortical plasticity. Neuroscience 2002; 111:815–835.

282. Juliano S, Ma W, Eslin D. Cholinergic depletion prevents expansion of topographic maps in somatosensory cortex. Proc Natl Acad Sci USA 1991; 88:780–784.

283. Juliano S. Mapping the sensory mosaic. Science 1998; 279:1653–1654.

284. Waelti P, Dickinson A, Schultz W. Dopamine responses comply with basic assumptions of formal learning theory. Nature 2001; 412:43–48.

285. Fried I, Wilson C, Morrow J, Cameron K, Behnke E, Ackerson L, Maidment N. Increased dopamine release in the human amygdala during performance of cognitive tasks. Nat Neurosci 2001; 4:201–206.

286. Granon S, Passetti F, Thomas K, Dalley J, Everitt B, Robbins T. Enhanced and impaired attentional performance after infusion of D1 dopaminergic receptor agents into rat prefrontal cortex. Neuroscience 2000; 20:1208–1215.

287. Volkow N, Wang G-J, Fowler J, Logan J, Gerasimov M, Maynard L, Ding Y, Gatley S, Gifford A, Franceschi D. Therapeutic doses of oral methylphenidate significantly increase extracellular dopamine in the human brain. J Neurosci 2001; 21: RC121 (1–5).

288. Paladini C, Fiorillo C, Morikawa H, Williams J. Amphetamine selectively blocks inhibitory glutamate transmission in dopmamine neurons. Nat Neurosci 2001; 4:275–281.

289. Badiani A, Oates M, Day H, Watson S, Akil H, Robinson T. Amphetamine-induced behavior, dopamine release, and c-fos mRNA expression: Modulation by environmental novelty. Neuroscience 1998; 18: 10579–10593.

290. Bao S, Chan V, Merzenich M. Cortical remodelling induced by activity in ventral tegmental dopamine neurons. Nature 2001; 412:79–83.

291. Coull J, Nobre A, Frith C. The noradrenergic a2 agonist clonidine modulates behavioural and neuroanatomical correlates of human attentional orienting and alerting. Cereb Cortex 2001; 11:73–84.

292. Usher M, Cohen J, Shreiber D, Rajkowski J, Jones G. The role of locus coeruleus in the regulation of cognitive performance. Science 1999; 283:549–554.

293. Kirkwood A, Rozas C, Kirkwood J. Modulation of long-term synaptic depression in visual cortex by acetylcholine and norepinephrine. J Neurosci 1999; 19:1599–1609.

294. Geyer M. Serotonergic functions in arousal and motor activity. Behav Brain Res 1996; 73:31–35.

295. Jacobs B, Fornal C. Serotonin and motor activity. Curr Opin Neurobiol 1997; 7:820–825.

296. Hasbroucq T, Rihet P, Blin O, Possamai C-A. Serotonin and human information processing: Fluvoxamine can improve reaction time performance. Neurosci Lett 1997; 229:204–208.

297. Stamford J, Davidson C, McLaughlin D, Hopwood S. Control of dorsal raphe 5-HT function by multiple 5-HT, autoreceptors: Parallel purposes or pointless plurality? Trends Neurosci 2000; 23:459–465.

298. Dinse H, Ragert P, Pleger B, Schwenkreis P, Tegenthoff M. Pharmacological control of short-term plasticity in human somatosensory cortex: Correlation betweeen cortical reorganization and discrimination performance. Soc For Neurosci Abstr 2001; 27:396.6.

299. Butefisch C, Davis B, Sawaki L, Waldvogel D, Classen J, Kopylev L, Cohen L. Modulation of use-dependent plasticity by d-amphetamine. Ann Neurol 2002; 51:59–68.

300. Kanwisher N. Domain specificity in face perception. Nat Neurosci 2000; 3:759–63.

301. Fuster J. The prefrontal cortex-an update: time is of the essence. Neuron 2001; 30:319–333.

302. Arshavsky Y. Role of individual neurons and neural networks in cognitive functioning: A new insight. Brain Cogn 2001; 46:414–428.

303. Cameron K, Yashar S, Wilson C, Fried I. Human hippocampal neurons predict how well word pairs will be remembered. Neuron 2001; 30:289–298.

304. Mesulam M. From sensation to cognition. Brain 1998; 121:1013–1052.

305. Mesulam M-M. Principles of Behavioral and Cognitive Neurology. New York: Oxford University Press, 2000.

306. Kourtzi Z, Kanwisher N. Cortical regions involved in perceiving object shape. Neuroscience 2000; 20: 3310–3318.

307. Varela F, Lachaux J-P, Rodriguez E, Martinerie J. The brainweb: Phase synchronization and large-scale integration. Nat Rev/Neurosci 2001; 2:229–239.

308. Damasio A. Category-related recognition defects as a clue to the neural substrates of knowledge. Trends Neurosci 1990; 13:95–98.

309. Stone J, Hunkin N, Hornby A. Predicting spontaneous recovery of memory. Nature 2001; 414:167–168.

310. Knowlton B, Squire L. The learning of categories: Parallel brain systems for item memory and category knowledge. Science 1993; 262:1747–1749.

311. Zola-Morgan S, Squire L. Neuroanatomy of memory. Ann Rev Neurosci 1993; 16:547–563.

312. Schacter D, Cooper L, Tharan M, Rubens A. Preserved priming of novel objects in patients with memory disorders. J Cogn Neurosci 1991; 3:117–130.

313. Marsolek C, Kosslyn S, Squire L. Form-specific visual priming in the right hemisphere. J Exp Psychol 1992; 18:492–508.

314. Schacter D. Memory and awareness. Science 1998; 280:59–60.

315. Poldrack R, Clark J, Pare-Blagoev E, Shohamy D, Moyano J, Myers C, Gluck MA. Interactive memory systems in the human brain. Nature 2001; 414:546–550.

316. Maddock R. The retrosplenial cortex and emotion: new insights from functional neuroimaging of the human brain. Trends Neurosci 1999; 22:310–316.

317. Anderson A, Phelps E. Lesions of the human amygdala impair enhanced perception of emotionally salient events. Nature 2001; 411:305–309.

318. Kim J, Lee H, Han J-S, Packard M. Amygdala is critical for stress-induced modulation of hippocampal long-term potentiation and learning. J Neurosci 2001; 21:5222–5228.

319. Eichenbaum H. A cortical-hippocampal system for declarative memory. Nat Rev/Neurosci 2000; 1:41–50.

320. Ojemann G, Ojemann S, Fried I. Lessons from the human brain: Neuronal activity related to cognition. Neuroscientist 1998; 4:285–300.

321. Krelman G, Koch C, Fried I. Imagery neurons in the human brain. Nature 2000; 408:357–361.

322. Kirchhoff B, Wagner A, Maril A, Stern C. Prefrontal-temporal circuitry for episodic encoding subsequent memory. J Neurosci 2000; 20:6173–6180.

323. Naya Y, Yoshida M, Miyashita Y. Backward spreading of memory-retrieval signal in the primate temporal cortex. Science 2001; 291:661–664.

324. Sara S. Retrieval and reconsolidation: Toward a neurobiology of remembering. Learn Mem 2000; 7:73–84.

325. Frankland P, O'Brien C, Ohno M, Kirkwood A, Silva A. a-CaMKII-dependent plasticity in the cortex is required for permanent memory. Nature 2001; 411: 309–312.

326. Shimizu E, Tang Y, Rampon C, Tsien J. NMDA receptor-dependent synaptic reinforcement as a crucial process for memory consolidation. Science 2000; 290:1170–1174.

327. Stickgold R, James L, Hobson A. Visual discrimination learning requires sleep after training. Nat Neurosci 2000; 3:1237–1238.

328. Maquet P, Laureys S, Peigneux P, Fuchs S, Petiau C, Phillips C, Aerts J, Del Fiore G, Degueldre C, Meulemans T, Luxen A, Franck G, Van Der Linden M, Smith C, Cleeremans A. Experience-dependent changes in cerebral activation during human REM sleep. Nat Neurosci 2000; 3:831–836.

329. Hardingham G, Arnold F, Bading H. Nuclear calcium signaling controls CREB-mediated gene expression triggered by synaptic activity. Nat Neurosci 2001; 4:261–267.

330. Shors T, Miesegaes G, Beylin A, Zhao M, Rydel T, Gould E. Neurogenesis in the adult is involved in the formation of trace memories. Nature 2001; 410:372–375.

331. van Praag H, Kempermann G, Gage F. Running increases cell proliferation and neurogenesis in the adult mouse dendate gyrus. Nat Neurosci 1999; 2:266–270.

332. van Praag H, Kempermann G, Gage F. Neural consequences of environmental enrichment. Neuroscience 2000; 1:191–198.

333. Gomez-Pinilla F, Dao L, So V. Physical exercise induces FGF-2 and its mRNA in the hippocampus. Brain Res 1997; 764:1–8.

334. Mizuno M, Yamada K, Olariu A, Nawa H, Nabeshima T. Involvement of brain-derived neurotrophic factor in spatial memory formation and maintenance in a radial arm maze test in rats. Neuroscience 2000; 20:7116–7121.

335. Tong L, Shen H, Perreau V, Balazs R, Cotman C. Effects of exercise on gene-expression profile in the rat hippocampus. Neurobiol Dis 2001; 8:1046–1056.

336. Cabeza R, Nyberg L. Neural bases of learning and memory: Functional neuroimaging evidence. Curr Opin Neurol 2000; 13:415–421.

337. Gabrieli J, Brewer J, Desmond J, Glover G. Separate neural bases of two fundamental memory processes in the human medial temporal lobe. Science 1997; 276:264–266.

338. Brown M, Aggleton J. Recognition memory: What are the roles of the perirhinal cortex and hippocampus? Nat Rev/Neurosci 2001; 2:51–61.

339. Eldridge L, Knowlton B, Furmanski C, Bookheimer S, Engel S. Remembering episodes: A selective role for the hippocampus during retrieval. Neuroscience 2000; 3:1149–52.

340. Stark C, Squire L. Functional magnetic resonance imaging (fMRI) activity in the hippocampal region during recognition memory. Neuroscience 2000; 20:7776–7781.

341. Wagner A, Schacter D, Rotte M, Rosen B. Building memories: Remembering and forgetting verbal experience as predicted by brain activity. Science 1998; 281:1188–1191.

342. Brewer J, Zhao Z, Desmond J, Glover G, Gabrieli J. Making memories: Brain activity that predicts how well visual experience will be remembered. Science 1998; 281:1185–1187.

343. Fernandez G, Weyerts H, Schrader-Bolsche M,

Tendolkar I, Smid H, Tempelmann C, Hinrichs H, Scheich H, Elger C, Mangun G, Heinze H. Successful verbal encoding into episodic memory engages the posterior hippocampus: A parametrically analyzed functional magnetic resonance imaging study. J Neurosci 1998; 18:1841–1847.

344. Jonides J, Schumacher E, Smith E, Koeppe R, Awh E, Lorenz-Reuter P. The role of parietal cortex in verbal working memory. J Neurosci 1998; 18:5026–5034.

345. Burgess P, Quayle A, Frith C. Brain regions involved in prospective memory as determined by positron emission tomography. Neuropsychologia 2001; 39:545–555.

346. Buckner RL, Koutstaal W. Functional neuroimaging studies of encoding, priming, and explicit memory retrieval. Proc Natl Acad Sci USA 1998; 95:891–898.

347. Poldrack R, Gabrieli J. Functional anatomy of long-term memory. Clin Neurophysiol 1997; 14:294–310.

348. Owen A. The role of the lateral frontal cortex in mnemonic processing: The contribution of functional neuroimaging. Exp Brain Res 2000; 133:33–43.

349. Smith E, Jonides J. Storage and executive processes in the frontal lobes. Science 1999; 283:1657–1661.

350. Petrides M, Pandya D. Dorsolateral prefrontal cortex: Comparative cytoarchitectonic analysis in the human and the macaque brain and corticocortical connection patterns. Eur J Neurosci 1999; 11:1011–1036.

351. MacDonald A, Cohen J, Stenger V, Carter C. Dissociating the role of the dorsolateral prefrontal and anterior cingulate cortex in cognitive control. Science 2000; 288:1835–1838.

352. Rao S, Rainer G, Miller E. Integration of what and where in the primate prefrontal cortex. Science 1997; 276:821–824.

353. Miller E. The prefrontal cortex and cognitive control. Nat Rev Neurosci 2000; 1:59–65.

354. Tomita H, Ohbayashi M, Nakahara K, Hasegawa I, Miyashita Y. Top-down signal from prefrontal cortex in executive control of memory retrieval. Nature 1999; 401:699–703.

355. D'Esposito M, Ballard D, Zarahn E, Aguirre G. The role of prefrontal cortex in sensory memory and motor preparation: An event-related fMRI study. NeuroImage 2000; 11:400–408.

356. Asaad W, Rainer G, Miller E. Task-specific neural activity in the primate prefrontal cortex. J Neurophysiol 2000; 84:451–459.

357. Passingham R, Toni I, Rushworth M. Specialisation within the prefrontal cortex: The ventral prefrontal cortex and associative learning. Exp Brain Res 2000; 133:103–113.

358. Dobkin B, Hanlon R. Dopamine agonist treatment of antegrade amnesia from a mediobasal forebrain injury. Ann Neurol 1992; 33:313–316.

359. Huber S, Shulman H, Paulson G, Shuttleworth E. Fluctuations in plasma dopamine level impair memory in Parkinson's disease. Neurology 1987; 37:1371–1375.

360. Mohr E, Fabbrini G, Ruggieri S, Fedio P, Chase T. Cognitive concomitants of dopamine system stimulation in Parkinsonian patients. J Neurol Neurosurg Psychiat 1987; 50:1192–96.

361. Rowe J, Toni I, Josephs O, Frackowiak R, Passing-ham R. The prefrontal cortex: Response selection or maintenance within working memory? Science 2000; 288:1656–1660.

362. Rowe J, Passingham R. Working memory for location and time: Activity in prefrontal area 46 relates to selection rather than maintenance in memory. NeuroImage 2001; 11:77–86.

363. Davidson R, Putnam K, Larson C. Dysfunction in the neural circuitry of emotion regulation-a possible prelude to violence. Science 2000; 289:591–594.

364. Lichter D, Cummings J. Frontal-subcortical circuits in psychiatric and neurological disorders. New York: Guilford Press, 2001.

365. Gross C, Graziano M. Multiple representations of space in the brain. The Neuroscientist 1995; 1:43–50.

366. Willmes K, Poeck K. To what extent can aphasic syndromes be localized? Brain 1993; 116:1527–1540.

367. Wise R, Scott S, Blank S, Mummery C, Murphy K, Warburton E. Separate neural subsystems within 'Wernicke's area'. Brain 2001; 124:83–95.

368. Ullman M. A neurocognitive perspective on language: The declarative/procedural model. Nature Rev Neurosci 2001; 2:717–726.

369. Dhond R, Buckner R, Dale A, Marinkovic K, Halgren E. Spatiotemporal maps of brain activity underlying word generation and their modification during repetition priming. J Neurosci 2001; 21:3564–3571.

370. Braun A, Guillemin A, Hosey L, Varga M. The neural organization of discourse. Brain 2001; 124:2028–2044.

371. Damasio A, Tranel D. Nouns and verbs are retrieved with differently distributed neural systems. Neurobiol 1993; 90:4957–4960.

372. Damasio H, Grabowski TJ, Tranel D, Ponto LLB, Hichwa RD, Damasio AR. Neural correlates of naming actions and of naming spatial relations. NeuroImage 2001; 13:1053–1064.

373. Naeser M, Gaddie A, Palumbo C, Stiassny-Eder D. Late recovery of auditory comprehension in global aphasia. Arch Neurol 1990; 47:425–432.

374. Alexander M, Naeser M, Palumbo C. Broca's area aphasias. Neurology 1990; 40:353–362.

375. Rossignol S, Barbeau H, Julien C. Locomotion of the adult chronic spinal cat and its modification by monoaminergic agonists and antagonists. In: Goldberger M, Gorio A, Murray M, eds. Development and Plasticity of the Mammalian Spinal Cord. Padova: Liviana Press, 1986:323–345.

376. Lovely R, Gregor R, Roy R, Edgerton V. Weight-bearing hindlimb stepping in treadmill-exercised adult spinal cats. Brain Res 1990; 514:206–218.

377. Edgerton V, Roy R, Hodgson J, Gregor R, deGuzman C. Recovery of full weight-supporting locomotion of the hindlimbs after complete thoracic spinalization of adult and neonatal cats. In: Wernig A, ed. Plasticity of Motoneuronal Connections. Vol. 5. Amsterdam: Elsevier, 1991:405–418.

378. Rossignol S, Chau C, Brustein E, et al. Pharmacological activation and modulation of the central pattern generator for locomotion in the cat. Ann N Y Acad Sci 1998; 860:346–359.

379. Edgerton V, Roy R, Hodgson J, Prober R, de Guzman C. Potential of the adult mammalian lumbosacral spinal cord to execute and acquire improved locomotion in the absence of supraspinal input. J Neurotrauma 1991; 9 (Suppl 1):S119–S128.

380. de Leon R, Hodgson J, Roy R, Edgerton V. Retention of hindlimb stepping ability in adult spinal cats after the cessation of step training. J Neurophysiol 1999; 81:85–94.

381. Tillakaratne N. Increased expression of glutamate decarboxylase (GAD67) in feline lumbar spinal cord after complete thoracic spinal cord injury. J Neurosci Res 2000; 60:219–230.

382. Bouyer L, Whelan P, Pearson K, Rossignol S. Adaptive locomotor plasticity in chronic spinal cats after ankle extensors neurectomy. J Neurosci 2001; 21: 3531–3541.

383. Merzenich M, Recanzone G, Jenkins W, Grajski K. Adaptive mechanisms in cortical networks underlying cortical contributions to learning and nondeclarative memory. Cold Spring Harbor Symposia on Quantitative Biology: 1990 Cold Spring Harbor Laboratory Press, 1990:873–887.

384. Lashley K. Temporal variation in the function of the gyrus precentralis in primates. Am J Physiol 1923; 65:585–602.

385. Nudo R, Jenkins W, Merzenich M, Prejean T, Grenda R. Neurophysiological correlates of hand preference in primary motor cortex of adult squirrel monkeys. J Neurosci 1992; 12:2918–2947.

386. Kano M, Ino K, Kano M. Functional reorganization of adult cat somatosensory cortex is dependent on NMDA receptors. Neuroreport 1991; 2:77–80.

387. Dykes R, Metherate R. Sensory cortical reorganization following peripheral nerve injury. In: Finger S, Levere T, Almli C, Stein D, eds. Brain Injury and Recovery. New York: Plenum Press, 1988:215–234.

388. Jenkins W, Merzenich M, Ochs M. Functional reorganization of primary somatosensory cortex in adult owl monkeys after behaviorally controlled tactile stimulation. J Neurophysiol 1990; 63:82–104.

389. Jenkins W, Merzenich M. Reorganization of neocortical representations after brain injury. In: Seil F, Herbert E, Carlson B, eds. Progress in Brain Research. Vol. 71. Amsterdam: Elsevier, 1987:249–266.

390. Jenkins W, Merzenich M, Recanzone G. Neocortical representational dynamics in adult primates: Implications for neuropsychology. Neuropsychologia 1990; 28:573–584.

391. Jacobs K, Donoghue J. Reshaping the motor cortical maps by unmasking latent intracortical connections. Science 1991; 251:944–947.

392. Pettit M, Schwark H. Receptive field reorganization in dorsal column nuclei during temporary denervation. Science 1993; 262:2054–2056.

393. Jog M, Kubota Y, Connolly C, Hillegaart V, Graybiel A. Building neural representations of habits. Science 1999; 286:1745–1749.

394. Laubach M, Wessberg J, Nicolelis M. Cortical ensemble activity increasingly predicts behavior outcomes during learning of a motor task. Nature 2001; 405:567–571.

395. Merzenich M, Recanzone G, Jenkins W, Nudo R. How the brain functionally rewires itself. In: Arbib M, Robinson J, eds. Natural and Artificial Parallel Computations. Cambridge, MA: MIT Press, 1990: 170–198.

396. Cheney P, Hill-Karrer J, Belhaj-Saif A, McKiernan B, Park M, Marcario J. Cortical motor areas and their properties: Implications for neuroprosthetics. In: Seil F, ed. Neural Plasticity and Regeneration. Amsterdam: Elsevier, 2000:136–160.

Chapter 2

Biologic Adaptations and Neural Repair

After an ischemic, hypoxic or traumatic injury to the central nervous system, physical and cognitive impairments and accompanying disabilities usually lessen over days, months, and even years. Remarkably mutable intrinsic biologic processes may enable these gains (Table 2–1). Clinically useful adaptations that follow an injury to the nervous system must proceed within the framework of its structures and functions. An injury may initiate molecular and cellular cascades for neuroplasticity, but activity-dependent plasticity is a more potent drive for functional adaptations in patients. Spontaneous improvements in impairments and disabilities may follow an injury over the very short term. Most gains are won, however, by patients who practice and extrinsically drive fundamental experience-dependent mechanisms (Table 2–2).

This chapter reviews the better understood intrinsic biologic mechanisms that may lessen impairments and disabilities during neurorehabilitation. I then explore the range of experimental manipulations for biologic repair before applying these potential clinical interventions specifically to the neural repair of spinal cord injury (SCI). This nascent research may lead to extrinsic strategies to rebuild, rewire, and retrain the brain and spinal cord after injury. By understanding some of these

Table 2–1. **Potential Intrinsic Biologic Mechanisms to Lessen Impairments and Disabilities**

A. NETWORK PLASTICITY

1. *Recovery of neuronal excitability*
   Resolve cell and axon ionic dysequilibrium
   Reverse edema, resorb blood
   Reverse transsynaptic diaschisis

2. *Activity in partially spared pathways*

3. *Representational plasticity within neuronal assemblies*

4. *Recruit a parallel network not ordinarily activitated by a task (e.g., unaffected hemisphere or ipsilesional prefrontal cortex)*

5. *Engage a subcomponent of a distributed network (e.g., a pattern generator for stepping)*

6. *Modulation of excitability by neurotransmitters (e.g., serotonin, dopamine)*

B. PRESYNAPTIC/POSTSYNAPTIC PLASTICITY

1. *Modulate neuronal intracellular signaling for trophic functions (e.g., neurotrophic factors, protein kinases)*

2. *Alter synaptic plasticity*
   Modulate basal synaptic transmission
   Neurotransmitter and peptide modulators alter excitability
   Denervation hypersensitivity of postsynaptic receptors
   Regulation of number or types of receptors (e.g., AMPA receptors)
   Activity-dependent unmasking of synaptic connections
   Experience-dependent learning (e.g., long-term potentiation)
   Dendritic sprouting onto denuded receptors of nearby neurons

3. *Axonal and dendritic collateral sprouting from uninjured neurons*

4. *Axonal regeneration*
   Gene expression for remodeling proteins
   Modulation by neurotrophic factors
   Actions of chemoattractants and inhibitors in the milieu

5. *Remyelination*

6. *Reverse conduction block; ion channel changes on axons*

7. *Neurogenesis*

AMPA, α-amino-3-hydroxy-5-methyl-4-isoxazoleproprionic.

promising mechanisms and the applicability of data drawn from animal models, rehabilitationists can talk to their patients about the near future prospects for neural repair with more insight, as well as assist in the development of clinical trials of biologic strategies. Neurologists, physiatrists, and neurosurgeons must also be knowledgeable enough to prepare guidelines for the ethical conduct of clinical trials in neural transplantation.

Table 2–2. **Potential Extrinsic Biologic Interventions for Central Nervous System Restitution and Substitution**

ACUTE NEUROPROTECTION STRATEGIES	
Block glutamate toxicity	Prevent free radical formation
Prevent edema	Modulate bystander injury from inflammatory
Remove hemorrhagic products	responses

PREVENT APOPTOSIS AND TRANSSYNAPTIC DEGENERATION	
Neurotrophins	Caspase inhibitors
Neurotransmitters	

PREVENT GLIAL SCAR FORMATION
Manipulate extracellular matrix molecules

NEUROPHARMACOLOGIC MANIPULATIONS	
Replace neurotransmitters and neuromodulators	Provide drugs that affect second messenger cascades

SPROUT AXONS AND DENDRITES FROM UNINJURED PATHWAYS	
Neurotrophin infusion	Implant neurotrophin-producing fibroblasts (BDNF, NT-3)

REGENERATE AXONS	
Drive intracellular signaling molecules for actin and cytoskeletal proteins (cAMP)	Increase permissive growth cues (netrins, immunoglobulin NCAMs and cadherins)
Promote presence of supportive cytokines (TGF-β)	Decrease inhibitory growth cone cues (proteoglycans)
Amplify adaptive immune responses	Provide antibodies to myelin-associated inhibitors (nogo, MAG)
Deliver neurotrophins to growth cone by infusion or fibroblast secreting factories of BDNF, NT-3, GDNF, NGF	Provide peptide growth factors (FGF, PDGF)
	Mechanically disrupt glial scar

GUIDE AXONS TO TARGETS AND FORM SYNAPSES	
Neurotrophins	Inhibit chemorepellants (semaphorins, collapsins)
Provide attracting extracellular matrix molecules (laminin, collagen, integrins)	Neurotransmitters (acetylcholine)

REMYELINATE AXONS	
Oligodendrocyte precursor implants	Schwann cell or oligodendrocyte implants

IMPROVE AXON CONDUCTION
Potassium channel blockers

REPLACE NEURONS AND GLIA		
Multipotent stem cells	Neuronal precursor cells	Olfactory ensheathing cells

SUPPORT CELL MIGRATION AND INCORPORATION	
Neurotrophin and peptide growth factors	Extracellular matrix molecules and glia
Immunosuppressants	

Continued on following page

Table 2–2.—*continued*

BRIDGE A CAVITY	
Embryonic tissue or cell slurry	Peripheral nerve conduits or artificial tubes
Alginate gels or biopolymers as porous scaffolds	Promote angiogenesis

PREVENT MUSCLE ATROPHY	
Resistance exercises	Hormonal and drug influences on myosin proteins

REPLACE A NEURAL NETWORK		
Biopolymer network	Silicon biochip	Micro/nanostimulators and sensors

BDNF, brain-derived neurotrophic factor; NT-3, neurotrophin-3; TGF-β, transforming growth factor-β; GDNF, glial-derived neurotrophic factor; NGF, nerve growth factor; NCAM, neural cell adhesion molecule; MAG, myelin-associated glycoprotein; FGF, fibroblast growth factor; PDGF, platelet-derived growth factor; cAMP, cyclic adenosine monophosphate.

TERMS FOR IMPROVEMENT AFTER INJURY

When considering how patients change over time after a lesion of the central (CNS) or peripheral (PNS) nervous system, we may find it difficult to distinguish between strict definitions of *recovery* and behavioral *compensation* (Table 2–3). Motor functions may appear to have recovered when, in fact, residual neural activity is actually supporting behavioral compensation. For example, after a unilateral pyramidal lesion in the rodent or monkey, reaching for a pellet of food gradually improves and at first glance may appear to have fully recovered. A closer analysis by slow motion videotaping of the movement reveals better control of the proximal than the distal limb. The animal reaches with a grasp, brings the pellet to its mouth without the normal supination of the hand and forearm, turns its head to chase after the food, and cannot easily release its grip.[1] The hand-to-mouth feeding pattern of the hemiparetic patient can be quite similar to the lesioned animal's combination of the use of an alternate strategy, within the limitations of residual sensorimotor networks, and training-induced plasticity. A more obvious compensatory behavior is to use the unaffected upper extremity for tasks, rather than incorporating the hemiparetic hand.

Compensation

Compensation aims to improve the mismatch between a patient's impaired skills and the demands of him- or herself or of the environment. This approach for rehabilitation is the heart of many interventions for functional and cognitive disabilities. Dixon and Backman have described the domains of compensation as follows.[2]

1. Remediation: Increase the time, effort, or amount of training to maintain or regain an affected skill.
2. Behavioral substitution: Use a latent skill already in the patient's repertoire or de-

Table 2–3. **Terminology for Postinjury Gains**

Term	Definition
Recovery	Complete return of identical functions that were impaired
Restitution	Neural network regains most of its activity as a consequence of internal, biologic events
Substitution	Functional adaptation of a defective or partially spared network or pathway that depends on external stimulation
Compensation	Behavioral adaptation for an impairment or disability

velop a new skill that replaces the defective one.

3. Accommodation: Adjust intentions or select new goals.
4. Assimilation: Adjust the expectations of others or modify the environment.

Restitution and Substitution

Another terminology considers two processes that interact to affect the level of gains during rehabilitation. The first, *restitution*, is considered to be relatively independent of external variables such as physical and cognitive stimulation. Restitution includes the biochemical and gene-induced events that take a turn for the better in restoring the functionality of neural tissue. The second, *substitution*, depends on external stimuli such as practice with the affected hemiparetic hand during rehabilitation. Substitution includes the functional adaptations of diminished, but partially restored neural networks that compensate for components lost or disrupted by the injury. Substitution may proceed through partially spared pathways.

These distinctions in terminology are often confounding, however, both for interpreting the behaviors we observe in patients and the biologic mechanisms that affect the behaviors. In most instances, recovery, restitution, substitution, and compensation intermingle. For example, when a patient awakened from obtundation after suffering a left thalamic parenchymatous and intraventricular hemorrhage, seen on the computerized tomographic (CT) scan in Figure 2–1A, he was found to have a right hemiplegia, hemianopia, hemianesthesia, and aphasia. Six months later, the magnetic resonance imaging (MRI) scan in Figure 2–1B shows encephalomalacia and shrinkage in the region of the left thalamus and internal capsule. The hemianopia and most language impairments had resolved by then. With rehabilitation efforts over much of that time, his self-care skills came to be performed with minimal assistance. He walked very slowly, taking 40 seconds to go 50 feet and this distance required hands-on assistance from another person. Over the next 3 months, a rehabilitation program that used a task-oriented approach with body weight-supported treadmill training led to his ability to walk independently in the community with an ankle-foot orthosis and cane, despite little selective movement in the right leg and no proprioception. His earliest gains, then, were associated with resolution of the toxic and compressive effects of the hematoma on neighboring tissue. He recovered vision and language. He made late progress in ambulation from repetitive practice using a particular approach to locomotor retraining. Were his gains owed to the good luck that critical tissue was spared and to success in finding behavioral ways to skirt his residual impairments? Can some credit be given to rehabilitation methods that modulated activity-dependent neuroplasticity? Clearly, restitution followed by substitution and some behavioral compensation combined to permit gains that improved the quality of his life after the stroke.

Impairment and Disability

The notion of recovery, which in common usage often means any measurable gains, also depends upon whether the clinician has in mind a neurophysiologic function, an impairment, a disability, or a handicap. Operationally, clinical efforts take into account *impairment*, such as a hemiparesis. Impairments include the loss or abnormality of sensorimotor and cognitive functions and imply physiologic and anatomic dysfunction. The clinical members of the rehabilitation team, however, primarily try to limit any associated *disability*, such as not being able to walk across a room without assistance because of the hemiparesis. Disabilities involve any restriction or lack of ability, resulting from an impairment, to perform daily activitities. In addition, rehabilitationists are concerned about resulting *handicaps*, such as no longer being able to make social visits because the hemiparesis impedes the person's ability to climb the steps to a friend's home. Handicaps are an individual's disadvantages, caused by impairments and disabilities, that limit the fulfillment of that person's desired roles and participation in activities. Disabilities are usually explained by premorbid and new neurologic impairments. Handicaps parallel impairments less directly. Society may inadvertently limit the participation of a paraplegic person who uses a wheelchair by failing to provide a wheelchair accessible ramp into public places. The most traditional aim of medical rehabilitation has been to try to decrease the limitations in participation in self-care, family, and community activities by improving the function of patients at the level of disability. We can aim, however, to draw upon new notions about neuroplasticity and consider ways to lessen impairments and improve motor and cognitive skills by manipulating mechanisms of substitution and restitution.

INTRINSIC BIOLOGIC ADAPTATIONS

The brain, spinal cord, and motor unit contain molecular mechanisms for experience-induced learning, representational plasticity, and structural modification. The CNS and PNS also contain the seeds of a predisposition toward structural plasticity that becomes apparent following an injury (Table 2–1). An understanding of some of these intrinsic mechanisms of spontaneous plasticity and self-repair provides the scientific basis for future attempts at manipulating cells, axons, and synapses for a restorative neurobiology.

Spontaneous Gains

Reversibly injured, edematous, and metabolically depressed nervous system tissue may regain its normal cell membrane properties over the first week or so after injury (Fig. 2–1). The homeostatic interactions between astrocytes and neurons, for example, must be restored. Anaerobic metabolism arising from ischemia acidifies extracellular fluid, causing a fall in synaptic transmission across GABA and NMDA receptors and a fall in calcium and sodium influx to neurons. This loss of signaling may have a partially protective effect in the presence of the excitotoxin glutamate, but normal intercellular transmission and learning suffer until these fluxes return to normal. Axonal impulse conduction may recover faster or more completely than cortical synaptic activity.[3]

Activity that returns in partially spared pathways may rapidly reconstitute functions, although behavioral retraining may also be needed. Spontaneous and experience-dependent plasticity evolves within the neuronal ensembles and networks discussed in Chapter 1.

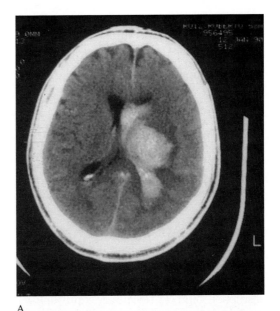

A

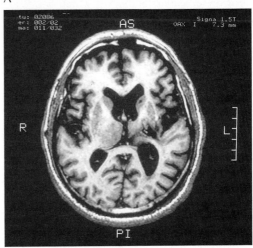

B

Figure 2–1. (*A*) Computerized axial tomography shows an acute left thalamic intracerebral hemorrhage with mass effect and intraventricular blood. (*B*) The magnetic resonance imaging (MRI) scan performed 6 months later shows encephalomalacia of the thalamus and subcortical tissue, including the internal capsule. The patient's initial aphasia and right hemianopia had resolved by spontaneous restitution of language and visual pathways.

Gains also arise from compensatory behavioral strategies that are learned through trial-and-error and rehabilitative efforts. Improvements after an acquired brain injury may also depend in part on the prior strength and density of synaptic connections in neural networks. For example, better outcomes after stroke and traumatic brain injury (TBI) are predicted by a higher premorbid level of education. Greater acquisition of experience-dependent synaptic plasticity may help protect against the loss of what was learned and affect how readily a subject can relearn. Other variables, such as age, the number of lesions, the timing of sequential lesions, and genetic factors contribute to a patient's final outcome.[4]

Spontaneous gains in function may also be driven by the expression of genes triggered by hypoperfusion, hypoxia, and trauma. Gene products protect cells, reequilibrate cells and their environment, and set off processes for repair. The most abundant gene expression may occur in stunned, but still viable tissue on the outskirts of the region of cell death and axonal disruption. Studies of local gene expression will provide an understanding of which genes are turned on, the course of their expression over the minutes, hours, and days post injury, and how these genes may be manipulated some day to enhance protective and repair processes.

ISCHEMIC PENUMBRA

For stroke, the ischemic penumbra has been defined as the potentially salvageable brain that surrounds infarcted, irreversibly damaged tissue. A similar zone may be present after cerebral trauma and possibly after traumatic and ischemic SCI. The size of a penumbra depends upon interacting factors. These include the delay between onset of the stroke and the evaluation for spared tissue, the technique of *in vivo* or *in vitro* analysis employed, the size and location of the stroke, collateral flow, and other factors. Positron emission tomography (PET) in human subjects defines the penumbra as a region of low blood flow, preserved cerebral metabolic rate for oxygen, and a high oxygen extraction fraction. The cerebral blood flow in the penumbra is approximately 16–22 mL/100 gm/minute, compared to approximately 50 mL in normal cortex. Protein synthesis may be suppressed in the penumbra, but adenosine triphosphate (ATP) stores ought to be about normal in this viable tissue. Outside of the penumbra, a surrounds of modest oligemia may exist at a lower risk for infarction. These regions offer an opportunity for acute neuro-

protective strategies to prevent extension of the infarction. To date, clinical trials using putative neuroprotective agents and carried out within 3, 6, 12, and 24 hours after onset of stroke have failed to improve outcomes. Reperfusion of the penumbra does protect the tissue. Remarkably, the penumbra may account for up to 50% of the final region of irreversible damage at 6 to 12 hours after onset of some forms of stroke.[5,6]

Diffusion-weighted and perfusion-weighted magnetic resonance imaging (MRI) may also detect tissue at risk in the penumbra.[7,8] These imaging techniques, for example, reveal that some patients with aphasia or hemineglect at onset of a subcortical stroke are likely to have cortical hypoperfusion as the cause.[8a] If cortical perfusion quickly recovers, e.g., by fibrinolysis of a middle cerebral artery thrombosis, the penumbra-like region recovers and the aphasia and neglect resolve.

Patients who preserve the ischemic penumbra may have better outcomes.[9] Is this due only to sparing of tissue? Studies in animal models suggest that the halo of penumbra and perhaps of oligemic tissue is a haven for the molecular changes necessary for synaptic learning and neural repair.[10] The former killing field expresses many genes for potential repair processes,[11] such as the production of neurotrophins for regeneration and focal angiogenesis,[12] and develops a high propensity for long-term potentiation (LTP).[13,14] This high potential for synaptic plasticity makes it imperative not only to rescue as much of the penumbra as possible, but also to find ways to drive its capacity for activity-dependent learning. Rehabilitation techniques ought to engage this tissue with training paradigms that incorporate peripenumbral neurons into the activities of their neighbors.

DIASCHISIS

Focal brain lesions depress the function of neurons at remote distances from the injury. The injured cortex may be connected to the remote region through one or more synapses in a network, by cortical association fibers or intracortical collaterals, and by connections across the corpus callosum. These noncontiguous regions appear hypometabolic when studied by PET. Color Figure 2–2 (in separate color insert) shows a stroke of the left caudate nucleus and anterior limb of the internal capsule that caused remote hypometabolism in the thalamus and frontal lobe via the region's transsynaptic connections. The subject was left with permanent cognitive impairments caused by inactivation of this frontal-subcortical circuit (see Chapter 1). Experimental Case Study 2–1 describes the behavioral effects of an acute decline in activation of the motor system, followed by partial restoration of synaptic connectivity. If synaptic drive to the network does not recover, transsynaptic degeneration, apoptotic neuronal death, and degeneration of fiber tracts may produce an irreversible decline in remote neuronal activity.

Neuromodulation by diffusely projecting neurotransmitters such as dopamine, serotonin, and norepinephrine (see Chapter 1) may contribute to diaschisis.[15] If so, then spontaneous restoration of activity in the brain stem neurons that project these neurotransmitters over wide regions of the cortex may lead to restitution of function. Efforts to diminish diaschisis by providing pharmacologic doses of a neuromodulator have been made in animal and human studies with modest success[16] to try to indirectly drive cortical synapses, just as clinicians try to activate the striatal neurons in Parkinson's disease with oral dopamine.

GENE EXPRESSION FOR REPAIR

After an injury such as ischemia, neural tissue expresses genes in a general relationship to the time from onset, intensity, and duration of ischemia. After the upregulation of immediate-early gene messenger ribonucleic acids (mRNAs) such as c-fos and junB,[17] various regions within, surrounding, and remote from the injury may express new mRNAs or downregulate the expression of other genes. Over time, various signaling mechanisms lead to the expression of many of the genes found during stages of embryonic development.

After experimental stroke,[11] focal cerebral trauma,[18] SCI,[19] and peripheral nerve injury,[20] fairly repeatable sequences of lesion-induced gene expression within each model have been demonstrated. The studies reflect degenerative and regenerative responses. Most studies find 60 or more genes expressed, usually including transcription factors, cytokines, neuropeptides, growth factors such as neurotrophins and interleukins and their receptors, cytoskeletal proteins and growth-associated proteins such as GAP-43 needed for regeneration, extracellular matrix and cell adhesion molecules and their receptors that can serve regeneration, and myelinating proteins. Each protein may rise

EXPERIMENTAL CASE STUDY 2–1:
Neuromaging Diaschisis-Related Recovery

Functional imaging in a primate model provides insight into the distributed networks associated with changes in motor function. Autoradiography was performed on the macaque monkey after unilateral ablation of cortical areas 4 and 6 on the left. Partial recovery of the local cerebral metabolic rate for ^{14}C-2-deoxyglucose in a number of subcortical structures accompanied partial motor recovery.[341] At 1 week, when the animal was hemiplegic, hypometabolism was found in the ipsilateral thalamus and the basal ganglia, structures that receive direct and indirect input from the motor cortex. Activity was diminished as well in the contralateral cerebellar cortex and, less so, in the thalamus and the bilateral brain stem and deep cerebellar nuclei. This hypometabolism was consistent with the unilateral and bilateral projections of the ablated cortex and with a decrease in transsynaptic activity. This deafferentation remote from the lesion is a functional depression called diaschisis. At 8 weeks, before maximal recovery, the animals used the affected hindlimb for ambulation and made incomplete extension movements for reaching with the right forelimb. The investigators found partial recovery of metabolic activity in some of the ipsilateral thalamic nuclei, complete recovery in the contralateral thalamus, and up to moderate restoration in the other regions. The vestibular nuclei increased their activity at 1 and 8 weeks, perhaps as a compensatory mechanism that increased extensor postural reflexes. The investigators suggested that connections from other cortical areas that project to the caudate and putamen may have accounted for the increase in glucose utilization and improved function. Other mechanisms that might have contributed include enhanced activity of interneurons within the affected striatal neuronal groups, increased activity from subcortical projections, and sprouting of fibers from undamaged axons within the caudate and putamen or from projections from other sites.[342]

and fall one or more times over the weeks and months following injury.

Microarray and other gene identification technologies will help investigators study and manipulate these cascades.[21] The chips for oligonucleotide and cDNA microarray analysis allow the investigator to identify the differences in tissues or cells in different states and monitor the expression of an enormous number of genes at any point in time.[21] The microarray technique will allow investigators to discern similarities and differences between rodent models of injury and repair and the sequences of gene changes in primates. For example, in a rodent stroke model, ischemia conditioned neurons and glia to turn on from 30 to 40 genes that have reparative potential (see Experimental Case Study 2–2). A future step

is to manipulate sustained expression of genes for neural repair and turn genes on and off as needed.

Activity in Spared Pathways

Bucy and colleagues reported an instructive clinicopathological correlation between corticospinal tract sparing and recovery.[22] To relieve a patient's hemiballismus, they made a 7 mm deep incision into the central 10 mm of the right cerebral peduncle just above the pons. Within 24 hours, the patient's flaccid hemiplegia began to improve. He regained hand grasp and toe movements. By the 10th day, he bore weight on the leg. By the 29th day, he ambulated with a walker and executed

EXPERIMENTAL CASE STUDIES 2–2:
New Patterns of Intracortical Connections and
Reparative Gene Expression After Stroke

In a rodent model of stroke, a thermocoagulatory lesion of the frontoparietal cortex induces axonal sprouting from the contralateral homologous cortex into the denervated striatum.[343] A nonischemic aspiration lesion of the same region does not. The two lesions share similar degrees of acute tissue injury, but differ in that only ischemia triggers the gene expression and molecular cascade for axonal sprouting. Similar signals produced by focal ischemia in the rodent also lead to proliferation and migration of neural progenitor cells into the perilesion region and striatum.[343a] These potential biologic consequences of ischemia are shown in Figure 2–5. If the signals for sprouting were understood, restorative manipulations may become available to patients.

Carmichael and colleagues found that ischemia, but not ablation injury, induced rhythmic slow waves with synchronized bursts of multi-unit action potentials in perilesion and contralateral homotypic cortex.[344] This likely thalamocortical activity peaked by 3 days postinjury in the region of cortex undergoing axonal sprouting. Positron emission tomography imaging[345] revealed that this activity was associated with a distinct metabolic change in the same contralateral cortical region. Using DNA microarray analysis of mRNA expression patterns[21] 3 days after injury, the investigators found 32 genes related to neurotransmitter receptors, activity-regulated kinases, growth factors, and proto-oncogenes differentially expressed in the cortex contralateral to the ischemic lesion. These genes were not present in rats with sham and aspiration lesions. Cortical lesions that are associated with axonal sprouting appear to trigger an early period of repetitive, synchronous neuronal activity in cortical networks accompanied by the expression of specific signal transduction proteins necessary for axonal sprouting. This process may represent a cellular program for the formation of new neuronal connections in the adult.

In another investigation, a cortical photochemically induced infarct in rodents produced acute hyperexcitability in the perilesional and homologous area of the contralateral hemisphere.[346] This model also reveals facilitation of electrical induction of LTP around the lesion.[14] The electrical and gene signals that reach the contralateral homologous cortex may explain some of the propensity for activity-dependent synaptogenesis found in the model of Jones, Schallert, and colleagues (see Experimental Case Studies 2–3).[89] An ischemic lesion, then, may cause both peri-infarct and connected regions to become especially adaptable as genes are signaled to make neurotrophins, cytoskeletal proteins, adhesion molecules, and other products for repair. The microarray analysis of both progenitor cells[347] and gene expression after ischemia or trauma[348] may reveal much about the new cells and molecules that may alter the balance between injury and repair.

fine movements of the fingers "fairly well." He plateaued by 7 months with a "very mild" hemiparesis, independent gait, and the ability to hop on the left leg almost as well as on the right. At autopsy $2^1/_2$ years later, the only intact corticospinal fibers were in the medial and lateral peduncle, descending from the frontal and parietal areas, respectively. Corticopontine fibers persisted in the upper lateral pons, which includes fibers of parietal origin. Only 17% of the axis cylinders in the right medullary pyramid persisted and an estimated 90% of the precentral giant cells of Betz showed retrograde degeneration. Thus, nonprimary motor cortices substituted for loss of S1M1.

Another study related the severity of a chronic hemiparesis in subjects who had suffered a stroke to the magnitude of shrinkage of the cerebral peduncle measured by CT. Sparing of more than 60% of the peduncle, including the medial portion, predicted the recovery of a precision grip and, to a lesser degree, the force of the grip.[23] The typical hemiplegic posture of elbow, wrist and finger flexion followed 60% shrinkage, which roughly corresponded to a loss of 88% of the descending fibers. For example, Figure 2–3 reveals Wallerian degeneration from a cortical infarction that extends through the internal capsule and pons, with approximately 30% to 40% shrinkage of the cerebral peduncle on the left. By 2 weeks after an acute right hemiparesis, the patient regained the ability to slowly grasp and release a cone and oppose his thumb to his fifth digit. Of course, studies of the pyramidal tract at the level of the peduncle may produce different results than studies of lesions of the internal capsule, where corticostriate, corticothalamic, corticopontine, and other corticofugal fibers may be damaged.

Sensorimotor Representational Plasticity

Do residual neurons and axons alone provide the structure for restitution and substitution or is training necessary? The evolutionary design of all animals is modified by experience and learning. Cortical representational changes follow paradigms of learning and the acquisition of specific skills. The greater the source of inputs onto neuronal representations for a skill

that are correlated by their timing, and the greater the convergence of inputs, the more likely a sensory or motor representation will show plasticity. This adaptivity is time-based rather than strictly anatomically based. For example, adjacent skin surfaces are represented in adjacent cortical regions especially because of the high probability that they are excited coincidentally.[24] Regions that work together enlarge their representations as they increase their synaptic efficacy. Indeed, it is reasonable to conclude that coupled assemblies of cortical neurons continually compete to dominate the neurons along their borders. Functional imaging studies reveal that the demand placed on a sensorimotor network expands its cortical territory, until greater synaptic efficacy is achieved with practice (see Chapters 1 and 3). Greater ability to perform the practiced task tends to accompany this more cohesive synaptic activity.

The improved hand functions and representational map changes in the primate studies of Merzenich and colleagues (see Experimental Case Studies 1–3 and 1–4) depend on use of the limb during a learning paradigm. Neighboring neurons come to adapt to the components of a task.[25] After an injury, neuronal groups have the potential to learn a sensory discrimination or movement if at least some nearby cells that were involved in representing the function regain their signal processing abilities.[26] This is an example of *vicariation*; neurons not usually involved in carrying out a behavior take over part of it.

Can rehabilitationists incorporate the modulation of cortical assemblies into treatment strategies? The studies of dynamic neuronal cell assemblies suggest that specific training paradigms and drugs that increase local synaptic activity may optimize remodeling and, in turn, improve sensorimotor and higher cognitive activities. If the task is simple and repetitive, such as repeatedly pronating and supinating the arm or flexing and extending the wrist, the sensorimotor area will briefly enlarge and then shrink. If the movement or sensory stimulation is part of an act that is important to the subject, such as supinating the arm to feed oneself, the relearned action is more likely to lead to widespread neuronal activation, to LTP that enlarges its representation, and to play a role in substitution of function. Task-specific, goal-

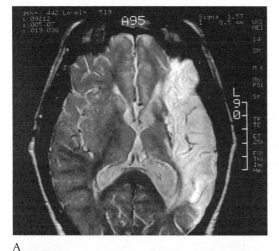

A

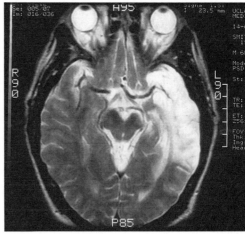

B

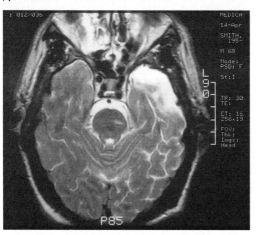

C

Figure 2–3. T$_2$-weighted magnetic resonance imaging (MRI) of a large, chronic left cerebral cortical infarction reveals partial involvement of the corticospinal tract by wallerian degeneration and relative sparing of subcortical tissue. (*A*) The MRI scan at the uppermost axial level shows hemi-ischemia in the distribution of the left middle cerebral artery. A linear area of demyelination is seen within the posterior limb of the left internal capsule. (*B*) The left cerebral peduncle is atrophic from loss of descending tracts. (*C*) A horizontal, linear region of wallerian degeneration appears within the belly of the left pons.

oriented training is one means to induce the activation of the distributed pathways that may participate in partial recovery of function.

Spasticity and the Upper Motor Neuron Syndrome

The latticework of interneurons and sensory and motor neurons, axons, and dendrites of the spinal cord make intrinsic adaptations when deafferented from supraspinal inputs. Spasticity is perhaps the most common clinical manifestation of spinal cord plasticity.

As a point of convergence, the interneuronal pools provide much greater flexibility for motor control than what simple spinal reflexes on motoneurons can provide (see Chapter 1). These pools, along with the mechanical properties of muscle and connnective tissue, contribute to normally flexible responses to active and passive muscle stretch.[27] The loss of descending pathways alters neurotransmitter release and membrane potentials, encourages dendritic sprouting and new synapses, and increases activity within previously ineffective synapses. Altered tone during passive and active movements arises from the combination of abnormal net modulation by residual descending and propriospinal excitatory and inhibitory inputs and by the effects of segmental peripheral sensory inputs that converge on interneurons. Loss of descending inhibitory control appears especially likely to cause hyperexcitability of the motor pools. The change also disrupts the orderly recruitment of motor units and of the modulation of the rate of a unit's discharges of action potentials.[28] Clinical manifestations include rapid fatigability and a lack of smoothness during movements.

More than M1 in BA4 and its descending tracts must be lesioned to produce spasticity. Incomplete spinal lesions are associated with the most clinically evident and most commonly treated manifestations of hypertonicity, clonus and flexor or extensor spasms (see Chapter 10). Another clinical example of activity-induced change is the rapid development of the dystonic flexor posture of the arm in hemiparetic patients who work out regularly doing strenuous resistive exercises. The neural circuitry that induces this spasticity has presumably been reinforced, perhaps by residual supraspinal drive on motoneurons and interneurons.[29]

In patients with spasticity, electrophysiological studies detail some of the changes that arise within the cord. Table 2–4, drawn from animal and human studies by many investigators, summarizes possible mechanisms of hypertonicity, clonus, and exaggerated cutaneous and withdrawal reflexes.[30,31] Experimental results vary, consistent with the amount of residual supraspinal input and the plasticity of the spinal cord. These studies are of interest to rehabilitationists because they provide insight into how drugs and noxious inputs may affect spinal mechanisms.

Hyperexcitability of alpha motoneurons, perhaps related to changes in their membrane properties from fewer or abnormal synaptic inputs, contributes to some signs of spasticity. In addition, decreased presynaptic inhibition of Ia primary muscle spindle endings, decreased reciprocal inhibition of antagonist motoneuron pools by Ia terminals, and decreased nonreciprocal inhibition have been found. No increased sensitivity of muscle spindle Ia endings or other pathologic increase of peripheral input to the cord and no decrease in Renshaw cell and group II afferent inhibition have been identified. In patients with spastic paraparesis, normal reciprocal inhibition from agonist to antagonist motoneurons is decreased during voluntary movements against resistance. On the other hand, antagonist to agonist inhibition may be present, which may help explain how drugs such as baclofen and tizanidine may reduce paresis during concentric muscle contractions.[32]

Dietz and colleagues performed serial electrophysiologic studies on patients with profound SCI from the time of the flaccidity and hyporeflexia of acute spinal shock through the evolution of hyperreflexia and then hypertonicity and spasms.[33] During shock, the excitability of F-waves and flexor reflexes in the legs was reduced, but the H-reflex was normal. The finding is explained by reduced excitability of the alpha motoneuron, perhaps from loss of tonic input. A decrease in presynaptic inhi-

Table 2–4. **Spinal Mechanisms That May Contribute to Spasticity and Hyperreflexia**

Mechanism	Activity	Neurotransmitter
Alpha MN excitability	Increase	—
Gamma MN excitability	No change	—
Excitatory interneuron		
Ia excitability	Increase	Glutamate
Flexor reflex afferents	Increase	NE, 5HT
Inhibitory interneuron		
Presynaptic Ia inhibition	Decrease	GABA
Recurrent Renshaw inhibition	Increase or decrease	Glycine
Nonreciprocal Ib inhibition	Decrease	
Reciprocal Ia inhibition	Decrease	Glycine
Group II inhibition	No change	
Renshaw cell inhibition	No change	

MN, motoneuron; NE, norepinephrine; 5HT, serotonin; GABA, γ-aminobutyric acid.

bition of Ia afferents may help explain the persistent excitability of the H-reflex. At the transition between spinal shock and the spastic state, an increase in the F-wave and flexor reflexes was found. This finding suggests recovery of alpha-motoneuron excitability and of gamma-motoneuron function. With hyperreflexia and spasms, the electrophysiologic findings changed little. In paraplegic patients, compared to tetraplegic patients, the M-wave and flexor reflex amplitudes decreased, suggesting additional loss of premotoneuronal circuitry or motoneurons. Some muscle and joint stiffness with passive movement also arises from mechanical alterations in muscle fibers and connective tissue. These studies, carried out at rest, may not reveal state-dependent changes associated with the loss of descending inputs during locomotion. Responses in H-reflexes and F-waves also may vary for different manifestations of the UMN syndrome. For example, a study found facilitation or reduced nonreciprocal Ib inhibition in spastic paretic subjects who also had spastic dystonia.[31] Patients with hyperreflexia without dystonia showed normal inhibition.

Other types of plasticity, possibly including sprouting of dendrites, may explain the finding that sensory stimulation of the feet in patients with high SCI produces brief, discrete muscle contractions of the hands and forearms. Subjects do not show these interlimb reflexes for at least 6 months after a SCI, suggesting that these connections between lower and upper extremity sensory inputs are not hard wired and must emerge from a biologic process.[31a]

These interacting mechanisms of spasticity are further complicated, especially after a SCI, by what remains of neurotransmitter projections. For example, the locus coeruleus tonically inhibits Renshaw cells and directly excites motoneurons. The loss of tonic inhibition of the Renshaw cell may explain how alpha-2 adrenergic agonists like clonidine reduce spasticity.

Clinicians tend to define spasticity in terms of a few manifestations of the neurologic examination. Muscle stretch reflex excitability is most commonly assessed by the briskness of the tendon jerk. This monosynaptic and oligosynaptic pathway does not reflect altered excitability as well as the more naturally elicited stretch reflex response derived from limb displacement.[34] In spastic patients, faster movements of an affected muscle evoke a reflex response that increases in proportion to the velocity of the stretch. Electromyographic activity persists throughout the movement, but ceases at whatever angle is reached, even when the stretch is maintained. The reflex contraction that opposes stretch is carried by the rapidly conducting Ia afferents from primary spindle endings into homonymous and synergistic motoneurons and interneurons. Reflex irradiation produces hyperreflexia. This arises from spread of the percussion wave or of a vibration along bone and muscle to the spindle endings of multiple muscle groups. The clasp-knife catch and giveway phenomenon appears to arise from disinhibition of interneurons that receive flexor reflex afferents (FRA).[35] Flexor and extensor spasms, particularly from cutaneous and nociceptive inputs, also seem to involve the short latency FRA pathways that are normally inhibited by the dorsal reticular and the noradrenergic and serotonergic mediated reticulospinal systems. The corticospinal and rubrospinal pathways facilitate these cells. In patients with paraparesis, electrical stimulation over the foot can generate a flexor response of the hip and knee via the FRAs that is strong enough to be of use during functional electrical stimulation-assisted gait. The interneuronal organization of the FRAs also plays a role in the generation of locomotor movements by the lumbar motor pools (see Chapter 1).

Spasticity is also the consequence of interactions between central and peripheral factors. The mechanical resistance to a passive change in the angle of a joint results from the elastic and viscous properties of muscle, tendons, and connective tissue, as well as reflexively mediated stiffness. With active contraction, the contractile properties of the muscle add to its mechanical impedance. Secondary changes in spastic muscle, such as an increase in connective tissue and loss of muscle fibers or change in their properties, explain at least some of the increased stiffness in patients.[36,37] For example, myosin crossbridges to actin filaments may produce stiffness.[38]

Thus, biologic changes after a CNS lesion may be clinically maladaptive. Flexor spasms and dystonic postures associated with central deafferentation of the spinal sensorimotor pools represent plasticity gone astray. Both positive and negative adaptations may arise from local synaptogenesis when neurons lose their ordinary inputs. The worst manifestations of spasticity are potentially preventable and, when necessary, treatable by physical and pharmacologic modulation of inputs to the spinal motor pools (see Chapter 8).

Synaptogenesis

Do spared neurons and axons and training-induced plasticity allow for restitution and substitution, or do new dendrites and dendritic spines, dendritic sprouts on residual neurons, and even new neurons have to be put in place through activity-dependent processes for behavior to improve?

Reactive synaptogenesis or collateral dendritic sprouting may be common intrinsic biologic sequelae of a CNS injury. The phenomenon has been demonstrated in many mammalian cortical pathways. For example, in the hippocampal circuits of rodents, one response to partial cell loss is the sprouting of fibers from the same or another converging population of neurons.[39] A small infarct in the somatosensory cortex of the rat leads to atrophy of the thalamus caused by loss of thalamocortical projections and new patterns of horizontal cortical connections around the infarct.[40] In other animal models, both use-dependent dendritic overgrowth and subsequent pruning have been observed in contralesional homologous cortex during recovery after experimental damage to ipsilateral sensorimotor cortex (see Experimental Case Studies 2–3). Reactive sprouting has also been observed in subcortical, brain stem, and spinal clusters of denervated neurons (see Experimental Case Studies 2–4). Figure 2–4 shows the generation of a basal axodendritic extension in a few pyramidal cells from a patient who died decades after undergoing a corpus callostomy for epilepsy. Loss of input from the opposite hemisphere may have led to signaling that activated this extension into gray and white matter.

Tuszynski and colleagues demonstrated structural plasticity of the corticospinal tracts in rats.[41] The investigators completely lesioned the rat's cervical corticospinal tract. This crossed tract is located in the dorsal column in rodents. The lesion led to spontaneous, compensatory sprouting from the uncrossed ven-

tral corticospinal tract onto motoneurons in the medial ventral horn. Skilled forelimb movements improved in association with this sprouting. When the ventromedial corticospinal tract was lesioned 4 weeks later, forelimb reaching for food pellets again deteriorated and did not recover, pointing to the importance of the ventral tract in restitution of function, at least in rodents. Of interest, a lesion of only the ventral tract, which accounts for approximately 5% of all corticospinal fibers, caused early behavioral impairment similar to lesioning only the dorsal tract, followed by good recovery. The impairment seemed related to a decline in proximal muscle control, as might be expected (see Chapter 1). After lesioning a lateral corticospinal tract in the low thoracic region in monkeys, hindlimb recovery was related, at least in part, to sprouting of the ventral uncrossed tract (M. Tuszynski, VR Edgerton, personal communication). After a low thoracic hemicordectomy in the monkey, lateral corticospinal tract fibers appeared to recross from the unaffected cord to the spinal gray matter of the hemisected side via axon collaterals.[42] Thus, both uncrossed and recrossing pyramidal tract fibers, which are a normal if modest spinal structural feature (Fig. 1–3), also evolve to play a role in motor recovery.

In patients with Parkinson's disease, striatal dopaminergic fibers sprout. Autopsy studies of this neurodegenerative disease suggest that the excitatory cholinergic terminals that contact nigral dopaminergic dendrites increase, as do the dendrites of surviving nigral neurons themselves.[43] Thus, even the elderly brain can reveal synaptic plasticity that is likely to have clinical effects. Large scale anatomic reorganization of thalamic and cortical somatosensory synaptic connections by sprouting finds support in primate studies after deafferentation by dorsal root lesions and by amputation of a forelimb (see Experimental Case Studies 2–5).

A few generalizations can be made about the potential contribution of sprouting in very young and adult mammals.[44] Partial damage to a system, such as a dorsal root injury at several levels, may elicit sprouting of inputs from spared dorsal root afferents from neighboring levels and lead to the recovery of a motor behavior close to the normal one. Damage to a descending system that deafferents neurons may elicit sprouting from interneurons and

EXPERIMENTAL CASE STUDIES 2–3:
Dendritic Sprouting in Contralesional Cortex After a Cortical Injury

Studies in animal models offer suggestive relationships between experience-dependent plasticity and mophological modifications such as axonal sprouting or dendritic spine proliferation in sensorimotor cortex. For example, normal motor learning can produce dendritic arborization and synaptogenesis in the cerebral and cerebellar cortex.[349,350]

A series of experiments with an electrolytic stroke model have offered insights into relationships between neural structural changes and behavioral demand after brain injury. After unilateral lesion of the forelimb sensorimotor cortex of adult rats, growth of neuronal dendrites in the sensorimotor cortex of the contralateral side was found within 18 days, followed by a partial reduction in dendritic branches 2 to 4 months later.[351] This plasticity was behaviorally associated with early disuse of the impaired forelimb and increased use of the normal one, followed by more symmetrical use of both. The increase in arborization was likely secondary to an increase in the compensatory activity of the normal limb. The partial elimination or pruning of processes probably reflected more symmetrical limb activity and less need for branches. Pruning may also have followed the typical developmental scheme of growth in which processes are overproduced at first, and then cut back. These possibilities were investigated further. When movements of the forelimb ipsilateral to the lesion were restricted by a cast during the period of dendritic overgrowth, the arborization process failed and greater sensorimotor impairments resulted.[352] Immobilization of the impaired limb during the period of pruning did not prevent pruning, so this process was not related only to recovery of more symmetrical limb movements.

In this model of use-dependent proliferation of dendritic processes, early use of a glutaminergic-NMDA receptor antagonist allows proliferation, but prevents pruning and impairs behavior.[353] Thus, although an early neuroprotective strategy for ischemic-hypoxic neurons with an NMDA receptor antagonist has facilitated early recovery, the same drug may have a detrimental effect during a later rehabilitative phase.

After the same injury, rats were trained for 28 days to carry out complex motor skills for balance and compared to rats that only ran on a treadmill. In addition to the increase in the synapse-to-neuron ratio in the intact cortex in layer II/III relative to the controls, the skills training increased the number of layer V synapses and spines in the opposite sensorimotor cortex for the forelimb and improved forelimb motor functions.[89] These dendritic spine increases were greater than the changes induced by nonskills motor training. Thus, a case can be made for the impact of signals that increase dendritic complexity of the undamaged, but not uninvolved connected cortex. This morphologic plasticity may contribute to overall functional recovery, as well as to compensatory behaviors.[86]

The injury model carries additional interest for rehabilitation. Very early intensive training of the affected limb, within 24 hours of the brain damage and for the first week after injury, led to greater cortical tissue injury.[354–356] A mild to moderate middle cerebral artery occlusion in a rodent model also led to greater sensorimotor impairment with equivocally greater anatomical injury when the animals were forced to overuse the affected limb immediately after the ischemia.[357] A more profound stroke induced in experiments by Grotta and colleagues did not increase the infact volume or severity of impairments, although perhaps no remaining tisssue was at risk; it was already irreversibly damaged. Moderate ischemia from a proximal middle cerebral artery occlusion that spares the cortex and damages the striatum does not increase tissue injury when followed by forced overuse.[333] Not using the forelimb with this injury, compared to overusing it, led to greater loss of several sensorimotor functions.

The intensity of overuse therapy with the rat's forelimb is not likely to be reproducible in humans, so concern for doing harm by early rehabilitation in human subjects is low.

other descending inputs. If this synaptic remodeling becomes a large change in organization, the adaptations may not partially restitute function. New connections may be anomalous and detrimental. For example, after a corticorubral pathway injury, sprouting of undamaged terminals onto partially deafferented red nucleus cells, say GABAergic interneurons within the red nucleus or inputs from the cerebellum, may inhibit the rubrospinal pathway from expressing its potential to mediate recovery of a motor function.

Denervation Hypersensitivity

Following the loss of some inputs, the receptors of postsynaptic neurons may become more sensitive to residual inputs. Denervation hypersensitivity, which has been demonstrated in many dopaminergic, serotonergic, and noradrenergic systems, may increase the responsiveness of a neuron to diminished input. This compensatory drive may improve function after a partial loss of homogeneous inputs. If several types of inputs were damaged, as happens when spinal motoneurons lose many of their descending inputs after a partial spinal cord injury, supersensitivity may worsen the function of a system, say, for motor control. Hypertonicity may arise from altered synaptogenesis and denervation hypersensitivity. When combined with reactive synaptogenesis, a very complicated reorganization of input weights makes predictions about the benefits and hazards of denervation hypersensitivity and synaptogenesis difficult to anticipate.

Axon Regeneration and Sprouting

PERIPHERAL AXONS

When a peripheral nerve is transected, the cell body of a spinal motoneuron does not degenerate, unless the injury occurs within a centimeter or so of its ventral root. Disruption of axon-glial contact is followed by calcium influx, caspase activation, and death of Schwann cells. Monocytes and macrophages from the blood remove myelin and other debris, which may clear away physical and chemical barriers to regeneration. The axon regenerates in a growth-promoting environment made fertile by acti-

EXPERIMENTAL CASE STUDIES 2–4:
Dendritic Sprouting After Hemispherectomy

Villablanca and colleagues related anatomic reorganization to a range of behavioral changes, including locomotion and reaching. The investigators used a hemispherectomy model in the neonatal and adult cat.[358] In the adult-lesioned cat, some corticorubral fibers that descended from the intact hemisphere developed novel axons that crossed the midline to innervate the red nucleus on the side of the hemispherectomy. Also, rubral terminals from the cerebellum on the ablated side expanded from the ventral to the dorsal aspect of the red nucleus. In the neonatal lesioned kittens, more extensive reinnervation was found in the red nucleus. In addition, corticospinal tracts from the intact side crossed to the thalamus on the ablated side and novel fibers terminated in the ipsilateral dorsal column nuclei and cervical spinal cord. Thalamic degeneration on the ablated side was also attenuated in the kitten compared to the adult.

The timing of the lesion in relation to normal development of these tracts is important, then, in determining the extent of morphologic plasticity. Presumably, the immature nervous system still expresses the growth factors, adhesion molecules, and other substances that nurture and guide normal axonal growth. The synaptic sprouting and axonal growth in the red nucleus raised the possibility that a change in the dominance of its control between relative cortical and cerebellar inputs altered the electrophysiological properties of its output, leading to some behavioral recovery in both the adult cat and kitten.[359] Although these sprouts appeared to make functional synaptic connections, it was not established that they accounted for recovery of motor behaviors.

Primates may not exhibit even the limited degree of morphological plasticity found within the cat's motor systems. For example, ablation studies of the motor or sensorimotor cortex of infant monkeys revealed very little evidence of a change in the subcortical projections of the contralateral cortex to replace lost connections.[360] The monkey brain's fiber systems are presumably too mature at birth to develop robust compensatory sprouting or to leave behind any of the anomalous connections of the immature brain that ordinarily retract by the time of maturity. The remarkable recovery of motor function that was found in these infant monkeys was felt to be related to the bilaterality of its cortical motor and extrapyramidal projections. Sprouting of residual ipsilateral fibers and of any of the other descending contralateral pathway fibers could have contributed to the primate's motor improvement and recovery of locomotion, which arose over several months.

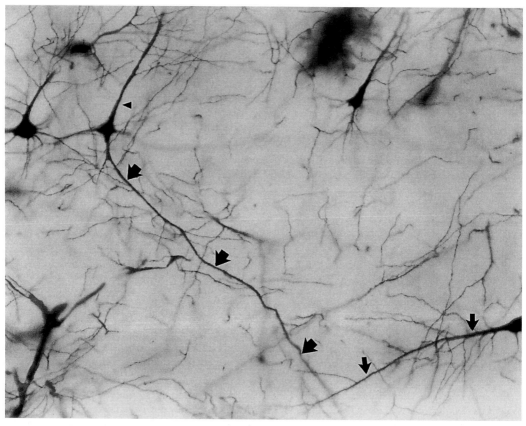

Figure 2–4. Photomicrograph of a Golgi stain of deep layer III pyramidal cells in Broca's area from a person who had a corpus callostomy several decades before death. The pyramidal cells in this layer may receive thalamic, association, and commisural fiber inputs. Their efferents most often end in layers 5 and 6, but some of the medium-sized neurons send out projection or association fibers. The apical dendrite (*small arrowhead*) that heads toward cortical layer 1 is typical of these neurons, but the "tap root" (*thicker arrows* from one cell and thinner arrows from another cell) is more typical of Betz and layer 6 cells that are projection or association fibers. The tap roots with visible spines appear to have grown up to several mm down into layer 6 or into the white matter as a consequence of loss of callosal input. Other pyramidal cells on either side of the one that sprouted an axodendrite do not have a tap root. (Source: Courtesy of Robert Jacobs, PhD and Arnold Scheibel, MD.)

vated Schwann cells and a Schwann-cell de-rived matrix that includes collagen, laminin, and fibronectin. With regrowth, the axon can recognize appropriate target cells, such as muscle fibers, and make functional connections.

For regeneration, cell bodies may require trophic supports such as BDNF and FGF. Schwann cells provide this support. A nerve injury also activates angiogenesis. Cells recruited through these new vessels of the endoneurium may support regeneration. Trophic factors such as BDNF and adhesion and guidance molecules such as the family of ephrins permit long distance growth of the axon. Electrical stimulation, intracellular signaling molecules, and gene induction foster extension of the axon.

Motor axons may sprout aberrantly. For example, a sprout may enter sensory branches, random motor reinnervation may put the axon into a branch going to the wrong muscle, and branches of a motoneuron may simultaneously reinnervate an agonist and antagonist muscle. Reinnervation of the wrong muscle fibers may not be a confounding problem. Practice may lead to functional adaptations and improved neuromuscular control.

CENTRAL AXONS

The dogma of regeneration in the CNS poses a sharp contrast to the PNS. Central nervous system neurons may die by apoptosis after ax-

EXPERIMENTAL CASE STUDIES 2–5:
Large Scale Anatomic Reorganization and Representational Plasticity

Somatotopic reorganization can occur at the earliest stages of somatosensory processing. Stimulation of peripheral afferents extends a cell's receptive field beyond the boundaries usually found in electrophysiologic studies. For example, after a peripheral nerve lesion, reorganization in the somatotopic map was shown in the ventroposterior lateral nucleus of the thalamus in adult monkeys that was as complete as what was found in the parietal cortex.[361]

Many other lines of research suggest that compensation after a central or peripheral injury can be caused by a functional shift to neighboring neurons. Pons and colleagues found an extensive amount of cortical reorganization 12 years after 4-year-old monkeys underwent peripheral deafferentation of the dorsal roots from C-2 to T-4.[362] The normal border of the face and hand representations in the somatosensory areas had been stretched along a line that was 10–14 mm long, the length of the deafferented zone. The expanded face area included the chin and lower jaw and met the adjacent normal trunk map. These distances are far greater than what one would expect if the mechanism were the unmasking of the synaptic arbors of thalamocortical axons. The investigators found transneuronal degeneration in the upper limb representation of the ventral posterior thalamic nucleus, presumably caused by loss of inputs from the deafferented cuneate nucleus.[363] A slower degeneration was found in the upper limb representation in the ventral posterolateral nucleus of the thalamus. Physiologic mapping of the thalamus revealed that the normally small representation of the face had expanded, comparable to the expansion in the cortex. The shrinkage may have contributed to a physical rearrangement of face and trunk neurons and sprouting may have reinnervated them together. Thus, the thalamus may be the primary site for reorganization after a dorsal root lesion and perhaps after a SCI that damages dorsal roots and ascending sensory tracts.

Kaas and colleagues showed that when the dorsal roots remain intact after a forelimb amputation, little or no neuronal degeneration occurs in the thalamus.[364] Representational remodeling in this instance was related to extensive and elaborate intracortical projections within and between somatosensory neurons in BA 3b and 1. Thalamocortical projections to these regions, however, appeared normal. Remarkably, the large-scale increases in divergent corticocortical sprouting was as great in a monkey that had injured its wrist and did not use the hand as in monkeys with a chronic amputation of the hand. Thus, the lack of functional activation of the cortical zones by a nonused and an amputated hand leads to similar representational adaptations. In addition to offering insights into mechanisms of plasticity, these investigations into deafferentation and amputation offer insights into potential mechanisms for phantom limb pain and chronic somatic pain.

otomy. Axonal regrowth is minimal and quickly aborted. Strategies of neural repair may put this dogma to rest.

Vertebrate experiments reveal the capacity of axons in adults to extend at least 1 to 2 mm, yet they rarely do so.[45] Indeed, central axons can be coaxed to extend long distances through the permissive environment of a peripheral nerve graft.[46] A variety of factors account for the difference between what is possible and what occurs. Central nervous system neurons may not continuously express the growth-promoting cytoskeletal and other proteins needed for regeneration. Another explanation relates to the barriers faced by an axon growth cone in its milieu.

1. A mechanical wall may be formed by the density and geometry of glia.

2. The glial scar includes molecules that stop a growth cone.
3. An excess of growth factors is within the area of gliosis, so axons are not attracted to pass beyond them.
4. Local cells make inhibitory molecules that repel a growth cone.

Axon growth cones have ameboid processes that require environmental cues and signals for genes to make actin, microtubules, and other cytoskeletal proteins. The advancing tentacles of microtubules stutter toward certain matrix molecules such as laminin, and turn away from inhibitory substances such as chondroitin sulfate. In tissue culture, the growth cone's tiny microtubular tentacles spread on a veil of actin also require cues from the milieu such as neurotrophins for guidance.

The environment of the growth cone must provide a rather specific spatial and temporal composition of attraction and guidance cues to permit axonal regeneration. Growth cone attraction and repulsion result from a complex interaction between molecules in the milieu that have differing abilities to raise and lower the concentration of cyclic nucleotides in the growth cone. The guidance molecules can be grouped according to the signal transduction machinery that they share in the growth cone.[47] The attractants include BDNF, acetylcholine, and netrin-1, which raise calcium levels and increase cAMP levels in the cell. The repulsants include myelin-associated glycoprotein (MAG), which decreases cAMP. Another neurotrophic factor attractant, NT-3, raises cyclic guanosine 3′,5′-monophosphate (cGMP) levels, whereas the repulsant semaphorin-3 decreases cGMP. Thus, attraction and repulsion are mechanistically related and can switch from one to the other depending on the cyclic nucleotide levels in the growth cone. One of the reasons embryonic and neonatal neurons grow axons may be the higher levels of cAMP in young neurons.[48] The switch in the ability of MAG to promote regeneration in the young CNS and inhibit growth in the adult is also regulated by endogeneous levels of neuronal cAMP. This switch from promotion to inhibition makes some sense in that the physiologic inhibition by myelin prevents spontaneous abnormal sprouting of axons late in development.

At least five cell types produce inhibitory molecules.[49] This chapter discusses only a few of the best studied molecules, but it is worth mentioning others in the context of potential targets for neural repair. Oligodendrocytes produce MAG, Nogo-A, and chondroitin sulfate proteoglycans. Oligodendrocyte precursors produce the proteoglycans phosphacan, neurocan and NG-2. Reactive astrocytes produce ephrins, proteoglycans including neurocan and NG-2, keratin, and tenascin-C. Meningeal cells such as fibroblasts provide keratan sulfate proteoglycans and NG-2, along with semaphorins and tenascin-C. Microglia produce tenascin, nitric oxide, and free radicals. The better known membrane-associated inhibitors in myelin that have been neutralized by antibodies to allow axonal growth in animal studies include MAG and at least one of its proteolytic fragments and Nogo, also present in several forms.[50]

Growth cone receptors, when activated, stimulate a cascade of signals that may elicit either growth cone extension or growth cone collapse with inhibition of the extension of neurites. The Rho family of GTPases, for example, destabilizes the actin cytoskeleton and inhibits the growth cone in the presence of MAG.[51] By inhibiting the Rho signaling pathway, a CNS axon may regenerate.

Axon Conduction

Functional integrity of the CNS also depends upon axonal conduction. After ischemia, overactivation of glial AMPA/kainate receptors contributes to the death of oligodendrocytes and disruption of axons.[52] Thus, glutamate excitotoxicity has a key role in the loss of neurons and glia. White matter regeneration, then, is another focus for biologic interventions. Injury-induced alterations in the location and types of sodium and potassium channels along axons may also interfere with conduction.

Growth Factors

The neurotrophins participate in axonal growth, synaptogenesis, and neurotransmission. These proteins promote the survival of mature neurons and axons, participate in synaptic plasticity and learning, and play a potentially critical role in mechanisms for neural repair. They also act on neuronal, astrocytic, and oligodendroglial precursors to mediate stem cell differentiation and proliferation. These growth factors are part of the complex system of chemical messengers and receptors that tie cells together depending on the context of the situation in the milieu. The story of these extraordinary molecules continues to unfold. Some of the cell properties that they help regulate are listed in Table 2–5.

An enlarging number of classes of growth factors have been identified during development and in adult PNS and CNS tissue. Table 2–6 lists the better characterized growth factors, their presynaptic and postsynaptic receptors, and some of the locations in which they have been detected. The signaling pathway for the classic neurotrophins, nerve growth factor (NGF), BDNF, neurotrophin-3 (NT-3), and

Table 2–5. **Neuronal Properties Affected by Neurotrophic Factors**

Proliferation, differentiation and survival of precursors.
Axon growth cone: cytoskeletal elements; collateral branching.
Synaptic modulation: formation, function, rearrangements; long-term potentiation and depression.
Membrane excitability by voltage-gated ion channels.
Calcium-binding proteins.
Neurotransmitter enzymes.

neurotrophin-4/5 (NT-4/5) involves receptors for one of the three forms of the proto-oncogene, tyrosine kinase (trk). In addition, a panneurotrophin, low affinity receptor called P75 is found on spinal motoneurons and other cells. Synaptic activity may help regulate the synthesis and transport of the neurotrophins and their receptors.[53]

Activation of the trk receptor leads to phosphorylation of tyrosine residues in the cytoplasmic domain of the receptor. The phosphotyrosine residues, in turn, serve as binding sites for signaling proteins in the cytoplasm. When these proteins are phosphorylated, a cascade of effectors modify gene expression and protein synthesis, making substances such as cytoskeletal proteins that allow axons to extend. The cytoplasmic effectors also have rapid actions on synaptic transmission and neuronal excitability that do not require genes to be turned on, such as the association of BDNF and LTP in learning, reviewed in Chapter 1. Thus, the neurotrophins are poised throughout the nervous system to contribute to cell processes that may contribute to recovery.

Other classes of growth factors also have rather specific distributions and complex actions in the PNS and CNS (Table 2–6). Some, such as leukemia inhibitory factor (LIF), upregulate another growth factor, in this instance NT-3. Others, such as the family of fibroblast growth factors or bone morphogenic proteins (BMPs), include from 15 to 20 members. Several, such as fibroblast growth factor (FGF), are powerful propagators of neural stem cells and progenitor cells. The immunophilins act on one type of FK-binding protein for immunosuppression and on other types that lead to neuroprotective and regenerative actions.[54] They bind cyclosporine and FK506, which are commonly used in people to prevent organ transplant rejection. FK506 acts on neurons af-

ter peripheral nerve axotomy to promote axonal regeneration, even 2 months after injury in rodents.[54a]

A growth factor present during development may reappear following an injury. For example, following a ventral rhizotomy, NGF receptors reappear on motoneurons after having disappeared early in the development of the motor unit; the receptors disappear when the axon rejoins its target. Such findings suggest that neurotrophins given exogenously may aid neural repair. Clinicians will soon be trying to translate the modest successes of researchers in using neurotrophic factors to manipulate stem cells into neurons and oligodendrocytes and regenerate axons through the hostile milieu of the white matter.

Neurogenesis

New neurons and glia are generated in the adult mammalian brain, including primates.[55] This iconoclastic finding began with studies on rodents in the 1960s by Joseph Altman and on birds that learn new songs carried out in the 1980s by Fernando Nottebohm.[56] By the 1990s, techniques that label proliferating cells, such as use of the synthetic thymidine analogue called bromodeoxyuridine (BrdU), with markers for specific cell types such as neurons and oligodendrocytes led to the identification of newly birthed cells and their progenitors.

STEM CELLS

Embryonic stem cells (ES cells) derived from the inner cell mass of embryos at the blastocyst stage include totipotent cells that may differentiate into all cell and tissue types. The term *neural stem cell* refers to cells of the nervous system that divide and self replicate

Table 2–6. **Localization of a Sample of Growth Factors**

Growth Factor	Receptor	PNS Neurons	CNS Neurons
		CLASSIC NEUROTROPHINS	
Nerve Growth Factor (NGF)	trkA, p75	Sympathetic, trigeminal, dorsal horn nociceptors	Cholinergic basal forebrain, medial septal, striatum
Brain-Derived Neurotrophic Factor (BDNF)	trkB, p75	Vestibular, auditory, retinal ganglion, mechanoreceptors	Cortex, hc, cholinergic basal forebrain, cortex, striatum, α-motoneurons
Neurotrophin-3 (NT-3)	trkC, p75	Nodose, enteric, trigeminal, auditory, proprioceptors	Cortex, hc, cholinergic basal forebrain, striatum; oligodendrocyte
Neurotrophin-4/5 (NT-4/5)	trk B, p75	Retinal ganglion, sensory	α-motoneurons
		CYTOKINES	
Ciliary Neurotrophic Factor (CNTF)	CNTF-α	Parasympathetic, sensory	Cholinergic basal forebrain, hc, α and cortical moto-neurons, striatum; oligodendrocyte precursor
Leukemia Inhibitory Factor (LIF)	LIF-α		Cortex, α and cortical motoneurons; glia
		FIBROBLAST GROWTH FACTORS	
FGF-1 (acidic)	trk FGF		Cortex, brainstem, cord
FGF-2 (basic)	trk FGF	Retinal ganglion	Cortex, cholinergic basal forebrain, dopaminergic; stem cell differentiation
		TRANSFORMING GROWTH FACTOR-β (TGF)	
Glial-Derived Neurotrophic Factor (GDNF)	trk RET	Sensory	α and cortical motoneurons; dopaminergic
Bone Morphogenic Proteins (BMP) Neurturin			Neuronal, cholinergic cell differentiation
		EPIDERMAL GROWTH FACTORS	
(EGF)	trk EGF		Cortex, hc; dopaminergic; stem cell differentiation
TGF-α	trk EGF	Schwann cell receptors	Dopaminergic; hc
Neuroregulins	trk Erb	Schwann cell; neuro-muscular junction	Glia; synapse
		INSULIN-LIKE GROWTH FACTORS (IGF)	
IGF-1	trk and ATP	Glucose utilization; sympathetic, trigeminal, dorsal root; muscle; Schwann cells	Cortex, α-motoneurons, hc; oligodendrocyte; hc neurogenesis
IGF-2	Glycine	Sensory, sympathetic	
PLATELET-DERIVED GROWTH FACTOR (PDGF)			Stem cell differentiation

Continued on following page

Table 2–6.—*continued*

Growth Factor	Receptor	PNS Neurons	CNS Neurons
IMMUNOPHILINS	FK506 binding proteins	Sensory, axon regeneration	Brain stem
INTERLEUKINS			Cholinergic basal forebrain
VASCULAR ENDOTHELIAL GROWTH FACTOR (VEGF)			Angiogenesis

trk, tyrosine kinase; hc, hippocampus; PNS, peripheral nervous system; CNS, central nervous system; ATP, adenosine triphosphate.

perhaps throughout life and serve as multipotential forebearers to cells other than themselves.[57] These cells may even be derived from bone marrow.[58] In response to different signals from the environment, neural stem cells commit to different lineages. Multipotential progenitor cells are a further step along the path of differentiation into cell lines with more restricted fates. They produce committed progenitor cells such as neuroblasts and glioblasts, which differentiate into neurons and glia, respectively.

Stem cells can be isolated *in vitro* and expanded with epidermal growth factor (EGF), LIF, and FGF into neurospheres. Proving that cells in the bunch-of-grapes-like neurosphere still have the traits of a stem cell can be difficult. *In vitro*, neurospheres can be differentiated by manipulations into the following cell types:

1. A neuronal lineage by exposure to NGF and BDNF.
2. An astrocyte lineage by ciliary neurotrophic factor (CNTF), some of the BMPs, and LIF.[59]
3. An oligodendrocyte lineage by platelet-derived growth factor (PDGF), insulin-like growth factor (IGF), and a transforming growth factor (TGF).[59] Oligodendrocyte precursor cells may also be converted back to multipotential neural stem cells,[60] which offers another potential source of cells for implantation.

Many other combinations of growth factors may also expand and differentiate stem cells and their lineages. Over time, neural stem cells can change their propensity to encode neurogenesis over gliogenesis and may respond differently to the same environment.[61] For example, many studies show that embryonic stem cells offer greater plasticity than adult stem cells taken from regions of the CNS.[62] Coaxing more than a small percentage of neural precursor cells toward a particular neural type such as a dopaminergic neuron has been much less reliable, so far, than coaxing dopamine neurons from embryonic stem cells. This issue is at the heart of the political and ethical debate about the use of embryonic cells in neural repair strategies. The difficulty in predetermining what a potentially mulipotent or precursor cell may be coaxed to become fuels the debate about the need to experiment with embryonic blastocyst or germinal cells.

Human neural progenitor cells have been isolated and expanded from fetal germ tissue ES cells and maintained for more than a year under the influence of neurotrophins (Geron Corp, CA.).[63] The cells form neurons, astrocytes, and oligodendrocytes. The neurons contain markers for GABA and tyrosine hydroxylase for monaminergic activity. The cells also produce BDNF, so they may have a tropic or trophic effect.

The identification of immunohistochemistry and other markers for what constitutes a stem cell sometimes seems to be about as definitive as the classification of plants by a 19th century botanist. The markers in multipotent cells or precursors for neurons, oligodendrocytes, and astrocytes are, for the most part, still at the level of descriptions of the shapes of petals and leaves, the colors of flowers, and the type of stem that identifies a rose as a rose. Until a definitive panel of genetic and protein markers is developed, the potential for *ex vivo* and *in vivo* manipulations of cells will not be realized.

PRECURSORS IN ADULT BRAINS

Self-renewing cells have been found in all mammals in discrete regions of the brain,[64] including the subgranular zone of the hippocampal dentate gyrus, the subventricular and ependymal zones of the lateral ventricles, and in the olfactory bulb.[65] Precursors have also been found in the periventricular region of the third and fourth ventricles and spinal cord, probably arising from the central canal. In rodents, one estimate is that one neuron is produced each day for every 2000 existing neurons.[66] Investigators identified a particular phenotype of neural stem cell in the ependymal and subventricular zone of mice, which accounted for approximately 60% of the total neural stem cell activity.[67] These cells differentiated, with chemical prods, into neural and muscle cell types. The methods used in studies like this may help identify the dominant functional neural stem cell types in humans and allow a better understanding of how to stimulate endogenous neuronal replacement.

Adult neurogenesis has also been conserved in primates in the hippocampus and subventricular zone. The progeny of neural stem cells may represent a programmed developmental strategy for homeostasis and repair.[68] Adult human temporal lobe tissue removed during surgery for epilepsy has, in tissue culture, revealed neuronal progenitor cells derived from the periventricular subependymal zone and adjacent white matter.[69] These precursors may produce one or more phenotype. At least some are self-renewing multipotential stem cells capable, given the right signals, of providing the CNS with specific types of neurons.[70] Human brain tissue removed at surgery for epilepsy or trauma also reveals the presence of multipotent precursors for neurons, astrocytes, and oligodendrocytes in the amygdala and frontal and temporal cortices.[71] Of interest, neurons, glia, and endothelial cells arise from the same niche in the subgranule zone of the hippocampus, suggesting that angiogenesis and neurogenesis may be linked by common signaling molecules such as FGF-2.[72] The precursor cells from this zone proliferate and migrate as neurons and glia. As many as 1.5% of the cells in the subgranular zone are neural

precursors. Hippocampal astrocytes may regulate as well as support neurogenesis by instructing adult stem cells to a fate as neurons.

Neuronal precursors were identified by one investigator in the association cortices of adult primates, including the prefrontal, inferior temporal, and posterior parietal cortices, but not in sensory areas.[73] Other investigators challenged this report and found no evidence for neocortical neurogenesis over the life span of macaque monkeys.[74] Newly generated neuroblasts were only found streaming from the subventricular zone to the olfactory bulb. The differences in reports of the ability of subventricular precursors to reach neocortex are related to methods of labeling new cells and distinguishing them microscopically from their overlapping neighbors.

Why does neurogenesis persist in adult mammals? Kempermann suggests that new granule cells move into the dentate gyrus of the hippocampus to provide strategically positioned neurons that enable the brain's gateway to memory to accommodate continued bouts of novelty and process greater levels of complexity, beyond what synaptic plasticity confers.[75] Neurons in the dentate gyrus are not needed for storage as much as for assisting new learning. New neurons are especially adaptable and exhibit robust LTP, so their contribution to memory processing may exceed their numbers.[76] Neurogenesis may also serve as a reservoir for replacement cells for the aging brain. Much work is yet to be done to figure out why neurogenesis persists in certain regions of the brain and how this structural plasticity affects cerebral functions.

One of the challenges in reconstructing a neural network with neuroblasts is the need to get the cells to their proper position. Cells usually migrate along radial glial processes. Cell–cell and cell–matrix interactions are mediated by cell adhesion molecules (CAMs). Neural (NCAM) and polysialylated (PSA-NCAM) CAMs assist in this function. These molecules also interact with neurotrophic factors including BDNF to help mediate activity-dependent aspects of synaptic remodeling,[77] so they may help new neurons integrate into a network. With this knowledge, researchers aim to manipulate the reservoir of progenitors in the adult brain into replacement cells and maneuver the cells chemically, or proliferate extracted cells and implant them where needed, and then manipulate the new neurons into a functioning network. This is no small task. Neuroblasts may be recruited, but not easily sustained. New cells may not migrate, integrate, or even survive outside of what their receptors perceive as a normal signaling environment. Neurogenesis is, however, an unexpected tool for neural repair, and one of many potential tools.

POTENTIAL MANIPULATIONS FOR NEURAL REPAIR

Clinicians may one day have methods to protect injured neurons and white matter, implant needed cells, regenerate axons, and manipulate the CNS environment to guide axons to targets. Researchers are still a long way from generating the cells and cues that may recreate the complex cytoarchitectonic structures for functional neuronal networks. Table 2–2 lists potential extrinsic manipulations for neural repair.

A plethora of acute neuroprotection interventions have reduced the volume of tissue destruction an average of 30% to 50% and improved behavioral outcomes in rodent models of stroke, TBI, and SCI. Unfortunately, the dramatic results of highly controlled experiments in homogenous animals, often carried out in ways that do not parallel ischemia and trauma in patients, have led to only one acute clinical intervention for spinal cord trauma and one for stroke. Lessons from trying to translate animal studies of neuroprotection into interventions for patients may help in the design of animal models for neural repair and their translation into clinical trials.

An analogy may help put the myriad potential manipulations for neural repair into perspective. The building blocks for early school achievement have been called the *3Rs*: Reading, wRiting, and aRithmetic. The brain's adaptations during childhood education in the *3Rs* can be thought of as a build up of functional wiring driven by cerebral maturation and learning. After a brain or spinal cord injury, a partial recapitulation of developmental and learning mechanisms includes the *3Rs of neural repair* that could promote functional rewiring:

Replace cells, neurotrophins and chemical messengers.

Regrow axons, dendrites, and synaptic connections.
Retrain circuits, networks, and behaviors.

These 3Rs evolved from nature, but they are coming within the grasp of the rehabilitation clinician's nurture. This section examines potential interventions. The following section offers traumatic SCI as a model for bringing together the range of strategies needed for the repair of a sensorimotor system.

Activity-Dependent Changes at Synapses

The storage of information in the brain and the development of neural circuits appear to depend upon enduring, activity-dependent changes in the efficacy of synaptic transmission (see Chapter 1). An accumulation of data points to the relationship between learning and memory with changes in synaptic strength induced by cellular mechanisms such as LTP and long-term depression (LTD) in the hippocampus and other regions of the brain.[78] Synaptogenesis itself is a major undertaking for the field of neural repair.[79] Axons must be guided to reach appropriate targets, must elaborate terminal arbors, and must form contacts with other dendritic shafts and spines to make functional connections. Signals from cells and the milieu will help support this morphologic feat, but activity-dependent processes, including rehabilitation, will consummate the new connections into functional units.

As knowledge grows, these mechanisms may come to be modulated by clinicians in ways that increase motor and cognitive learning within uninjured or partially injured cortical networks. Manipulations may combine a task-specific training paradigm and pharmacologic activation of a cascade that produces dendritic sprouting and strengthens synapses. Chapter 3 provides examples from functional imaging studies of cortical representational plasticity that parallels changes in impairment and disability.

EFFECTS OF PRACTICE

One of the binding themes of this text is the need to incorporate rehabilitation strategies that will drive mechanisms of use-dependent plasticity for specific tasks in brain and spinal circuits. Just as an enriched environment may lead to synaptogenesis in rodent cortex, an enriched environment and task-specific behavioral learning after a cortical injury may lead to growth of dendrites and dendritic spines and improved behavior.

Representational Plasticity

Nudo and colleagues have developed a cortical injury model in the squirrel monkey that allows the study of aspects of plasticity and the effects of rehabilitation training. The model is less a duplication of changes associated with stroke than a method to drive cortical representational plasticity in a state of partial reduction of critical neurons. The investigators perform tedious cortical microstimulation with glass electrode penetrations into layer 5 of M1 or related regions. They delineate the movement representations for the digits, wrist, and proximal arm of the monkeys. Such studies show that motor skills training with the digits as the monkeys grasp pellets in a small well leads to an expansion of the representation for the wrist and digits and a reduction in the representation for the arm in M1 (see Chapter 1).

The investigators induced a small infarct, less than 1–2 mm wide and 2–3 mm deep in M1, within the representation for the digits. The lesion aims to destroy 30% to 50% of the digit representation. Animals that do not receive any specific retraining to use the hand to pick up food pellets evolved a 30% smaller representational map for the hand.[80] Approximately 5 days after inducing the infarct, the investigators instituted motor skills training that emphasized wrist and finger extension to grasp food pellets. From 10 to 12 hours of training and greater success in pellet retrieval was associated with reorganization of the cortical representations in M1 for the fingers and wrist.[26] The representation became considerably larger compared to the baseline map and the map of spontaneous recovery. When practice for grasping food pellets was delayed for 2 months after the digit region infarct, the hand map in the monkeys was larger than after spontaneous recovery, but smaller than baseline.[81] In addition, general daily use of the affected limb did not induce representational plasticity after an M1 infarct. When the

unaffected forelimb of the monkey was kept in a sleeve to force the animal to use its affected hand (see Chapters 5 and 9 about forced use strategies for hemiparetic patients), the representation for the digits and wrist still decreased in size compared to when the affected hand trained to learn the skilled pellet grasping task.[82] Thus, repetitive, task-oriented practice is critical for inducing representational plasticity with rehabilitation.

The degree of functional improvement in successful pellet grasping in the monkeys in these experiments often did not differ substantially from the level of success in hand-grasping skill achieved by animals that did not train and did not show reorganization in M1. The gains in both groups may have been represented in yet another portion of the sensorimotor cortices, probably the ventral premotor area or cingulate motor cortex or both. In preliminary work by Nudo and colleagues, the ventral premotor region for digital and wrist movements also expands in relation to the percentage of loss of the digital area in M1. Indeed, an increase in synaptogenesis is also found despite the loss of M1 inputs to the ventral premotor area, perhaps arising from added inputs from S1 or BA 7, which participate in hand preshaping as the hand reaches for an object. Other investigators have found a reinstatement of hand weakness in a similar model of partial M1 ablation in rats when the premotor region is injected to block neurotransmission. Thus, evidence is accumulating to suggest that neuronal assemblies in spared regions of the motor network that make synaptic connections with residual neurons near the lesion are likely sites to reorganize to help carry out retrained movements. Functional neuroimaging in poststroke patients adds to this evidence (see Color Figure 3–5 in separate color insert).

Using a similar approach, Kleim and colleagues trained rats rather than monkeys in a skilled forelimb movement, made a small infarct in the caudal forelimb region of motor cortex, and retested the representational movement map after the animals were given either skilled, unskilled, or no retraining for the task.[83] The skill-trained group had significant sparing of distal and proximal representations to microstimulation of the peri-injury cortex. The unskilled group spared only proximal movement representations. The untreated group lost the motor map for both proximal and distal representations. Thus, in animal models, behavioral and neural compensation are influenced by the type of rehabilitation experience. This representational plasticity with skills relearning is accompanied by parallel changes, such as an increase in the number of synapses per neuron.[84]

Studies of nonhuman primates are important, but the control of upper limb function is probably not identical to human motor control of reaching and grasping. The basic features of prehension kinematics of an item in space are similar.[85] Nonhuman primates, however, have climbing muscles not present in humans that extend the elbow and adduct the upper arm simultaneously, larger cross-sectional area of muscles to produce greater forces, less range at the shoulder from a more laterally placed scapula, much more forward stoop as they use a hand, and they display other variations in morphology and biomechanics especially at the wrist. The nonhuman primate's forelimbs also serve locomotion, so they may be more dependent on spinal mechanisms such as pattern generation for synergistic movements rather than on corticospinal pathways. How neural network differences between a macaque and a human may differ in reaching to pinch a raisin is uncertain. More important, the Nudo and Kleim models may have limited application to the human pathologic condition, in which many, but not all patients suffer lesions large enough to destroy the entire upper extremity representation.

Morphologic Plasticity

Morphologic changes have been found in ipsilateral cortex following a corticostriatal infarct in rats. An enriched environment improved some behaviors, but did not improve the motor function of the impaired forelimb and digits.[86] When a task-specific activity, such as reaching with the affected forelimb to obtain food pellets was added to the social group and toys of an enriched environment, the function of the forelimb on reaching for pellets and foot placing tasks did improve compared to the animals living in standard conditions. Of interest, the gains did not generalize to weight-bearing movements on the affected forelimb. The training in this study began 15 days after the

stroke and continued for up to 9 weeks. The layer 5 pyramidal cells of the forelimb motor cortex on the nonlesioned side had greater numbers of basilar dendritic arbors. In addition, perilesional sprouting and synaptogenesis occur when a cortical infarct in a rodent is followed by general training, and after injection of d-amphetamine.[87,88] Use-dependent synaptogenesis in the uninjured hemisphere has also been demonstrated after a small cortical infarct followed by extensive training in rodents (see Experimental Case Studies 2–3.[89,90] Nonuse of an affected or unaffected limb in rodent models of stroke leads to poor outcomes in terms of morphologic signs of plasticity and sensorimotor functions of the affected limb.

Stimulate Axonal Regeneration

Inhibitory proteins in myelin and other matrix barriers, along with a lack of trophic factors and other molecules that signal genes and intracellular cascades for growth cone extension, must be managed if axons are to regenerate in the CNS. The patchwork of substances that attract, repel, and modulate axonal regeneration has grown so complex that the clinician may have difficulty seeing the whole fabric. The potential to manipulate some of these substances for neural repair, however, puts some clinical importance on knowledge of the following experimental studies in animal models.

One of the first examples of the reconstruction of a CNS circuit (Table 2–7) was the growth of retinal ganglion cell axons into the superior colliculus through the nonneuronal environment provided by a peripheral nerve bridging graft.[91] In the model of Aguayo and colleagues, approximately 10% to 20% of the retinal ganglia cells survived an induced injury. Their axons regrew approximately 4 cm to make functional connections that permitted a response to light. The Schwann cells of the peripheral nerve protected and sustained the retinal growth cones. This study pointed to the inhibitory aspects of the CNS milieu compared to the PNS. Oligodendrocytes, for example, produce Nogo, the inhibitor of axon regeneration, but Schwann cells do not. Peripheral nerve bridges and Schwann cells embedded in artificial matrices are still, 20 years after the first experiments by Aguayo and colleagues, a

Table 2–7. **Criteria for Confidence in the Experimental Regeneration of a Central Circuit**

Survival of axotomized neurons	Synapses made with proper targets
Axonal regeneration over a long distance	Electrophysiologic demonstration of functional connectivity
Penetration of gray matter	Behavioral effects of circuit
Form synapses with arbors and boutons	Loss of behavioral effects with experimental disruption of regenerated path

potentially powerful means to direct long distance CNS axonal growth. This group also showed that neurons from the adult rodent brain send axons from cortex, striatum, substantia nigra, and other regions into peripheral nerve conduits implanted near these regions.[92] Manipulations to get the axons to exit the favorable environs of the conduit are still a work in progress.

Reactive astrocytes in the region of an injury inhibit axonal sprouting, although these cells do protect nearby neurons and protect the blood-brain barrier.[93] Oligodendrocytes and, more so, myelin degradation products especially inhibit regeneration. Myelin-associated glycoprotein[94] and Nogo-A[95] inhibit axonal regeneration in the adult CNS. MAG is found in uncompacted myelin and in the innermost membrane of myelin, where it contacts its axon. Nogo-A is a protein associated with the endoplasmic reticulum, so it too is exposed only after an injury. Both proteins inhibit the growth cone, perhaps especially when released from damaged oligodendrocytes.[96] Thus, intact myelin may be less inhibitory than first considered. Indeed, Davies, Silver, and colleagues showed that in the absence of scar, normal and degenerating white matter in adult rats permitted rapid growth of axons from implanted embryonic neurons and from adult spinal dorsal root ganglia sensory neurons over long distances.[97,98] Thus, the external leaflet of intact myelin may be a permissive substrate for regeneration. Indeed, the outer leaflet of myelin contains another myelin-associated protein called oligodendrocyte-associated glycoprotein, which may promote axonal regeneration.

To permit axon regeneration, antibodies have been directed against several of the growth cone inhibitors. Immunodepletion may come into greater use as the components of inhibitory molecules are characterized. For example, cells that make an antibody to Nogo were placed near a spinal cord injury site in rodents, resulting in greater axon growth compared to not inhibiting Nogo.[99] In a rodent model of a middle cerebral artery occlusion, cells that make the monoclonal antibody called IN-1 to Nogo were injected near the infarction.[99a] Corticorubral fibers from the contralesional cortex sprouted into the ipsilesional red nucleus, associated with modest improvement in use of the affected forelimb. Immunization against specific myelin-associated inhibitors may also produce a favorable milieu for the growth cone after a CNS injury.[100]

Another approach would block the initial production of inhibitory molecules by the five cell types that secrete them. For example, several proteoglycans and semaphorins would be less available to inhibit axonal sprouting and growth after meningeal irradiation or by instilling a drug that limits fibroblast migration. Inhibitory matrix substances such as chondroitin sulfate proteoglycans can be dissolved with local infusions of protein enzymes.[101]

Potential inhibitors of the axon growth cone in adults, based on their inhibitory function during CNS development, include members of the netrin, ephrin, semaphorin, and slit families of axon guidance proteins. Specific proteases cleave molecules such as the semaphorins. Another approach to the injury site would alter the gene expression for a semaphorin or its receptor by introducing antisense constructs into scar-associated cells or neurons.[49] These oligonucleotides, which then block protein synthesis of the inhibitory substance or of its receptor, can be delivered by viral vectors. Another approach is to block the intracellular messenger that inhibits, for example, the formation of structural proteins such as actin and microtubules. The C-3 toxin from Clostridia botulinum is an antagonist to Rho, which is one such inhibitor. The drug inactivated Rho, promoted axonal growth, and had a neuroprotective effect in a crush model of the optic nerve in rats and in the spinal cord of mice.[51]

In addition to trying to improve the environment for regeneration, researchers may manipulate the intrinsic properties of neurons. Studies suggest that by increasing α-integrin levels in cells, especially dorsal root ganglion neurons, regeneration regains much of the vitality of young neurons.[102] The integrins enable axons to interact with growth-promoting substrates such as laminin and fibronectin. Another clever approach would place plasmids with DNA that encode for neurotrophins in the proximal and distal stumps of an injured nerve or tract.[103] The DNA is taken up by axons and transported retrograde to the axotomized neurons to signal regeneration. Gene-activated matrices may contain other promotors of cell health and axon growth.

Inosine and other purines may also switch on the growth program for axons by either affecting cAMP, an intracellular kinase, or by stimulating neurotrophins.[104] Following a lesion of the corticospinal tract in the medulla of rodents, inosine by mini pump into the nonaxotomized sensorimotor cortex produced sprouting of axon collaterals from uninjured pyramidal cells into the denervated spinal cord white matter. A derivative of the purine hypoxanthine, AIT-082 (NeoTherapeutics, CA), increases NGF-mediated neurite outgrowth and neurotransmitter release.[105] An oral preparation is in trials for Alzheimer's disease and SCI.

The most likely first-line approach for patients will include pharmacologic manipulation of intracellular cAMP and cGMP. By increasing endogeneous levels of cAMP by, for example, priming the milieu of injured axons with neurotrophins or other peptides and hormones, the inhibition of axonal regeneration by myelin can be overcome.[106] A drug that inhibits the breakdown of cAMP, such as the phosphodiesterase inhibitor rolipram, also encourages the axon growth cone to extend its filapodia in the presence of MAG.[107] In addition, one consequence of an increase in cAMP to overcome the inhibition of MAG is the upregulation of arginase I and polyamine synthesis. These substances may also be manipulated by drugs and gene therapies.[48] Neurotrophins and other molecules that turn on the production of cytoskeletal proteins for regeneration are available for use in patients. Several spe-

cific inteventions are discussed in the section on repair of SCI.

Deploy Neurotrophins

Many of the neurotrophins have both trophic and tropic effects. Their trophism supports the survival and proliferation of cells and axons. Their tropism attracts growing axons and dendrites.

Reports point to the survival of neurons injured by ischemia or axotomy after treatment with NGF, NT-3, NT-4/5, and BDNF. For example, NGF was infused into the lateral ventricles of adult rats that had received bilateral lesions of all cholinergic axons projecting from the medial septum to the dorsal hippocampus, an important pathway for memory. A 350% increase in survival of the axotomized septal cholinergic neurons was found, presumably related to the effects of the NGF on the cells after it was taken up by NGF receptors and transported in retrograde fashion.[108] Intracerebral grafts of fibroblasts that were genetically engineered by a retroviral vector to express NGF also sustained axotomized cholinergic septal neurons and promoted axon regeneration and reinnervation.[109] Nerve growth factor secreting cells are being implanted into people with Alzheimer's disease to attempt to lessen cholinergic neuron loss in a safety trial (Mark Tuszynski, University of California San Diego).

Apoptosis of neurons and glia contribute to the pathology of stroke, TBI, SCI, and degenerative neurologic diseases. The cascades to cell death involve a shift in the balance between pro-apoptotic and anti-apoptotic proteins.[109a] Although a variety of interventions have been proposed to prevent delayed cell death, apoptosis cells activate genes that may induce in the milieu immune responses, axonal sprouting, and neuronal differentiation from endogenous precursors in adult rodents. Thus, apoptosis may have proregenerative actions.

Brain lesions can result in delayed degeneration of neurons remote from the site of injury, such as the thalamus. Fibroblast growth factor prevented this degeneration after infusion in an animal injury model.[110] Much evidence points to the potential for neurotrophins to prevent apoptosis or delayed cell death.[111] Apoptosis in animal models may also be prevented by providing antiapoptotic proteins such as bcl-2 to a

Human studies for cell replacement ought to be carried out with a rather clear, experimentally derived expectation of the capabilities of the precursors and what they are expected to do after recruitment or implantation. Are the new cells to provide a trophic function, integrate locally to help bridge a cortical injury between two regions that have functioning neurons, make corticocortical neuronal connections, or send out projecting axons to nearby or distant targets (see Color Fig. 2–5 in separate color insert)? Can we really expect the finely organized structure of, say, the striatum to be rebuilt by a slurry of implanted neuroblasts? Can precursors remyelinate, regenerate, and direct axon collaterals to brain stem or spinal targets in patients with hemiplegia owing to small deep infarctions of the internal capsule? Can cells placed in Wernicke's area in an aphasic patient be coaxed to reconnect long distances through the arcuate fasciculus to contact cells in Broca's area and, with training, restore verbal communication and comprehension in patients with damage to the posterior superior temporal gyrus? Different strategies will be needed for different clinical aims.

STIMULI FOR NEUROGENESIS

Neurogenesis of granule cells in the dentate gyrus, studied mostly in rodents, is diminished by aging, by glutamate, and by stress-induced glucocorticoid production.[116] Cell proliferation is augmented by estrogens, seizures, environmental enrichment, exercise, and associative learning tasks that require hippocampal activation.[116,129] Such learning seems to enhance the survival of neurons that had been generated prior to the training. Training apparently aids incorporation into the hippocampal circuit. Thus, neurogenesis may participate in creating hippocampal-dependent memory.[130] Physical activity may affect neurogenesis by mechanisms that include increases in neurotrophin levels and altered gene expression. Brain-derived neurotrophic factor,[131] FGF,[132] and IGF-1[133] increase with exercise. These neurotrophins augment proliferation and differentiation of neuronal precursor cells from the subependyma of human temporal lobes,[134] pointing to their potential effects on neurogenesis in humans. In rats, exercise increases blood levels of IGF-1 and its uptake into the hippocampus, leading to the formation of new granule cells.[133] The growth factor may increase both the proliferation and survival of precursor cells.

The level of neurogenesis in adult mice dramatically increased after a subcutaneous injection of FGF-2.[135] After one injection of adenoviral BDNF into the wall of a cerebral ventricle in rodents, increased numbers of subependymal precursor cells and neuroblasts were found.[117] The precursors, which usually migrate to the olfactory bulb, also streamed into the adjacent striatum and evolved into the spiny neurons usually found in the striatum, but the neuroblasts did not migrate into the cortex.

Focal cerebral ischemia in a rodent model of stroke generates new cells within 24 hours. Approximately 10% of these cells have neuronal markers.[136] The cells were especially prominent at the boundary of the ischemic and uninjured cortex (see Color Fig. 2–5 in separate color insert). Forebrain ischemia stimulated proliferation of neuronal progenitor cells from the subgranular zone of the hippocampus, as well as from the subventricular zone in rats, but the stroke was more effective in stimulating neurogenesis in younger than older rats.[137] In senior rats, newborn cells were less likely to survive. Unfortunately, in the abnormal milieu of peri-infact tissue, the majority of the neuronal precursors that migrate do not survive. A few survivors appear to send out dendrites, but their functionality is uncertain. Traumatic brain injury may also induce neurogenesis. Following a fluid percussion injury in rodents, new neurons appear in the granule cell layer of the dentate gyrus neurons.[18]

CELL IMPLANTS

Both fetal and adult-derived neural stem cells from rodents and from human brain tissue can survive when implanted in intact and damaged brain and spinal cord (see Color Fig. 2–5 in separate color insert and Fig. 2–6). Their activity and usefulness for transplantation will be determined especially by their intrinsic genetic differentiation programs and by the availability of external cues such as the diffusible neurotrophins in the milieu and the cell contacts they make. The milieu at the time of implantation can destroy the graft. The release of cytokines near the time of an acute injury, for example, may make the environment unsafe for new cell survival, proliferation or migration, as well as set off a series of cellular cues that lead to delayed cell death or inhibition of axonal regeneration. On the other hand, some immune responses provide regenerative cues. Intracerebral grafts have partially restored a variety of sensorimotor and cognitive skills in animal models of injury, but methodologies must take into account many factors (Table 2–8).[138] Early experience with implants into animal models suggests that stem cells and progenitors may be able to take on the cell type characteristics of their neighbors. Given that they can proliferate and migrate, they may also serve as transport vehicles for a variety of genetically engineered proteins (Table 2–9).

Most successful transplantation attempts have used embryonic tissue, dissociated stem cells from blastocysts, precursors of neurons and glia, or genetically engineered fibroblasts. Multipotent adult progenitor cells from fat stores and bone marrow offer an intriguing source for investigation. Embryonic stem cells, so far, seem more flexible than stem cells found in adult tissues, but the gap appears to be closing. The way the donor material is prepared strongly influences the ability of the cells to proliferate, survive, and incorporate into their new home. These techniques are improving, but the results of transplantation are rather unpredictable. For example, neural stem cells from the subventricular zone preferentially migrate to the olfactory bulb and form interneu-

rons. When the stem cells were transplanted into the striatum, cortex, hippocampus, and olfactory bulb of adult mice, the cells migrated and differentiated extensively only in the bulb.[139] Most of the grafted cells in other regions became astrocytes. In contrast, embryonic neuronal precursors and adult precursors that were grown *in vitro* before transplantation have been more efficient at migration and differentiation, perhaps because these cells are more plastic in their gene expression and responsiveness to the environment. Neural progenitor cells from embryonic human forebrain tissue have remarkable potential for adaptability in a new environment. When implanted into the hippocampus and subventricular zone of the adult rat, they migrate and differentiate into typical neural and astrocytic phenotypes for the region.[140] Transplantation of fetal tissue or dissociated fetal cells requires further efforts to enhance survival of the grafted tissue. Many immunosuppression and neuroprotection strategies are being tried. For example, a cocktail of the growth factor GDNF was combined with a caspace inhibitor of apoptosis to enhance the survival of dopamine neurons from fetal ventromesencephalic tissue.[141]

Immortalized neural progenitor cells provide a genetically homogenous neural population that has been rapidly expanded to supply as many cells as needed.[142,143] On the other hand, neural precursor cells, such as human mesencephalic precursors that make dopamine, may require a cocktail of growth factors, cy-

Table 2–9. Neural Stem or Precursor Cells as Delivery Vehicles

POTENTIAL CAPABILITIES	
Cell replacement in a circuit	Provide extracellular matrix products
Contact with intact cells, altering their activity	Provide anti-inhibitory molecules for axonal growth cone extension
Myelination	
Provide diffusable molecules (e.g., neurotrophins)	Carry viral vectors for gene expression
Provide nondiffusable molecules (e.g., neurotransmitters)	Replace deficient enzymes or other proteins in degenerative diseases

POTENTIAL PROBLEMS	
Tissue source for stem cells	Tumorigenesis
Variability in manufacturing processes	Commitment to the cell type needed once in tissue environment
Consistency of gene expression of implanted cells	
Migration beyond region where needed	Control of the quantity and timing of delivered molecules

tokines, and striatal tissue to promote their replication into the neurons of choice in large numbers. Genes can also be delivered directly into neurons by infecting them with a virus that carries the message for cells to produce a neurotransmitter, growth factor, or other substance.[143] Multipotent cell lines from mice that can differentiate into neurons and glia have been genetically engineered to transport specific genes or cells into the nervous system.[144] These donor cell lines act as stem cells, much like they would during development. Such constructs may provide the substances missing in genetic diseases that affect the CNS. Multipotent cells are potentially useful for repairs, replacements, and to transport genes for trophic factors, proteins, and neurotransmitters.

Fibroblasts are rather easily transfected with genes that produce specific neurotrophins or other molecules that can diffuse toward cells in need of nurture and toward axons that may be coaxed to regenerate. Sophisticated techniques for gene therapy allow both direct and cell-mediated transfer of therapeutic genes into the CNS.

Olfactory ensheathing cells (OEC) are a unique class of glia derived from the olfactory nerve fiber layer. They can differentiate into astrocyte-like and Schwann-like cell types.[145] When placed into white matter or a graft-host boundary, they migrate better than Schwann cells,[146] elicit axonal regeneration in rat spinal cord,[147] and form a thin layer of myelin over axons.[145] Olfactory ensheathing cells have been identified in humans and have many of the same properties of rodent OECs, so these cells may find an important place in transplantation strategies for both axonal regeneration and re-myelination.[148] Commercial sources are available and attempts to use them in human subjects have started.

Stem cell research, using cells derived from human embryos, carries a great deal of political and ethical concern.[149] Human stem cells from a blastocyst can be expanded in large numbers, maintained, and manipulated into many types of cells and tissues. The developmental signals that lead to neural stem cells are becoming better understood.[150] Thus, the human progenitors can respond to *in vivo* guidance cues and molecular signals. Clinicians can do a great service for stem cell research by making sure that lay people understand just what comprises a blastocyst from which ES

cells are derived. Clinicians can also help put the potential of stem cell research for mollifying neurologic disease into the context of the disabilities caused by these diseases in millions of people.

These experiments point to the potential for driving intrinsic neurogenesis and for manipulating stem cells and progenitors. The remarkable effects of exercise have implications for rehabilitation strategies, although the relationships found in animal models will be technically difficult to show in humans. It is difficult enough to show an exercise-dose to neurogenesis-response curve in rodents. Also, reducing stress-induced glucorcorticoids and adding growth factors may lead to greater proliferation of progenitors or better survival and migration. Basic researchers must still pursue how the myriad genetic, molecular, and environmental factors that continue to be identified come to regulate proliferation, migration, differentiation, and incorporation of newly minted neurons. At the moment, the state-of-the-art cannot quite define the identity of in situ multipotent cells or describe what these cells can do or may do.[151] Precursor cells and their progeny, for example, may not have to incorporate by dendritic contacts. The cells may simply provide trophic substances for the region. Greater knowledge of the endogenous regulators of natural neurogenesis may eventually lead to proactive self-repair strategies manipulated by clinicians.

PARKINSON'S DISEASE

Parkinson's disease has been a ripe target for cell implants because of the seeming simplicity of restoring striatal dopamine by replacing degenerated dopaminergic neurons. In addition to the growing clinical data in Parkinson's disease that support transplants of fetal tissue containing dopaminergic cells,[152,153] the evidence for graft survival, fiber outgrowth, neurotransmitter activity, and positive clinical effects in Parkinsonian monkeys enhanced the rationale for this approach.[154] Grafted striatal neurons in the rodent even showed rather normal responses to cortical stimulation.[155] Cells have come from a variety of sources.[156,157] These include adrenal medulla autotransplantation, dopaminergic neurons from human fetuses, a human teratocarcinoma cell line, committed dopaminergic neurons from embryonic midbrain expanded *in vitro*, immortalized progenitor cells given a gene or other factor for dopaminergic differentiation, and other clever manipulations. Reports suggested that graft survival in animal models of induced Parkinson's disease increased when fibroblasts engineered to make basic FGF were added to the dopamine-producing neurons. Viral vectors that lead to the production of GDNF have diminished the degeneration of dopaminergic cells in a Parkinson's model.[126] Grafts are most often placed directly into the primary target for dopamine in the striatum. Some grafts in rodents have been placed in the substantia nigra where a small percentage of neurons have sent axons into the striatum.

The first prospective, randomized, placebo-controlled clinical trial of 40 patients with severe Parkinson's disease tested the efficacy of cultured mesencephalic tissue cells from 4 embryos implanted into each putamen.[158] The investigators did not immunosuppress their subjects. A modest, but statistically significant improvement in function was found by the end of the first year in those treated with implants who were under 60 years of age. In retrospect, the patients who were clinically responsive to L-dopa prior to surgery with at least a 30% improvement were the subjects most likely to benefit from the transplant. Fiber outgrowth from the transplant, demonstrated by PET scanning, occurred in most of these cases. At postmortem examination of two subjects, the dopamine neurons generated dendrites from 2 to 3 mm from the cell body. Unfortunately, 15% of these subjects developed dystonia and dyskinesias.

The results point to some of the potential difficulties in translating preclinical studies in rodents or nonhuman primate models into human trials. Effects of age, severity of disease, and behaviors cannot be matched in animal models. Differences in responses to injury and to biologic interventions are inherent. In the Parkinson's implant trial, the number of implanted cells and the location of their surgical placement may have contributed to the dopamine excess that led to the head and upper body movement disorder. That problem had not been appreciated in animal studies. Most importantly, the number of surviving fetal cells continues to be too modest.

In the Swedish experience of Bundin, Bjorkland and colleagues over the past 20 years, less than 10% of human fetal substantia nigral cells survive grafting; approximately 25% are damaged by manipulation, and another 25% are dead before implantation, even when the surgeon immediately deploys the cells. Using 4–8 fetuses per patient will not allow the survival of this technique. If fetal tissue is somehow permissible in the United States, measures to increase cell survival, such as adding GDNF or basic FGF to the cell slurry, hypothermia of the recipient, immunosuppression, or other methods will be needed. A promising way to gather large numbers of cells came from the apparent success of implanting fetal pig cells into rodents and then into humans.[159] A minimally reported experiment used embryonic xenografts to obtain up to 48 million nigral cells for bilateral grafting into patients (Diacrin and Gemzyme Corporations, 2000). No clinical gains were described 18 months later. In one patient who died, only 600 out of 12 million implanted cells had survived.

HUNTINGTON'S DISEASE

Huntington's disease (HD) is a progressive autosomal dominant degeneration that produces disorders of movement, cognition, and behavior. The apparent success of transplanting fetal precursor cells, striatal cells, and human donor cells from the lateral ventricle of fetuses into rats and primate models of HD has led to human trials. Hopes have been high, in part because the dominant region of pathology in this neurodegenerative disease, which is caused by increased cytosine, adenine, guanidine (CAG) repeats in the huntingtin gene, is within the circumscribed medium spiny projection neurons in the putamen and caudate nucleus. Nine patients each received two to eight donors of embryonic striatal tissue. These grafts were implanted into the postcommisural putamen, which is associated with motor function, and some subjects also received tissue in the caudate and precommissural putamen, which are associated with cognitive activities.[160] Three subjects suffered subdural hematomas, two requiring drainage. One subject died 18 months later for unrelated causes. Six of ten graft tracts in that patient survived and appeared to have typical striatal cell morphology with host-derived dopaminergic inputs, but less than 10% of the striatal region was occupied by graft material. No improvements in motor and cognitive scores were appreciated in the patients. Another transplant study suggested some motor and cognitive gains when the grafts were placed more anteriorly in the putamen.[161] One drawback to the transplantation strategy is that other regions of the brain, especially the cortex, are also affected by HD. The pattern of cortical degeneration varies across patients and seems to be a primary event related to the gene defect, rather than to a transsynaptic phenomenon from loss of striatal input.[162] Thus, grafts into the striatum alone, and especially not to just 10% of this tissue, are unlikely to halt the disease and will not prevent the cortical degeneration.

APOPTOSIS

Table 2–7 lists some of the key requirements for demonstrating the success of biologically reconstituting a new circuit. Maklis and colleagues met many of these conditions in a model of focal apoptosis of cortical projection neurons. In this model of disease, structural integrity is maintained, unlike what happens after ischemic and traumatic lesions. Induced apoptotic degeneration of corticothalamic neurons in a mouse model led to neurogenesis.[163] When cortical BrdU-labeled neurons were again labeled retrograde from the thalamus, a modest number were shown to have taken the place of the degenerated neurons. Thus, long distance connections were made when the death of cortical projection neurons reactivated a program of developmental gene expression for cell replacement and axonal regeneration. When these investigators induced apoptotic degeneration of cortical callosal projection neurons, they achieved functional integration of implanted neuroblasts.[164] The exogenous neuroblasts migrated into the cortical layer in which neurons had been induced to degenerate, then differentiated into mature neurons of the appropriate phenotype. The new cells sent axons to the contralateral cortex, made synaptic contacts, and gradually, over approximately 3 months, expressed the neurotransmitters and receptors typical of callosal projection neurons. The investigators also replaced corticospinal pyramidal neurons with exogenous precursors after inducing apoptosis. The new cells projected to the cervical spinal cord.

These rodent studies are a remarkable success story for cell replacement therapy, although under quite special experimental conditions. Knowledge about the signals in the milieu needed to create successful cortical projection neurons, however, may be derived from these sorts of experiments. If so, neural repair strategies may include techniques to entrain the signaling needed by endogenous or exogenous neuroblasts and their environmental supports for the successful long range projection of cortical cells. The specific approach may be most applicable to certain degenerative diseases, such as amyotrophic lateral sclerosis.

STROKE

Fetal neocortex grafted into an infarcted area of adult rat cortex may establish functional connections with the host.[165] Such grafts may fuse with the host parenchyma within the infarcted tissue (see Color Fig. 2–5 in separate color insert). In this model, improvements in behavioral tests accompanied the combination of transplantation within a week of the experimental stroke, plus housing in an enriched environment.[166] Behavioral improvements were also found for the rats that were not implanted but lived in the enriched enviroment. The cortical implants in infarcted tissue also prevented transsynaptic thalamic atrophy. This injury and repair model further establishes the interactions between ischemic tissue injury, neurotrophins, and environmental and rehabilitative influences. The effect of environment and experience is consistent with other data showing increased cortical thickness, greater dendritic branching, greater neurotransmitter content, larger synaptic contact area, and more astrocytes in normal animals exposed to a complex housing environment.[167] It is worth noting that normal housing and activity for rodents in cages is profoundly less stimulating than what wild rodents experience.

As in normal development, the growth and connectivity of implanted cells may depend in part on their physiological activity. In another rat model, for example, the volume and number of cells from neocortical grafts placed into ablated somatosensory cortex was reduced by sensory deprivation, which also caused permanent morphological and functional isolation of the cells.[168] Striatal cell injury has been used as a model for stroke and Huntington's disease. Explicit postoperative retraining was a critical component for the success of relearned stimulus-response associations in rats after embryonic neural cells were implanted into the damaged striatum.[169] Learning to use the transplant may be as essential as the maturation and integration of the implant. Activity-dependent plasticity is an important concept for both experimental models and human clinical trials. *Grafting strategies may require the experience of commensurate rehabilitation strategies if these implanted cells are to help patients.*

Other sources of cells have found experimental use in models of stroke and cerebral trauma. Human neural stem cells transplanted into the ischemic brain of rats led to differentiation into neurons and glia and some level of incorporation into normal adjacent parenchyma within 10 days of the infarct.[170] Bone marrow mesenchymal stem cells are multipotent and can differentiate into neurons. They pass through the blood–brain barrier and take on the characteristics of the cells in their new environment. When directly implanted into ischemic tissue in a rat stroke model, however, no effect was detected. When infused intravenously, the cells tended to migrate into the lesioned hemisphere and some modest behavioral improvements were noted.[171] Intravenously administered human umbilical cord blood may also provide stem cells and progenitors. When injected 24 hours after a stroke or trauma in rats, donor cells appear throughout the body. The number of cells in the injured hemisphere is greater than those in the uninjured hemisphere. The cells express markers for neurons and glia. Possible mechanisms of action of mesenchymal and umbilical cells include the production of trophic factors and endothelial progenitor cells, but apparently not by new neurons becoming incorporated into host networks. The injured hemisphere does attract potentially useful cells.

Conditionally immortalized murine stem cells have been expanded and grafted into the somatosensory and striatal regions of the normal hemisphere several weeks after an induced stroke.[172] Approximately one-third of the cells migrated across the corpus callosum and approximately half of these cells had marker proteins for neurons. Some behaviors improved in grafted animals. The investigators suggested that the gains arose from a plasticity influence provided by the new cells, rather than direct cell replacement.

Studies with various types of stem cells point to an approach for repair that aims to enhance intrinsic neuroplasticity, rather than fill a hole and try to create new circuits. Some stem cell lines may be able to migrate into cerebral tissues when injected into the ventricles or into the normal or infarcted hemisphere by responding to molecular signals near and far from the injury. The cells, if implanted soon after a stroke, could limit secondary damage around the infarct, as well as participate in reorganizational processes. Just where the cells migrate, what they differentiate into, and how they come to integrate into the substrates of plasticity will determine what behaviors they may improve. Thus, any study of tranplantation of progenitor and stem cells will have to examine a variety of sensorimotor and cognitive outcomes. Future studies will aim to reveal the best timing, location, and signaling cues for implanted cells and the best rehabilitative techniques to aid their functional incorporation.

Human Studies

Cultured neuronal cells derived from a human teratocarcinoma cell line and from porcine fetal brain cells have been injected into subcortical tissue such as the infarcted striatum. A clinical trial with a line of porcine cells (from the Diacrin Corporation) was halted in 2001. Little information was made public, which is a growing problem in failed transplant clinical trials sponsored by biotechnology companies. The teratocarcinoma NT2 human precursor cell line (Layton BioScience Corporation) caused no toxicity or tumors when injected into monkeys and rodents. The neuronal cells appeared to integrate with host brain. The cells produced axons, released neurotransmitters, and contained neuronal marker proteins.[173] In a safety and feasibility trial, 12 subjects with chronic hemiplegic stroke and deep lesions involving the basal ganglia and internal capsule were injected with 2 to 6 million cells into the medial wall of the infarct cavity.[174] Subjects were immunosuppressed with cyclosporine for 8 weeks. No rehabilitation intervention was provided. Six months after implantation, approximately half of the subjects showed very modest clinical improvements, gains that clinicians often see in patients who become more motivated after a brief pulse of rehabilitation. Positron emission tomography scans in 6 of 11 revealed flurodeoxyglucose uptake at the implant site. This activity could have been from the neurons or from glia or inflammatory cells. A randomized phase 2/3 trial was initiated in 2001.

DEMYELINATING DISEASES

Embryonic stem cells and ES-derived neural precursors, as noted earlier, can be cued to form oligodendocytes. When these cells were placed into the CNS of myelin-deficient rats in an animal model of Pelizaeus-Merzbacher disease, they myelinated brain and cord axons.[175] In a similar disease model, oligodendrocyte progenitors that were injected intrauterine into the ventricles of myelin-deficient rat embryos produced myelin over much of the brain.[176] Oligodendrocyte progenitor cells have also been used to remyelinate an area of induced focal demyelination in an animal model.[177]

Precursors exist in normal adult humans and around the plaques of multiple sclerosis lesions.[178] The number of oligodendrocyte precursors declines as the plaque ages and few precursors appear to migrate into a plaque from normal adjacent tissue.[179] Strategies for remyelination in patients with MS will require methods to stimulate proliferation and differentiation of precursors. Implanted OECs and Schwann cells may also remyelinate CNS axons. Human trials have been initiated using OECs.

SUMMARY

These preliminary advances increase the chance that tissue grafts or cells grown in tissue culture will some day replace a particularly needed cell line or trophic or neurotransmitter substance. Stem cells may require an increasingly feasible genetic engineering approach to push them in a desired direction. The reconstitution of a neural network to repopulate tissue lost to a stroke, however, will demand a greater understanding of the developmental signals that manipulate progenitor cells and allow them to integrate into the environs of a damaged host. In addition, any neuronal cell graft will need to experience a training paradigm to incorporate it into a functioning circuit. Indeed, training may compensate for some imprecision in the targeting of implanted cells. The ability of researchers to create, *in vivo*, a complex neural circuit with cells that receive and send synaptic signals in a way that recapitulates normal regulation of excitation,

inhibition, and modulation of neuronal ensembles and distant connections has, however, enormous requirements.

Pharmacologic Potentiation

Animal studies and small clinical trials have provided preliminary evidence that a variety of pharmacologic agents may facilitate or inhibit the rate or degree of gains after a cerebral injury (see Experimental Case Studies 2–6). Although studies of neurotransmitter manipulations in animal lesion models are intriguing, the results may not readily apply to clinical trials in patients undergoing rehabilitation.

Just how a drug affects restitution or substitution is often speculative. A reduction of diaschisis, promotion of collateral sprouting, denervation supersensitivity to neurotransmitters,[180] the unmasking of latent connections, and facilitation of the cellular bases for new learning have been suggested.[15,181] Other possible mechanisms include replacement of a normally present transmitter, provision of a mediator of synaptic plasticity for cortical representational adaptations, stimulation of a pattern generator, and modulation of substances such as growth factors. A variety of agents appear to enhance sprouting of dendrites and dendritic spines. Inosine and AIT-082 were mentioned earlier and nicotine and amphetamine may expand dendrites in frontal regions (see Experimental Case Studies 2–6). Some drugs will have more clear-cut mechanisms of action. For example, 4-aminopyridine may partially restore the conduction of action potentials along demyelinated axons. The drug blocks potassium channels, prolongs action potentials, and improves impulse conduction.[182,183]

In most instances, drug studies of small molecules, neuromodulators, and neurotransmitters in patients will pose confounding problems. What has to be determined includes:

1. the type, location, extent, and age of the lesion to be treated
2. the specific drug, its dosage, time of initiation, duration of use, and adverse effects
3. the accompanying physical or cognitive therapy that adds to a drug's effectiveness in inducing activity-dependent plasticity

An augmentation strategy with a medication may find an inverted U-shaped curve for dosing in which minimally higher doses reverse

EXPERIMENTAL CASE STUDIES 2–6:
Pharmacologic Interventions for Plasticity

After being given *d*-amphetamine, both rats and cats that underwent a unilateral or bilateral ablation of the sensorimotor or frontal cortex have exhibited an accelerated rate of recovery, but not necessarily a greater degree of recovery of the ability to walk across a beam. This improvement endured well past the single or intermittent dosing schedule of the drug.[365] After a primary somatosensory cortex infarction in rodents, *d*-amphetamine augmented the rate and completeness of recovery in a T-maze sensorimotor integrative task.[366] In these instances, the drug worked only when combined with physical activity and practice, the equivalent of training and motor experience. A dopamine blocker, haloperidol, prevented this recovery in the animal studies. Yohimbine, an alpha-2 noradrenergic antagonist accelerated recovery. Both the alpha-1 noradrenergic antagonist prazosin and the alpha-2 noradrenergic agonist clonidine reinstated deficits in recovered rats.[367] Clonidine inhibits locus coeruleus neuronal activity, reducing norepinephrine synthesis and release. The drug did not delay early recovery as had been expected. However, clonidine has at least one other potential effect. In young rats, the drug can activate the lumbar neural circuitry for stepping. In this cortical injury model then, norepinephrine played a role in both the promotion and maintenance of recovery, although not always in a predictable fashion. The investigators suspected that the noradrenergic drug alleviated a functional depression, or diaschisis, in remote, transsynaptically connected regions of the brain.

Other neurotransmitters, including acetylcholine, dopamine, GABA and serotonin have enhanced motor recovery. Nicotine upregulates nicotinic receptors and improved performance in some human studies and improved performance in rats after a basal forebrain lesion of the cholinergic system. Nicotine improved performance on the Morris water maze when the drug was given before or after a medial frontal lesion, although gains were not up to the level of sham-operated rats.[368] Nicotine, amphetamine, and cocaine increase the length of some dendrites and the density of spines on neurons of the nucleus accumbens and medial frontal cortex.[369]

Phenytoin, scopolamine, clonidine, neuroleptics, and benzodiazepines have retarded gains in specific experimental designs in animals. In the rat sensorimotor cortex lesion model described in Experimental Case Study 2–3, treatment with a benzodiazepine led to ipsilateral loss of neurons in the striatum and substantia nigra and interfered with behavioral recovery of the affected limb.[370] As noted earlier, acetylcholine may play a key role in modulating the reorganization of the somatosensory representational map and serotonergic and noradrenergic agents enhance the lumbar neural circuits for stepping. Some drugs could enhance one function, but reinstate or cause another type of motor or cognitive dysfunction.[371]

any efficacy. Pharmacologic replacement may miss the form of the chemical messenger that acts on a specific receptor, such as the D1 versus D2 dopamine receptor.

In subsequent chapters, we look at agents that, in specific settings, can help ameliorate disorders of cognition, behavior, and mood. What is clear is that clinicians should select medications with special care in the months following a cerebral injury, so they do not iatrogenically impede the course toward improvement.

MUSCLE PLASTICITY

Muscle is highly adaptable. Methods to strengthen muscle and to limit atrophy pose a challenge to therapists and patients when neural control falters. Muscle atrophy may evolve from an upper or lower motor neuron lesion, as well as from a catabolic state and disuse. The reduction in muscle mass is proportional to the reduction in force output, so atrophy may aggravate neural causes of weakness and impaired motor control. Ordinary walking activates only a small proportion of the motor units within a given motor pool. For the quadriceps, walking requires approximately 20% of the muscle's maximum force output. Following the atrophy of 50% of that group, recruited motor units generate half the normal force that would have been generated without atrophy, so subjects would have to recruit 40% of the motor units of the quadriceps rather than 20% to generate the forces needed to step. This additional recruitment may require the activation of motor units with higher thresholds than normal. Such units quickly fatigue. Loss of muscle mass, then, may prevent a hemiparetic or para-paretic subject from walking.

Skeletal muscle has dynamic functional and molecular properties. The molecular diversity of the fiber population is reflected in the many phenotypes that have been characterized.[184] Although the functional significance of this diversity is uncertain for the more subtle fiber type differences, the factors that create diversity are becoming clear. Genetic programs, hormones, trophic substances, usage patterns, and levels of resistance exercise act on phenotypic expression. In addition to exercise, methods to augment plasticity include electrical stimulation of muscle, transplants, and pharmacologic interventions.

Exercise

Normal exercise utilizes the oxidation of carbohydrates and fats to generate ATP for muscle contractions. Reflex actions adjust ventilation and circulatory requirements to deliver oxygen and remove carbon dioxide. The maximum oxygen consumption serves as a good measure of exercise capacity and fitness. Low cardiovascular fitness reduces the maximal capacity to deliver fuels to working muscle and reduces the mass of mitochondria and the enzymatic machinery needed for high rates of oxidative phosphorylation. Patients with an acute debilitating neurologic illness become deconditioned rather quickly and their tolerance for exercise drops off.

Human skeletal muscle is categorized histologically as type I and type II fibers. Type I fibers have high levels of oxidative metabolic enzymes that enable relative resistance to fatigue. This phenotype dominates in antigravity muscles. Type II fibers have larger axons, rapidly fatigue and slowly recover, and use glycogen for anaerobic metabolism. Many myosin isoforms exist between these two broad categories. Skeletal muscle adapts to mechanical stress by hypertrophy of its fibers. This adaptation reflects the highly plastic expression of myosin heavy chain (MHC) units, which are controlled by a multi-gene family.[185] Actin and MHC represent 60% of the proteins in muscle. The MHC units provide considerable structural and functional diversity for the performance of ordinary motor activities, which will vary in skill, economy of energy, and power requirements over the course of an activity. Mechanical loading, for example,

leads to fiber enlargement and a net transformation in contractile protein phenotype toward slower-twitch, low ATPase MHC isoforms. Resistance training also remodels the neuromuscular junction by increasing axon terminal branches and muscle receptors.[186] Loading and unloading a muscle affects other organelles within the fiber, such as the cell's oxidative machinery and components needed for calcium sequestering and release.

In human studies of strength training, protocols focus on the use of free weights or devices designed to perform shortening concentric and elongating eccentric muscle contractions. Subjects usually train for 3–4 sessions per week for 12–15 weeks. Muscle mass increases from 7% to 10%, along with increments in strength that generally exceed the gains in muscle mass. Some of the incremental gains come from greater skill in carrying out the resistance exercise. Dynamic strength training with a focus on either concentric or eccentric contractions often is said to produce greater gains in strength and mass compared to isometric programs, but the data are difficult to interpret because of confounding variables across studies. Programs for exercise are not standardized, so studies differ in factors such as (1) the number of contractions performed per session; (2) the relative loads imposed on the muscle groups; (3) the number of training sessions performed each week; (4) the duration of the training program; and (5) the pretraining history of the participants.

An isometric contraction offers the simplest form of biomechanical stress to activate the contractile apparatus of muscle. Isometric exercise may be best, especially for patients with diseases affecting the motor unit. Compared to activities that require a high eccentric contractile component, isometric exercise tends not to produce muscle injury and may cost less energy. For the rehabilitation of people with limited mobility, isometric paradigms provide the most energy efficient means of maintaining muscle mass and strength. Specific methods for improving fitness and strength that are relevant to the disabled subject are discussed in Chapters 5 and 12.

Atrophy

Approximately half of people over 60 years of age have a significant relative reduction in muscle mass, called sarcopenia. About 10% fall more than two standard deviations below the values of muscle mass of younger adults, which is an independent risk factor for functional impairments and disabilities.[184a] With onset of a neurologic disease affecting the motor system and as patients age with chronic motor impairments, muscle is likely to atrophy in both young and old persons. The latter, however, may have significantly less reserve.

Chronic unloading of skeletal muscle, as occurs during bed rest, exposure to microgravity in outer space, and in the rat model of hindlimb suspension, produces marked atrophy in muscles used primarily for standing and locomotion.[185,187,188] During the initial stages of unloading, the synthetic rate of proteins abruptly decreases and degradation gradually increases, until a new steady state of smaller muscle mass is reached. Protein synthesis and degradation eventually come into balance. Closely paralleling the net loss of muscle mass is a corresponding loss of proteins for the contractile machinery, particularly MHC. The slow-twitch type I MHC is preferentially reduced, whereas a concomitant upregulation of faster MHC isoforms may create hybrid fibers composed of a combination of fast and slow MHCs of varying proportion. These alterations leave patients with less muscle mass to perform activities that require a sustained force output, especially in the antigravity, extensor muscle groups. In addition, an inverse relationship has been found between energy expenditure or exercise economy and the intensity of exercise after the equivalent of bed rest. Skeletal muscle becomes less economical as its force production increases. The decrease in metabolic economy may be related to an increased dependence on type II fibers.[189] At the systems and molecular levels, one of the goals for neurorehabilitation is to devise countermeasures to conserve muscle mass and maintain the contractile phenotype in muscles used especially for antigravity support and locomotion.[190,191]

TROPHIC INFLUENCES

The subcellular events that regulate contractile protein turnover during muscle hypertrophy and atrophy pose a work in progress. Autocrine and paracrine processes involving muscle-derived IGF-1 may play a pivotal role in linking the mechanical stimulus to the muscle's mor-phologic and biochemical adaptations.[192] Muscle produces an isoform of IGF-1 in response to stretch or increased mechanical activity that is directly linked to the expression of genes necessary for muscle repair, maintenance, and remodeling. Insulin-like growth factor is also involved in satellite cell proliferation and differentiation processes. Skeletal muscles contain multiple pathways for protein degradation, including lysosomal, calcium dependent, and ubiquitin-ATP-dependent proteolysis systems. Skeletal muscle protein degradation is instigated by many states associated with neurologic illnesses other than bed rest and paresis, including aging, sepsis, uremia, uncontrolled diabetes, and starvation, primarily from accelerated proteolysis via the ubiquitin-proteosome pathway. Insulin-like growth factor levels are affected by all of these events. The trophic agent activates several intracellular signaling pathways in muscle, including the mitogen-activated protein kinase cascade, which participates in catabolic and anabolic actions.[193] Indeed, local injection and viral-mediated expression of IGF-1 has restored the proliferation of satellite cells and reversed the loss of muscle in aged rats.[194,195]

A cytokine, tumor necrosis factor, contributes to skeletal muscle degeneration associated with illnesses that cause cachexia.[196] This cytokine may play a role in the clinical entity, critical illness neuropathy and myopathy. Inhibition of the cytokine-mediated pathway of muscle loss by pharmacologic means may help prevent atrophy.

Muscle activity directly influences the formation and maintenance of synaptic sites and sprouting after denervation. For example, NT-4 is produced by active muscle. Levels diminish after neuromuscular blockade. NT-4 has an activity-dependent influence on motoneuron survival and axonal sprouting onto muscle fibers.[197] Proteins secreted by motoneurons, such as neuregulin for the synthesis and agrin for the clustering of postsynaptic acetylcholine receptors, are synthesized by retrograde signaling from muscle BDNF, NT-3, and NT-4/5.[53] Agrin, after being released into the synaptic cleft, binds to the basal lamina and triggers the muscle fiber to aggregate acetylcholine, acetylcholinesterase, and other postsynaptic components. Muscle-secreted neurotrophins may also act on themselves in an autocrine fashion to modify acetylcholine receptors. Thus, resistance exercises trigger a cascade of remodeling proteins that restore the motor unit, so exercise serves as a critical component of any neurologic rehabilitation prescription.

NEURAL INFLUENCES

Biopsies of affected muscle after hemiplegic stroke and paraplegic SCI in humans reveal atrophy of type I fibers. Although mostly related to the molecular sequelae of inactivity of the muscle, the pattern of fiber type grouping may also arise from loss of supraspinal inputs onto spinal motoneurons.

Following an upper motor neuron lesion in patients, muscle fiber type grouping and end-plate changes have been described, raising the possibility of collateral sprouting and reinnervation by the spinal motoneuron pools. Neurogenic changes in paralyzed muscles have also been suggested by the finding of fibrillation potentials and positive sharp waves by electromyography. These signs of lower motoneuron denervation peak at 4 to 10 weeks after a stroke or cervical SCI and have been reported even a year later.[198,199] Nerve conduction studies do not identify any peripheral nerve injury as the cause of these findings. Transsynaptic degeneration of anterior horn cells has been invoked as the cause.

Pathological studies reveal no loss of anterior horn motoneurons after stroke. However, the cross-sectional area of lower motoneurons on the affected side is significantly less in hemiparetic patients, compared to the motoneurons on the opposite side and in controls.[200] Indeed, the degree of degeneration of the medullary pyramid and of muscular weakness parallel the decrease in the size of the motoneurons. The decrease in cell area may follow the loss of a transsynaptic trophic influence from the upper motor neuron, from the atrophied muscle target, or from both. Motoneuron and muscle fiber atrophy is also evident after denervation of muscle.

Motor unit firing rates have been related to contractile properties and the myosin composition of muscle fibers. Hemiparetic subjects with severely weak tibialis anterior muscles had low rates of motor unit firing during walking and 99% of the fibers were type I.[201] The tibialis muscle of the unaffected leg, which tends to fire far more than it would in a normal subject, contained 75% type I fibers, a bit more than control subjects. The maximal tension in the paretic muscle was low as well, suggesting the combination of fiber atrophy, a reduced number of myosin cross bridges, and lower force generation per cross bridge. A better understanding of the interactions of each element of the motor unit should lead to hypothesis-driven interventions to maintain muscle morphology and forces.

NONUSE

Muscle wasting can be attributed more to changes in muscle length and loading experiences than to a fall in neuromuscular activity. Disuse atrophy tends to be most pronounced in paralyzed, slow fatigue-resistant muscle fibers that normally bear weight and cross single joints.[202] The most severe atrophy is found in unloaded muscles that are immobilized in a shortened state. Muscle in humans at complete rest is said to initially atrophy at the rate of 1% to 6% daily for the first week and strength in an immobilized limb can fall 30% to 40% in 6 weeks.[203] A change from fast to slow type of activity pattern leads, over 1 to 3 weeks, to changes in capillary density, sarcoplasmic reticulum ATPase, hexokinase, oxidative and anaerobic metabolism, and alteration of the myosin molecule.[204] No simple, linear relation exists between inactivity and consequent changes in mass, force, and endurance. Recent data offer clues about possible interventions for disabled patients.

Many of the properties of skeletal muscle can be modulated by the pattern and level of both active and passive mechanical activity. Passive stretch, alone, can induce some muscle enlargement. A number of cellular signals transduce mechanical stretch.[205] When neuromuscular activation was reduced in animal experiments by suspension of the hindlimbs, by thoracic transection of the spinal cord, by isolation of the cord by transection and deafferentation of lumbar roots, or by spaceflight, a number of observations were made that are relevant to rehabilitation of the suddenly bedridden patient.[188] Atrophy is greatest in the slow extensor muscles and in the deeper portions of muscles that contain the greatest proportion of slow twitch and high oxidative fibers. Nonpostural muscle fibers are less affected by a lack of weight bearing. Limb unloading, as in the hindlimb suspension model, led to a rapid phase of atrophy in the first 1 to 2 weeks, so countermeasures are perhaps most important in this phase after onset of paresis and bedrest. For a muscle fiber to maintain or increase its usual size, it had to produce some minimum level of force for some minimum time each day. In rats whose hindlimbs were suspended so they bore no load, a modest isometric training program, amounting to 150 contractions per week, attenuated atrophy by 25% and decelerated the bias from slow to fast MHCs.[188] Mechanical loading was better than electrical stimulation of muscle, perhaps because the protocol for stimulation did not allow the development of enough tension.

HORMONES AND DRUGS

Receptors for hormones are present on the muscle membrane and contribute to plasticity. Fiber features are altered by thyroid and growth hormones, testosterone, and other anabolic steroids,[206] and beta-2 agonists.[207] Each may stimulate muscle fiber growth or prevent disuse atrophy. For example, experimental animal models show that hypothyroidism can prevent the loss of slow MHC mRNA in the nonweight bearing soleus, whereas hyperthyroidism prevented the switch of fast MHC protein types.[208] Growth hormone with exercise may have a synergistic effect on limiting muscle atrophy and increasing muscle mass and strength in the elderly subject,[209] but can cause adverse side effects. Indeed, all hormone replacement strategies include some risk for medical complications (see Chapter 12). The beta-2 adrenergic agonists metaproterenol and clenbuterol have increased muscle mass and strength in patients with atrophy from a chronic SCI.[210] Albuterol had modest effects in patients with a muscular dystrophy.[211] These drugs probably exert an anabolic effect on protein structures in muscle,[212] but may have to be combined with exercise.

An observational study suggested that older, somewhat disabled women who took an angiotensin-converting enzyme (ACE) inhibitor for hypertension walked faster and had greater quadriceps strength than women who did not use these agents.[212a] The ACE inhibitors shift the MHC of skeletal muscle toward slow, aerobic, more fatigue-resistant isoforms and increase insulin sensitivity, among other factors. If shown to be valid in a clinical trial, the ACE inhibitors may lessen the decline of muscle loss in older persons and enhance recovery of

strength in patients with neurologic disease. Genetic studies suggest that healthy people with a gene polymorphism that reduces the expression of ACE have greater muscular efficiency and a higher anabolic response to exercise training.[212b] Thus, some drugs that are already in the medical armamentarium may help clinicians reverse muscle wasting and augment the effects of strengthening therapies.

Regeneration

The identification of myogenic precursor cells and stem cells points to the possibility of developing techniques to reverse atrophy and the effects of aging on muscle, as well as repair injured muscle and treat hereditary and acquired myopathies. Myoblasts have been derived from satellite cells and other cells within muscle, as well as from marrow and mesenchymal tissues.[213] A variety of gene markers, some of them still controversial and less reliable than others, identify satellite and other myoblast cells, so they can be collected and cultured.

Growth factors, including IGF-1, LIF, FGF and hepatocyte growth factor have been used alone or with transplanted myoblasts to enhance regeneration.[214] Genes can be directly injected into muscle as a regional genetic engineering approach to aid myogenesis. Synthetic polymers that imitate heparan sulfates and other extracellular matrix molecules may accelerate regeneration and reinnervation.[215] The ephrins and other molecules help specify the topographic location of axons at the neuromuscular junction, so manipulations of these muscle genes may lead to better guidance for reinnervation.[216]

As the genetic defects for muscle diseases come to be recognized, specific interventions such as myoblast implants, dystrophin gene insertions, and other gene replacement therapies may offer ways to modulate neuromuscular plasticity.[217]

Combined Approaches

The most critical clinical situation for preventing loss of muscle arises in the patient who is unable to move against gravity or is paralyzed, but is likely to regain better motor control over several weeks or months. When chronic complete and incomplete SCI subjects who could not walk were trained with manual assistance and partial body weight support to step on a treadmill belt, they modestly increased the mass of antigravity leg muscles, presumably from mechanical loading and intrinsic spinal neural influences.[218] A combination of early weight bearing, even modest isometric strength training, hormones and trophins, beta blockers or ACE inhibitors, and electrical stimulation of muscle using optimal stimulation parameters[219,220] could limit atrophy until greater volitional activity recovers. Noninvasive techniques that include CT and MRI imaging of muscle volume,[221,222] Positron-emission tomography, studies of amino acid uptake, and magnetic resonance spectroscopy[223] can help monitor the effects of interventions to limit atrophy and induce hypertrophy. For less affected muscles, isometric resistance exercise and conditioning exercises ought to be instituted as soon as possible to prevent disuse atrophy and loss of overall fitness.

Although sometimes neglected, basic and clinical research on the impact of mechanical loading and various types of resistance exercise may add a critical dimension to motor recovery and neural repair strategies. Clinical trials of drug and exercise paradigms will reveal the level and type of activity necessary to prevent protein degradation over synthesis and to slow the transition from slow to fast MHCs. Whether in animal models of neural repair or in day to day rehabilitation of patients, the maintenance or restoration of muscle mass may be a critical component for successful motor gains.

EXPERIMENTAL INTERVENTIONS FOR REPAIR OF SPINAL CORD INJURY

Some of the more promising applications of biologic interventions for reconstituting networks and diminishing disability derive from animal models of neural repair for SCI. A growing number of provocative studies describe interventions to enhance recovery of a forepaw for grasping and of the hindlimbs for locomotion.[177,224–229] The potential for implantation of stem cells, neural and myelinating precursor cells, and cells genetically modified to produce neurotrophins and other

molecules for regeneration has been an especially intriguing development.

Spinal repair strategies fall into approximately 5 general categories (Fig. 2–6): (1) promote regrowth of lesioned ascending and descending fiber tracts or promote collateral sprouting of intact axons by providing factors that stimulate the axon growth cone or suppress inhibitors of growth; (2) provide a bridge of substrate such as neurotrophins and scaffolds to guide axons from one side of the cord lesion to the other side; (3) induce intrinsic precursor cells from the central canal into serving as the bricks and mortar for spinal repair or implant bridging neurons within the cavity; (4) remyelinate axons with implanted cells; (5) use training and pharmacologic techniques to enhance activity-dependent plasticity within spared representations and newly functioning circuits. So far, however, *no published experiments have demonstrated growth of new cells and axons by morphologic or anatomic labeling techniques along with physiologic evidence of connectivity between the cells and their targets, and proof that the presumed reconnectivity accounts for restitution of important behaviors.*

We can begin to imagine how a combination of neurobiologic interventions may increase functional connections postinjury. This research is especially applicable to SCI, where clinicopathologic studies show that as little as 10% of residual supraspinal motor input is needed for the recovery of walking.[230,231] Similarly, to regain one more level of useful upper extremity function, even to go from C-5 to C-6 quadriplegia, would greatly improve the independence of a patient. What follows is a selection of highly controlled experimental manipulations in specific animal models. These experiments serve as stepping stones to a mix of repair strategies. Their applicability as standalone interventions for larger and more complex human injuries is moot. Clinical trials that make use of a singular intervention, however, are growing in number (see www.sciwire.com). A potpourri of manipulations may soon find applications in patients.

Prevent Cell Death

Neuroprotection in rodent models with methylprednisolone led to positive clinical trials sup-

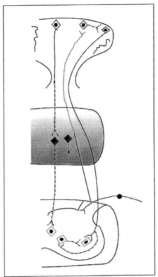

- Representational plasticity

- Acute neuroprotection
- Block axonal growth cone inhibitors
- Bridge injury site
- Harness neurotrophins

- Guide regenerating axons to targets
- Manipulate neurogenesis

- Make functional connections
- Optimize control of surviving and regenerated axon/dendrite connections for sensorimotor functions, e.g., walking

Figure 2–6. The drawing shows potential biologic responses to a spinal cord injury (*gray middle*). A cortical pyramidal neuron (*top*) partially retracts from the injury and then extends its axon (*dashed line*) to an transplanted neural precursor, which in turn sends its axon to a motoneuron in the ventral horn. An injured ascending fiber extends through the implanted milieu to reconnect to a cortical neuron. In response to deafferentation, that cortical neuron had sent out a dendritic contact to a neighboring neuron (*far right*). The cortical neuron on the far right had its descending axon spared. In response to motoneuron denervation in the cord, the cortical cell sprouted a dendritic connection to another spinal motoneuron in the ventral horn. One of the implanted neural precursors extended an axon a short distance, but made a connection only within the milieu of the transplant.

porting infusion of the drug within 8 hours of human SCI.[232] Although many other drug interventions have worked well in rodents to lessen injury, the efficacy of these pharmacologic interventions has not transferred to successful human clinical trials. Trials with 21-aminosteroids and antioxidants such as tirilizad have been disappointing. Trials with T-cells and vaccines directed against CNS myelin-associated proteins such as myelin basic protein[233] and spinal cord irradiation to limit gliosis are being assessed as interventions.

To try to enhance supraspinal input after a SCI, spinal motoneurons at the level of and below the lesion may need to be protected from transsynaptic injury. After a cervical SCI in rats, axonal retraction of reticulospinal and rubrospinal tracts was less than 1 mm. The investigators detected no progression of dying back beyond the first 4 weeks after the injury.[234] Thus, a neurotrophin placed within the lesion puts the factor within its diffusable range for reaching injured axons.

More remarkably, the rubrospinal neurons of rats whose axons were cut in the cervical cord 1 year before, causing profound atrophy

(seemingly dying of apoptosis), recovered size and protein synthesis when BDNF was applied to the cell bodies in the midbrain.[234a] Thus, regenerative competence may be manipulated even in chronic SCI.

Neurotrophins do have a sparing effect on motoneurons when placed within the injury site.[235] Several neurotrophic factors prevent retrograde neuronal injury.[236] A preventative measure may be especially important at the time of a neural repair strategy. Reinjury of axons during a surgical manipulation to place cells into the wall of a cavity in the cord, for example, may activate genes for regeneration, but may also damage additional axons and their neurons.[111] Brain-derived neurotrophic factor and CTNF protected brain stem neurons and their axons when infused near the SCI. In addition, perilesion apoptosis occurs for up to 8 weeks after an experimental spinal cord contusion in a rodent.[237] Oligodendrocytes and microglia also progressively die in regions of wallerian degeneration, so apoptosis may contribute to further demyelination. Therapeutic approaches include interrupting the cascade of apoptosis, such as blocking the release of cytokines, providing caspace inhibitors, and perhaps providing neurotrophins to perilesional cells.[237,238]

Increase Axonal Regeneration

The major barriers to axonal regeneration include glial scar, molecules in the milieu that inhibit growth cones or are not available to attract growth cones, and a core of necrosis and dead space that cannot be traversed. Following a SCI in rodents, lesioned corticospinal tract axons from layer V pyramidal cells have regenerated into implants of neurotrophins, fetal tissue, peripheral nerve, and Schwann cell grafts, but tend not to extend beyond these stimuli into distal white matter. Olfactory ensheathing cells have led to greater growth into white matter. Inosine enabled uninjured axons to sprout collaterals into normal white matter. Other axons, especially serotonergic and noradrenergic fibers, have traversed longer distances after injury.

LIMIT GLIAL SCAR

Immediately after a spinal cord contusion, petechial hemorrhages and tissue damage spread and enlarge in centripetal and rostrocaudal directions for up to several days. Resident and activated inflammatory cells infiltrate an increasingly necrotic cavity. Neutrophils, microglia, and proinflammatory chemokines and cytokines initiate macrophage phagocytosis. Within a week, T-lymphocytes and circulating monocytes enter the region of injury. These cells move throughout the perilesional area for more than a month postinjury and contribute to further axonal damage by creating free radicals, cytokines, proteolytic enzymes, and other toxins.[239] In addition, extracellular matrix molecules contribute to the glial scar. Cystic cavities within the central core of injury add a further barrier to the penetration of surviving axons. Injured axons retract.

Researchers have tried to block the acute and bystander damage inflicted by natural and autoimmune inflammatory responses. Drugs that block cytokines have not had clinical efficacy. Focal irradiation within several days of a contusion may quench the influx of inflammatory cells. This intervention in rodents has modest effects on behavior and histology.[240] Activated macrophages, however, may have proregenerative actions and autoimmune T cells against one or more myelin components may have neuroprotective effects, so irradiation may backfire. Macrophages transplanted into the acutely contused tissue produce neurotrophins and inhibit extracellular matrix molecules in the rat.[239] Trials of synthetic peptides and vaccines with peptides derived from Nogo and myelin basic protein for antiself immunity and neuroprotection have had modest success in rodent models of SCI.[241] The vaccines may find their way into trials for patients with acute SCI. Vaccinations designed to enhance autoreactive lymphocyte responses after CNS trauma may cause greater injury in patients who are genetically predisposed to autoimmune diseases.[241a]

MOLECULES FOR ATTRACTION AND REPULSION

Around a SCI contusion and cavity, axons retract less than 1 cm and then may sprout. Bresnahan and colleagues found corticospinal tract sprouting between 3 weeks and 3 months after a moderate SCI in rodents.[242] Collateralization and penetration of reticulospinal tracts into the matrix of the lesion started by 3 months. Thus, a modest percentage of injured axons may regenerate into the trabecular tissue that thinly bridges the cavity, as well as into residual gray and white matter around the cyst for a long time after the injury.

Antibodies to specific myelin-associated inhibitors of neurite growth have been given to rats after a partial SCI to prevent the milieu's inhibition of axonal regeneration.[243] Schwab and colleagues first implanted hybridomas of plasma cells that made myelin-associated neurite inhibitors into the ventricular system of newborn rats lesioned with a hemicordectomy. The primary inhibitor was later characterized as Nogo-A.[95,244] The antibodies increased axonal growth, although the fibers mostly skirted the surgical scar. Neurotrophin-3, but not BDNF injected into the lesioned rat spinal cord increased the regenerative sprouting of the transected corticospinal tract; neutralizing the myelin-associated neurite growth inhibitory proteins resulted in regeneration of up to 20 mm.[245] The axons generally did not pass through the cord lesion itself. Under the influence of anti-Nogo antibodies, axons have also sprouted and regenerated from the rubrospinal tract and other descending tracts at approximately 1 mm per day.[246] Although the regenerated tracts seem to enhance aspects of locomotor gains in the dorsal hemisection model,[246–248] which is the location of the corticospinal tracts in rats, stepping depends largely upon residual reticulospinal and vestibulospinal tracts in the ventral cord. Multiple inhibitors of axonal outgrowth are being identified on the surface of oligodendrocytes and myelin layers adjacent to axons. So far, they seem to exert their effects through the same signaling pathway as Nogo-A and can be neutralized by antibodies or by antagonists to the Nogo receptor.[248a,248b] The value of neutralizing myelin-associated inhibitors of neurite growth needs to be demonstrated in a nonhuman primate.

Other approaches to neutralizing inhibitors derived from oligodendrocytes and myelin have shown similar success. A vaccine against extracts of myelin, for example, appeared to block MAG, Nogo, and other less well-defined inhibitors of the growth cone in mice.[100] The immunizations started 3 weeks before a corticospinal tract lesion was induced, however. Axons in the treated mice did penetrate the scar and regenerate.

Another target for regeneration would be to block the primary transduction pathway in the growth cone that the inhibitory proteins set off. Potential means to increase cAMP, block Rho, and neutralize semaphorins were described earlier for animal models. For example, microinjection of an analog of cAMP in dorsal root ganglia regenerates central sensory axons.[248c]

Myelin-associated inhibitors may be no more harmful than proteoglycans such as chondroitin sulfate and keratan sulfate and tenascin, which suffuse scar tissue. Perilesional infusion of chondroitinase may degrade proteoglycans and make the milieu more conducive to regeneration of axons.[101] Such interventions are especially critical for transplantation strategies. Proteoglycans, for example, formed at the gray and white matter interface between a graft of Schwann cells embedded in Matrigel-filled channels and the host spinal cord.[249] The inhibitory proteoglycans prevented the outgrowth of axons from the transplant into the host.

PROMOTE AXONAL GROWTH

Different neuronal populations vary in the ease with which they have been induced to regenerate. The goal is to get critical supraspinal and propriospinal axons to sprout and reach targets in the gray matter of the cord. Unmyelinated monaminergic and serotonergic axons seem most able to traverse around a cavity or hemisection of the spinal cord. Regeneration of myelinated axons has posed greater difficulties. One of the most encouraging interventions in animal models has been the ability of implanted OECs to migrate and serve as guides for regenerating axons.[226,228] The OECs appear effective even at a distance from the site of implantation into a spinal cord cavitation. In addition, they myelinate regenerating axons with a patch of peripheral-type myelin.[250] Ramon-Cueto and colleagues showed that by 7 months after a transplant of OECs into a rat model of spinal cord transection, regenerated corticospinal, raphespinal, and coerulospinal axons were associated with improved hindlimb sensation and motor function.[228] Similar hindlimb locomotor gains were reported when OECs from the rat's olfactory mucosa were implanted 4 weeks after the transection at T-10.[251] Ten weeks later, axons from the brainstem raphe nucleus and serotonergic axons regenerated through the OEC graft.

Olfactory ensheathing cells may produce substances that degrade proteoglycans and limit the growth cone's exposure to reactive astrocytes and their inhibitory products. Also, OECs secrete at least a few varieties of adhesion molecules and growth factors. Of interest, corticospinal axons after exposure to OECs in the rat model used by Ramon-Cueto regenerated on the surface of the cord through the pia mater, suggesting that meningeal fibroblasts may also play a role. Further experiments with these cells will determine the reproducibility and level of efficacy of behavioral outcomes.

Other clever interventions, including gene therapies, have enticed axonal regeneration. Fibroblasts genetically engineered to express neurotrophic factors, including NT-3, LIF, and BDNF, have been placed below the lesioned cord in rats to enhance regeneration of corti-

for intracerebral grafts of CNS tissue. Technical factors, the effects of endogenous and exogenous neurotrophic factors, immunosuppression, and pharmacologic modulation of the expression of the graft will interact with task-oriented practice to affect graft survival and its physiologic and behavioral function. Still, transplants and supportive manipulations after a profound SCI offer promise as a means to permit the development of some descending and intersegmental control for movement. The following studies suggest that by combining several interventions, a modest amount of descending input to the L-1 motor pools below the SCI, enough to provide some trunk control and some supraspinal and propriospinal drive to the lumbar locomotor pools, will restore rather functional quadripedal walking. This finding needs to be demonstrated in a nonhuman primate.

EMBRYONIC TISSUE

Intraspinal transplants of supraspinal neurons and embryonic spinal cord have mostly aimed to restore locomotor abilities in rodent models of SCI. These studies, which began to show a variety of regenerative processes in the late 1970s, can be divided into two general categories.[275] Some experimenters transplant supraspinal neurons to provide a particular neurotransmitter. Others implant spinal cord tissue to provide a favorable milieu for regeneration. The optimal milieu includes cells for a synaptic relay, a favorable substrate for axonal elongation, and new cells that may migrate. Figure 2–6 shows how a bridge or relay may reconfigure after a SCI.

Transplantation of fetal noradrenergic neurons from the locus coeruleus was associated with the recovery of stepping in adult rats after spinal transection, presumably by replacing lost noradrenergic projections.[276] Midbrain and medulla raphe serotonergic neurons implanted into the caudal part of the spinal hole have grown axons for up to 2 cm into host cord, where the new fibers formed axodendritic and axosomatic synapses within the gray matter's ventral, dorsal, and intermediolateral regions.[277] Brain stem raphe cells restored locomotion on a treadmill better when placed into the T-11 level than the T-9 level of the transected cord, suggesting that reinnervation of the L-1–L-2 region restores an important serotonergic influence on the sublesional spinal cord's central pattern generators for stepping (see Chapter 1). Many studies have pointed to the beneficial effect of serotonergic input to locomotor neurons, including the use of a direct 5-hydroxytryptophan agonist combined with an embryonic transplant.[278] Overground locomotion in these rats may require some additional propriospinal or other supraspinal input.

After the thoracic cord was more than hemisected in another rat model, spinal embryonic transplants supported the regeneration of brain stem–spinal and segmental dorsal root projections, associated with recovery of hindlimb placement and aspects of locomotion; this growth was enhanced by providing neutralizing antibodies to neurite inhibitors.[279] Descending serotonergic, noradrenergic, and corticospinal fibers traversed the transplant only in neonates. In adults, the implant seemed to serve as a relay, rather than as a bridge. Propriospinal neurons sent axons into the embryonic tissue, providing segmental and intersegmental input that could account for the locomotor gains in the adults.

Clinicoanatomical correlations between behavioral gains and the regeneration of axons have improved as investigator experience has increased, especially with the addition of behavioral training and other repair strategies.[224,280,281] Overall results have been promising, but not behaviorally robust. A more recent study in adult rats by Bregman and colleagues showed that the transplantation of fetal rat spinal cord tissue, plus the administration of BDNF or NT-3, improved outcomes when delayed for a few weeks after a low thoracic spinal transection.[282] The growth of axons across the transplant into host cord and improvements in hindlimb motor function were more robust than after giving only neurotrophins or only fetal tissue shortly after a hemisection. Brainstem nuclei, propriospinal neurons, and scattered corticospinal neurons were among the cells that contributed the modest number of regenerating axons. A reinjury of the wall at the site of transection at the time of delayed implantation may contribute to gene expression for regeneration in this model.[283]

The feasibility and safety of embryonic spinal cord tissue transplants is being assessed in eight patients who had a progressively enlarging syrinx after SCI.[284] The investigators used from 4 to 8 human embryos that were 6 to 9 weeks gestational age. The implants appear to have filled a portion of each syrinx and probably interact with the host tissue. No safety problems and no clear clinical benefits have been found in up to 3 years of follow-up.

Transplantation with human embryonic tissue is not likely to be acceptable in the United States. Xenografts or stem cells grown in culture appear to be more feasible approaches.

EMBRYONIC STEM CELLS

Embryonic stem cells from mice were manipulated into a neural lineage and transplanted into rats 9 days after a spinal cord contusion.[285] Although many cells died, some divided. Others migrated probably through the central canal and into gray and white matter via radial glia, traveling up to 1 cm by 2 weeks after implantation. Approximately 60% became oligodendrocytes, 10% neurons, and the rest astrocytes. Their presence was associated with some axonal growth and improved hindlimb activity, suggesting that remyelination played a role in the modest behavioral gains. With grafting after a SCI, most studies show that neural stem cells are primarily restricted to a glial lineage. With a variety of *in vitro* manipulations, however, stem cells from embryonic spinal cord can be made to differentiate into many classes of neurons that synthesize and respond to different neurotransmitters.[286] Hippocampal-derived neurospheres may also differentiate and migrate into host spinal cord.[287] Experiments are in progress to determine whether neural lineage cells or specific precursor cells will offer better results in specific models of SCI.

VENTRAL HORN NEURONS AND ROOTS

Approximately 20% of traumatic SCIs occur at the level of the conus and cauda equina, producing a lower motor neuron injury. Traumatic and ischemic SCI invariably affect ventral and dorsal horn roots and neurons. Trauma often tears or avulses proximal nerve roots, which, if proximal enough to the cord, leads to motoneuron death. The motoneuron operates within both the CNS and PNS, so its regenerative ability to make a new axon depends on features of both environments. Although a variety of biologic differences exist between a normal spinal motoneuron, its axon, and its neuromuscular junctions compared to a motor unit that regenerates after injury in the adult,[288] these differences should not interfere with the promise of motoneuron reinnervation strategies for repair.

Embryonic motoneurons have been implanted into the anterior horn under very special experimental conditions to successfully take the place of lost motoneurons.[289] Neural precursors could some day replace damaged motoneurons after SCI and perhaps in diseases such as ALS. Human progenitor cells from fetal germ tissue have partially repopulated spinal tissue after injection into the spinal fluid of rats and monkeys following a viral-induced motor neuronopathy.[290]

Following an intramedullary axotomy or ventral root avulsion, up to 90% of motoneurons will die from apoptosis within a month of disconnection from their proximal axons. Surviving motoneurons may develop supernumerary axons originating from the soma.[291] These new axons can establish normal synaptic contacts with spinal neurons and grow into a piece of implanted peripheral nerve. The motoneuron may also generate one or more axons into the white matter from distal dendrites.

Other interventions may help motoneurons survive and regenerate after a proximal root injury. Antagonists to L-gated calcium channels such as nimodipine and 21-aminosteroid inhibitors of lipid peroxidation, along with glutamate blockers, have shown some success in animal models when given at the time of injury. As noted earlier, however, these same neuroprotection strategies have generally not succeeded when put into clinical trials. In addition to neurotrophins such as BDNF, NT-3, IGF-1, and GDNF that provide trophic support for motoneurons, suprathreshold electrical stimulation at 20 Hz better than doubled the rate of axonal regeneration into a femoral nerve in the rat.[292] The nerve stump had to be stimulated proximally, suggesting that electrical input to motoneurons may have upregulated gene expression for cytoskeletal proteins and neurotrophins.

ROOT IMPLANTATION

Dorsal and ventral roots may avulse or tear with traumatic SCI. In studies of rats, cats, and nonhuman primates, ventral roots have been avulsed and reimplanted back into the ventro-lateral cord. Regenerating axons from motoneurons that lose their connection to their roots will grow into a reimplanted ventral root and grow until the axons reinnervate muscles.[293,294] Although synkinetic contractions are common at first, selective movements evolve over time, presumably related to practice. Over 80% of motoneurons and preganglionic parasympathetic neurons in rats survive, regenerate axons, and remyelinate new fibers into the ventral roots, if the roots are reimplanted within a week.[295]

In 10 patients who suffered intraspinal brachial plexus injuries, a neurosurgeon reimplanted the avulsed roots into the cervical cord from 10 days to 9 months later.[296] Signs of reinnervation appeared by 9 to 12 months. Proximal muscles were more likely to be reinnervated. Half the patients improved in motor function and three patients had useful movement by 2 years later. Initial cocontractions tended to resolve over time. A reimplanted ventral root with intact Schwann cells probably contains trophic substances that diffuse into the remains of the rootlets of motoneurons within the white matter along the circumference of the cord.

The neurotrophins, primarily BDNF, have been infused into the subarachnoid space after experimental ventral root avulsion in rats. Brain-derived neurotrophic factor also limited apoptosis of motoneurons when the conus and cauda were focally damaged in the rat.[297] Brain-derived neurotrophic factor, compared to control infusions, led to greater numbers of surviving motoneurons and a dramatic increase in axons that extended from these cells to the surface of the cord.[298] In related experiments, investigators showed that BDNF preserved the dendritic architecture of the motoneurons that did not undergo retrograde degeneration. Brain-derived neurotrophic factor also restored some of the synaptic covering of the motoneurons, at least for inhibitory boutons. Without reimplantation of the avulsed root, the effects of BDNF persist for about a month after discontinuing it. The combination of reimplantation and a neurotrophin infusion may augment the benefits of each. Orally given immunophilins may also serve as an adjunct for enhancing peripheral nerve regeneration.[299]

Another surgical approach in rodents interposed a peripheral nerve autograft between a limb muscle and the ventral cord[300] or between the distal end of a root and the ventral cord. In a study with marmosets, the lumbar roots were sectioned on one side of the cord. One end of an autograft was implanted into the ventral thoracic cord at T-10 and the other was fused with transected L-3 and L-4 roots.[301] Control animals showed no motor function in the quadriceps and no histological evidence for regeneration. The animals with a bypass graft developed motor control of the muscle as the thoracic motoneurons regenerated into the graft and reinnervated the quadriceps. This surgical and retraining approach should reach human trials to provide patients after a conus/cauda injury with new proximal motor control for walking.

A rather remarkable example of axonal regeneration and plasticity may come into use to restore micturition in patients with SCI. In a cat model, the L-7 ventral root, which innervates hindlimb muscles, was anastomosed to the S-1 ventral root, which innervates the bladder.[302] By 4 to 9 months later, scratching the L-7 dermatome (which corresponds to S-1 in humans) initiated bladder contractions and voiding. This reflex voiding was demonstrated in the intact cat and after a high lumbar spinal transection. Motoneurons had innervated bladder parasympathetic ganglion cells, making nicotinic and muscarinic synapses, to create a cross-wired somato-autonomic reflex.

The loss of motor axons after a partial peripheral nerve or root injury leads to changes that may affect the approach to the rehabilitation of reinnervated muscle. The remaining motoneurons in one model of a partial peripheral nerve ligation were found to have a decrease in their conduction velocity and prolongation in the duration of the afterhyperpolarization when they reinnervated muscle.[303] Such changes may alter the functional properties of available motor units. The effects of lower motoneuron activity on sprouting adds further complexity. During the acute phase of sprouting after partial denervation in a rat model, high levels of neuromuscular activity induced by electrical stimulation were detrimental to sprouting and reduced the enlargement of motor units.[304] The effect was greatest in more severely denervated muscle where fewer than 20% of motor units remained. Physical activity that exceeds these physiologic levels may be detrimental. Studies in humans must determine whether limits for the intensity and level of resistance exercise apply to patients with reinnervating muscle.

Given the remarkable plasticity demonstrated by these experiments, a surgical approach to reinstating proximal leg movement and bowel and bladder control may be feasible after a conus or cauda equina lesion. For example, at the time of surgery after an L-1 burst fracture to clean out bone fragments and stabilize the spine, the neurosurgeon could open the dura and reimplant one or more lumbar and sacral roots that have been torn or avulsed back into the ventrolateral cord. If the animal studies are correct, the motoneurons will regenerate axons into the implant and out to the periphery to the hip and knee flexor and extensor muscles and to the bladder. The peripheral nerve and its Schwann cells are still intact and will offer regenerative signals for these growing axons. An avulsed cervical root could be reimplanted as well, placed just above the level of the SCI.

Conceivably, reimplanting an L-4 or S-2 ventral root into the ventrolateral cord above the spinal lesion will sprout axons from the local motoneurons and restore some supraspinal control over the hip flexors and knee extensors and some bladder contractile function after training. In this scenario, a conditioning lesion of the motoneurons above the SCI, at the level of the implant, will be necessary to help stimulate growth of axons from the spinal neurons into the graft. An autologous nerve graft or polymer conduit from the torn lumbar or sacral root may also be needed to reach above the lesion.[304a] A biologically more adventuresome repair strategy for lesions that destroy the somatic and preganglionic parasympathetic neurons of the conus is to put autologous neural precursors into the cystic lesion and coax them to send axons into existing or implanted ventral roots, and to make connections with regenerating supraspinal inputs. If lumbar root implants were shown to be efficacious in a clinical trial, cervical implants of ventral roots into the cord above the lesion to muscles below the SCI may be seen as worth the potential risks for patients.

DORSAL HORN NEURONS

Most experiments relevant to the regeneration of dorsal horn neurons with their inputs and outputs have been devoted to understanding mechanisms of pain (see Chaper 8). In the presence of central pain associated with a SCI, experimental interventions often aim to diminish regeneration and sprouting in the dorsal horn. This approach may also prevent autonomic dysreflexia. For example, antibodies to NGF prevented small-diameter afferents from sprouting in the dorsal horn below a thoracic SCI in the rat.[305] The intervention prevented a colonic stimulus from inducing hypertension.

Axons from dorsal root ganglia will spontaneously regenerate within their peripheral nerve segment after a lesion, but stop at the CNS border of the dorsal root entry zone. Embryonic transplants of both spinal cord and brain tissue from rats, when placed between the lumbar cord and a transected dorsal root stump, provide cues that allow dorsal ganglia axons to regenerate into the host gray matter.[281] The embryonic transplants also induce axons to arborize with motoneurons. The graft may supply neurotrophins and other molecules of a friendly mileu.

Large myelinated dorsal horn neurons express trk C receptors. Neurotrophin-3 had a greater effect than other neurotrophins in regenerating ascending fibers in one model.[306] This neurotrophin also promoted regeneration across the dorsal root entry zone, where the central axon from the ganglion enters the cord, but only if infused within 1 week of dorsal rhizotomy.[307] Injections into the dorsal cord of an adenovirus that encodes for FGF and NGF induced considerable regeneration of axons into the dorsal horn 2 weeks after a dorsal root avulsion in adult rats.[308] In this model, NGF also caused uninjured sensory axons to sprout, which could cause pain. Tenascin and proteoglycans are among the inhibitors at the dorsal root entry zone.[309] These substances can be neutralized as discussed earlier. Immunophilins also may increase root entry zone penetration by sensory axons.[310]

SPINAL NEURONS AS TARGETS

Some fundamental questions about the pools of neurons within the ventral and dorsal horns have yet to be answered. Which spinal neurons should neural repairists target with the new axons they coax down white matter columns of the cord? One of the remarkable chasms in knowledge about spinal cord anatomy and physiology is that very little is known about how and where descending inputs to the dorsal and ventral horns make their connections. Over what expanse, rostrocaudal and mediolateral, do incoming axons normally join interneurons and sensory and motoneurons? How many targets can one axon effectively reach and activate? What are the neurotransmitters that drive and inhibit these pools? Which descending inputs and which target cells would give new axons the greatest behavioral effects for restoration of movement, sensation, and bowel and bladder control? Which inputs would prevent or eliminate at-level spinal pain? The mechanisms that regulate target recognition within the cord have been shown in a few studies of the injured CNS to be intact, so regenerating axons may recognize appropriate attractive and inhibitory signals once axons penetrate the gray matter.[311] Behavioral retraining strategies may aid target recognition, as well as the functional incorporation of new axonal inputs.

Retraining the Spinal Motor Pools

The spinal neuronal pools become a new playing field when descending inputs and segmental afferents are withdrawn by injury. If neural repair strategies are to produce functional benefits to patients, biologic interventions will require motor learning and rehabilitation interventions to help train the new networks.

A growing number of studies point to the augmented effectiveness of residual supraspinal, corticospinal, and afferent activity after SCI on the spinal and cortical regulation of facilitation and recruitment.[312,313] These alterations may expand the cortical and subcortical representations for the sensorimotor activities of the limbs and trunk after a SCI. Cortical representations for the hand and trunk have shown considerable plasticity in people with complete SCI.[314,315] The PET scans performed in people with complete SCI reveal an expansion of the hand's topographic map toward the leg area during hand movements and greater bilateral activation of the thalamus and cerebellum.[315] This representational plasticity may derive from altered spinothalamic and spinocerebellar inputs to primary motor cortex. The spinocerebellar pathway runs along the outer rim of spinal cord white matter, so it may be partially spared by a central contusion, as may the sacral portion of the spinothalamic tract, which is out-

ermost in this tract at all spinal levels. Changes in representational maps were also found by intracortical microstimulation of the leg area after amputation of a hindlimb in monkeys.[316] Cortical representations in M1 for the hindlimb region that had been deafferented and deefferented evoked hip stump, trunk, and tail movements.

Spinal locomotor-related neurons and interneurons offer an important target for biological interventions that reinstate some supraspinal input, even if only as caudal as the T-11 to L-1 levels. New inputs may not have to reach lumbar neuronal targets in the specific fashion they had prior to the SCI to elicit functional flexor and extensor movements. Inherent mechanisms of plasticity will help incorporate new inputs, if driven to do so. The model of the spinal transected cat and rat demonstrates the plasticity of the flexor and extensor motor pools in relation to their pattern generating properties and their facilitation by step training.[317] The lumbar spinal organization for synergistic movements in the workspace of the leg, as well as the propriospinal connections of the thoracolumbar columns of motor pools for stepping contribute further to truncal and leg activity for locomotion (see Chapter 1). Segmental sensory feedback from locomotor-related proprioceptive and cutaneous afferents has a powerful modulating effect on locomotor networks in patients (Fig. 1–7).[10,317–319] A facsimile of normal sensory inputs to the lumbosacral spinal cord, cerebellum, thalamus, brainstem, and sensorimotor cortex (Figure 1–1) from physical therapy that entrains stepping with these inputs will drive the locomotor network at all levels (Color Figs. 3–5 and 3–8, in separate color insert). Such facilitation may lead to functional incorporation of new motoneurons and ascending and descending axons that bridge a SCI.

Task-oriented practice (see Chapter 5) for upper and lower extremity activities that optimizes the sensory cues recognized by the nervous system as being relevant to skills such as reaching and locomotion appears to be critical for normal learning and plasticity. Repetitive practice under a variety of conditions may induce many of the neurochemical, trophic, and morphologic changes in the spinal cord that underpin proposed neural repair strategies. Optimal training strategies need to be married to repair strategies if clinicians are to turn a modest number of new and residual connections and networks into circuitry that lessens the disabilities of patients.

RELEVANCE OF ANIMAL MODELS OF REPAIR TO CLINICAL TRIALS

The number of failed phase 2 and phase 3 human trials of acute interventions for stroke, TBI, and SCI have left many scientists and clinicians wondering whether translational research from the laboratory bench to the bedside is feasible. Despite marvelous results in rodent models of injury,[320–324] as of the year 2002, at least 65 randomized clinical trials in stroke, 25 in cerebral trauma, and 8 in SCI have not led to better outcomes for patients. Only one or two acute interventions for each type of disease have proved their value. Investigators and pharmaceutical companies have tried to find ways to explain the failures to translate rodent studies into successful clinical trials.[325] Researchers in neural repair may benefit from considering questions about the intersections of animal and human research.

Table 2–10 lists some of the animal models and outcome measures used in studies of neural repair.[324,326] Some consideration of these may help clinicians understand the promise and limitations of the experimental studies published by journals. These experiments are often given a breathless sound byte by the media, which raises expectations about an imminent cure for paralysis.

Research laboratories most often rely upon tissue culture and small rodent studies to study singular mechanisms of neural injury and repair. Are such studies likely to lead to interventions for patients? Clinicians often express the misconception that basic research with animals is easier to carry out, more scientifically rigorous, and permits the measurement of more clearcut outcomes than any possible design for a clinical trial in patients. Can interventional studies in animal models have systematic flaws that may mislead clinicians about the potential for efficacy in human trials? Clinicians and clinical and basic scientists must face these important and complex issues if preclinical work in neural repair is to point to worthy human trials. The ethical clinician who looks to

Table 2–10. Overview of Animal Models of Neural Repair for Spinal Cord Injury

MODELS	
Rodents	
Standard drop weight contusion	Focal demyelination
Focal compression	Root avulsion
Hemisection—dorsal or lateral cord	Transgenic mouse gene manipulation
Tract ablation	
Nonhuman primates	
Tract ablation	Root avulsion

MEASURED OUTCOMES	
Gross tissue preservation	
Histology	
Label and count new axons, growth cones, boutons	Morris water maze
Label and count new neurons	Activity meter
Behaviors (often videotaped evaluations)	*Robotic device measures—kinematics, torques*
Forepaw use—feeding, locomotion, climbing	*Sensation—tail flick analgesia*
Hindlimb use—BBB scale for qualitative locomotion; footprint placement; grid, beam or ladder walk	

BBB, open-field Basso, Beattie, Bresnahan score.

the literature for ideas about how to help patients or wants to put highly publicized animal
studies in perspective for desperate patients
and families needs to be aware of potential pitfalls in translational animal research.

Eight Potential Pitfalls of Animal Models

1. What is the study population? In animal research, vendors provide healthy, highly inbred
rats and mice. The rodents are the same species
and strain, same age, weight, and gender.
Males tend to be used most often to avoid the
hormonal fluxes of the estrous cycle. The experiments are usually carried out on neonates
and young adults, approximately 3–6 months
old (an old rat is 2 years old). The CNS of a
neonate may still be developing, allowing for
far greater opportunity for morphologic adaptations than may evolve in an adult. In human
trials, the study population has great variability in genes, age, sex, medication taken, and
premorbid health. Such heterogeneity in humans may not be overcome by simply using
large sample sizes and some obvious inclusion
and exclusion criteria in randomized clinical
trials. Indeed, large sample sizes will not be
practical for trials of neural repair strategies.
Even in rats, significant interspecies and in-
trastrain variablity may foil the results of studies carried out in different laboratories. For example, when several American research
laboratories at universities on the east and west
coasts shared a uniform brain percussion
method, the outcomes were far worse for the
rats in the West (personal communication,
Anat Biegon, PhD). Although the rodents
came from the same strain, different vendors
provided rats to each coast. When all labs used
the same vendor, the injury model became
more uniform.

Species differences are even more pronounced. Some rodents are much less likely
than others to develop a glial scar after the
same SCI that produces a large barrier to axonal regeneration in another species. Differences in injury-induced T-cell responses and in
other not so readily appreciated genetic sus-
ceptibilities of a particular strain also account
for possible differences in the responses between some rodents and humans.[327] In SCI
models, the choice among Wistar, Long-Evans,
and Sprague-Dawley strains of rat has a great
impact on the likelihood of locomotor recovery
after the same contusion injury.[328] Skilled
movements for manipulating food are suppos-
edly highly conserved across species and genetically wired.[329] Whishaw and colleagues,
however, showed that proper reaching movements with a forepaw have been breeded out
of Fischer-344 rats. Also, microstimulation of
the motor cortex that represents the paw and
distal arm reveals a much smaller representation for the wrist in Fischer rats than in Long-
Evans rats. Intensive training of paw reaching
for food pellets does not enlarge the representation in the Fischer rats the way training affects other rats.

Mice have come to monopolize mammalian
genetic studies of trauma and ischemia. A single gene mutation permits the study of a specific phenotype, such as absence of an inhibitory molecule in the matrix of the cord or
excessive production of a particular neurotrophin. Different inbred murine strains respond quite differently to ischemia or trauma
and most mice respond differently than most
rats in terms of injury and regenerative cascades.[330] Given this confounding difference
among animals, the researcher and clinician
cannot assume that a human subject will have
responses similar to any one species of rodent.

Laboratory rodents are kept in separate
cages in most instances, so they do not injure
each other with aggressive territorial defenses.
The amount of stimulation and intensity of
learning opportunities provided by housing
conditions for rodents may strongly affect important interactions between the environment
and genetic factors.[331] The responses made by
animals depend largely upon rules that evolved
from interactions with natural environments.
Isolation can cause odd, stereotyped behaviors.
Changes between the postnatal and adult environment can also disrupt habitat-dependent
adaptations. Standard laboratory rearing is
quite unnatural. Indeed, although highly inbred transgenic mice are wonderful tools for
the study of the effects of specific genes, environmental conditions have led to a reversal of
those gene effects.[331]

Dramatic consequences may follow seemingly innocuous variations in daily rodent life,
such as the amount of sleep, handling by the
research staff, and nutrition in one group compared to another. The biologic effects of an in-

tervention and its behavioral outcomes have, for example, been repeatedly confounded by differences in caloric intake, whether spontaneous or secondary to the experimental manipulation.[332]

Even without an injury, the laboratory search for repair mechanisms may yield results in rats that are not clearly relevant to people. For example, I discussed trials in which running in an enriched environment increased production of a variety of neurotrophins, as well as neurogenesis, in the hippocampus.[332a] Would this happen in people? Rodents in natural environments evolved to find food and shelter by scurrying about as they vigilantly attend to details in their surroundings. Aimless exercise, such as jogging on a treadmill or wandering in a shopping mall, may be much less of an inducement for the stimulation of BDNF and other growth factors, genes that promote plasticity, memory molecules, or neurons in patients with neurologic diseases. If such stimulation is part and parcel to human learning, as it seems, learning paradigms will need to be designed for rehabilitation that stimulate genes and cells.

2. Is the model of injury and repair in rodents similar enough to what happens to people? Scooping out cortex in an ablation model for stroke may produce the same amount of tissue injury as a vascular occlusion, but the cascade of molecules and gene expression that follow injury will differ between ablation and ischemia, as described in Experimental Case Studies 2–2. The milieu for mechanisms of repair will differ as well with the type of lesion induced. A cortical infarct will not elicit the same responses as a subcortical infarct.[333] The commonly employed fluid percussion model of TBI in rodents most often induces a focal, mild to moderate cortical injury that resolves in several days. A human injury may include contusions, white matter axonal injury, ischemia, bleeding, edema, and raised intracranial pressure. These differences in pathology and the persistence of injury-induced cascades in humans make interventions for neuroprotection and repair in humans a large leap of faith when built upon the typical rat model. Very different mechanisms and outcomes may unfold in humans over time as molecular cascades interact.

Researchers are inclined to use an established acute injury model to study repair. Since the injury model was originally developed to produce a uniform lesion with particular features that represent a partial equivalent to human damage, the model may not serve a study of repair. For example, most stroke and trauma models produce little or no white matter damage. Some injury models originally aimed to evaluate NMDA receptor-mediated neuronal injury in the cortex or hippocampus. Most human lesions from stroke or TBI do not even involve the hippocampus, unless global hypoperfusion or hypoxia develop. Of equal importance, human trauma and ischemia involve white matter destruction. The AMPA receptors of oligodendrocytes mediate cytotoxic injury, not NMDA receptors. Such basic variations across tissues help account for the failure of human clinical trials of interventions for NMDA receptor-mediated injury. Differences in receptor types within regions of the brain and spinal cord and further changes brought on by injury will also have to be reckoned with in the translation of models to human neural repair. Among other queries, the reader of an experiment carried out with animals or cell cultures must always wonder how similar the results would be if another SCI or stroke model had been used and how applicable the particular model of injury and repair will be to the majority of clinical injuries and of mechanisms of restitution or substitution.

3. Is the brain and spinal cord of a rat or mouse simply a thimble-sized version of the human brain? The surface area of the brain of a mouse is $1/1000^{th}$ that of the human brain. Studies of axonal regeneration in rats and mice consider an extension of axons for a few millimeters to a centimeter as exuberant growth. Clinicians may not realize how small the rodent brain and spinal cord are compared to the human CNS (Fig. 2–7). Axons in human brain or spinal cord may have to grow from several centimeters to over a meter to reach targets. Neural progenitors may need to migrate 10 cm or more to repopulate gray or white matter. Signaling molecules that fashioned the CNS during embryogenesis and development never had to manage such long distance tours.

Can rodent models give insight into the effective dose-response curve for biologic interventions in man? A repair intervention in mice probably requires a lot less regeneration of axons compared to the number of connections humans will need to produce complex behaviors such as goal-directed walking and manip-

22. Bucy P, Keplinger J, Siqueira E. Destruction of the "pyramidal tract" in man. J Neurosurg 1964; 21: 385–398.

23. Warabi T, Inoue K, Noda H, Murakami S. Recovery of voluntary movement in hemiplegic patients. Brain 1990; 113:177–189.

24. Merzenich M, Recanzone G, Jenkins W, Allard T, Nudo R. Cortical representational plasticity. In: Rakic P, Singer W, eds. Neurobiology of Neocortex. John Wiley, 1988:41–67.

25. Nudo R, Milliken G, Jenkins W, Merzenich M. Use-dependent alterations of movement representations in primary motor cortex of adult squirrel monkeys. J Neurosci 1996; 16:785–807.

26. Nudo R, Wise B, SiFuentes F, Milliken G. Neural substrates for the effects of rehabilitative training on motor recovery after ischemic infarct. Science 1996; 272:1791–1794.

27. Davidoff R. Skeletal muscle tone and the misunderstood stretch reflex. Neurology 1992; 42:951–963.

28. Heckman C. Alterations in synaptic input to motoneurons during partial spinal cord injury. Med Sci Sports Exerc 1994; 26:1480–1490.

29. Denny-Brown D. The Cerebral Control of Movement. Liverpool: Liverpool University Press, 1966.

30. Pierrot-Deseilligny E. Electrophysiological assessment of the spinal mechanisms underlying spasticity. In: Rossini P, Mauguiere F, eds. New Trends and Advanced Techniques in Clinical Neurophysiology (EEG Suppl. 41). Amsterdam: Elsevier, 1990:264–273.

31. Young R. Spasticity. Neurology 1994; 44(suppl 9):S12–S20.

31a. Calancie B, Molano M, Broton J. Interlimb reflexes and synaptic plasticity become evident months after human spinal cord injury. Brain 2002; 125:1150–1161.

32. Knutsson E, Martensson A, Gransberg L. Influences of muscle stretch reflexes on voluntary, velocity-controlled movements in spastic paraparesis. Brain 1997; 120:1621–1633.

33. Hiersemenzel L-P, Curt A, Dietz V. From spinal shock to spasticity. Neurology 2000; 54:1574–1582.

34. Fellows S, Ross H, Thilmann A. The limitations of the tendon jerk as a marker of pathological stretch reflex activity in human spasticity. J Neurol Neurosurg Psychiatry 1993; 56:531–537.

35. Burke D. Spasticity as an adaptation to pyramidal tract injury. In: Waxman S, ed. Functional Recovery in Neurological Disease. New York: Raven Press, 1988:401–423.

36. Hufschmidt A, Mauritz KH. Chronic transformation of muscle in spasticity. J Neurol Neurosurg Psychiatry 1985; 48:676–685.

37. Dietz V, Quintern J, Berger W. Electrophysiological studies of gait in spasticity and rigidity. Brain 1981; 104:431–449.

38. Carey J, Burghardt T. Movement dysfunction following central nervous system lesions: A problem of neurologic or muscular impairment? Phys Ther 1993; 73:538–547.

39. Cotman C, Anderson K. Synaptic plasticity and functional stabilization in the hippocampal formation: Possible role in Alzheimer's disease. In: Waxman S, ed. Functional Recovery in Neurological Disease. New York: Raven Press, 1988.

40. Carmichael ST, Wei L, Rovainen C, Woolsey T. New patterns of intracortical projections after focal cortical stroke. Neurobiol Dis 2001; 8:910–922.

41. Weidner N, Ner A, Salimi N, Tuszynski MH. Spontaneous corticospinal axonal plasticity and functional recovery after adult central nervous system injury. Proc Natl Acad Sci USA 2001; 98:3513–3518.

42. Aoki M, Fujito Y, Mizuguchi A, Satomi H. Recovery of hindlimb movement after spinal hemisection and collateral sprouting from corticospinal fibers in monkeys. In: Shimamura M, Grillner S, Edgerton V, eds. Neurobiological Basis of Human Locomotion. Tokyo: Japan Scientific Societies Press, 1991:401–405.

43. Anglade P, Tsuji S, Agid Y. Plasticity of nerve afferents to nigrostriatal neurons in Parkinson's disease. Ann Neurol 1995; 37:265–272.

44. Goldberger M, Murray M. Patterns of sprouting and implications for recovery of function. In: Waxman S, ed. Functional Recovery in Neurological Disease. Vol. 47. New York: Raven Press, 1988:361–385.

45. Bahr M, Bonhoeffer F. Perspectives on axonal regeneration in the mammalian CNS. Trends Neurosci 1994; 17:473–479.

46. David S, Aguayo A. Axonal elongation into peripheral nervous system 'bridges' after central nervous system injury in adult rats. Science 1981; 214:931–933.

47. Caroni P. Driving the growth cone. Science 1998; 281:1465–1518.

48. Cai D, Qiu J, Cao Z, McAtee M, Bregman B, Filbin M. Neuronal cyclic AMP controls the developmental loss in ability of axons to regenerate. J Neurosci 2001; 21:4731–4739.

49. Pasterkamp J, Verhaagen J. Emerging roles for semaphorins in neural regeneration. Brain Res Rev 2001; 35:36–54.

50. Tang S, Qiu J, Nikulina E, Filbin M. Soluble myelin-associated glycoprotein released from damaged white matter inhibits axonal regeneration. Mol Cell Neurosci 2001; 18:259–269.

51. Lehmann M, Fournier A, Selles-Navarro I, Dergham P, Sebok A, Leclerc N, Tigyi G, McKerracher L. Inactivation of Rho signaling pathway promotes CNS axon regeneration. J Neurosci 1999; 19:7537–7547.

52. Tekkok S, Goldberg M. AMPA/kainate receptor activation mediates hypoxic oligodendrocyte death and axonal injury in cerebral white matter. J Neurosci 2001; 21:4237–4248.

53. Poo M. Neurotrophins as synaptic modulators. Nat Rev Neurosci 2001; 2:24–32.

54. Guo X, Dillman J, Dawson V, Dawson T. Neuroimmunophilins: Novel neuroprotective and neuroregenerative targets. Ann Neurol 2001; 50:6–16.

54a. Sulaiman O, Voda J, Gold BG, Gordon T. Fk506 increases peripheral nerve regeneration after chronic axotomy but not after chronic Schwann cell denervation. Exp Neurol 2002; 175:127–137.

55. Kornack D, Rakic P. The generation, migration, and differentiation of olfactory neurons in the adult primate brain. Proc Natl Acad Sci USA 2001; 98:4752–4757.

56. Gross C. Neurogenesis in the adult brain: Death of a dogma. Nat Rev/Neurosci 2000; 1:67–73.

57. McKay R. Stem cells in the central nervous system. Science 1997; 276:66–71.

58. Mezey E, Chandross K, Harta G, Maki R, McKercher S. Turning blood into brain: Cells bearing

neuronal antigens generated in vivo from bone marrow. Science 2000; 290:1779–82.

59. Lee J, Mayer-Proschel M, Rao M. Gliogenesis in the central nervous system. Glia 2000; 30:105–121.

60. Kondo T, Raff M. Oligodendrocyte precursor cells reprogrammed to become multipotential CNS stem cells. Science 2000; 289:1754–1756.

61. Morrison S. The last shall no be first: the ordered generation of progeny from stem cells. Neuron 2000; 28:1–9.

62. Watt F, Hogan B. Out of Eden: stem cells and their niches. Science 2000; 287:1427–1430.

63. Carpenter M, Inokuma M, Denham J, Mujtaba T, Chiu C, Rao M. Enrichment of neurons and neural precursors rom human embryonic stem cells. Exp Neurol 2001; 172:383–397.

64. Goldman S. Neuronal precursor cells and neurogenesis in the adult forebrain. The Neuroscientist 1995; 1:338–50.

65. Lois C, Alvarez-Buylla A. Long-distance neuronal migration in the adult mammalian brain. Science 1994; 264:1145–1148.

66. Gage F. Mammalian neural stem cells. Science 2000; 287:1433–1438.

67. Rietze R, Valcanis H, Brooker G, Thomas T, Voss A, Bartlett P. Purification of a pluripotent neural stem cell from adult mouse brain. Nature 2001; 412:736–739.

68. Ourednik V, Ourednik J, Flax J, Zawada W, Freed C, Snyder E. Segregation of human neural stem cells in the developing primate forebrain. Science 2001; 293:1820–1824.

69. Kirschenbaum B, Nedergaard M, Goldman S, Preuss A, Barami K, Fraser R. In vitro neuronal and glial production by precursor cells derived from the adult human forebrain. Ann Neurol 1994; 36:322–323.

70. Johansson C, Svensson M, Wallstedt L, Janson A, Frisen J. Neural stem cells in the adult human brain. Exp Cell Res 1999; 253:733–736.

71. Arsenijevic Y, Villemure J-G, Brunet J-F, Bloch J, Déglon N, Kostic C, Zurn A, Aebischer P. Isolation of multipotent neural precursors residing in the cortex of the adult human brain. Exp Neurol 2001; 170:48–62.

72. Palmer T, Willhoite A, Gage F. Vascular niche for adult hippocampal neurogenesis. J Comp Neurol 2000; 425:479–494.

72a. Song H, Stevens C, Gage F. Astroglia induce neurogenesis from adult neural stem cells. Nature 2002; 417:39–44.

73. Gould E, Reeves A, Graziano M. Neurogenesis in the neocortex of adult primates. Science 1999; 286:548–552.

74. Kornack D, Rakic P. Cell proliferation without neurogenesis in adult primate neocortex. Science 2001; 294:2127–2130.

75. Kempermann G. Why new neurons? Possible functions for adult hippocampal neurogenesis. J Neurosci 2002; 22:635–638.

76. Gould E, Gross C. Neurogenesis in adult mammals: some progress and some problems. J Neurosci 2002; 22:619–623.

77. Kiss J, Troncoso E, Djebbara Z, Vutskits L, Muller D. The role of neural cell adhesion molecules in plasticity and repair. Brain Res Rev 2001; 36:175–184.

78. Malenka R. LTP and LTD: Dynamic and interactive processes of synaptic plasticity. The Neuroscientist 1995; 1:35–42.

79. Benson D, Colman D, Huntley G. Molecules, maps and synapse specificity. Nat Rev/Neurosci 2001; 2:899–909.

80. Nudo R, Milliken G. Reorganization of movement representations in primary motor cortex following focal ischemic infarcts in adult squirrel monkeys. J Neurophysiol 1996; 75:2144–2149.

81. Barbay H, Plautz E, Friel K, Frost S, Nudo R. Delayed rehabiliative training following a small ischemic infarct in nonhuman primate primary motor cortex. Soc Neurosci Abstr 2001; 27:931.4.

82. Friel K, Heddings A, Nudo R. Effects of postlesion experience on behavioral recovery and neurophysiologic reorganization after cortical injury in primates. Neurorehabil Neural Repair 2000; 14:187–98.

83. Goertzen C, Yamagishi K, VandenBerg P, Kleim J. Neural and behavioural compensation following ischemic infarct within motor cortex is dependent upon the nature of motor rehabilitation experience. Soc For Neurosci Abstr 2001; 27:761.10.

84. Kleim J, Barbay S, Cooper N, Hogg T, Reidel C, Remple M, Nudo R. Motor learning-dependent synaptogenesis is localized to functionally reorganized motor cortex. Neurobiol Learn Mem 2002; 77:63–77.

85. Roy A, Paulignan Y, Frarne A, Jouffrais C, Boussaoud D. Hand kinematics during reaching and grasping in the macaque monkey. Behav Brain Res 2000; 117:75–82.

86. Biernaskie J, Corbett D. Enriched rehabilitative training promotes improved forelimb function and enhanced dendritic growth after focal ischemic injury. J Neurosci 2001; 21:5272–5280.

87. Stroemer R, Kent T, Hulsebosch C. Neocortical neural sprouting, synaptogenesis, and behavioral recovery after neocortical infarction in rats. Stroke 1995; 26:2135–2144.

88. Stroemer R, Kent T, Hulsebosch C. Enhanced neocortical neural sprouting, synaptogenesis and behavioral recovery with d-amphetamine therapy after neocortical infarction in rats. Stroke 1998; 29:2381–2395.

89. Jones T, Chu C, Grande L, Gregory A. Motor skills training enhances lesion-induced structural plasticity in the motor cortex of adult rats. J Neurosci 1999; 19:10153–10163.

90. Jones T, Kleim J, Greenough W. Synaptogenesis and dendritic growth in the cortex opposite unilateral sensorimotor cortex damage in adult rats: A quantitative electron microscopic examination. Brain Res 1996; 733:142–148.

91. Aguayo A, Rasminsky M, Bray G. Degenerative and regenerative responses of injured neurons in the central nervous system of adult mammals. Phil Trans R Soc Lond 1991; 331:337–343.

92. Benfey M, Aguayo A. Extensive elongation of axons from rat brain into peripheral nerve grafts. Nature 1982; 296:150–152.

93. Bush T, Puvanachandra N, Ostenfeld T, Sofroniew M, Horner C, Polito A, Svendsen C, Mucke L, Johnson M. Leukocyte infiltration, neuronal degeneration, and neurite outgrowth after ablation of scarforming, reactive astrocytes in adult transgenic mice. Neuron 1999; 23:297–308.

94. McKerracher L. Spinal cord repair: strategies to promote axon regeneration. Neurobiol Dis 2000:1–8.

95. Chen M, Huber A, van der Haar M, Frank M, Schnell L, Spillman A, Christ F, Schwab M. Nogo-A is a myelin-associated neurite outgrowth inhibitor and an antigen for monoclonal antibody IN-1. Nature 2000; 403:434–439.

96. Tessier-Lavigne M, Goodman C. Regeneration in the Nogo zone. Science 2000; 287:813–814.

97. Davies S, Fitch M, Memberg S, Hall A, Raisman G, Silver J. Regeneration of adult axons in white matter tracts of the central nervous system. Nature 1997; 390:680–683.

98. Davies S, Silver J. Adult sensory neurons regenerate axons through adult CNS white matter: Implications for functional restoration after SCI. Top Spinal Cord Inj Rehabil 2000; 6:27–41.

99. Karim F, Dietz V, Schwab M. Improving axonal growth and functional recovery after experimental spinal cord injury by neutralizing myelin-associated inhibitors. Brain Res Rev 2001; 36:204–212.

99a. Papadopoulos C, Tsai S-Y, Alsbiei T, O'Brien T, Schwab M, Kartje G. Functional recovery and neuroanatomical plasticity following middle cerebral artery occlusion and IN-1 antibody treatment in the adult rat. Ann Neurol 2002; S1:433–441.

100. Huang D, McKerracher L, Braun P, David S. A therapeutic vaccine approach to stimulate axon regeneration in the adult mammalian spinal cord. Neuron 1999; 24:639–647.

101. Moon L, Asher R, Rhodes K, Fawcett J. Regeneration of CNS axons back to their target following treatment of adult rat brain wth chondroitinase ABC. Nat Neurosci 2001; 4:465–466.

102. Condic M. Adult neuronal regeneration induced by transgenic integrin expression. J Neurosci 2001; 21:4782–4788.

103. Berry M, Gonzalez A, Clarke W, Greenlees L, Baird A, Barrett L, Tsang W, Seymour L, Bonadio J, Logan A. Sustained effects of gene-activated matrices after CNS injury. Mol Cell Neurosci 2001; 17:706–716.

104. Benowitz L, Goldberg D, Madsen J, Soni D, Irwin N. Inosine stimulates extensive axon collateral growth in the rat corticospinal tract after injury. Proc Natl Acad Sci USA 1999; 96:13486–13490.

105. Middlemiss P, Glasky A, Rathbone M, Werstuik E, Hindley S, Gysbers J. AIT-082, a unique purine derivative, enhances nerve growth factor mediated neurite outgrowth from PC12 cells. Neurosci Lett 1995; 199:131–134.

106. Cai D, Shen Y, De Ballard M, Tang S, Filbin M. Prior exposure to neurotrophins blocks inhibition of axonal regeneration by MAG and myelin via a cAMP-dependent mechanism. Neuron 1999; 22:89–101.

107. Filbin M. Overcoming inhibitors or regeneration in myelin. J Rehabil Res Develop 2001; 38(Suppl):S14.

108. Kromer L. Nerve growth factor treatment after brain injury prevents neuronal death. Science 1987; 235:214–216.

109. Kawaya M, Rosenberg M, Yoshida K, Gage F. Somatic gene transfer of nerve growth factor promotes survival of axotomized septal neurons and the regeneration of their axons in adult rats. J Neurosci 1992; 12:2849–2864.

109a. Raghupathi R, Graham D, McIntosh T. Apoptosis after traumatic brain injury. J Neurotrauma 2000; 17:927–938.

110. Yamada K, Kinoshita A, Kohmura E, Sakaguchi T, Taguchi J, Kataoka K, Hayakawa T. Basic fibroblast growth factor prevents thalamic degeneration after cortical infarction. J Cereb Blood Flow Metab 1991; 11:472–478.

111. Houle J, Ye J-H. Survival of chronically-injured neurons can be prolonged by treatment with neurotrophic factors. Neuroscience 1999; 94:929–936.

112. Henderson C, Phillips H, Pollock R, Davies AM, Lemeulle C, Armanini M, Simmons L, Moffet B, Vandlen RA, Simpson L. GDNF: A potent survival factor for motoneurons present in peripheral nerve and muscle. Science 1994; 266:1062–1064.

113. Sendtner M, Kreutzberg G, Thoenen H. Ciliary neurotrophic factor prevents the degeneration of motor neurons after axotomy. Nature 1990; 345:440–441.

114. Louis J, Magal E, Takayama S, Varon S. CNTF protection of oligodendrocytes against natural and tumor necrosis factor-induced death. Science 1993; 259:689–692.

115. McAllister K, Katz L, Lo D. Opposing roles for endogenous BDNF and NT-3 in regulating cortical dendritic growth. Neuron 1997; 18:767–778.

116. Gould E, Beylin A, Tanapat P, Reeves A, Shors T. Learning enhances adult neurogenesis in the hippocampal formation. Nat Neurosci 1999; 2:260–265.

117. Benraiss A, Chmielnicki E, Lerner K, Roh D, Goldman S. Adenviral brain-derived neurotrophic factor induces both neostriatal and olfactory neuronal recruitment from endogenous progenitor cells in the adult forebrain. J Neurosci 2001; 21:6718–6731.

118. Apfel S, Schwartz S, Adornato B, et al. Efficacy and safety of recombinant human nerve growth factor in patients with diabetic polyneuropathy. JAMA 2000; 284:2215–2221.

119. Miller R, Group. ACTS. A placebo-controlled trial of recombinant human ciliary neurotrophic (rhCNTF) factor in amyotrophic lateral sclerosis. Ann Neurol 1996; 39:256–260.

120. Kawamata T, Dietrich W, Schallert T, Gotts J, Benowitz L, Finkelstein S. Intracisternal basic fibroblast growth factor enhances functional recovery and up-regulates the expression of a molecular marker of neuronal sprouting following focal cerebral infarction. Proc Natl Acad Sci USA 1997; 94:8179–8184.

121. Snyder S, Sabatini D, Lai M, Steiner J, Hamilton G, Suzdak P. Neural action of immunophilin ligands. Science 1998; 19:21–26.

122. Kordower J, Palfi S, Chen E, Ma S, Comella C, Sendera T, Cochran E, Mufson E, Penn R, Goetz C. Clinicopathological findings following intraventricular glial-derived neurotrophic factor treatment in a patient with Parkinson's disease. Ann Neurol 1999; 46:419–424.

123. Zurn A, Widmer H, Aebischer P. Sustained delivery of GDNF: Towards a treatment for Parkinson's disease. Brain Res Rev 2001; 36:222–229.

124. Woerly S. Restorative surgery of the central nervous system by means of tissue engineering using NeuroGel implants. Neurosurg Rev 2000; 23:59–77.

125. Ooboshi H, Ibayashi S, Takada J, Yao H, Kitazono T, Fujishima M. Adenovirus-mediated gene transfer to ischemic brain. Stroke 2001; 32:1043–1047.

126. Kordower J, Emborg M, Bloch J, Ma S, Chu Y, Lev-

enthal L. Neurodegeneration prevented by lentiviral vector deliver of GDNF in primate models of Parkinson's disease. Science 2000; 290:767–724.

127. Turner D, Noordmans A, Feldman E, Boulis N. Remote adenoviral gene delivery to the spinal cord: Contralateral delivery and reinjection. Neurosurgery 2001; 48:1309–1316.

128. Rakic P. Neurocreationism—making new cortical maps. Science 2001; 294:1011–1012.

129. van Praag H, Kempermann G, Gage F. Running increases cell proliferation and neurogenesis in the adult mouse dentate gyrus. Nat Neurosci 1999; 2:266–270.

130. Shors T, Miesegaes G, Beylin A, Zhao M, Rydel T, Gould E. Neurogenesis in the adult is involved in the formation of trace memories. Nature 2001; 410:372–375.

131. Neeper S, Gomez-Pinella F, Choi J, Cotman C. Physical activity increases mRNA for brain-derived neurotrophic factor and nerve growth factor in rat brain. Brain Res 1996; 726:49–56.

132. Gomez-Pinilla F, Dao L, So V. Physical exercise induces FGF-2 and its mRNA in the hippocampus. Brain Res 1997; 764:1–8.

133. Trejo J, Carro E, Torres-Aleman I. Circulating insulin-like growth factor I mediates exercise-induced increases in the number of new neurons in the adult hippocampus. J Neurosci 2001; 21:1628–1634.

134. Pincus D, Keyoung H, Restelli C. Fibroblast growth factor-2/brain-derived neurotrophic factor-associated maturation of new neurons generated from adult human subependymal. Ann Neurol 1998; 43:576–585.

135. Wagner J, Black I, Bloom E. Stimulation of neonatal and adult brain neurogenesis by subcutaneous injection of basic fibroblast growth factor. J Neurosci 1999; 19:6006–6016.

136. Jiang W, Gu W, Brannstrom T, Rosqvist R, Wester P. Cortical neurogenesis in adult rats after transient middle cerebral artery occlusion. Stroke 2001; 32:1201–1207.

137. Yagita Y, Kitagawa K, Ohtsuki T, Takasawa K, Miyata T, Okano H, Hori M, Matsumoto M. Neurogenesis by progenitor cells in the ischemic adult rat hippocampus. Stroke 2001; 32:1890–1896.

138. Fisher L, Gage F. Grafting in the mammalian central nervous system. Physiol Rev 1993; 73:583–616.

139. Herrera D, Garcia-Verdugo J, Alvarez-Buylla A. Adult-derived neural precursors transplanted into multiple regions in the adult brain. Ann Neurol 1999; 46:867–877.

140. Fricker R, Carpenter M, Winkler C, Greco C, Gates M, Bjorklund A. Site-specific migration and neuronal differentiation of human neural progenitor cells after transplantation in the adult rat brain. J Neurosci 1999; 19:5990–6005.

141. Helt C, Hoernig G, Albeck D, Gerhardt G, Ickes B, Reyland M, Quissell D, Strömberg I, Granholm AC. Neuroprotection of grafted neurons with a GDNF/caspace inhibitor cocktail. Exp Neurol 2001; 170:258–269.

142. Mehler M, Kessler J. Progenitor cell biology: Implications for neural regeneration. Arch Neurol 1999; 56:780–784.

143. Snyder E. Neural stem-like cells: Developmental lessons with therapeutic potential. The Neuroscientist 1998; 4:408–425.

144. Snyder E, Deltcher D, Walsh C, Cepko C. Multipotent neural cell lines can engraft and participate in development of mouse cerebellum. Cell 1992; 68:33–51.

145. Franklin R, Barnett S. Olfactory ensheathing cells and CNS regeneration: The sweet smell of success. Neuron 2000; 28:15–18.

146. Iwashita Y, Blakemore W. Areas of demyelination do not attract significant numbers of Schwann cells transplanted into normal white matter. Glia 2000; 31:232–240.

147. Ramon-Cueto A, Plant G, Avila J, Bunge M. Long-distance axonal regeneration in the transected adult rat spinal cord is promoted by olfactory ensheathing glia transplants. J Neurosci 1998; 18:3803–3815.

148. Barnett S, Alexander C, Iwashita Y, Gilson J, Crowther J, Clark L, Dunn L, Papanastassiou V, Kennedy P, Franklin R. Identification of a human olfactory ensheathing cell that can affect transplant-mediated remyelination of demyelinated CNS axons. Brain 2000; 123:1581–1588.

149. MacLaren A. Ethical and social considerations of stem cell research. Nature 2001; 414:129–131.

150. Temple S. The development of neural stem cells. Nature 2001; 414:112–117.

151. Anderson D. Stem cells and pattern formation in the nervous system: The possible versus the actual. Neuron 2001; 30:19–35.

152. Freed C, Breeze R, Mazziotta J, Rosenberg NL, Schneck SA, Kriek E, Qi JX, Lone T, Zhang YB, Snyder JA, Wells TH. Survival of implanted fetal dopamine cells and neurologic improvement 12 to 48 months after transplantation for Parkinson's disease. N Engl J Med 1992; 327:1549–1555.

153. Spencer D, Robbins R, Naftolin F, Marek KL, Vollmer T, Leranth C, Roth RH, Price LH, Gjedde A, Bunney BS. Unilateral transplantation of human fetal mesencephalic tissue into the caudate nucleus of patients with Parkinson's disease. N Engl J Med 1992; 327:1541–1548.

154. Lindvall O, Sawle G, Widner H, Rothwell J, Bjorklund A, Brooks D, Brundin P, Frackowiak R, Marsden C, Odin P. Evidence for long-term survival and function of dopaminergic grafts in progressive Parkinson's disease. Ann Neurol 1994; 35:172–180.

155. Xu Z, Wilson C, Emson P. Synaptic potentials evoked in spiny neurons in rat neostriatal grafts by cortical and thalamic stimulation. J Neurophysiol 1991; 65:477–493.

156. Dunnett S. Repair of the damaged brain. Neuropathol Appl Neurobiol 1999; 25:351–362.

157. Bjorklund A, Lindvall O. Cell replacement therapies for central nervous system disorders. Neuroscience 2000; 3:537–544.

158. Freed C, Greene P, Breeze R, Tsai W, DuMouchel W, Kao R, Dillon S, Winfield H, Culver S, Trojanowski J, Eidelberg D, Fahn S. Transplantation of embryonic dopamine neurons for severe Parkinson's disease. New Engl J Med 2001; 344:710–719.

159. Deacon T, Schumacher J, Dinsmore J, Thomas C, Isacson O, Palmer P, Kott S, Edge A, Penney D, Kassissieh S, Dempsey P. Histological evidence of fetal pig neural cell survival after transplantation into a patient with parkinson's disease. Nat Med 1997; 3:350–353.

160. Hauser R, Furtado S, Cimino C, Delgado H, Eich-

ler S, Schwartz S, Scott D, Nauert G, Soety E, Sossi V, Holt D, Sanberg P, Stoessl A, Freeman T. Bilateral human fetal striatal transplantation in Huntington's disease. Neurology 2002; 58:687–695.

161. Bachoud-Levi A, Remy P, Nguyen J, Brugieres P, LeFaucher JP, Bourdet P, Baudic B, Gaura V, Maison P, Haddad B. Motor and cognitive improvements in patients with Huntington's disease after neural transplantation. Lancet 2000; 356:1975–1979.

162. Rosas H, Liu A, Hersh S, Glessner M, Fischl B, Ferrante R, Salat D, Van der Kouwe A, Jenkins B, Dale A. Regional and progressive thinning of the cortical ribbon in Huntington's disease. Neurology 2002; 58:695–701.

163. Magavi S, Leavitt B, Macklis J. Induction of neurogenesis in the neocortex of adult mice. Nature 2000; 405:951–955.

164. Shin J, Fricker-Gates R, Perez F, Leavitt B, Zurakowski D, Macklis J. Transplanted neuroblasts differentiate appropriately into projection neurons with correct neurotransmitter and receptor phenotype in neocortex undergoing targeted projection neuron degeneration. J Neurosci 2000; 20:7404–7416.

165. Grabowski M, Brundin P, Johansson B. Functional integration of cortical grafts in brain infarcts of rats. Ann Neurol 1993; 34:362–368.

166. Mattsson B, Sorensen J, Zimmer J, Johansson B. Neural grafting to experimental neocortical infarcts improves behavioral outcome and reduces thalamic atrophy in rats housed in enriched but not in standard environments. Stroke 1997; 28:1225–1232.

167. Klintsova A, Greenough W. Synaptic plasticity in cortical systems. Curr Opin Neurobiol 1999; 9:203–208.

168. Bragin A, Vinogradova O, Stafekhina V. Sensory deprivation prevents integration of neocortical grafts with the host brain. Rest Neurol Neurosci 1992; 4:279–283.

169. Brasted P, Watts C, Robbins T, Dunnett S. Associative plasticity in striatal transplants. Proc Natl Acad Sci USA 1999; 96:10524–10529.

170. Takahashi A, Honmou O, Sasaki M, Oka S, Uede T, Hashi K. Transplantation of human neural stem cells repairs the ischemic lesions in the rat middle cerebral occlusion model. Soc Neurosci Abstr 2001; 27:371.6.

171. Chen J, Li Y, Wang L, Zhang Z, Lu D, Lu M, Chopp M. Therapeutic benefit of intravenous administration of bone marrow stromal cells after cerebral ischemia in rats. Stroke 2001; 32:1005–1011.

172. Veizovic T, Beech J, Stroemer R, Watson W, Hodges H. Resolution of stroke deficits following contralateral grafts of conditionally immortal neuroepithelial stem cells. Stroke 2001; 32:1012–1019.

173. Borlongan C, Tajima Y, Trojanowski J. Transplantation of cryopreserved human embryonal carcinoma-derived neurons (NT2N cells) promotes functional recovery in ischemic rats. Exp Neurol 1998; 149: 310–321.

174. Kondziolka D, Wechsler L, Goldstein S, Meltzer C, Thulborn K, Gebel J, Janetta P, Decesare S, Elder E, McGrogan M, Reitman M, Bynum L. Transplantation of cultured human neuronal cells for patients with stroke. Neurology 2000; 55:565–569.

175. Brustle O, Jones K, Learish R. Embryonic stem cell-derived glial precursors: A source of myelinating transplants. Science 1999; 285:754–756.

176. Learish R, Brustle O, Zhang S. Intraventricular transplantation of oligodendrocyte progenitors into a fetal myelin mutant results in widespread formation of myelin. Ann Neurol 1999; 46:716–722.

177. Keirstead H, Hur T, Rogister B. Polysialylated neural cell adhesion molecule-positive CNS precursors generate both oligodendrocytes and Schwann cells to remyelinate the CNS after transplantation. J Neurosci 1999; 19:7529–7536.

178. Chang A, Nishiyama A, Peterson J, Prineas J, Trapp B. NG2-positive oligodendrocyte progenitor cells in adult human brain and multiple sclerosis lesions. Neuroscience 2000; 2000:6404–6412.

179. Wolswijk G. Oligodendrocyte precursor cells in the demyelinated multiple sclerosis spinal cord. Brain 2002; 125:338–349.

180. Boyeson M, Jones J, Harmon R. Sparing of motor function after cortical injury. Arch Neurol 1994; 51:405–414.

181. Goldstein L. Pharmacology of recovery after stroke. Stroke 1990; 21(suppl III):139–142.

182. Davis F, Stefoski D, Rush J. Orally dministered 4-AP improves clinical signs in multiple sclerosis. Ann Neurol 1990; 27:186–192.

183. Waxman S, Ritchie J. Molecular dissection of the myelinated axon. Ann Neurol 1993; 33:121–136.

184. Pette D, Staron R. Cellular and molecular diversities of mammalian skeletal muscle fibers. Rev Physiol Biochem Pharmacol 1990; 116:1–76.

184a. Janssen I, Heymsfield S, Ross R. Low relative skeletal muscle mass (sarcopenia) in older persons is associated with functional impairment and physical disability. J Am Geriatr Soc 2002; 50:889–896.

185. Baldwin K. Effects of altered loading states on muscle plasticity: what have we learned from rodents? Med Sci Sports Exerc 1996; 28:S101–S106.

186. Deschenes M, Judelson D, Kraemer W, Meskaitis V, Volek J, Nindl B, Harman F, Deaver D. Effects of resistance training on neuromuscular junction morphology. Muscle Nerve 2000; 23:1576–81.

187. Edgerton V, Roy R, Hodgson J, Day MK, Weiss J, Harkema S, Dobkin B, Garfinkel A, Konigsberg E, Koslovskaya I. How the science and engineering of spaceflight contribute to understanding the plasticity of spinal cord injury. Acta Astronautica 2000; 47:51–62.

188. Roy R, Baldwin K, Edgerton V. The plasticity of skeletal muscle: Effects of neuromuscular activity. In: Holloszy J, ed. Exercise and Sports Reviews. Baltimore: Williams and Wilkins, 1991:269–312.

189. Hunter GR, Newcomer BR, Larson-Meyer DE, Bamman MM, Weinsier RL. Muscle metabolic economy is inversely related to exercise intensity and type II myofiber distribution. Muscle Nerve 2001; 24:654–661.

190. Baldwin K. Research in the exercise sciences: Where do we go from here? J Appl Physiol 2000; 88:332–336.

191. Edgerton V, Roy R. Gravitational biology of the neuromotor systems: A perspective to the next era. Appl Physiol 2000; 89:1224–31.

192. Goldspink G. Changes in muscle mass and phenotype and the expression of autocrine and systemic growth factors by muscle in response to stretch and overload. J Anat 1999; 194:323–334.

193. Singleton J, Feldman E. Insulin-like growth factor-

1 in muscle metabolism and myotherapies. Neurobiol Dis 2001; 8:541–554.

194. Barton-Davis E, Shoturma D, Musaro A, Rosenthal N, Sweeney H. Viral mediated expression of insulin-like growth factor I blocks the aging-related loss of skeletal muscle function. Proc Natl Acad Sci USA 1998; 95:15603–15607.

195. Chakravarthy M, Davis B, Booth F. IGF-I restores satellite cell proliferative potential in immobilized old skeletal muscle. Appl Physiol 2000; 89:1365–79.

196. Guttridge D, Mayo M, Madrid L, Wang C, Baldwin A. NF-kappaB-induced loss of myoD messenger RNA: Possible role in muscle decay and cachexia. Science 2000; 289:2363–2365.

197. Funakoshi H, Belluardo N, Arenas E, Yamamoto Y, Casabona A, Persson H, Ibanez C. Muscle-derived neurotrophin-4 as an activity-dependent trophic signal for adult motor neurons. Science 1995; 268: 1495–1499.

198. Aisen M, Brown W, Rubin M. Electrophysiologic changes in lumbar spinal cord after cervical cord injury. Neurology 1992; 42:623–626.

199. Brown W, Snow R. Denervation in hemiplegic muscles. Stroke 1990; 21:1700–1704.

200. Qiu Y, Wada Y, Otomo E, Tsukagoshi H. Morphometric study of cervical anterior horn cells and pyramidal tracts in medulla oblongata and the spinal cord in patients with cerebrovascular diseases. J Neuro Sci 1991; 102:137–143.

201. Frontera W, Grimby L, Larsson L. Firing rate of the lower motoneuron and contractile properties of its muscle fibers after upper motoneuron lesion in man. Muscle Nerve 1997; 20:938–947.

202. Gordon T, Mao J. Muscle atrophy and procedures for training after spinal cord injury. Phys Ther 1994; 74:50–60.

203. Hakkinen K. Neuromuscular adaptation during strength training, aging, detraining, and immobilization. Crit Rev Phys Rehabil Med 1994; 6:161–198.

204. Vrobova G. The concept of neuromuscular plasticity. J Neuro Rehab 1989; 3:1–6.

205. Booth F, Thomason D. Molecular and cellular adaptation of muscle in response to exercise: perspectives of various models. Physiol Rev 1991; 71:541–585.

206. Dobs A. Is there a role for androgenic anabolic steroids in medical practice. JAMA 1999; 281:1326–1327.

207. Gupta K, Shetty K, Agre J, Cuisinier M, Rudman I, Rudman D. Human growth hormone effect on serum IGF-I and muscle function in poliomyelitis survivors. Arch Phys Med Rehabil 1994; 75:889–894.

208. Booth F, Tseng B. Molecular and cellular approaches to understanding muscle adaptation. NIPS 1993; 8:165–169.

209. Yarasheski K, Zachwieja J. Growth hormone therapy for the elderly. JAMA 1993; 270:1694–1698.

210. Signorile J, Banovac K, Gomez M, Flipse D, Caruso F, Lowensteyn I. Increased muscle strength in paralyzed patients after spinal cord injury: Effect of beta-2 adrenergic agonist. Arch Phys Med Rehabil 1995; 76:55–58.

211. Kissel J, McDermott M, Mendell J, King W, Pandya S, Griggs R, Tawil R. Randomized, double-blinded, placebo-controlled trial of albuterol in facioscapulohumeral dystrophy. Neurology 2001; 57:1434–1440.

212. Kjaer M, Mohr T. Substrate mobilization, delivery, and utilization in physical exercise: Regulation by hormones in healthy and diseased humans. Crit Rev Phys Rehabil Med 1994; 6:317–336.

212a. Onder G, Pennix B, Balkrishnan R, Fried L, Chaves P, Guralnik J, Pahor M. Relation between use of angiotensin-converting enzyme inhibitors and muscle strength and physical function in older women. Lancet 2002; 359:926–930.

212b. Williams AG, Rayson M, Jobb M. The ACE gene and muscle performance. Nature 2000; 403:614–615.

213. Grounds M. Muscle regeneration: Molecular aspects and therapeutic implications. Curr Opin Neurol 1999; 12:535–543.

214. White J, Bower J, Kurek J, Austin L. Leukemia inhibitory factor enhances regeneration in skeletal muscles after myoblast transplantation. Muscle Nerve 2001; 24:695–697.

215. Desgranges P, Barbaud C, Caruelle J-P, Barritault D, Gautron J. A substituted dextran enhances muscle fiber survival and regeneration in ischemic and denervated rat EDL muscle. FASEB J 1999; 13: 761–766.

216. Feng G, Laskowski M, Feldheim D, Wang H, Sanes J, Lewis R, Frisen J, Flanagan J. Roles for ephrins in positionally selective synaptogenesis between motor neurons and muscle fibers. Neuron 2000; 25:295–306.

217. Fletcher S, Wilton S, Howell J. Gene therapy and molecular approaches to the treatment of hereditary muscular disorders. Curr Opin Neurol 2000; 13: 553–60.

218. Harkema S, Dobkin B, Requejo P, Edgerton V. Effect of assisted treadmill step training on EMG patterns and muscle volumes in spinal cord injured subjects. J Neurotrauma 1995; 12:121.

219. Kramer J. Muscle strengthening via electrical stimulation. Crit Rev Phys Rehabil Med 1989; 1:97–133.

220. Pette D, Vrbova G. What does chronic electrical stimulation teach us about muscle plasticity? Muscle Nerve 1999; 22:666–677.

221. Fleckenstein J, Weatherall P, Bertocci L, Haller R, Greenlee R, Bryan W, Peshock R. Locomotor system assessment by muscle magnetic resonance imaging. Magnetic Res Quart 1991; 7:79–103.

222. Fukunaga T, Roy R, Edgerton V, Shellock F, Hodgson J, Day M, Lee P, Kwong-Fu H. Physiological cross-sectional area of human leg muscles based on magnetic resonance imaging. J Orthop Res 1992; 10:926–934.

223. Durozard D, Gabrielle C, Baverel G. Metabolism of rat skeletal muscle after spinal cord transection. Muscle Nerve 2000; 23:1561–1568.

224. Bregman B, Diener P, McAtee M, Dai H, James C. Intervention strategies to enhance anatomical plasticity and recovery of function after spinal cord injury. In: Seil F, ed. Neural Regeneration, Reorganization, and Repair. Philadelphia: Lippencott-Raven Publishing, 1997:257–275.

225. Grill R, Murai K, Blesch A, Gage F, Tuszynski M. Cellular delivery of neurotrophin-3 promotes corticospinal axonal growth and partial functional recovery after spinal cord injury. J Neurosci 1997; 17:5560–5572.

226. Li Y, Field P, Raisman G. Repair of adult rat corticospinal tract by transplants of olfactory ensheathing cells. Science 1997; 277:2000–2002.

227. Z'Graggen W, Metz A, Kartje G, Thallmair M, Schwab M. Functional recovery and enhanced corticofugal plasticity after unilateral pyramidal tract lesion and blockade of myelin-associated neurite growth inhibitors in adult rats. J Neurosci 1998; 18:4744–4757.

228. Ramon-Cueto A, Cordero M, Santos-Benito F, Avila J. Functional recovery of paraplegic rats and motor axon regeneration in their spinal cords by olfactory ensheathing glia. Neuron 2000; 25:425–436.

229. Ramer M, Priestley J, McMahon S. Functional regeneration of sensory axons into the adult spinal cord. Nature 2000; 403:312–316.

230. Blight A. Cellular morphology of chronic spinal cord injury in the cat: Analysis of myelinated axons by line-sampling. Neuroscience 1983; 10:521–543.

231. Kaelan C, Jacobsen P, Morling P, Kakulas B. A quantitative study of motoneurons and corticospinal fibres related to function in human spinal cord injury (abstract). Paraplegia 1989; 27:148–9.

232. Bracken M, Shepard M, Holford T, Leo-Summers L, Marshall L, Young W. Administration of methylprednisolone for 24 or 48 hours or tirilazad mesylate for 48 hours in the treatment of acute spinal cord injury. JAMA 1997; 277:1597–1604.

233. Schwartz M, Kipnis J. Protective autoimmunity: regulation and prospects for vaccination after brain and spinal cord injuries. Trends Mol Med 2001; 7: 252–258.

234. Houle J, Jin Y. Chronically injured supraspinal neurons exhibit only modest axonal dieback in response to a cervical hemisection. Exp Neurol 2001; 169: 208–217.

234a. Kwon BK, Liu J, Messerer C, Kobayashi N, McGraw J, Oschipok L, Tetzlaff W. Survival and regeneration of rubrospinal neurons 1 year after spinal cord injury. PNAS 2002; 99:3246–3251.

235. Gimenez y Ribotta M, Privat A. Biological interventions for spinal cord injury. Curr Opin Neurol 1998; 11:647–654.

236. Nishi R. Neurotrophic factors: Two are better than one. Science 1994; 265:1052–1053.

237. Beattie M, Farooqui A, Bresnahan J. Review of current evidence for apoptosis after spinal cord injury. J Neurotrauma 2000; 17:915–925.

238. Yuan J, Yankner B. Apoptosis in the nervous system. Nature 2000; 407:802–809.

239. Popovich P. Immunological regulation of neuronal degeneration and regeneration in the injured spinal cord. In: Seil F, ed. Neural Plasticity and Regeneration. Amsterdam: Elsevier, 2000:43–58.

240. Zeman R, Feng Y, Peng H, Vistainer P, Etlinger J, Moorthy C, Couldwell W. X-irradiation of the contusion site improves locomotor and histological outcomes in spinal cord-injured rats. Exper Neurol 2001; 172:228–234.

241. Schwartz M, Moalem G. Beneficial immune activity after CNS injury: Prospects for vaccination. J Neuroimmunology 2001; 113:185–192.

241a. Jones TB, Basso DM, Sodhi A, Pan J, Hart R, Popovich P. Pathological CNS autoimmune disease triggered by traumatic spinal cord injury. J Neurosci 2002; 22:2690–2700.

242. Hill C, Beattie M, Bresnahan J. Degeneration and sprouting of identified descending supraspinal axons after contusive spinal cord injury in the rat. Exp Neurol 2001; 171:153–169.

243. Schnell L, Schwab M. Axonal regeneration in the rat spinal cord produced by an antibody against myelin-asociated neurite growth inhibitors. Nature 1990; 343:269–272.

244. GrandPre T, Nakamura F, Vartanian T, Strittmatter S. Identification of the Nogo inhibitor of axon regeneration as a reticulon protein. Nature 2000; 403:439–444.

245. Schnell L, Schneider R, Schwab M, Kolbeck R, Barde Y. Neurotrophin-3 enhances sprouting of corticospinal tract during development and after adult spinal cord lesion. Nature 1994; 367:170–173.

246. Merkler D, Metz G, Raineteau O, Dietz V, Schwab ME, Fouad K. Locomotor recovery in spinal cord-injured rats treated with an antibody neutralizing the myelin-associated neurite growth inhibitor Nogo-A. J Neurosci 2001; 21:3665–3673.

247. Brosamle C, Huber A, Fiedler M, Skerra A, Schwab M. Regeneration of lesioned corticospinal tract fibers in the adult rat induced by a recombinant, humanized IN-1 antibody fragment. J Neurosci 2000; 20:8061–8068.

248. Bregman B, Kunkel-Bagden E, Schnell L, Dai H, Gao D, Schwab M. Recovery from spinal cord injury mediated by antibodies to neurite growth inhibitors. Nature 1995; 378:498–501.

248a. GrandPre T, Li S, Strittmatter S. Nogo-66 receptor antagonist peptide promotes axonal regeneration. Nature 2002; 417:547–551.

248b. Wang KC, Koprivica V, Neve R, Ho Z. Oligodendrocyte-myelin glycoprotein is a Nogo receptor ligand that inhibits neurite outgrowth. Nature 2002; 417:941–944.

248c. Neumann S, Bradke F, Tessier-Lavigne M. Aegeneration of sensory axons within the injured spinal cord induced by intraganglionic cAMP elevation. Neuron 2002; 34:885–893.

249. Plant G, Bates M, Bunge M. Inhibitory proteoglycan immunoreactivity is higher at the caudal than the rostral Schwann cell graft-transected spinal cord interface. Molec Cell Neurosci 2001; 17:471–487.

250. Li Y, Field P, Raisman G. Regeneration of adult rat corticospinal axons induced by transplanted olfactory ensheathing cells. Neuroscience 1998; 18: 10514–10524.

251. Lu J, Feron F, Mackay-Sim A, Waite P. Olfactory ensheathing cells promote locomotor recovery after delayed transplantation into transected spinal cord. Brain 2002; 125:14–21.

252. Liu Y, Kim D, Himes T. Transplants of fibroblasts genetically modified to express BDNF promote regeneration of adult rat rubrospinal axons and recovery of forelimb function. J Neurosci 1999; 19: 4370–4387.

253. Fehlings M, Tator C. The effect of direct current field polarity on recovery after experimental spinal cord injury. Brain Res 1992; 579:32–42.

254. Borgens R. Electrically mediated regeneration and guidance of adult mammalian spinal axons into polymeric channels. Neurosci 1999; 91:251–264.

254a. McCraig C, Rajnicek A, Song B, Zhao M. Has electrical growth cone guidance found its potential? Trends Neurosci 2002; 25:354–359.

255. Faissner A. Glial derived extracellular matrix components: Important roles in axon growth and guidance. The Neuroscientist 1997; 3:371–380.

256. Cheng H, Cao Y, Olson L. Spinal cord repair in adult

paraplegic rats: Partial restoration of hind limb function. Science 1996; 273:510–514.

257. Wang M, Gold B. FK506 increases the regeneration of spinal cord axons in a predegenerated peripheral nerve autograft. J Spinal Cord Med 1999; 22:287–296.

258. Bamber N, Li H, Aebischer P. Fetal spinal cord tissue in mini-guidance channels promotes longitudinal axonal growth after grafting in to hemisected adult rat spinal cords. Neural Plast 1999; 6:103–121.

259. Chauhan N, Figlewicz H, Khan T. Carbon filaments direct the growth of postlesional plastic axons after spinal cord injury. Int J Devl Neurosci 1999; 17: 255–264.

259a. Teng YD, Lavik E, Qu X, Park K, Ourednik J, Snyder EY. Functional recovery following traumatic spinal cord injury mediated by a unique polymer scaffold seeded with neural stem cells. Proc Natl Acad Sci USA 2002; 99:3024–3029.

260. Loh N, Woerly S, Bunt SM, Wilton S, Harvey A. The regrowth of axons within tissue defects in the CNS is promoted by implanted hydrogel matrices that contain BDNF and CNTF producing fibroblasts. Exp Neurol 2001; 170:72–84.

261. Lee K, Peters M, Anderson K, Mooney D. Controlled growth factor release from synthetic extracellular matrices. Nature 2000; 408:998–1000.

262. Hadlock T, Sundback C, Koka R. A novel, biodegradable polymer conduit delivers neurotrophins and promotes nerve regeneration. Laryngoscope 1999; 109:1412–1416.

263. Schlosshauer B, Brinker T, Muller H-W, Meyer J-U. Towards micro electrode implants: in vitro guidance of rat spinal cord neurites through polyimide sieves by Schwann cells. Brain Res 2001; 903:237–241.

264. Blight A. Remyelination, revascularization, and recovery of function in experimental spinal cord injury. In: Seil F, ed. Spinal Cord Injury. New York: Raven Press, 1993:91–104.

265. Bunge R, Puckett W, Becerra J. Observations on the pathology of human spinal cord injury. In: Seil F, ed. Spinal Cord Injury. Vol. 59. New York: Raven Press, 1993:75–89.

266. Segal J, Pathak M, Hernandez J. Safety and efficacy of 4-aminopyridine in humans with spinal cord injury: a long-term, controlled trial. Pharmacotherapy 1999; 19:713–723.

267. Prineas J, Barnard R, Kwon E, Sharer L, Cho E. Multiple sclerosis: Remyelination of nascent lesions. Ann Neurol 1993; 33:137–151.

268. McTigue D, Horner P, Stokes B, Gage F. Neurotrophin-3 and brain-derived neurotrophic factor induce oligodendrocyte proliferation and myelination of regenerating axons in the contused adult rat spinal cord. J Neuroscience 1998; 18:5354–5365.

269. Liu S, Qu Y, Stewart T, Howard M, Chakrabortty S, Holekamp T, McDonald JW. Embryonic stem cells differentiate into oligodendrocytes and myelinate in culture and after spinal cord transplantation. Proc Natl Acad Sci USA 2000; 97:6126–6131.

270. Pinzon A, Calancie B, Oudega M, Noga B. Conduction of impulses by axons regenerated in a Schwann cell graft in the transected adult rat thoracic spinal cord. J Neurosci Res 2001; 64:533–541.

271. Honmou O, Felts P, Waxman S, Kocsis J. Restoration of normal conduction properties in demyeli-

nated spinal cord axons in the adult rat by transplantation of exogenous Schwann cells. J Neurosci 1996; 16:3199–3208.

272. Weidner N, Blesch A, Grill R, Tuszynski M. Nerve growth factor-hypersecreting Schwann cell grafts augment and guide spinal cord axonal growth and remyelinate central nervous system axons in a phenotypically appropriate manner. J Comp Neurol 1999; 413:495–506.

273. Compston A. Development, Injury, and Repair of CNS Glia, 119th Annual Meeting of the American Neurological Association, San Francisco, CA, 1994.

274. Akiyama Y, Honmou O, Kato T, Uede T, Hashi K, Kocsis J. Transplantation of clonal neural precursor cells derived from adult human brain establishes functional peripheral myelin in the rat spinal cord. Exp Neurol 2001; 167:27–39.

275. Tessler A. Intraspinal transplants. Ann Neurol 1991; 29:115–123.

276. Yakovleff A, Roby-Brami A, Guezard B, Mansour H, Bussel B, Privat A. Locomotion in rats transplanted with noradrenergic neurons. Brain Res Bull 1989; 22:115–121.

277. Gimenez y Ribotta M, Provencher J, Feraboli-Lohnherr D, Rossignol S, Privat A, Orsal D. Activation of locomotion in adult chronic spinal rats is achieved by transplantation of embryonic raphe cells reinnervating a precise lumbar level. J Neurosci 2000; 20:5144–5152.

278. Kim D, Adipudi V, Shibayama M, Giszter S, Tessler A, Murray M, Simansky K. Direct agonists for serotonin receptors enhance locomotor function in rats that received neural transplants after neonatal spinal transection. Neuroscience 1999; 19:6213–6224.

279. Bregman B, Reier P, Kunkel-Bagden E, Reier P, Dai H, McAtee M, Gao D. Recovery of function after spinal cord injury: Mechanisms underlying transplant-mediated recovery of function differ after spinal cord injury in newborn and adult rats. Exp Neurol 1993; 123:3–16.

280. Giszter SF, Kargo WJ, Davies M, Shibayama M. Fetal transplants rescue axial muscle representations in M1 cortex of neonatally transected rats that develop weight support. J Neurophysiol 1998; 80:3021–3030.

281. Itoh Y, Miozi K, Tessler A. Embryonic central nervous system transplants mediate adult dorsal root regeneration into host spinal cord. J Neurosurg 1999; 45:849–858.

282. Coumans J, Lin T, Dai H, MacArthur L, Bregman B, McAtee M, Nash C. Axonal regeneration and functional recovery after complete spinalcord transection in rats by delayed treatment with transplants and neurotrophins. J Neurosci 2001; 21:9334–9344.

283. Ye J, Houle J. Treatment of the chronically injured spinal cord with neurotrophic factors can promote axonal regeneration from supraspinal neurons. Exp Neurol 1997; 143:70–81.

284. Wirth E, Reier P, Howland D, Anderson D. Fetal grafting in animal models of spinal cord injury. Top Spinal Cord Inj Rehabil 2000; 6:52–64.

285. McDonald J, Liu X-Z, Qu Y, Liu S, Mickey SK, Turetsky D, Gottlieb DI, Choi DW. Transplanted embryonic stem cells survive, differentiate, and promote recovery in injured rat spinal cord. Nat Med 1999; 5:1410–1412.

286. Kalyani A, Piper D, Mujtaba T, Lucero M, Rao M. Spinal cord neuronal precursors generate multiple

neuronal phenotypes in culture. J Neurosci 1998; 18:7856–7868.

287. Wu S, Suzuki Y, Kitada M, Kitaura M, Nishimura Y. Migration, integration, annd differentiation of hippocampus-derived neurosphere cells after transplantation into injured rat spinal cord. Neurosci Lett 2001; 312:173–176.

288. Bowe C, Beale R, Carlsen R. Long-term changes in spinal motor neurons after injury. In: Seil F, ed. Neuronal Regeneration, Reorganization, and Repair. Philadelphia: Lippincott-Raven, 1997:201–215.

289. Clowry G, Sieradzan K, Vrbova G. Transplants of embryonic motoneurones to adult spinal cord: survival and innervation abilities. Trends Neurosci 1991; 14:355–357.

290. Rothstein J, Llado J, Teng Y, Kerr D, Snyder E. Transplantation of embryoid body-derived cells in motor neuron lesioned African green monkeys. Soc Neurosci Abstr 2001; 27:369.14.

291. Havton L, Kellerth J-O. Regeneration of supernumerary axons with synaptic terminals in spinal motoneurons of cats. Nature 1987; 325:711–714.

292. Al-Majed A, Neumann C, Brushart T, Gordon T. Brief electrical stimulation promotes the speed and accuracy of motor axonal regeneration. J Neurosci 2000; 20:2602–2608.

293. Hallin R, Carlstedt T, Nilsson-Remahl I, Risling M. Spinal cord inplantation of avulsed ventral roots in primates; correlation between restored motor function and morphology. Exp Brain Res 1999; 124:304–310.

294. Hoffmann C, Marani E, Dijk J. Reinnervation of avulsed and reimplanted ventral rootlets in the cervical spinal cord of the cat. J Neurosurg 1996; 84:234–243.

295. Nieto J, Hoang T, Tillakaratne N, Havton L. Avulsed lumbosacral ventral roots implanted into the spinal cord promote survival of lesioned preganglionic parasympathetic neurons. Soc Neurosci Abstr 2001; 27:829.11.

296. Carlstedt T, Anand P, Hallin R, Misra P, Noren G, Seferlis T. Spinal nerve root repair and reimplantation of avulsed ventral roots into the spinal cord after brachial plexus injury. J Neurosurg 2000; 93:237–247.

297. Aldrich E, Dobkin B, Kim B, Edgerton V. A new model of experimental lumbar spinal cord injury and treatment with intrathecal BDNF. Exp Neurol 1998; 51:158.

298. Novikov L, Novikova L, Kellerth J-O. Brain-derived neurotrophic factor promotes axonal regeneration and long-term survival of adult rat spinal motoneurons in vivo. Neuroscience 1997; 79:765–774.

299. Gold B, Zeleny-Pooley M, Chaturvedi P, Wang M. Oral administration of a nonimmunosuppressant FKBP-12 ligand speeds nerve regeneration. Neuroreport 1998; 16:553–558.

300. Rhrich-Haddout F, Kassar-Duchossoy L, Bauchet L, Destombes J, Thiesson D, Butler-Brown G, Lyoussi B, Baillet-Derbin C, Horvat JC. Alpha-motoneurons of the injured cervical spinal cord of the adult rat can reinnervate the biceps brachii muscle by regenerating axons through peripheral nerve bridges: Combined ultrastructural and retrograde axonal tracing study. J Neurosci Research 2001; 64:476–486.

301. Liu S, Aghakhani N, Boisset N, Said G, Tadie M. Innervation of the caudal denervated ventral roots and their target muscles by the rostral spinal motoneurons after implanting a nerve autograft in spinal cord-injured adult marmosets. J Neurosurg 2001; 94:82–90.

302. Xiao C, de Groat W, Godec C, Dai C, Xiao Q. "Skin-CNS-bladder" reflex pathway for micturition after spinal cord injury and its underlying mechanisms. Urology 1999; 162:936–942.

303. Havton L, Hotson J, Kellerth J-O. Partial peripheral motor nerve lesions induce changes in the conduction properties of remaining intact motoneurons. Muscle Nerve 2001; 24:662–666.

304. Tam SL, Archibald V, Jassar B, Tyreman N, Gordon T. Increased neuromuscular activity reduces sprouting in partially denervated muscles. J Neurosci 2001; 21:654–667.

304a. Stieglitz T, Ruf H, Gross M, Schuettler M, Meyer JU. A biohybrid system to interface peripheral nerves after traumatic lesions: design of a high channel sieve electrode. Biosens Bioelectron 2002; 17:685–696.

305. Krenz N, Meakin S, Krassioukov A. Neutralizing intraspinal nerve growth factor blocks autonomic dysreflexia caused by spinal cord injury. J Neurosci 1999; 19:7405–7414.

306. Bradbury E, Khemani S, King V. NT-3 promotes growth of lesioned adult rat sensory axons ascending in the dorsal columns of the spinal cord. Eur J Neurosci 1999; 11:3873–3883.

307. Ramer M, Duraisingam I, Priestly J, McMahon S. Two-tiered inhibitiion of axon regeneration at the dorsal root entry zone. J Neurosci 2001; 21:2651–2660.

308. Romero M, Rangappa N, Garry M, Smith G. Functional regeneration of chronically injured sensory afferents into adult spinal cord after neurotrophin gene therapy. J Neurosci 2001; 21:8408–8416.

309. Zhang Y, Tohyama K, Winterbottom J, Haque NSK, Schachner M, Lieberman AR, Anderson PN. Correlation between putative inhibitory molecules at the dorsal root entry zone and failure of dorsal root axonal regeneration. Mol Cell Neurosci 2001; 17:444–459.

310. Sugawara T, Itoh Y, Mizoi K. Immunosuppressants promote adult dorsal root regeneration into the spinal cord. Neuroreport 1999; 10:3949–3953.

311. Wizenmann A, Thies E, Klostermann S, Bonhoeffer F, Bahr M. Appearance of target-specific guidance information for regenerating axons after CNS lesions. Neuron 1993; 11:975–983.

312. Davey N, Smith H, Savic G, Maskill D, Ellaway P, Frankel H. Comparison of input-output patterns in the corticospinal system of normal subjects and incomplete spinal cord injured patients. Exp Brain Res 1999; 127:382–390.

313. Jain N, Catania K, Kaas J. Deactivation and reactivation of somatosensory cortex after dorsal spinal cord injury. Nature 1997; 386:495–498.

314. Cohen L, Topka H, Cole R, Hallett M. Paresthesias induced by magnetic brain stimulation in patients with thoracic spinal cord injury. Neurology 1991; 41:1283–1288.

315. Bruehlmeier M, Dietz V, Leenders K, Roelcke U, Missimer J, Curt A. How does the human brain deal

with a spinal cord injury? Euro J Neurosci 1998; 10:3918–3922.

316. Wu C, Kaas J. Reorganization in primary motor cortex of primates with long-standing therapeutic amputations. J Neurosci 1999; 19:7679–7697.

317. Edgerton V, de Leon R, Harkema S, Hodgson J, London N, Reinkensmeyer D, Roy R, Talmadge R, Tillakaratne N, Timoszuk W, Tobin A. Retraining the injured spinal cord. J Physiol 2001; 533:15–22.

318. Harkema S, Hurley S, Patel U, Dobkin B, Edgerton V. Human lumbosacral spinal cord interprets loading during stepping. J Neurophysiol 1997; 77: 797–811.

319. Dobkin B. Overview of treadmill locomotor training with partial body weight support: A neurophysiologically sound approach whose time has come for randomized clinical trials. Neurorehabil Neural Repair 1999; 13:157–165.

320. Soblosky J, Song J-H, Dinh D. Graded unilateral cervical spinal cord injury in the rat: evaluation of forelimb recovery and histological effects. Behav Brain Res 2001; 119:1–13.

321. McAuley M. Rodent models of focal ischemia. Cerebrovasc Brain Metab Rev 1995; 7:153–180.

322. Ginsberg M, Busto R. Rodent models of cerebral ischemia. Stroke 1989; 20:1627–1642.

323. Dixon C, Hayes R. Fluid percussion and cortical impact models of traumatic brain injury. In: Narayan R, Wilberger J, Povlishock J, eds. Neurotrauma. New York: McGraw-Hill, 1996:1337–1346.

324. Blight A. Animal models of spinal cord injury. Top Spinal Cord Inj Rehabil 2000; 6:1–13.

325. Roundtable. STAI. Recommendations for standards regarding preclinical neuroprotective and restorative drug development. Stroke 1999; 30:2752–2758.

326. Schallert T, Fleming S, Leasure J. CNS plasticity and assessment of forelimb sensorimotor outcome in unilateral rat models of stroke, cortical ablation, parkinsonism and spinal cord injury. Neuropharmacology 2000; 39:777–787.

327. Kipnis J, Yoles E, Schori H, Hauben E, Shaked I, Schwartz M. Neuronal survival after CNS insult is determined by a genetically encoded autoimmune response. J Neurosci 2001; 21:4564–4571.

328. Mills C, Hains B, Johnson K, Hulsebosch C. Strain and model differences in behavioral outcomes after spinal cord injury in rat. J Neurotrauma 2001; 18: 743–756.

329. Iwaniuk A, Whishaw I. On the origin of skilled forelimb movements. Trends Neurosci 2000; 23:372–376.

330. Steward O, Schauwecker P, Guth L, Zhang Z, Fujiki M, Inman D, Wrathall J, Kempermann G, Gage F, Saatman K, Raghupathl R, McIntosh T. Genetic approaches to neurotrauma research: Opportunities and potential pitfalls of murine models. Experi Neurol 1999; 157:19–42.

331. Wurbel H. Ideal homes? Housing effects on rodent brain and behavior. Trends Neurosci 2001; 24:207–211.

332. Bruce-Keller A, Umberger G, McFall R, Mattson M. Food restriction reduces brain damage and improves behavioral outcome following excitotoxic and metabolic insults. Ann Neurol 1999; 45:8–15.

332a. Cotman CW, Berchtold N. Exercise: a behavioral intervention to enhance brain health and plasticity. Trends Neurosci 2002; 25:295–301.

333. Bland S, Pillai R, Aronowski J, Grotta J, Schallert T. Early overuse and disuse of the affected forelimb after moderately severe intraluminal suture occlusion of the middle cerebral artery in rats. Behav Brain Res 2001; 126:33–41.

334. Muir G, Webb A. Assessment of behavioural recovery following spinal cord injury in rats. Eur J Neurosci 2000; 12:3079–3086.

335. D'Hooge R, Deyn P. Applications of the Morris water maze in the study of learning and memory. Brain Res Rev 2001; 36:60–90.

336. Gonzalez C, Kolb B, Whishaw I. A cautionary note regarding drug and brain lesion studies that use swimming pool tasks. Behav Brain Res 2000; 112:43–52.

337. Ramos J. Training method dramatically affects the acquisition of a place response in rats with neurotoxic lesions of the hippocampus. Neurobiol Learning Memory 2002; 77:109–118.

337a. Loy D, Magnuson D, Zhang YP, Onifer S, Mills M, Whittemore S. Functional redundancy of ventral spinal locomotor pathways. J Neurosci 2002; 22:315–323.

338. Benes F, Lange N. Two-dimensional versus three-dimensional cell counting: A practical perspective. Trends Neurosci 2001; 24:11–17.

339. Oorschot D. Are you using neuronal densities, synaptic densities or neurochemical densities as your definitive data? Prog Neurobiol 1994; 44:233–244.

340. Bhardwaj A, Castro A, Alkayed N, Hurn P, Kirsch J. Anesthetic choice of halothane versus propofol. Stroke 2001; 32:1920–1925.

341. Shimoyama I, Dauth G, Gilman S, Frey K, Penney J. Thalamic, brainstem and cerebellar glucose metabolism in the hemiplegic monkey. Ann Neurol 1988; 24:718–726.

342. Gilman S, Dauth G, Frey K, Penney J, JB. Experimental hemiplegia in the monkey: Basal ganglia glucose activity during recovery. Ann Neurol 1987; 22:370–376.

343. Napieralski J, Butler A, Chesselet M-F. Anatomical and functional evidence for lesion-specific sprouting of corticostriatal input in the adult rat. J Comp Neurol 1996; 373:484–497.

343a. Zhang RL, Zhang ZG, Zhang L, Chopp M. Proliferation and differentiation of progenitor cells in the cortex and the subventricular zone in the adult rat after focal cerebral ischemia. Neurosci 2001; 105:33–41.

344. Carmichael ST, Chesselet M-F. Synchronous neuronal activity is a signal for axonal sprouting after cortical lesions in the adult rat. J Neurosci 2002; 22:6062–6070.

345. Kornblum H, Araujo D, Annala A, Tatsukawa K, Phelps M, Cherry S. In vivo imaging of neuronal activation and plasticity in the rat brain by high resolution positron emission tomography (microPET). Nat Biotechnol 2000; 18:655–660.

346. Buchkremer-Ratzmann I, August M, Hagemann G, Witte O. Electrophysiological transcortical diaschisis after cortical photothrombosis in rat brain. Stroke 1996; 27:1105–1111.

347. Geschwind D, Ou J, Easterday M, Jackson R, Kornblum H. A genetic analysis of neural progenitor differentiation. Neuron 2001; 29:325–339.

348. Jin K, Mao X, Eshoo M, Nagayama T, Minami M, Simon RP, Greenberg DA. Microarray analysis of

hippocampal gene expression in global cerebral ischemia. Ann Neurol 2001; 50:93–103.

349. Connor J, Diamond M. A comparison of dendritic spine number and type on pyramidal neurons of the visual cortex of old adult rats from social or isolated environments. J Comp Neurol 1982; 210:99–106.

350. Black J, Isaacs K, Anderson B, Alcantara AA, Greenough WT. Learning causes synaptogenesis, whereas motor activity causes angiogenesis, in cerebellar cortex of adult rats. Proc Natl Acad Sci USA 1990; 87:5568–5572.

351. Jones T, Schallert T. Overgrowth and pruning of dendrites in adult rats recovering from neocortical damage. Brain Res 1992; 581:156–160.

352. Jones T, Schallert T. Use-dependent growth of pyramidal neurons after neocortical damage. J Neurosci 1994; 14:2140–2152.

353. Kozlowski D, Jones T, Schallert T. Pruning of dendrites and restoration of function after brain damage: Role of the NMDA receptor. Restor Neurol Neurosci 1994; 7:119–126.

354. Humm J, Kozlowski D, James D, Gotts J, Schallert T. Use-dependent exacerbation of brain damage occurs during an early post-lesion vulnerable period. Brain Res 1998; 783:286–292.

355. Kozlowski D, von Stuck S, Lee S, Hovda D, Becker D. Behaviorally-induced contusions following traumatic brain injury: Use-dependent secondary insults. Soc Neurosci abstr 1996; 22:1905.

356. Kozlowski D, James D, Schallert T. Use-dependent exaggeration of neuronal injury after unilateral sensorimotor cortex lesions. J Neurosci 1996; 16: 4776–86.

357. Bland S, Schallert T, Strong R, Aronowski J, Grotta J. Early exclusive use of the affected forelimb after moderate transient focal ischemia in rats. Stroke 2000; 31:1144–1152.

358. Villablanca J, Hovda D. Developmental neuroplasticity in a model of cerebral hemispherectomy and stroke. J Neurosci 2000; 95:625–637.

359. Burgess J, Villablanca J. Recovery of function after neonatal or adult hemispherectomy in cats: II. Limb bias and development, paw usage, locomotion and rehabilitative effects of exercise. Behav Brain Res 1986; 20:1–18.

360. Sloper J, Brodal P, Powell T. An anatomical study of the effects of unilateral removal of sensorimotor cortex in infant monkeys. Brain 1983; 106:707–716.

361. Garraghty P, Kaas J. Functional reorganization in adult monkey thalamus after peripheral nerve injury. Neuroreport 1991; 2:747–750.

362. Pons T, Garraghty P, Ommaya A, Mishkin M. Massive cortical reorganization after sensory deafferentation in adult macaques. Science 1991; 252: 1857–1860.

363. Jones E, Pons T. Thalamic and brainstem contributions to large-scale plasticity of primate somatosensory cortex. Science 1998; 282:1121–1125.

364. Florence S, Taub H, Kaas J. Large-scale sprouting of cortical connections after peripheral injury in adult macaque monkeys. Science 1998; 282:1117–1120.

365. Sutton R, Hovda D, Feeney D. Amphetamine accelerates recovery of locomotor function following bilateral frontal cortex ablation in cats. Behav Neurosci 1989; 103:837–841.

366. Hurwitz B, Dietrich W, McCabe P, Ginsberg M, Alonso O, Watson BD, Schneiderman N. Amphetamine promotes recovery from sensory-motor integration deficit after thrombotic infarction of the primary somatosensory rat cortex. Stroke 1991; 22: 648–654.

367. Sutton R, Feeney D. Alpha-noradrenergic agonists and antagonists affect recovery and maintenance of beam walking ability after sensorimotor cortex ablation in the rat. Restor Neurol Neurosci 1992; 4:1–11.

368. Brown R, Gonzalez C, Kolb B. Nicotine improves Morris water task performance in rats given medial frontal cortex lesions. Pharm Biochem Behav 2000; 67:473–478.

369. Brown R, Kolb B. Nicotine sensitization increases dendritic length and spine density in the nucleus accumbens and cingulate cortex. Brain Res 2001; 899:94–100.

370. Jones T, Schallert T. Subcortical deterioration after cortical damage: Effects of diazepam and relation to recovery of function. Behav Brain Res 1992; 51: 1–13.

371. Barth T, Grant M, Schallert T. Effects of MK801 on recovery from sensorimotor cortex lesions. Stroke 1990; 21(suppl III):153–157.

372. Classen J, Knorr U, Werhahn K. Multimodal output mapping of human central motor representation on different spatial scales. J Physiol 1998; 512:163–179.

373. Redmond D, Freeman T. The American Society for Neural Transplantation and Repair: Considerations and guidelines for studies of human subjects. Cell Transplant 2001; 10:661–664.

Chapter 3

Functional Neuroimaging of Recovery

Neurophysiologic imaging follows structure and function. Unlike the traditional model in which the clinician associates an impairment with a focal lesion, functional neuroimaging offers insights that go beyond the region of damaged tissue. A systems level approach can be taken to identify sites of dysfunction even in the absence of structural damage. Spared tissue can be identified physiologically, rather than based on an anatomic guess.

The diagnostic and therapeutic potential of monitoring brain activity *in vivo* in behaving people has opened a vision for rehabilitation that only a Ray Bradbury could have believed possible just 20 years ago. The rapid pace of change from computerized axial tomography of the brain, offered by most hospitals by the late 1970s, to magnetic resonance imaging (MRI), available in the mid 1980s, has been followed by increasingly practical functional imaging techniques, each with its own virtues and fallabilities (Table 3–1).[1] The more demanding functional imaging techniques, such as positron emission tomography (PET) and magnetoencephalography (MEG) require highly specialized and expensive equipment. Others, such as functional MRI (fMRI) and transcranial magnetic stimulation (TMS), have spread throughout the world, although mostly within university centers.

These techniques serve as unique windows on the resting and experimentally activated brain. They allow researchers to test theories

Table 3–1. **Techniques For Functional Neuroimaging**

INDIVIDUAL METHODS	
Positron emission tomography (PET)	High Resolution Electroencephalography (HREEG)
Functional magnetic resonance imaging (fMRI)	Magnetoencephalography (MEG)
Single photon emission computerized tomography (SPECT)	Near-infrared spectroscopy (NIRS)
	Transcranial doppler (TCD)
Magnetic resonance spectroscopy (MRS)	Optical imaging of intrinsic signals (IOS)
Transcranial electrical and magnetic stimulation (TES, TMS)	

INTEGRATED METHODS	
PET, SPECT, or fMRI superimposed upon MRI	TMS immediately followed by PET or fMRI
EEG or MEG superimposed upon MRI, fMRI, or PET	

regarding cerebral functional specialization and integration. Each demands and provides perspectives on normal functional anatomy, the effects of a CNS or PNS injury, and on spontaneous and rehabilitation-induced plasticity. Each varies in its sensitivity for resolving neural events in time and space. One of the drawbacks across most techniques is that experimental paradigms generally cannot test movements as they are carried out in daily activities. Despite the technical problems posed by these young neuroscientific tools, myriad uses of functional imaging are feasible.

Table 3–2 lists some of the potential benefits of imaging functional anatomy for neurologic rehabilitation. In this chapter, we examine whether resting and activated functional imaging patterns can serve as surrogate markers for predicting behavioral gains; whether physical, cognitive, and pharmacologic interventions can be aimed at inducing activations at key sites to achieve gains by restitution or substitution; and whether elicited activations can serve as a physiologic marker of the adequacy of the intensity and duration of a rehabilitative intervention. For neurologic rehabilitationists, the goal will be to harness mechanisms of plasticity to drive or restrict changes in functional anatomy that enhance behavioral outcomes.

Future functional imaging techniques and multicenter data bases[2] may permit map making at every level of function, from the neural networks of behaviors to released neurotransmitters, and to cell responses such as gene expression and protein synthesis. Positron emission tomography can already detect some molecular events. In this new field, for example, a reporter gene for an enzyme, given to the subject by injection of an adenovirus, and a reporter probe for a radiolabeled substance given intravenously that stays in the cell if acted on by the enzyme, produce a signal in the cell that is imaged.[3] This detail will open additional windows on the poorly lighted box of cerebral responses to rehabilitation efforts.

NEUROIMAGING TECHNIQUES

Positron Emission Tomography

Positron emission tomography and fMRI provide a view of the distributed functional and anatomical network engaged by a task. The ability of PET to reveal rCBF and metabolism was the first solid advance in functional imaging for understanding specific operations within the distributed neural systems for movement, language, attention, memory, perception, and other aspects of cognition.[4,5] The technique allows quantification of absolute physiologic variables such as rCBF, oxygen extraction and utilization, glucose metabolism, protein synthesis, and the binding of molecules to receptors on neurons. Positron emission tomography is a rather direct measure of synaptic activity, although glial activity may account for some tracer uptake. The energy demands of glutaminergic neurons account for approximately 85% of total glucose utilization in studies performed with ^{18}F-fluorodeoxyglucose

Table 3–2. **Potential Uses of Functional Neuroimaging for Rehabilitation**

1. Characterize the natural history and relationship of resting metabolic activity (PET, SPECT) to changes in impairment and disability.

2. Relate rCBF and metabolic patterns, at rest or by an activation study for a specific task, to readiness for rehabilitation (PET, fMRI). Determine whether functional prerequisites within a neural network, especially for attention, encoding and retrieval, must be fulfilled before effective adaptive change can occur, and before rehabilitation can affect outcomes.

3. Characterize predictors of recovery using activation studies (PET, fMRI, HREEG, NIRS, MEG) for specific movements and cognitive functions. Determine whether or not specific nodes in a network, such as the thalamus, must be spared to allow useful gains in function.

4. Correlate changes in representational plasticity and perilesional activations with gains or lack of gains over the course of specific sensorimotor and cognitive interventions.

5. Determine whether a particular rehabilitation intervention engages areas that usually need to be activated for success in carrying out a task, such as those for working memory during problem solving. Develop treatments based upon the ability of the intevention to activate necessary nodes. If another region participates in an alternate strategy for accomplishing a task, develop an intervention that engages the alternative node.

6. Correlate activation patterns over the time of an intervention with variations in the type, duration, and intensity of physical and cognitive therapies. Use fMRI, TMS or NIRS changes in the size and location of representational activations over time as a physiologic marker of optimal intensity of a therapy.

7. Assess strategies to modulate interhemispheric competition and cooperation, for example, for hemiinattention or aphasia, in which engaging or suppressing the activity of the uninjured hemisphere may improve function.

8. Map the initial response to a particular training intervention for a new patient. Compare the results to a data bank of prospective studies that have correlated pathology, behavior, and early patterns of activation in response to the intervention with long-term functional gains. Use the patient's initial activation to predict whether or not that intervention is likely to be of benefit.

9. Study the effects of medications on levels of activation and changes in patterns of engaged regions. Combine the use of drugs that alter an activation with specific training and compare to efficacy training alone.

10. Use early activation paradigms to establish subsets of patients who are most likely to respond to a particular intervention. This strategy may help reduce the number of subjects needed to study the efficacy of a new intervention.

11. Understand how the nodes in a network dynamically interact in their connectivity. New analytic models may be needed to interpret the effect one region of activity has on others.

12. Monitor the effects of biological interventions over time to determine whether or not implanted cells and regenerating axons are incorporated into a network.

PET, positron emission tomography; SPECT, single photon emission computerized tomography; rCBF, regional cerebral blood flow; fMRI, functional magnetic resonance imaging; HREEG, high resolution electroencephalography; MEG, magnetoencephalography; NIRS, near-infrared spectroscopy.

(PET-FDG). The most dominant factor of cortical oxygen and glucose consumption is the resetting of ionic concentrations via the sodium-potassium ATPase after synaptic activity.[6]

Positron emission tomography measures the concentration of radioactivity in a volume of tissue after injection of a specifically labeled substrate such as water or glucose. Positron emitting isotopes, which must be made at the time of a study, include fluorine-18, oxygen-15, nitrogen-13, and carbon-11. More biologically important radiopharmaceuticals are available for PET compared to single photon emission computerized tomography (SPECT). Future PET labeling techniques may allow studies of enzymatic reactions, protein synthesis, and neurotransmitter receptors in addition to the dopamine and benzodiazepine receptors labeled today. Spatial resolution for PET is approximately 125 mm^3. Whole brain samples and isotopes that have half-lives of several minutes, such as $^{15}O_2$, allow 30-second activation or rest studies to be repeated every 10 minutes.

Positron emission tomography is expensive and not generally available even within university facilities. Scanning equipment and a cyclotron to manufacture the radiotracers are becoming less cumbersome, but still require a dedicated team of physicists and other scientists. The technique has other limitations. Hemodynamic responses follow synaptic activity by at least several hundred milliseconds, so tightly coupled physiologic studies are not feasible. Scanning during the rest or active periods must last for approximately 30 seconds when using an oxygen tracer to detect a change in perfusion of as little as 5%. Thus, an activation task must be brief. Repeated studies during the same session are limited by the total radiation exposure and the time it takes the radiotracer to no longer be detectable in the structures of interest. For example, PET-FDG studies require considerably longer times to carry out, up to 30 minutes after injection. For an activation study, the subject would have to continue performing a task over that interval. Newer techniques allow repeat studies with small doses of tracer, but in general, oxygen tracers are cleared faster and permit several injections for repeated activation studies within a session. Another limitation is that the uptake of tracer does not allow the investigator to view the temporal sequence of regional activations. Also, both inhibition and excitation at synapses produce the same level of activation, so these processes cannot be separated. Finally, PET inherently cannot distingush between an activation that arises directly from motor programming or output and the activation induced by sensory inputs from joints and muscles into motoneurons. This limits the ability to interpret the effects of sensory drive for motor reorganization, especially within the primary sensorimotor cortex.

A variety of technical approaches have been taken for data acquisition, image processing, and statistical analysis of voxels of activation. Experimental Case Study 3–1 describes the most commonly used data manipulation and analysis technique for PET, called Statistical Parametric Mapping.

Single Photon Emission Computerized Tomography

Single photon emission computerized tomography (SPECT) is performed with radiophar-maceuticals that are given intravenously or by inhalation. Radioisotopes that emit gamma rays include xenon-133, iodine-123, and technetium-99m. Single photon emission computerized tomography does not directly assess neuronal function. The procedure measures cerebral perfusion, blood volume, and the distribution of several receptors, which indirectly reflect metabolism and network activity.[7] Early after stroke, SPECT tends not to differentiate between viable and irreversibly ischemic tissue, because the uptake of the radiotracer is not linearly related to perfusion. For postacute ischemia studies applicable to rehabilitation interventions, SPECT's spatial resolution is just under 1 cm^3. Ionizing radiation, nonuniform spatial resolution, low temporal resolution, and the relativity of measures from one region of interest to another limit its usefulness in the functional imaging of plasticity. Many of the pitfalls of SPECT are found among the methods and paradigms of components of functional imaging listed in Table 3–3.

Functional Magnetic Resonance Imaging

Functional magnetic resonance imaging (fMRI) does not require the preparation of radiopharmaceuticals or expose patients to irradiation. Functional magnetic resonance imaging indirectly detects increases in neuronal activity. The fMRI signal arises when neuronal activity increases local arterial blood flow and volume with little change in oxygen consumption. The blood flow increases the oxygen content of local venous blood and decreases its concentration of deoxyhemoglobin, which increases the intensity of the so-called blood oxygenation level dependent (BOLD) signal.[8] Thus, BOLD fMRI employs hemaglobin as an endogenous contrast agent. The amount of BOLD signal observed by a scanner depends on the strength of the magnetic field, the echo time (TE), and the imaging technique. For example, a 1% BOLD signal at an echo time of 30 ms is equivalent to 2% at TE 60 ms, even if the hemodynamic response is constant.[6] To properly interpret the meaning of a BOLD study, the clinician must keep in mind that the signal in a voxel that makes a pretty map colored in reds, yellows, and blues are statistics, not measures (Experimental Case Study 3–1).

The precise relationship between the BOLD signal and underlying neuronal activity appears best explained by the local field potential, which is the aggregate activity of a local population of neurons.[9] The local field potential reflects changes in the excitatory and inhibitory membrane potentials related to synaptic activity at the dendrites and soma of neurons, as

Table 3–3. Components of a Functional Neuroimaging Activation Study Data Acquisition

METHODS	
Sensitivity	*Repeatability*
Signal to noise	Single or multiple trials in same session
Contrast with background activity	Reliability for repeated sessions over days or weeks
Relative (fMRI) or absolute (PET) physiologic response	
	Accuracy
Resolution	Gold standard (PET for cerebral blood flow, none for fMRI)
Spatial, temporal	
Field of view	*Precision*
Contrast with background activity	

PERSONAL DECISIONS
Availability of method, cost, accessibility of the site
Invasiveness
Risks: radiation (PET), toxic contrast, seizure (TMS), craniectomy (OIS)
Environment for subject: tolerance of gantry, duration of study, movement artifact
Types of paradigms: inside or outside of a device, view videoscreen, wear goggles with screen, use manipulanda

PARADIGMS	
Hypothesis	*Control versus task activity*
	Percent of time doing task compared to imaging time
Entry criteria	Rest or other comparison activity
Age, handedness, gender	
Healthy or representative control subjects	*Monitoring task*
Features of history and examination	Assess strategy of subject
Cerebral anatomy; site and volume of lesion	Muscle movement (EMG)
Duration of disease or impairment; stable or dynamic condition	Video movements
Medications: neuromodulators, sedatives	Ocular movements
Habits for sleep, caffeine, nicotine, alcohol, drugs	EEG
Cycles: menstrual, diurnal, seasonal	Debrief subject about tasks
Mood: anxiety, depression	
	Assessment
Patient training for task	Follow-up at particular time or at certain behavioral milestones
Introduction to technique and environment	Relevant behavioral outcome measures
Responses during novel compared to habituated activity	
	Subclinical events
Implicit or explicit learning	Attention, imagery, inaudible vocalization, sleep
Order effect of tasks	

Continued on following page

Table 3–3.—*continued*

DESIGN STRATEGIES	
Comparisons within or between subjects	*Response requirements*
Choice of control condition	Speed, accuracy, or relative to normal or to affected population's skill
Choice of task(s)	
One or more levels of task difficulty	*Number of subjects to power study*
Set difficulty based on relative success of performance	*Number of trials*
Skilled, fluent, practiced versus unskilled, nonfluent, unpracticed	*Block design or random event-related design*
	Use of more than 1 modality
Rate of stimulus presentation	

DATA ANALYSIS	
Analysis of artifact	*Subtraction studies*
Movements: head motion, heart beat, chest wall	Validity of comparisons across tasks
Radiofrequency inhomogeneities (fMRI), scatter (PET)	*Statistical tests*
Electrode dysfunction	Assumptions
Changing mental states	Data interpolation, resampling, repeated tests
	Assess differences between noise and predicted activation
Data smoothing and correction	A priori choices
Potential differences across software packages	Post hoc analyses
Registration onto anatomical map; linear transormation or other approach	
Attentuation	
Motion	
Normalize for spatial and intensity parameters	
Choose onset and offset of task-related responses	

fMRI, functional magnetic resonance imaging; PET, positron emission tomography; TMS, transcranial magnetic stimulation; OIS, optical imaging of intrinsic signals; EMG, electromyography; EEG, electroencephalography.

well as local action potentials. In visual cortex, for example, an estimated 0.4 spikes per second per neuron accounts for each 1% fMRI signal change in area V1.[6] Inhibition may be less metabolically demanding than excitation,[10] so the BOLD signal may owe much of its origin to excitatory inputs, but the contributions of excitatory and inhibitory influences are controversial. The mechanism of BOLD contrast, then, may be better ascribed to the input and intracortical processing of an activated region, rather than its spiking output. Blood oxygenation level dependent signals and neural responses have a fairly linear relationship for brief stimuli.[9]

After the start of a task, fMRI signals peak within several seconds followed by a ramp-like incline for 6 to 12 seconds to a plateau, if neural activation remains constant. Once the stimulus stops, blood inflow and the BOLD signal return to baseline by 6 to 12 seconds in a ramp-like decline.[9] A small, brief pre- and poststimulus undershoot of the signal may be seen as well. The small early dip appears to represent an increase in oxygen consumption, which is followed by an increase in blood flow.[11] During visual, motor, sensory, and cognitive activation studies, fMRI signals can be resolved to 1 to 2 mm.[12] Given the origin of the BOLD signal, its spatial resolution is limited by capillary microvascular density, which is quite a bit greater than the size of the neurons represented by the signal. The signal also derives from larger draining veins that are consider-

EXPERIMENTAL CASE STUDY 3–1:
Analysis of Functional Magnetic Resonance Imaging Data

Many methodologies have been used to capture and assess functional activation data.[203,204] I briefly re-view several that seem most reliable for repeated rehabilitation-related motor and cognitive studies. Overall, an fMRI time series activation paradigm must place the blood oxygenation level dependent (BOLD) signal into the subject's anatomical space and evaluate the statistical meaning of the location, number, and level of activation of each BOLD signal voxel.[205] Transformations are needed to realign the data and remove movement-related signal components that persist after realignment. Images are then warped to match a template of the brain that conforms to a standard anatomical space. After smoothing, the General Linear Model is often used to estimate the parameters of the model and to de-rive the appropriate univariate statistic for each voxel in the brain matrix. Then, statistical inferences can be made about the activations in relation to the behavior that evoked changes in the BOLD signal.

Image Acquisition

An initial shimming procedure captures alterations in the magnetic field associated with putting the head in the field. Distortions are corrected and the power needed to perform the scans is determined. Regions of poor shim are near the sinuses, anterior temporal lobes, and inferior frontal lobes when us-ing a gradient echo sequence, but this can be corrected. An error in this procedure will alter the align-ment and location of a voxel. Distortions can occur in only one plane and not others, so the images ought to be reviewed before proceeding with the activation paradigm.

An anatomic T1: or T2:-weighted image of the patients is acquired. The detail of the image may be bet-ter with a 1.5 Tesla than a 3.0 Tesla magnetic field. Software figures out how to match and transform the 4 mm slices chosen from the sagittal anatomic brain image to the resliced image acquired during func-tional imaging. Talaraich or affine rigid body linear transformation approaches may be used to transform the data. A 1.5 or a 3.0 Tesla magnet and either gradient echo-pulse (GRE) sequence or spin echo (SE) sequence and echo-planar imaging (EPI) are most commonly employed for fMRI studies. Gradient hard-ware permits echo planar imaging for multislice imaging with GRE and SE. Gradient echo-pulse is more affected by motion but more sensitive to BOLD-based signal changes. Both are sensitive to the BOLD signal in veins and venules, which must be distinguished from regions of activation. A higher field strength magnet produces a greater percentage of signals that arise from capillaries and cerebral tissue.

Typical parameters for a motor activation trial include an EPI GRE study with a TR (time between pulses or repetition rate that remagnetizes and realigns protons) 2.5 seconds, TE (echo time which is the time of magnetic pulse excitation) 45 ms, voxel size 3.125 × 3.125 × 5 mm, field of vision of 20 cm, and 16 axial slices 4–5 mm thick with 1 mm skip between slices.

Activation Paradigm

Many of the concerns and pitfalls are listed in Table 3–3. An experiment may compare active, passive, and rest conditions or conditions at differing speeds and forces, usually in blocks of, e.g., active wrist extension for 30 seconds alternating with 30 seconds of rest. Cognitive tasks often work best using an event-related design. This approach can take into account the levels of difficulty of a language, work-ing memory, or other cognitive task for a subject. For example, to study working memory, the N-back test can be performed with 0, 1, 2, or 3 previously shown numbers or letters to be held in mind.[206,207] Task difficulty needs to be determined before the patients get into the scanner. The activation task then can include levels of difficulty that can be accomplished at, e.g., a level of 80% correct responses. In a scanner, the brain does not rest. Patients may be imagining, thinking, or talking to themselves. Thus, 2 or 3 conditions may need to be included along with rest. Because a change in the hemodynamic re-sponse may lag behind a movement or thought, the rate of stimulus presentation and response time cannot exceed the hemodynamic response. The novelty of the scanner environment may increase the level or distribution of the BOLD signal, so initial acclimation is important for serial session studies.

Controlling for effort during a motor task can be accomplished by using a self-paced task that is less difficult for subjects and does not produce associated or overflow movements. In general, a motor task can only involve the elbow, wrist, fingers or ankle to prevent head motion artifact. Passive limb move-ments are just as restricted.

free of metals such as bullets, pacemakers, and some prosthetic heart valves. Motor activities that require active movement of the shoulder or hip cause excessive head motion. Commonly used drugs may alter the signal. For example, caffeine acts as a vasoconstrictor that decreases cerebral perfusion without a change in performance and decreases the BOLD signal at rest. During activation, the vasculature responds from below the normal baseline, producing an overall increase in the BOLD signal with performance, a sort of contrast enhancer.[13] Dose-response curves that take into account body weight and blood levels of caffeine, theophylline, and other vasoactive agents will shed light on this phenomenon.

Event-related fMRI allows the responses to a single stimulus or task to be imaged, much as an evoked potential is stimulated electrophysiologically. A single experimental trial may free the response from such difficult–to–assess matters as attention and the context in which the stimulus is presented. A singular action or cognitive task may also permit the study of the spatial and temporal dynamics of a neural network. Thus, fMRI and its variations could become a key method for evaluating the topographic organization and reorganization of the brain. Indeed, the technique has rapidly become the best noninvasive tool for 3-dimensional localization of distributed processing networks. Experimental Case Study 3–1 provides more details about methodologies for the benefit of the reader of activation studies.

Transcranial Magnetic Stimulation

Magnetic scalp stimulation techniques apply a transient clockwise current from a stimulating coil placed on the scalp in an optimal position to induce a counterclockwise current in the brain (Fig. 3–2). The brief, intense electric field induced by magnetic coils shaped as a figure-of-

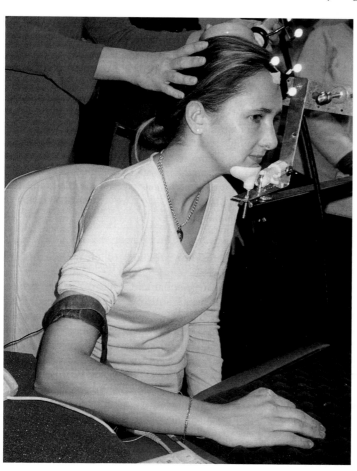

Figure 3–2. Transcranial magnetic stimulation over primary motor cortex causes a twitch of the finger muscles. When the subject contracts the extensor propius indicis slightly, this muscle is preferentially excited. The markers are stereotactically matched to an MRI scan of the subject's brain using *Brain Site Software*. This procedure allows the site of maximal stimulation to be overlaid precisely on the cerebral anatomy for localization.

eight is more focal, but weaker than the field induced by circular coils. Transcranial magnetic stimulation (TMS) painlessly activates corticospinal neurons transsynaptically through their horizontal afferent connections. The horizontal projections extend only a few millimeters. The focal point of the stimulation is within a few millimeters of cortex and peaks around 300 ms after onset of the stimulus. Thus, the investigator needs a good a priori hypothesis about the structure involved and behavioral effects of a stimulus at a focal location. Single pulses are repeated at no more than 5-second intervals. Direct electrical stimulation has a history that goes back to 1875, when Ferrier mapped cortical responses in monkeys. Transcranial electrical stimulation (TES) bypasses cortical interneurons and stimulates pyramidal tract neurons. The brain stem and spinal cord can be directly stimulated over the occiput and posterior spine, although this may cause discomfort.

The minimal spatial resolution of TMS, meaning the smallest distance at which a difference in amplitude of the evoked potentials can be recognized, is approximately 5 mm.[14] Transcranial magnetic stimulation, then, may not reliably resolve the overlapping mosaic of M1 representations for the upper extremity. Also, mapping that aims to demonstrate motor plasticity may not distinguish between organizational adaptations and changes in cortical excitability. The technique can be used to stimulate the leg muscles, but many bilateral muscles will be activated. Medial and subcortical structures are generally too deep and at a difficult angle for TMS activation. Motor potentials evoked from a single muscle, such as the abductor pollicus brevis, are more easily elicited if a subject contracts the muscle slightly.

Transcranial magnetic stimulation has been used increasingly by investigators to make maps of cognitive[15] and sensorimotor[16] activity, to detect representational plasticity caused by pain[17] and brain tumors,[18] to investigate motor system plasticity after peripheral nerve injury, stroke and spinal cord injury,[19] and to assess the effects of practice and neuropharmacologic agents on simple motor learning.[20] By combining TMS and TES results at the same cortical site, along with TES of the brain stem and spinal cord, the site of motor reorganization after, for example, a lower limb amputation, can be deduced.[21]

Variables measured include the threshold and amplitude of an evoked muscle response, central conduction time, the number of excitable positions on the scalp, the positions that give the highest amplitude of evoked muscle response, and the center of gravity, meaning the amplitude-weighted location of the motor map. Thus, the direction and size of a change in representational plasticity can be determined for a motor map, most commonly for an evoked response of a single finger muscle. The TMS-induced map can be coregistered on an MRI scan. Voluntary contraction of a muscle with a 20% or less of maximum contraction shortens the latency by several milliseconds. The absolute amplitude depends on many factors that reflect the sum of activity of the upper and lower motoneurons. Measures of peak to peak amplitude vary so much that an absolute measure has little clinical meaning, although a side-to-side difference of over 50% in patients with an upper motoneuron lesion suggests a disease state on the affected side.[22]

A paired-pulse technique, often at approximately 1 Hz, allows testing of intracortical inhibition (short interval repetition) and excitation (longer interval repetition in which the first stimulus primes the second one). Paired-pulse inhibition can be used to interrupt a cognitive process as well. The area of cortex that evokes a motor response can be tested over time to examine the size and location of changes in representational plasticity.

Transcranial magnetic stimulation is the only functional technique that can temporarily disrupt a pathway by inducing disorder in neuronal firing which, in turn, creates a transient virtual lesion. For example, stimulation of the primary visual cortex impaired the ability of subjects to imagine stimuli, just as it interrupted their ability to see the stimuli.[23] Repetitive pulse TMS (rTMS) is especially effective at creating disruptions using very brief pulses at rates of 2–50 Hz. The technique did not induce a seizure when rTMS trains at 20 Hz for 1.6 seconds were carried out at intervals of 5 seconds.[24] At 1-second intervals, safety was compromised in normal subjects. Greater care may be needed for stimulation of patients with stroke or other structural brain lesions.

Memory, language, perception, attention, and other cognitive tasks have been studied with rTMS.[25] Trains of stimulis at 15 Hz over the left frontal and parietal cortex impaired picture-word matching in healthy subjects.[26]

Twenty minutes of rTMS at 1 Hz over the left or right parietal lobe extinguished the detection of visual stimuli in the opposite hemifield during double simultaneous visual stimulation.[27] Attention to ipsilateral targets improved, suggesting disinhibition of structures in the hemisphere that did not receive rTMS. The study supports interhemispheric competition in the network for spatial attention with dominance in the right parietal cortex (see Chapter 1). Repetitive pulse TMS may possibly be used to inhibit the unlesioned hemisphere during a retraining approach for hemineglect (see Chapter 9). Unlike metabolic neuroimaging studies of cognition, which show regions of interconnected activation, TMS interruption reveals whether a region is needed for performance of the task.

Repetitive pulse TMS can also be used to excite cortex. Some studies show that frontal lobe rTMS may lessen depression. For rehabilitation, coupling rTMS with a specific cognitive or motor therapy may improve the targeted function. For example, low intensity rTMS at 5 Hz over the left prefrontal region led to an decrease in the response time of normal subjects to complete a reasoning task.[28] Could it do so in a patient with TBI or stroke who has a prefrontal injury or another lesion connected to this node of a cognitive network?

Magnetoencephalography

Magnetoencephalography (MEG) reveals changes in magneto-electrical fields with precise 3-dimensional localization of the activated neuronal pool within milliseconds. Subjects wear a helmet-shaped neuromagnetometer array with up to 122 planar gradiometers. The technique records the tangential component of dipoles in the depth of gyri and sulci.[29] It also measures the strength and orientation of a dipole generator source, so MEG can detect changes in activity-dependent plasticity and changes in the size and location of a representation. The MEG is usually coregistered with MRI anatomy. An estimated 30,000 neurons must be simultaneously activated for detection of an extracranial field. High resolution EEG is often simultaneously recorded to confirm the detection of electrical events.

The procedure takes considerable time to sample the entire brain and requires a room isolated from external magnetic interferences. Equipment is expensive. Interpretation of dipole measures depends on the chosen mathematical model. Analytic methods to correct for motion artifact are in development, such as blind source separation and independent component analysis. In good hands, studies have revealed changes in representational plasticity after stroke[30] and adaptations in amputees with phantom limb pain[17] and chronic back pain.[31]

Magnetoencephalography can detect source currents in S1. In a pilot study, the median nerve was stimulated and somatosensory evoked magnetic fields recorded.[32] Subjects who had a stroke and improved in the ability to do 2-point discrimination over the thenar eminence showed an improvement in the second deflection after the stimulus, called P1m, in S1. The first deflection reflects excitatory postsynaptic potentials generated by thalamocortical afferents to layer IV pyramidal cells in BA 3b. The second deflection probably reflects inhibitory postsynaptic potentials near the somata of the cells.[32] To maintain small receptive fields in the cortical sensory representation requires strong lateral inhibition. Presumably, inhibition was reestablished in subjects who had clinical improvement, although other cortical regions may have played a role as well.

This technique may be useful in monitoring somatosensory changes induced by rehabilitation interventions. Optimal sensory feedback appears to be a pivotal requirement for motor gains in hand function and walking (see Chapter 1). Magnetoencephalography may also help researchers understand the bridge between the sensorimotor internal dynamics of the cortex and movement behavior.[33]

High Resolution Electroencephalography

Electroencephalography (EEG) with frequency analysis and topographical displays, sometimes referred to as EEG brain mapping or quantitative EEG, uses signal averaging and statistical approaches to assess EEG field potentials and evoked potentials such as the P300 of an event-related potential (see Chapter 4). The technique reflects the activity of cortical surface dipoles. It offers high temporal resolution, but limited spatial resolution. Greater numbers of electrodes, up to 128 in various configurations over the scalp, improve spatial sensitivity. Also, EEG and MRI data have been combined to provide a 3-dimensional map in experiments that seek greater temporal and spatial resolution for functional imaging.[34] Movement-related motor potentials, arising in M1, have been analyzed with the technique. Studies find ipsilesional and contralesional activation during finger movements in some subjects after stroke.[35] This technique, then, may assess aspects of cerebral reorganization over time. The technique has not been validated for use after a concussion, although it has found favor in some medico-legal circles to try to prove objective evidence of brain adaptations after injury[36] or of excessive distractability.[36a]

In special circumstances, such as preoperative evaluations for epilepsy, tumor, and arteriovenous malformation surgery, cortical electrode grids and electrodes placed deep into cerebral tissue achieve spatial resolution of approximately 100 μm^3 over a small region of interest. Functional localization and rapid plasticity can be studied under this unique circumstance.[37,38] Chapter 4 describes other field and neuronal spike potentials that have been processed for brain-machine interface technologies.

Intrinsic Optical Imaging Signals

High resolution intrinsic optical imaging signals (IOS) of human cortex at the time of a craniotomy may aid investigations of the cortical organization of sensorimotor and cognitive processes.[39] White light shined on a patch of cortex is reflected at specific wavelengths that are a function of the neuronal activity of the illuminated tissue, associated with parameters such as blood flow and volume, the oxidative state of the tissue, and any cell swelling. These changes occur during a behavioral task in awake subjects. A charge-coupled device camera captures the images. The video signal is digitized and converted into pixels. The signals represent changes in the optical properties of brain tissue, such as light scattering, absorption or transmittance, and reflectance.[40]

An IOS offers high temporal (milliseconds) and spatial (micrometers) resolution over a confined intraoperative site. In studies that combined direct neuronal unit recordings to IOS in monkeys as they observed objects, regional clustering of neurons that responded to similar object features were found in patches just 0.5 mm in diameter.[41] Human studies suggest a time-course curve of activation peak between 1 and 3 seconds after stimulation and detection sensitivity of 0.5 to 1 cm^2 for activation of somatosensory cortex.[42] During neurosurgical tissue resections, language studies that included visual and auditory naming, word discrimination, and orofacial movements detected response profiles within Broca's and Wernicke's areas that depended upon the task.[43] Other topographical distinctions have been described for sensorimotor representations.[42,44]

Near-Infrared Spectroscopy

Near-infrared spectroscopy (NIRS) is an optical method for measuring changes in the concentration of oxyhemoglobin and deoxyhemoglobin in cortical vessels. The technique uses near-infrared light directed into the skull through a fiberoptic bundle. Multiple optodes attached to the scalp over regions of interest capture reflected light to measure both rCBF and oxygenation. Spatial and metabolic correlations between NIRS and PET and fMRI have been reported for functional activations in cognitive, language,[45] sensorimotor,[46] and locomotor[47] studies using 2 optodes or up to 24 optodes 3 cm apart with 12 light sources and 12 detector fibers in a 36-channel recording system that covered the regions of interest. Although NIRS is not as spatially precise as PET and fMRI, initial reports suggest that it readily distinguishes each of the motor regions. A single light-emitting probe was used over the frontal region to successfully monitor changes in cerebral oxygenation associated with simple tasks while standing.[48] Multiprobe studies that segment regions of interest are far more likely to be of value.

Near-infrared spectroscopy (NIRS) offers a major advantage for some rehabilitation studies. Subjects can walk on a treadmill or use their arms for functional activities during a NIRS study without inducing the head motion artifacts that limit fMRI and PET activation paradigms that assess plasticity and whether a task or practice engages a network.

Magnetic Resonance Spectroscopy

Magnetic resonance imaging is based on the nuclear magnetic resonance (NMR) signal from water protons. Magnetic resonance spectroscopy (MRS) uses high field magnets to detect intracellular NMR signals from carbon-13, phosphorus-31, sodium-23, and fluorine-19.[49] This biochemical assay, which compares regions of interest, has a spatial resolution of 1–2 cm^3 and requires rather long imaging times. It measures compounds found in gray and white matter. The more interesting ones for neurorehabilitation include N-acetylaspartate (NAA), found only in neurons and axons, as well as choline, creatine, and myo-inositol. Choline compounds are involved in membrane metabolism and often increase in brain tumors. Inositol is asociated with glial cells and glial swelling. Lactate is associated with ischemia. Creatine levels are usually stable, so the other compounds may be described as a ratio of the creatine peak.

Volumes of interest can be compared to regions that are not involved in the pathological process. The extent or reversibility of axonal injury can be compared to changes in regional activation by fMRI with the same MR equipment. For example, in a patient with multiple sclerosis who had an exacerbation with a hemiparesis, serial MRS revealed a reversible decrease in the NAA concentration. The change from presumed greater to lesser tissue injury was associated with a decrease in the number of pixels activated in primary sensorimotor cortex during an fMRI study of finger tapping and by less disability.[50] In normal appearing frontal lobe white matter, based on MRI after cerebral trauma, proton MRS abnormalities such as a low NAA suggest diffuse axonal injury.[51] Magnetic resonance spectroscopy has been combined with MEG and MRI to relate physiology to chemistry in ischemic brain.[52]

Transcranial Doppler

Another technique, transcranial doppler ultrasonography, assesses the velocity of blood flow through large arteries such as the middle, anterior, and posterior cerebral arteries. Although primarily used to detect atherostenoses and vasospasm, a few studies have evaluated changes in CBF in both middle cerebral arteries during movements of the recovered hand after a stroke[53] and associated with a language activation paradigm in aphasic patients.[54] Thus, the technique may inexpensively complement other physiologic data.

Combined Methods

An integration of techniques allows the integration of structural and physiological information about where and under what circumstances neuronal assemblies and networks are engaged. For example, TMS stimulation over a region of interest, such as the dorsolateral prefrontal cortex during a working memory task, can be combined with a simultaneous injection of $H_2^{15}O$ for a PET scan to see the regions that are connected to this prefrontal site. Making a virtual lesion with rTMS followed by PET is a strategy to test the treatment efficacy of exciting or inhibiting a node in a network after a brain injury. Multimodal investigations have generally demonstrated overlapping maps and good reproducibility for sensorimotor tasks.[14,18,29]

In the near future, the anatomic, cytologic, neurochemical, physiologic, and functional architecture of the brain will be correlated into multidimensional atlases built upon data from thousands of subjects who were studied in depth. In addition, information about changes in structure and function and statistical correlations will be incorporated to account for age, gender, race, pertinent genetic data about populations, and types of diseases and lesions. A clinician may be able to "warp" an individual patient's brain after MRI and standardized fMRI studies onto this multilevel statistical map and predict the best approaches to enhance recovery, based on the experience of similar patients in the database. The Human Brain Mapping Project intends to create this database.[2] The effort is as important for neurorehabilitation as the Human Genome Project is to medicine.

LIMITATIONS OF FUNCTIONAL NEUROIMAGING STUDIES

Table 3–3 lists many of the components of a functional neuroimaging study. Whether reading an experiment or planning one, the clinician needs to decide what approaches are most applicable to the experiment. All of these issues may affect the clinical and statistical interpretation of the data. Imaging studies can mislead the clinician.[55]

General Limitations

Regions selectively activated by a particular sensorimotor or cognitive task are interconnected areas that represent components of the task. These connections, however, are especially sensitive to the context of the task. Chapter 1 examined the cartography of connections likely to be of interest to rehabilitationists. Functional neuroimaging studies such as PET and fMRI infer functional integration on the basis of correlations with a measure of neuronal activity, such as rCBF or metabolism. Most of the models used to evaluate functional imaging data and most statistical approaches to the data do not take into account the level of modulation that one region has on another, but approaches to do so are feasible.[56] In addition, instructions to subjects about a task, the amount of practice, habituation, level of difficulty, attentional demands, emotional state, rate and order of stimuli in an activation task, and other features of experimental design all affect metabolic localization.

Other limitations for mapping rapid cognitive processes with PET or fMRI include the relative slowness of scanning, which is measured in seconds rather than in milliseconds; relative insensitivity of detecting changes in regional perfusion that are in the range of a few percent; the adequacy of statistical methods used to compare two or more activation states; spatial resolution and signal-to-noise strength of activated pixels; and errors in mapping a PET, fMRI, or MEG result onto an MRI image to combine exact anatomy with physiologic activity. Anatomic differences among subjects must be handled with sophisticated software. That anatomy may be altered by the brain lesion and degrade the relationship between a patient's brain and the template brain used by the software package. Of course, regional brain activity measures in a clinical setting cannot fully reflect the fine details of local neural activity and connectivity.

Even when the activation paradigm, data acquisition, and data analysis appear reliable, the results may produce misinformation. Unrecognized subconscious processes may be at work during the activation task. For example, anterior language areas can be activated merely by preparation for speech, in the absence of articulation. The investigator often cannot be sure that the subject is carrying out the process of interest, such as silent speech or no intended speech to engage the intended network. For motor tasks, greater physical effort may produce subtle mirror movements that cause activation, usually in the hemisphere of the unaffected limb, when none is expected[57] or produce overflow movements with associated head motion artifacts. These problems are managed by configuring the task in a way that lessens the effort required of the subject.

Motor and cognitive activations may change with aging, perhaps related to changes in strategies or effort and associated with degenerative changes over time such as dopaminergic cell loss. Thus, healthy subjects and patients must be carefully matched for age, since aging alters cerebral responses during performance. For example, an fMRI study compared performances during a reaction time task in which subjects under the age of 35 years and over age 50 years pressed one of four buttons to a visual stimulus.[57a] The older subjects had relatively larger regions of activation in the contralateral S1M1, lateral premotor area, SMA, and ipsilateral cerebellum. In addition, ipsilateral S1M1, bilateral putamen, and contralateral cerebellum were activated. Relatively larger and more bilateral frontal activations are found in older subjects performing the same cognitive tasks as younger people as well, especially in the dorsal and lateral prefrontal cortices. Recruitment of additional regions does not necessarily imply any decline in task performance, however. Indeed, when younger subjects attempt more demanding motor or cognitive tasks, similar bilateral motor or frontal regions may also be activated.

Prescribed medications may alter excitation and inhibition of functional activations (Color Figure 3–9 in separate color insert). Ovarian steroids that vary with the menstrual cycle more clearly do this. TMS studies show greater excitatory responses when estradiol is high and inhibition when progesterone increases.[57b] These hormones act on a variety of neurotransmitters. The entry criteria in Table 3–3 mention other potentially important variables,

sensorimotor, insular and dorsolateral pre-frontal cortices, the left cerebral peduncle, and the ipsilateral right cerebellum.[70] This pattern corresponds to the circuits between the basal ganglia, thalamus, and cortical projections (see Color Fig. 3–3 in separate color insert). The remote effects of the striatocapsular lesions were postulated to be related to either a transsynaptic functional deactivation (see Diaschisis below) or to structural changes from transsynaptic or retrograde degeneration. Also, rCBF was increased in the left posterior cingulate and premotor cortices and ipsilateral caudate. The investigators speculated that a loss of the functional inhibition of these areas by homotopic regions of the opposite hemisphere had developed. No premotor cortex was deactivated. This finding was consistent with the bilateral connections of premotor cortex and with studies in normal subjects that show that these homologous areas are bilaterally activated during a unilateral motor task.

VASCULAR DEMENTIA

Resting metabolic studies have also demonstrated cortical hypofunctioning in patients with multiple subcortical strokes (see Chapter 9) and diffuse axonal injury after trauma (see Chapter 11). For example, global glucose metabolism and regional metabolism in the right dorsolateral frontal lobe were lower in subjects with a vascular dementia compared to subjects who had subcortical infarcts and no dementia.[71] Involvement of the cortico-striato-thalamo-cortical loop by lacunes and small strokes may contribute to the pathology of vascular dementia. Color Figure 3–3 (in separate color insert) shows a PET scan from a patient who was told by his family physician that he may have had a minor stroke, but could return to work. The patient was bland, passive, and indifferent, even when confronted about his new cognitive impairments. Neuropsychologic measures of attention, word list generation, and verbal memory showed poor scores. He performed the Wisconsin Card Sort in a random, perseverative fashion. Visuospatial skills were excellent. His affect and ability to interact with family improved moderately with 20 mg of methylphenidate every morning compared to holidays off the drug, but overall cognition did not improve. One critical disconnection, then, had caused profound memory and executive

dysfunction. Vascular dementia implies many such disconnections.

Frontal hypometabolism may correlate with vascular dementia as well as temporoparietal hypometabolism correlates with Alzheimer's disease.[72,73] These disconnection-induced global and regional abnormalities reveal what may limit or prevent functional gains in some patients.

SPARED TISSUE AND PATHWAYS

Magnetic resonance imaging and PET can also reveal spared tissue that accounts for subsequent partial restitution. For example, some patients with blindsight have been shown to have an island of spared striate cortex appreciated only by PET.[74] Functional imaging holds the greatest promise for identifying spared architecture in the neural networks for specific tasks.

Subcortical lesions that only partially damage the corticospinal and other motor tracts are especially likely to participate in gains (see Chapter 2). This sparing may not be appreciated by clinical examination. Predictions about improvement in hand strength and function have been made by early poststroke TMS studies aimed at detecting subclinically intact corticospinal pathways.[75,76] In a modest number of cases, an initial TMS response in a subject who offers no movement or twitch movement is accompanied by subsequent recovery of hand function. Transcranial magnetic stimulation in subjects with pyramidal lesions suggests 3 mechanisms in spared corticospinal pathways that cause weakness.[77]

1. When the number of corticospinal fibers that synapse with a motoneuron falls too short to generate adequately sized excitatory postsynaptic potentials (EPSPs), a descending volley will not excite the spinal neuron.
2. The conduction velocity of a demyelinated corticospinal fiber may be slow, which could delay and disperse its excitatory stimuli to the point where the spinal neuron is not excited.
3. A dysfunctional descending pathway allows one impulse to pass, but the next volley finds the fiber to be refractory. A subsequent volley may pass, but the relative blocking of the required train of volleys impedes spinal neuron excitation. This

mechanism could also cause fatigability with repetitive attempts to use a paretic muscle group.

DIASCHISIS

Positron emission tomography and SPECT reveal the phenomenon of diaschisis and transneuronal hypometabolism. Tissue remote from the ischemic injury can be hypometabolic due to loss of afferent input from the damaged neural network or from disconnection from the input of one of the several diffuse neurotransmitter systems, such as noradrenergic or serotonergic modulators from the brainstem (see Chapter 2). Remote hypometabolism is most often reported in the contralesional cerebellum and ipsilesional thalamus and frontal cortex following a subcortical lesion. Color Figure 2–2 (in separate color insert) reveals the transsynaptic effects of an infarction of the caudate and anterior limb of the internal capsule. The patient had no sensorimotor impairments, but had poor working memory and could no longer manipulate information or think creatively. Color Figure 3–3 (in separate color insert) reveals the remote metabolic sequelae of a small infarct in the anterior thalamus. Color Figure 3–4 (in separate color insert) reveals the profound clinical and transsynaptic effects of an anterior inferior corpus callosal infarct, also involving the septal region. The patient could not form new memories and confabulated. The PET scans of both patients included hypometabolism of the frontal lobes, basal ganglia, and thalamus.

In a PET study of patients approximately 6 months after a cortical stroke who recovered the ability to make sequential finger movements with the recovered hemiparetic hand, lesion-induced remote metabolic changes at rest overlapped the territory of some of the recovery-related activity during finger tapping.[78] The study used a data reduction analytical technique called principal components analysis to allow a comparison between the extent of a lesion with connectivity patterns and to identify the cerebral areas that participated in finger tapping with the affected hand, the unaffected hand, and at rest. The contralesional lateral thalamus and visual association cortex were the only regions involved both by a passive metabolic effect and an increase in recovery-related activity for the task. Diaschisis fol-

lowed by recovery of thalamic activity is described in Experimental Case Study 2–1. Of interest, thalamic activation has correlated with better motor outcomes.[79] Visual imagery and guidance for movement, or attention to motion, may explain the change in visual association cortex in this study of patients with cortical stroke. Also, the thalamus and extrastriate cortex may participate in cross-modal visuomotor plasticity after stroke.[78]

Other resting metabolic studies, using less sophisticated analytic methods, suggest that regions of diaschisis in the contralesional hemisphere, which are found soon after a stroke, may not participate in recovery. Within 18 hours of onset, no proportional relationship was discerned between regional oxygen metabolism of the contralateral hemisphere and neurologic recovery using the Orgogozo scale when these studies were repeated 3 weeks later.[80] Oxygen consumption decreased in the contralesional cortex by the second scan, suggesting degeneration of transcallosal connections from the infarcted hemisphere.

Resting metabolic studies that show transsynaptic hypometabolism in cortex may not mean that the tissue is not functional. Thalamic lesions often cause hypometabolism of their cortical connections (see Color Fig. 3–3 in separate color insert and see Fig. 9–6.) This decrease in rCBF is relative. Subjects with chronic infarcts in the ventroposterior nucleus of the thalamus who had contralateral impairment of hand sensation were compared to normal controls and to subjects with infarcts in the anteromedial thalamus.[81] Positron emission tomography revealed a significant decrease in rCBF in the primary sensorimotor cortex ipsilateral to the stroke, which correlated best to the score of decreased appreciation of vibration and proprioception. A vibratory stimulus to the hand, however, produced no difference in the cortical rCBF responses of all subjects and controls. Subjects with sensory impairment had a decrease in sensory perception, but preserved awareness of sensory stimuli. Partial deafferentation with the partial sparing of inputs and outputs in the thalamic nucleus or input from other thalamic vibratory pathways could explain the findings. The bilateral thalamic nuclei have connections that may enhance plasticity after unilateral damage.[82] Thus, a sensory or pharmacologic drive may make use of spared projections in the presence of diaschisis and become part of a rehabilitative strategy.

Most functional imaging studies after stroke and traumatic brain injury have not shown clearly that the presence of transneuronal hypometabolism limits functional recovery or that some level of clinical restitution accompanies the resolution of apparent diaschisis.[83,86] Such clinical and imaging correlations could have a potential impact on making decisions about when to start rehabilitation efforts if certain instances of diaschisis were accompanied by failure to make functional gains.

Aphasia

Mimura and colleagues[84] made comparisons of resting CBF using SPECT for single brain slices. Regions of interest were restricted to the frontal operculum and Rolandic area, thalamus, and superior temporal gyrus. The initial mean CBF in the left hemisphere, but not the CBF in the right hemisphere, correlated with language test scores in scans performed 3 months after stroke. Lower initial mean CBF was associated with poorer scores. Six months later, improved scores correlated with higher left hemisphere CBF in those who had a good recovery. In a retrospective study, recovery patterns of another group of aphasic subjects at a mean of 7 years poststroke were significantly higher in the right hemisphere in the frontal and thalamic regions and in the left frontal region for those subjects who showed a good compared to a poor recovery in the language test. These findings suggest that when the language skills of aphasic patients improve over a long period, some of the physiologic and structural underpinnings of gains come to be managed by the right hemisphere. The study revealed lower than normal CBF bilaterally in the group with poor recovery of language and did not reveal higher than normal resting regional or mean CBF in the right hemisphere in subjects whose aphasia scores had improved. These studies suggest, then, that the patterns of CBF in relation to clinical recovery will be more than simple unchanging ones over time. Also, recovery of metabolic activity in the left cortical language areas may be most critical to gains.

Traumatic Brain Injury

Imaging CBF and metabolism at rest reveals the cortical deafferentation that accompanies diffuse axonal injury (DAI). These studies cannot always distinguish between loss of inputs from corticocortical damage and from afferents that ascend through cerebral white matter. Identification of metabolically affected neural networks will provide insight into the causes of attentional, memory, and other cognitive and behavioral problems of patients with TBI. Resting metabolic studies that correlate rCBF with behavioral outcomes will help determine the likelihood of recovery at a particular point in time. In addition, activation studies can be designed to assess whether or not a patient is able to learn novel information or likely to benefit from a particular rehabilitative intervention.

Positron emission tomography has revealed focal and diffuse cortical hypometabolism in areas remote from, but transsynaptically connected to subcortical regions affected by DAI. Hyperglycolysis accompanies severe TBI in the first days,[85] followed by a reduction in global glucose metabolism. Metabolic rates improve by 1 month after injury regardless of initial severity of injury, but functional outcomes do not necessarily improve, at least in a group of patients that did not have serial PET studies.[86] Thus, PET scans of glucose metabolism may be rather unrevealing within a month of TBI, perhaps because of a ceiling effect of the measure in relation to severity of behavioral impairments.

Single photon emission computed tomography measures of diminished CBF show some general relationships to executive dysfunction and neurobehavioral impairments in more chronic TBI.[87] Low flow in the thalamus correlates with greater cognitive and neurologic impairment. Low frontal CBF occurs with disinhibited behavior. Improvements in neuropsychologic test scores during rehabilitation correlates with increases in CBF by SPECT,[88] although associations between rCBF changes and impairments are not demonstrated consistently. Hypometabolism in the limbic and paralimbic areas, when MRI showed no lesion, correlated with poorer outcome on the Glasgow Outcome Scale (see Chapter 7).[89]

Regional cerebral glucose metabolism at rest and scores on a range of neuropsychologic tests were compared in 13 subjects who had a severe TBI a mean of 150 days earlier.[90] No subjects had focal brain lesions. At the time of testing, only two had a good recovery on the Glasgow Outcome Scale. Cognitive and behavioural disorders correlated with decreased metabolism in the prefrontal cortex and cingulate gyrus. Impairments in memory and executive functions occurred with hypometabolism in the mesial and lateral prefrontal cortex and cingulate gyrus. Behavioral deficits correlated with mesial prefrontal and cingulate hypometabolism. As expected, BA 9 and 10 were most involved (see Chapter 1), especially in the left hemisphere for subjects with impaired verbal memory and attention/executive impairments. The bilateral dorsolateral prefrontal cortices were most hypometabolic in the most impaired subjects. Anterior cingulate dysfunction, which is essential for executive aspects of attention and goal-directed behavior, was prominent in the most disabled subjects. The investigators found no significant correlations between neuropsychologic scores and metabolism in the temporal, parietal, and occipital cortices or in subcortical regions.

Persistent Vegetative State

Arousal without awareness may follow TBI, hypoxia, carbon monoxide poisoning, and other global cerebral insults (see Chapter 11). After closed-head injury, recovery from a vegetative state is less likely in patients who suffer injuries to the corpus callosum and dorsolateral brain stem.[91] ^{18}F-fluorodeoxyglucose-PET studies point to altered connectivity of association cortices and hypometabolism in prefrontal, premotor, parietotemporal, and posterior cingulate regions.[92] Global metabolic rates are often 30%–50% of normal, but islands of relatively normal glucose metabolism associated with fragments of behavior have been identified.[92a]

ACTIVATION STUDIES: FUNCTIONAL REORGANIZATION AFTER INJURY

The neuroimaging literature implies that spontaneous reorganization in resting metabolic and activation studies may differ from what transpires in regions activated in normal subjects or in patients after rehabilitative training. As described in Chapters 1 and 2, the CNS does have a remarkable capacity for reorganization at the cellular level and within its neuronal assemblies and networks. Rapid changes occur with unmasking of relatively latent synapses. Slower changes are related to induction of LTP and dendritic sprouts. Some of the drive for these changes derives from intrinsic properties of cells and circuits. Much of so-called spontaneous plasticity, however, derives from extrinsic influences such as experience and learning, which induce a range of activity-dependent adaptations over acute, subacute, and long-term intervals.

Spontaneous plasticity should not imply that gains in behavior and regional adaptations in brain activity arise in patients who have done nothing to lessen their disabilities. Studies of subjects with CNS and PNS lesions cannot lock subjects in a dark closet and keep them totally dependent on others. The term, if not removed from the rehabilitation literature, ought to be limited to passive recovery mechanisms that depend, for example, on the reversal of the cellular and network effects of acute ischemia or other cause of injury. If stated clearly, spontaneous reorganization might be attributed to changes that cannot be related to a defined form of practice or to formal rehabilitative interventions. Researchers, however, rarely measure the amount and sorts of practice carried out by subjects throughout a day of ordinary self-care and community activities. The plasticity associated with a defined training paradigm and assessed by serial neuroimaging and behavioral studies is most reliably considered as training-induced reorganization.

Functional activation studies track some of the changes in connectivity among regions, such as recruitment of areas remote from the lesion or of cell assemblies that do not usually become activated by a task. Imaging also reveals the changing representational map of a functionally specialized Brodmann's area. The interpretation of functional activation experiments usually includes the notion that differences in subjects with CNS lesions compared to controls have some causative relationship to behavioral gains or lack of gains. Consequential relationships, however, have not been demonstrated convincingly. Plausible associations have been made in a few studies that directly tested an intervention's behavioral and imaging sequela.

Sensorimotor Reorganization After Central Nervous System Lesion

HEMIPARETIC STROKE

Positron emission tomography, fMRI, and TMS have been most useful in revealing plasticity at various times poststroke and in association with levels of improvement in motor skills. The following general observations have held across most studies.

1. Recruitment of remote regions evolves over time with a reweighting of the contributions from other regions of the network. The ipsilateral sensorimotor cortex, for example, shows a much larger activation than normal, even when mirror movements of the unaffected hand can be excluded. Mechanisms include activity of the uncrossed corticospinal tract, transcallosal activation or disinhibition, polysynaptic activity and feedback through other parts of the motor network in the cortex and brain stem, and sensory drives from bilateral thalamic or callosal inputs. This activity is suppressed as skilled use of the affected hand improves.

   The ipsilesional premotor cortex is also often activated during simple tapping with the affected fingers. Brief suppression of the dorsal premotor area by single pulse TMS contralateral to the hemiparetic hand may prolong the simple reaction time, whereas stimulation of the ventral premotor area does not; a TMS pulse over M1 also delays the reaction time in the contralateral hand in patients and healthy contols.[93] A decrease in the level of premotor activation is associated with better hand function. Thus, this region with its corticospinal projections plays an important substitutive role.

2. The primary representation for a movement, such as M1 for hand movement, may expand if spared and later contract as movements regain some of their skill (see Color Fig. 3–5 in separate color insert). This evolution parallels changes in S1M1 observed during normal motor learning of a complex finger sequence.[94,95]

3. Activation along the rim of the infarct is common, especially within M1 and premotor areas (see Color Fig. 3–5 in separate color insert). This activity likely reflects a representational expansion for the movement and local reorganization within the periinfarcted tissue.

4. Patients who recover good hand movement evolve higher activation in the cerebellar hemisphere ipsilateral to the hemiparetic fingers, which is opposite the affected corticospinal tract.[95a]

5. Finger tapping often activates the ipsilateral as well as contralateral precentral gyrus in control and in hemiparetic subjects. The ipsilateral representation, however, is more anterior, lateral, and ventral compared to the site activated by the opposite hand (see Color Fig. 3–5 in separate color insert).[96]

6. The balance of bilateral activation tends to shift over time in a highly variable fashion, depending in part on the location of a lesion and the level of gains in the behavior. Greater shift of activation toward the uninjured hemisphere during tasks with the affected hand tends to correlate with worse behavioral outcomes, at least for subcortical infarcts.[96a] Persistent recruitment of M1 ipsilateral to the affected hand is associated with greater damage within injured M1. If M1 is spared, activation with movement of the affected hand tends to focus there over time.[96b] Primary sensorimotor cortex for the representation of the affected hand probably increases its synaptic efficacy. Behavioral gains, however, seem better in relation to the relative sparing of the corticospinal tract, determined by less Wallerian degeneration, than by the balance of activation in ipsilateral compared to contralateral M1. The other cortical constituents of the spared corticospinal tract, along with M1, probably come to play a greater role.

7. Regions usually associated with attention, planning, sequencing complex movements, and other higher level cognitive aspects of movement may be drawn into the network when patients perform a simple action. Ordinarily, only a novel or complex action would have activated these regions. The level of activation may rise or fall, depending on the demands of

the task for a subject. The contralesional dorsolateral premotor cortex and bilateral SMA participate in the acquisition of new complicated finger movement and upper extremity reaching skills. Many, but not all functional imaging studies of recovered hand movements[78] demonstrate activation of these regions by the time of recovery of even simple movements. The medial wall of BA 6 contains four separable motor areas[99] that may become activated with increasing task difficulty, as well as during recovery of hand function in patients with hemiparetic stroke. The SMA activation enlarges on the affected side or bilaterally (see Color Fig. 3–5 in separate color insert), especially when finger tapping is carried out by the affected hand without an external cue, such as a metronome. Most studies of recovery reveal rostral BA 24 activation for even simple hand movements, rather than its activation with only complex hand movements.[70]

8. Differences between individuals in the location and strength of nodes in a network or in the strategies that subjects used before or employ after the brain injury can account for some differences across subjects in regional activations. Neurologic impairments often change just how an action is performed, which may also change the pattern of activation during a voluntary movement.

Active Movements

Many movement paradigms have lighted the sensorimotor network, including individuated simple or complex sequential finger tapping, simultaneous finger and wrist extension, gripping, sequential wrist or elbow flexion and extension, toe or ankle dorsiflexion or plantarflexion, and tracing or following the movement of an object. The motor task chosen influences the level and location of network activation. The choice depends in part on the capability of the study group. Some tasks, however, may be more sensitive to defining differences between subjects and normal controls. Also, switching tasks in a serial study from a flexion-only grip to an individuated index finger tapping paradigm as motor control improves may confound interpretation of the data.

A few studies have examined differences in activations across hand movement paradigms. An fMRI study compared right-handed index finger tapping, four-finger tapping, and squeezing at 1–2 Hz.[100] The level of activation increased across these tasks in controls. Recovered hemiparetic patients showed a larger volume of activation during right index finger tapping compared to controls in the right sensorimotor and left SMA cortices. A serial study of two hemiparetic subjects showed that simultaneous bilateral gripping soon after stroke produced a larger activation in primary sensorimotor cortex in the affected hemisphere than did use of the affected hand alone. With improved hand function, the bilateral grip activation decreased to the same level as activation induced by grip with the affected hand.[101] When feasible, bilateral manual tasks may have some advantages in triggering plasticity. Some therapies do incorporate this approach.[102]

One of the larger serial studies of recovery from a recent stroke that was monitored by the same movement paradigm by PET was reported by Baron and colleagues.[103] At a mean of 7 and 30 weeks (with a wide range) after a striatocapsular infarct, 5 patients performed thumb-to-index finger tapping at 1 Hz to an auditory cue. The activations were compared to healthy controls. The first scan coincided with the time at which patients reacquired the ability to perform the task. Although the lesions were quite similar in extent, greater activations than in control subjects were found with the first scan in differing parts of the bilateral sensorimotor system. Significantly larger activation for the group was found in M1 and bilateral SMA. A global reduction in the magnitude and extent of activations followed at the second scan in the cerebellum, premotor area, S1M1 and SMA, as well as in the superior and inferior parietal cortices and insula. A contralesional premotor activation persisted.

Light, brief grasping of a sponge ball resting on the abdomen has been useful for serial evaluations of my patients who are studied soon after a severe hemiparesis. The movement may be synergistic at first. Care must be taken to prevent associated movements. As motor control improves, the force and speed of grasping ought to be kept constant during scanning. Other paradigms can be added. For patients who have fair function, a serial paradigm that employs repetitive finger and wrist exension of 10°–20° provides large activations that decline over time as motor control returns. This movement is a critical component for reaching to grasp. Lightly grasping and releasing a cup without moving the the forearm gives similar activations. Each task is performed at 0.5 Hz. For serial studies in subjects who cannot voluntarily make the requested movement, passive wrist movement activates the contralateral sensorimotor network.

Passive Movements

In patients with a plegic hand or leg or who can offer only extensor or flexor synergistic movements, a passive movement testing strategy may serve as a useful paradigm to study treatment-induced plasticity. Active proximal arm and leg movements often cause head motion artifacts during PET and fMRI scanning, so a passive motion paradigm is also a practical approach. Passive movements of the fingers, wrist, or elbow can be employed to activate the motor network. The contralateral M1, SMA, and bilateral inferior parietal cortices (BA 40) process this input.[97,98] As discussed in Chapter 1, BA 40 is the secondary somatosen-

sory cortex SII and connects to area 3b, posterior parietal, and prefrontal cortex. BA 40 is usually activated bilaterally by passive proprioceptive inputs. Passive proprioceptive movement studies of the wrist or fingers produce consistent contralateral activity in the associated region of M1 and S1.[104] Sometimes, the stimulus activates the SMA, premotor cortex, and cerebellum.

We have used passive ankle dorsiflexion to monitor representational plasticity over the time of training in patients with initially profound paraparesis or hemiparesis. Healthy subjects activate M1S1, SMA, bilateral SII in BA 40, and sometimes cingulate cortex (Fig. 3–6). As noted in Chapter 1, the dorsal spinocerebellar tract carries passive ankle movement to the cerebellum and eventually to M1S1. The cortex is clearly interested in this information. The primary motor cortex is quite active during voluntary dorsiflexion of the ankle during ambulation, so both active and passive ankle movements ought to elicit the representational changes in motor control that evolve during the practice of ambulation. Indeed, this approach has provided insights that parallel for the leg what active and passive finger and wrist movements reveal about changes in motor control of the hand.

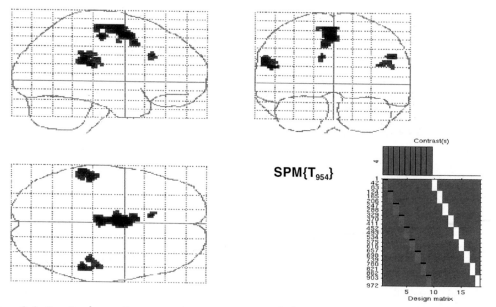

$$SPM\{T_{954}\}$$

Figure 3–6. Functional magnetic resonance imaging activation study during passive ankle and toe dorsiflexion of 20° at 0.5 Hz for 30 seconds is compared to rest in healthy subjects. Passive motion elicited significant voxels primarily in contralateral M1, S1, SMA, cingulate cortex, and bilateral secondary sensory connections in BA 40.

Passive wrist flexion-extension at 1 Hz over a 60° arc activates the contralateral primary sensorimotor cotex, SMA, cingulum, BA 40, and ipsilateral cerebellum, much as voluntary movements would. In a test-retest paradigm of passive movement that did not involve training, habituation caused some decrease in the size of regional activations, although this was partially reversed at a subsequent fMRI session.[105] Repeated proprioceptive training for 4 weeks in normal subjects led, rather surprisingly, to an increase in activation in posterior SMA and contralateral primary sensorimotor cortex for the hand.[106] Chollet and colleagues concluded that a learning effect can evolve with passive movements in normal subjects, perhaps associated with memory for the amplitude and frequency of the movement and related to the context of activity in the novel environment of an MRI scanner.

Passive movement paradigms have identified regions of the brain that participate in functional recovery. Passive movement of the elbow during PET was performed in subjects with severe upper extremity paresis up to 3 weeks after a subcortical stroke.[107] Patients received general rehabilitation therapies for 3 weeks. Regional cerebral blood flow increased primarily in the ipsilateral premotor cortex. Activations decreased over the 3 weeks in BA 7, perhaps as sustained attention to passive movement lessened. No correlations were made in this small trial between the changes in activation and functional gains. In another report, 12 subjects with hemiplegic stroke who could not use the affected hand had PET studies in the first week after stroke and 3 months later.[108] Activations accompanied passive elbow movements in the contralateral primary sensorimotor cortex or, if the area was infarcted, along its rim. Other regions, such as SMA, BA 40, ipsilateral M1, dorsolateral prefrontal cortex, and thalamus, varied in their activity across subjects. The investigators found a correlation between reorganization in the first week, including ipsilateral primary sensorimotor cortex activation, and recovery of hand function at 3 months. Thus, passive movement paradigms and other sensory inputs offer a potentially rich tool for the evaluation of representational and network plasticity. This finding is also another example of the potential impact of optimizing sensory inputs such as proprioception during skills relearning.

Contralesional Control of the Hemiparetic Hand

In adults with an acquired hemiplegia, TMS and metabolic imaging studies have described activation of ipsilateral sensorimotor cortex during movements of the affected hand. Transcranial magnetic stimulation produces an ipsilateral motor response in the hand in a minority of normal adults. Does this prove that uncrossed corticospinal projections provide a measure of substitution for finger movements? The anatomical basis for bilateral inputs from projections in the corticospinal tract is discussed in Chapter 1 (see Fig. 1–3).

Evoked responses are more commonly reported in subjects with poor recovery of the hemiparetic hand who exhibit mirror movements of the unaffected hand.[109] Thus, the corticospinal projections from M1 in the unaffected hemisphere may not be a basis for functional recovery of motor control in most patients. Another fMRI study, however, using sequential finger-to-thumb movements, found that contralesional cortex in patients with subcortical lesions was more highly activated than ipsilesional cortex soon after a stroke.[110] The ipsilesional cortex became more active over time, as hand function improved. In addition, the bilateral prefrontal and contralesional posterior parietal cortices shifted from greater activation acutely to lesser activation by 3 to 6 months poststroke. Six of the eight patients, however, had a plegic hand at the time of the first fMRI and showed mirror movements, so it is not so certain that the uninjured hemisphere's corticospinal tract played a primary role in recovery of hand function. Simply imagining the movement of plegic fingers can activate bilateral S1M1. An overflow of activation brought about by the great effort that goes into attention, planning, and monitoring a newly difficult action by a paretic hand may also drive frontal and cingulate cortices and feed back into the bilateral motor network.

A PET study of patients who recovered finger tapping after lesions within the striatocapsular complex found activations in ipsilateral S1M1 to be greater than in control subjects only in patients who exhibited associated movements of the unaffected hand during the finger opposition task by the recovered hand.[111] Again, mirror movements make it difficult to draw conclusions about contributions to motor control by the hemisphere on the side of the paretic hand. Some TMS studies suggest that premotor cortex and SMA provide bilateral output projections to spinal motoneurons and contribute to movement of the affected hand upon stimulation of the unlesioned cortex.[112] Any of the origins of descending corticospinal projections can also activate bilateral cortico-reticulospinal and corticopropriospinal pathways. These contralesional cortical neurons may be more excitable when they are less inhibited by callosal inputs that no longer project from the injured cortex.[113] Most likely, some adults, perhaps those with the most robust uncrossed corticospinal pathways, can divert these projections to enhance gains in motor control. Functional imaging studies can only point to this possibility.

Network and Representational Plasticity

In a series of groundbreaking studies by Weiller and colleagues, PET was performed in normal control subjects and patients who recovered hand function after a striatocapsular infarction.[70] Subjects were tested under the conditions of rest, repeated thumb-to-finger opposition of the recovered hand, and the same movement for the unaffected hand. The motor task with either hand activated the contralateral motor cortices and ipsilateral cerebellum to the same degree as in healthy subjects. Subjects with recovered hand function had greater rCBF compared to the control subjects in the bilateral ventral premotor (BA 6), SMA, anterior insula, and parietal (BA 40) cortices, as well as in the ipsilateral premotor cortex and basal ganglia, and in the contralateral cerebellum. These nonprimary cortical motor areas apparently served a substitutive function. The bilateral recruitment may also explain the associated or mirror movements in the left hand that often accompanied a right-handed task.

Sites of activation differed in relationship to the precise localization of the subcortical lesion. For example, one subgroup of patients with lesions limited to the posterior limb of the internal capsule showed a 1 cm extension of activation in S1M1 of the affected hemisphere. This corresponded to a spread from the hand area into the cortex for the face. The patient whose fMRI study is shown in Color Figure 3–5 (in separate color insert) not only transiently expanded the representation for the lower face into the hand representation, but his lower chin moved in synchrony with movements of the paretic thumb. Indeed, studies of healthy subjects suggest dendritic connnections between the face and hand representations[114] and a hand-to-mouth synergistic movement elicited by microstimulation of motor cortex,[70a] which may hark back to prenatal activity-dependent connectivity created by the fetal thumb-in-mouth position. Lesions confined to the anterior limb of the capsule in Weiller's series did not show this pattern of face-hand representational plasticity, perhaps because the disrupted frontopontine or corticostriatal fibers that initially caused the hand paresis recovered or compensated by a parallel motor pathway.

These PET studies of recovery offer other insights. Opposition of the fingers of the normal left hand activated the right insula, anterior cingulate, striatum, and the lateral prefrontal, premotor, and inferior parietal (area 40) cortices more than normal. Mild impairment of movements of the ipsilateral upper extremity has been reported with cerebral infarcts and is perhaps related to bilateral changes in pathway function induced by a unilateral lesion.[115–117] The experiments also showed that the lateral prefrontal and cingulate cortices and the angular gyrus were activated by a simple task after the stroke. These interconnected areas for selective attention and intention come into play when an automatic movement reorganizes. Thus, these pioneering studies with PET revealed at least three mechanisms for recovery: sparing of pathways in the case of anterior limb capsular lesions, representational expansion, and activation of distributed pathways that would not ordinarily have been as metabolically active. The imaging studies were not designed to determine whether representational changes and the recruitment of remote regions played a role in recovery.

Imaging with fMRI has been remarkably successful, given the complexity of the technique. The small number of cases in each study, the wide variations in the type and location of stroke, differences in clinical outcomes, and the limited range of imaging paradigms and analyses employed leave much yet to be learned. These investigations have yielded some additional insights into plasticity after stroke, especially in regard to S1M1. Contralesional S1M1 is the most common region of interest to rapidly reveal an increased number of activated voxels during movement of the affected hand.[118,119] The activation seen in ipsilesional S1M1 tends to center more posteriorly over time compared to controls, consistent with greater activity in the postcentral gyrus.[120]

Functional imaging studies may not appreciate shifts of less than 5 mm, depending on the data acquisition parameters. Also the data processing technique of spatial smoothing to optimize signal-to-noise may obscure a small shift. Metabolic imaging studies have, however, yielded other instances of shifts in neuronal networks, especially in primary sensory and association cortex. These movements of the center of activation are most evident as the paretic subject carries out and monitors difficult motor activities.[121] Increased attention for a task enhances both primary and secondary somatosensory cortical activations in healthy subjects as well.[122] Associative sensory inputs, which can be provided by rehabilitation interventions, have profound effects on long-term potentiation and representational plasticity (see Chapter 2).

Sensorimotor Integration

The influence of sensory input to M1 appears to be an especially important part of the restorative process. The specific mechanisms for adaptations, such as changes in synaptic efficacy and long-term potentiation, are discussed in Chapters 1 and 2. The impact of sensory inputs that are relevant to carrying out a task should not be underestimated. Primary somatosensory cortex provides a true representation of body surface. Primary motor cortex acts to bring together functionality across the joints of a limb.[123] Primary motor cortex has an overlapping somatotopy. Primary somatosensory cortex cannot. Thus, a sensory region may gain voxels (greater neuronal assembly representation) in a PET or fMRI study as sensory inputs, especially proprioceptive inputs, reorganize within S1 with repetitive practice. On the other hand, M1 may enlarge from input about a movement coming from S1, then shrink toward normal as the skill is reacquired. When the sensory inputs and motor outputs came closer to normal, S1 may also shrink to normal.

Although the hippocampus and association cortices such as the posterior parietal, inferior temporal, and prefrontal regions are most often thought of as storage areas for sensory information, S1 is also involved in storage and retrieval.[124] As noted in Chapter 1, each functional region of cortex that encodes information for storage seems to use the same population of neurons for retrieval, which ensures the fidelity of the information processed. *Thus, changes in level of activation and size of a representation in M1S1 implies that the neurons in these Brodmann's regions remember the sensory features of an action.* Retraining a skill may, then, require optimizing the sensory feedback for the desired task-related movement, which integrates sensorimotor contributions for the movement. Success in accomplishing a skill may be reflected by serial functional imaging studies as a patient learns a task.

Regional neural responses show adaptations over the course of multiple repetitions of the same stimulus when associated with learning. The activation, for example, in a specialized cortical region decreases over time by what has been called *repetition suppression.* In an fMRI study of associative learning of the locations of visually presented objects, repetition suppression occurred in parallel to the functional integration of the dynamic neuronal assemblies activated and to an increase in the effective connectivity between cortical areas involved in the learning.[125] For cognitive and sensorimotor tasks, an enlargement or refining of an activation within its representation may reflect a time-dependent change in the effective connectivity of interacting regions that drives greater synaptic efficacy within a region.

The chief theoretical limitation to assessing the degree of representational plasticity is that the size of a functional unit for performing a task is not known. What percentage of a maximal regional activation is required under differing circumstances, such as the representation's role in carrying out a simple task, a similar but more difficult task, and either of these tasks after varying degrees of injury?

MIRROR MOVEMENTS IN CEREBRAL PALSY

Attempts at unilateral or isolated movements may produce contralateral mirror movements or a general overflow of associated movements from any part of the body. Imaging studies after stroke have attempted to understand whether or not these movements, which are often transient in adults, represent a phase of reorganization. Onset of a brain injury early in life is associated with corticospinal tract adaptations. The capacity for functional reorganization has been especially apparent in infants and children after hemispherectomy for epilepsy[126] and after early stroke (Color Figure 12–3 in separate color insert). Ipsilateral cortical efferent pathways can come to subserve hand movements.[127] This plasticity correlates with the maturational changes of human sensorimotor cortex through age 15, prior to the natural, perhaps activity-dependent regression of neurons and synapses in the developing brain.[128]

The short-latency muscle compound action potentials that are typical of fast fiber conduction in corticospinal pathways have been elicited bilaterally in some children with infantile hemiplegia, suggesting a spared function of the ipsilateral ventral tract. They have generally not been observed after adult onset hemiparesis.[129,130] The presence of a hand response to ipsilateral TMS activation of the motor cortex of subjects with hemiplegic cerebral palsy correlated with a prenatal injury prior to 32 weeks gestation and intense mirror movements.[131] Corticospinal axons apparently branched from the normal hemisphere to bilateral homologous spinal motoneuron pools during the time of normal developmental growth of axons.

Another study pointed to a potential problem in sensorimotor integration in subjects with hemiplegic cerebral palsy. An active and passive movement fMRI study and TMS produced contralateral activation for the unaffected hand in seven subjects.[132] For the affected hand, TMS produced either an ipsilateral or bilateral hand movement. Passive movement of the affected hand caused only a contralateral activation, however, creating an apparent dissociation in some subjects between the hemisphere that received kinesthetic inputs and the hemisphere that provided the motor output.

SPINAL CORD INJURY

Paraplegic and tetraplegic subjects reorganize their primary sensorimotor cortical representations for movements. Transcranial magnetic

stimulation evoked larger motor responses in the abdominal muscles rostral to a thoracic spinal cord lesion and from a greater number of scalp positions than were evoked in the abdominal groups of normal subjects.[133] This finding suggests that the cortical motor map had expanded after the injury. The investigators could not exclude a change at the level of the affected spinal motoneurons, such as an increase in their excitatory response to a descending volley or to sprouting of corticospinal axons. Another group of paraplegic subjects had PET studies with ^{15}O-H_2O as their hands moved a joystick in different directions. The investigators found enhanced bilateral activity in the thalamus and cerebellum and expansion of the hand region medially toward the activity-deprived leg representation.[134] Magnetoencephalography showed that 20 of 24 tetraplegic subjects and 9 of 20 paraplegic subjects, including all 5 who could move their toes, had a posterior displacement of the evoked motor potential, suggesting plasticity-related somatosensory cortex adaptation to deafferentation and deefferentation.[135]

Cortical representations were mapped using fMRI with self-paced tongue and wrist movements in patients with motor complete cervical lesions graded ASIA A or B (see Table 10–1). The cortical activation for the tongue shifted medially and superiorly about 13 mm, compared to healthy subjects.[136] Indeed, the focus of maximum activation shifted more as the level of the lesion moved higher in the patients. No shift was found, surprisingly, for the wrist representation. The findings are consistent with other studies revealing that a disconnected, but available cortical representation may come to cofunction with neighboring active cortex, either by physiologic unmasking of latent synapses or growth of new dendritic connections.

TRAUMATIC BRAIN INJURY

Activation paradigms after mild to moderate TBI may provide insights into the effects and management of a postconcussion syndrome, focal brain injuries, and diffuse axonal injury. Twelve subjects who had a mild TBI 1 month before testing were compared to controls in the auditory n-back task (see Experimental Case Study 3–1) for assessing working memory (see Chapter 1).[137] The subjects described more cognitive symptoms, especially in concentration and recall of recent events, than did the controls. Activity in the bilateral dorsolateral prefrontal and superior parietal cortices was similar for the 0-back (simple vigilance) compared to 1-back (low demand) condition. A much more extensive activation was found in these regions on the right in patients with TBI for the 1-back to 2-back comparison, although performance did not differ. Both groups had a similar magnitude of task-related increase in activation when the 0-back and 2-back were compared. Functional imaging, then, revealed a difference in the ability of the TBI subjects to modulate or allocate resources with an increase in working memory demand. The clinical symptoms of the patients suggested difficulties in the maintenance and manipulation of verbal information. A study of patients who were recovering from more severe TBI used the paced auditory serial addition test to assess working memory (see Chapter 7). Compared to healthy subjects, the patients made more errors and the pattern of cerebral activations was more dispersed and lateralized to the right frontal lobe.[138] As in studies of progressive Alzheimer's disease,[139] greater demands on an impaired network may require larger or more widespread network activity to successfully carry out cognitive tasks.

Another PET activation study examined one of the consequences of diffuse axonal injury. The number of perseverative errors made on the Wisconsin Card Sorting Test was compared to results of FDG-PET in eight subjects with chronic behavioral symptoms after a closed-head injury.[140] The patients performed an auditory task that activates the dorsolateral prefrontal cortex. Perseverative errors were significantly and inversely related to metabolism in the right, but not the left dorsolateral prefrontal cortex and caudate nucleus. This relationship was independent of any individual differences in global brain metabolism, general cognitive ability, or overall performance on the test. No relationship was found between perseverative errors and the presence of prefrontal lesions on MRI. Functional imaging tests of this frontal-subcortical circuit, then, may help clinicians measure the impact of diffuse axonal injury in frontal white matter and serve as physiologic markers for the evaluation of cognitive and pharmacologic interventions aimed at modulating the circuit.

A growing number of PET and fMRI activation paradigms that emphasize planning (Tower of London task), switching from one aim to another during a task (Stroop Test), aspects of memory,[141,142] expectation and receipt of rewards,[143] and emotional responses to stimuli[144] can be used to compare normal subjects to people who remain disabled by the typical sequelae of TBI (see Chapter 11). One underlying hypothesis is that patients process information less efficiently after TBI. In addition, the effects of repetition and priming on memory processing can be monitored by functional imaging, which may aid the development of cognitive rehabilitation approaches.[145]

MULTIPLE SCLEROSIS

The partial remissions after exacerbations of multiple sclerosis (MS) and the progression over long periods of time lead to the speculation that partial restitution and substitution may evolve from lesion-induced and practice-related network and representational plasticity, improved axonal conduction,[146] remyelination, and of course, recovery from the effects of local inflammation. By the same logic, exhaustion of reorganizational plasticity as the burden of axonal lesions grows may contribute to functional declines.

An fMRI study employed simultaneous flexion-extension movements of 4 fingers at 10% and 75% of each MS subject's maximum rate.[147] The region of interest analysis was limited to the precentral and postcentral gyri and SMA. Supplementary motor area activation was higher in patients than in healthy controls. Lower activation in contralateral S1M1 and higher ipsilateral activation accompanied greater functional impairment in patients compared to controls. Also, with increasing T2-weighted MRI lesion load of MS plaques, the center of the activation shifted posteriorly in the sensorimotor representation contralateral to the hand that moved, especially as the volume of the MS lesions increased within the corticospinal projection. The center of activation moved approximately 8 mm, from the posterior wall of the precentral gyrus to the anterior wall of the postcentral gyrus in 15 of 24 subjects. As in the studies of patients with stroke described earlier, this posterior migration may point to a greater representational drive by the somatosensory region. A study of patients with primary progressive MS who had normal function of an upper extremity also revealed a different pattern of cortical activation than healthy control subjects during flexion-extension movements of the unaffected hand.[148] Moderate correlations were found between greater activations in regions for sensorimotor control and multimodal integration and the burden of MS lesions, especially in the cervical cord. In addition, functional imaging has revealed evidence for motor reorganization after a single bout of MS[148a] and adaptive changes during a sustained attention task in patients who performed normally.[148b]

Functional reorganization over the course of other chronic diseases has also been shown in patients with amyotrophic lateral sclerosis and cerebral autosomal dominant arteriopathy with subcortical infarcts and leukoencephalopathy (CADASIL). Nine patients with CADASIL, for example, were more likely to have bilateral S1M1 activations on an fMRI task of hand tapping than healthy control subjects.[149] As subcortical white matter injury increased, based on the relative concentration of N-acetyl asparate by MR spectroscopy, the ipsilateral activation increased.

Color Figure 3–7 (in separate color insert) shows the impact of a U-fiber plaque underneath M1 that partially disconnects its projections, leading to fatigue and functional reorganization of the leg region. Fatigue may be associated with impaired functionality between cortical and subcortical components of a network in patients with MS (see Chapter 12). Fifteen patients with MS and fatigue were compared to 14 patients with MS and no fatigue and to healthy controls as they performed repetitive flexion-extension of 4 fingers of a clinically normal hand.[150] Patients with fatigue showed significantly less activation in regions for motor planning and execution and in the thalamus. Thus, disruption of corticosubcortical circuits is associated with central fatigue.

Peripheral Nerve Transection

Experimental studies in monkeys that had a limb amputation or peripheral nerve injury show that sensory deprivation leads to contralateral somatosensory reorganization in the thalamus and cortex.[151–154] Limb amputation in humans also leads to sensorimotor representational changes as assessed by TMS, MEG, PET, and fMRI. Transcranial magnetic stimulation reveals a lower threshold, greater number of stimulation sites, and higher evoked amplitude for the muscles most proximal to the stump; the pattern of response varies over time.[155]

TRAINING-INDUCED REORGANIZATION

Although the number of pilot studies of patients with CNS lesions is still relatively few, the evidence is rather convincing that specific task practice leads to behavioral gains associated with changes in brain activations in the networks and representations evoked by the task.

The ideal serial study compares performance-related activations before, during, and after completion of training. The task performed during PET, fMRI, or another technique ought to include an important component of the practiced motor or cognitive skill. For example, if a patient practices repetitive functional use of the upper extremity under a variety of circumstances, the task during imaging ought to include grasp and release of an object or simultaneous extension of the fingers and wrist. These movements accompany typical reaching and may include preforming the hand in the shape of the item to be grasped. The success of training ought to be measured by tools that are relevant to the skills practiced by the patient. Too often, investigators choose an outcome tool such as the Functional Independence Measure that does not require the incorporation of the affected upper extremity into ADLs. Finally, *to most clearly demonstrate training-induced plasticity, practice ought to continue not for an arbitrary number of sessions, but until patients achieve an important behavioral milestone or no longer resculpt network activations.* Color Figure 3–8 (in separate color insert) shows the consequences of this strategy. Learning-dependent plasticity is a function of the intensity, duration, and specificity of what is practiced (see Chapters 1 and 2).

Serial measures of the behaviors to be learned and of the effects of learning on neuronal assemblies and networks, then, give the investigator tools to assess the progress and best-of-possible outcomes for the training strategy. This investigational strategy allows the clinician to study patients at any point in time after onset of a persisting impairment and disability. The critical component is the need for a well-defined and testable rehabilitative intervention. *This paradigm may allow investigators to use functional neuroimaging as a physiologic marker of the adequacy of interventions for rehabilitation.*

Activation patterns at a given time may also have predictive meaning. For example, a poor performance in discriminating the size of objects with the recovering hand after a striatocapsular infarct correlated with low rCBF in the contralateral sensorimotor cortex at rest and bilateral activation during the task.[156]

Normal motor learning, as discussed in Chapters 1 and 2, tends to focus the sensorimotor representation for the movement as practice and skill progress. In general, training after a CNS or PNS lesion augments the activity in local and remote regions. The representational enlargement and distribution is followed by activation suppression over time, presumably as synaptic connectivity becomes more effective with learning and the acquired motor skill is established within a corticocerebellar network for motor routines and cognitive strategies for their use.

Sensorimotor Training

USE OF THE UPPER EXTREMITY

Massed practice with the affected upper extremity (see Chapters 5 and 9) has led to sensorimotor representational plasticity over time in patients with subacute and chronic stroke. One technique, constraint-induced movement therapy (CIMT), which aims to reverse chronic nonuse of a paretic hand, is the most frequently studied intervention. Subjects selected for this intervention have at least 20° of voluntary wrist extension and 10° of finger extension. Thirteen patients who had been hemiparetic for over 4 years, 10 from a lacunar infarct in the internal capsule, spent 12 days in therapy for 6 hours a day and used only the affected hand for daily activities.[157] Liepert and colleagues performed serial TMS studies to map the evoked motor response from the abductor pollicis brevis of the affected hand. Before the intervention, the sensorimotor representation of the affected

muscle was smaller than in the unaffected hand. Behavioral outcomes for the upper extremity significantly improved with training. The gains were associated with an expansion of the scalp areas *that evoked a thumb muscle* response. Indeed, after one day of therapy, stimulation sites over the infarcted hemisphere changed from about 40% less than those on the normal side to about a 40% increase compared to the normal side. This rapidly induced representational plasticity suggests that much latent function of the hand had been present. A prior study by the same investigators found a significant decline in the number of activation sites for the unaffected hand after therapy, but this larger study did not.[158] By 4 weeks after the end of treatment, the number of sites became equal (having nearly doubled for the affected hemispere) and stayed this way 5 months later. Functional gains in terms of active use of the affected arm were stable over that period. The amplitude-weighted center of activated sites shifted to a more medial or lateral position, suggesting a representational change. The motor thresholds that evoked thumb responses did not change, but the thresholds were higher over the affected hemisphere.

The mechanism for this short-term plasticity may have been greater synaptic efficacy in M1, possibly through a decrease in interneuronal inhibition associated with previous nonuse of preexisting neuronal connections. Reorganization in M1, at another sensory or motor cortical area, or at a subcortical level may also have accounted for the findings. Continued greater use of the affected hand after the intervention presumably accounted for the reduction in area of cortical excitability by 4 weeks.

Serial PET scans revealed changes in the pattern of activation in a small randomized trial of task-oriented upper extremity training.[159] The 10 subjects, all approximately 3 weeks postonset, had subcortical strokes in the basal ganglia or pons and no movement of the forearm and distal joints. The experimental group primarily trained their proximal muscle groups for 45 minutes a day for 3 weeks. Their rCBF was measured during passive elbow flexion-extension from 0° to 90° before and after therapy. The small study was not powered to test for efficacy and the intervention was modest in its intensity. In the rest versus passive movement

cortex has been partially usurped by another modality, such as visual, somatosensory, or other afferents associated with, lip reading for example. Greater hypometabolism in primary auditory cortex by resting PET was associated with less likelihood of cross-modal input and, after training, higher hearing capability after cochlear implantation.[182] Large-scale reorganization of sensory maps may be feasible in young children undergoing rehabilitation. Some cross-modal plasticity may be accessible in adults.

NEUROPHARMACOLOGIC MODULATION

For rehabilitationists, a major goal for functional neuroimaging is to use techniques to visualize the physiologic activity of medications and their potential for modulating cerebral reorganization. A few tantalizing studies in highly selected patients with stroke or TBI suggest that a monaminergic, serotonergic, or cholinergic medication, especially when combined with practice, may hasten or incrementally improve motor,[183–186] language,[187] and cognitive[188] outcomes. Well within the experiences of rehabilitationists are the adverse actions of certain drugs on aspects of cognition, especially anticonvulsants such as phenytoin, phenobarbital and topiramate. Other common drugs also may have a negative, although less obvious, impact on functional outcomes.[189]

The ability to screen drugs for potential positive and negative effects on the rehabilitation of individual patients could have a profound impact on patient management. A few studies have shown that available medications can influence functional networks. Responses to a drug may be state dependent. For example, flenfluramine, which releases serotonin, increased the regional metabolic rate in anterior cingulate and lateral prefrontal cortex in a PET-FDG study of normal young subjects.[190] This response is blunted in people diagnosed with an aggressive, impulsive personality disorder.[191] Thus, after TBI, patients with a similar phenotypic behavior may respond to a serotonergic agent in different ways, depending on lesion location. Actions of neurotransmitters and modulators (see Chapter 1) can be studied by functional neuroimaging and cortical stimulation techniques.

Monaminergic Agents

Fluoxetine 20 mg, a selective serotonin reuptake inhibitor, and fenozolone (20 mg), an amphetamine-like drug that increases monamine transmission, was given to healthy subjects during an fMRI task that compared rest to two fist closings then touching the thumb to each digit.[192] The drug, compared to a placebo, focused the activity in the contralateral primary sensorimotor cortex and increased the activation of the posterior SMA, while decreasing bilateral cerebellar activation. The executive motor regions are rich in monaminergic receptors (see Chapter 1). Serotonin activates both pyramidal cells and GABAergic inhibitory interneurons. The neurotransmitter may inhibit Purkinje cell firing. Using the same task, another SSRI, paroxetine 20 mg, but not 60 mg, produced the same fMRI change in activation and improved hand speed modestly for the 9-Hole Peg Test.[193] Other SSRIs have also improved performance time.[194] A small controlled trial of fluoxetine in a single dose given to patients with stroke and pure motor hemparesis included an active and passive finger and wrist fMRI study carried out 5 hours after the drug was taken.[195] Finger tapping speed and hand strength improved while on the drug, associated with an increase in contralateral M1 activation during voluntary movement of the paretic hand. No modulation of cortical activation was found for passive movement. Thus, increasing brain concentrations of monamines may promote motor learning.

Color Figure 3–9 (in separate color insert) shows the effect of a single dose of fluoxetine on the S1M1 response during active ankle dorsiflexion in a healthy subject. The decrease in regional activation in S1M1 and SMA suggests greater synaptic efficacy induced by the SSRI. Further studies will examine whether a drug-induced alteration in activation in patients with hemiparesis or paraparesis can augment the training effects of a training intervention such as BWSTT.

As noted in Chapter 2, dextroamphetamine and dopamine agonists may have favorable effects on cognitive function and metabolic activity after a brain injury. The propensity for responsiveness to a medication may be predicted by regional fMRI activation studies.[196,197] Trials are in progress. A PET study using [^{11}C]raclopride, which labels extracellular dopamine, showed that rTMS of the left dorsolateral prefrontal cortex releases endogenous dopamine into the left dorsal caudate nucleus, which is a major projection for corticostriatal fibers.[198] Transcranial magnetic stimulation, then, may find a use during rehabilitation in asessing specific neurotransmission pathways.

Other Agents

Piracetam is a γ-aminobutyric acid derivative, or nootropic agent, available in Europe and Asia. A PET study showed that 2400 mg of the drug twice a day increased rCBF during a word-repetition task in mildly to moderately impaired aphasic subjects at the end of 6 weeks of language therapy.[199] Activations were greater than in the placebo group in Broca's and Wernicke's areas and in Heschl's gyrus. The drug group also improved in more subtests of language function. The mechanism of action is uncertain, but presumably piracetam aids learning in subjects with spared nodes in the language pathways. A larger study is needed to make that determination.

In a series of TMS experiments, Cohen and colleagues evaluated the effects of drugs with differing actions on rapidly induced motor plasticity.[20] In the paradigm described earler, they activated the corticocortical connections of pyramidal neurons of the motor cortex to elicit either a thumb flexor or an extensor movement. The subjects then practiced making movements in the opposite direction, until TMS over the same scalp location elicited a response in that direction. Most, but not all subjects had the kinematics reversed within 30 minutes of repetitive practice. The investigators then gave subjects drugs to help enhance or block the reversal in the direction of the movement. Lorazepam, which acts on GABA receptors, and dextromethophan, which blocks NMDA receptors and decreases cortical excitability,[200] reduced the activity-dependent plasticity. Amphetamine enhanced the practice time required for reversal of direction. The reversals lasted approximately an hour, but were not achieved uniformly in all subjects. This technique of short-term induction and testing of representational plasticity may prove useful in screening the effects of drugs on skills and declarative learning.

Positron emission tomography can map an increasing number of neurotransmitters and proteins. For example, a measure of acetylcholinesterase activity[201] may prove useful in understanding deficiencies not only in Alzheimer's disease, but after stroke and TBI. If abnormal, the response to oral anticholinesterase inhibitors or the potential value of cholinergic agonists could be tested *in vivo*. Functional magnetic resonance imaging and TMS also may demonstrate the negative impact of certain drugs. For example, some alcoholics show unusual activation patterns as they carry out working memory tasks.[202] Given that drug abuse is seen frequently especially among patients with TBI and spinal cord injury, the impact may be appreciated through brain mapping paradigms.

SUMMARY

The strength of the relationships between practice by patients with brain and spinal lesions, mechanisms of activity-dependent plasticity, and alterations in the maps acquired by techniques of functional imaging is not fully understood. More work, to date, has gone into demonstrating plasticity than in trying to extract the elements of training that best induce plasticity that furthers a patient's gains. As maps of cognitive and sensorimotor tasks are defined for healthy subjects and patients with a CNS or PNS injury, however, rehabilitationists will better recognize the pathways that subserve recovery and the effects of physical, cognitive, and pharmacologic interventions on behavioral learning and associated plasticity. Functional imaging's index of synaptic activity and connectivity can detect the evolution of functional reorganization within and between nodes of reverberating networks as clinician's manipulate a patient's sensorimotor and cognitive experience. Imaging may reveal how specific pharmacologic agents affect motor and mental processes. Perhaps more importantly, clever paradigms allow clinicians to use these tools as physiologic measures of the effects of intensity and duration of an intervention. When is enough therapy or drug enough?

Imaging studies can also serve as teaching tools. By seeing the brain's responses to how practice alters a representation or by showing how a lesion in one region, e.g., the thalamus, affects remote areas, such as the frontal lobe, patients and families may better understand therapeutic approaches and the nature of impairments and disabilities. Transcranial magnetic stimulation, fMRI, NIRS, and other techniques can become the tools of rehabilitationists for the study of hypotheses about training and recovery. Carefully designed experiments and clinical trials that incorporate these tools will provide insights for a scientific approach to neurorehabilitation.

REFERENCES

1. Mazziotta J. Imaging: Window on the brain. Arch Neurol 2000; 57:1413–1421.
2. Cohen J, Dale A, Evans A, Mazziotta J, Roland P. Neuroimaging databases. Science 2001; 292:1673–1676.
3. Phelps M. PET: The merging of biology and imaging into molecular imaging. J Nucl Med 2000; 41:661–681.
4. Mazziotta J, Gilman S. Clinical Brain Imaging: Principles and Applications. Philadelphia: FA Davis, 1992.
5. Posner M, Petersen S, Fox P, Raichle M. Localization of cognitive operations in the human mind. Science 1988; 240:1627–1631.
6. Arthurs O, Boniface S. How well do we understand the neural origins of the fMRI BOLD signal? Trends Neurosci 2002; 25:27–31.
7. Masdeu J, Brass L, Holman L, Kushner M. Brain single-photon emission computed tomography. Neurology 1994; 44:1970–1977.
8. Turner R. Magnetic resonance imaging of brain function. Ann Neurol 1994; 35:637–638.
9. Logothetis N, Pauls J, Augath M, Trinath T, Oeltermann A. Neurophysiological investigation of the basis of the fMRI signal. Nature 2001; 412:150–157.
10. Waldvogel D, van Gelderen P, Muellbacher W, Ziemann U, Immisch I, Hallett M. The relative metabolic demand of inhibition and excitation. Nature 2000; 406:995–998.
11. Vanzetta I, Grinvald A. Increased cortical oxidative metabolism due to sensory stimulation: Implications for functional brain imaging. Science 1999; 286:1555–1558.
12. Cohen M, Bookheimer S. Localization of brain function using magnetic resonance imaging. Trends Neurosci 1994; 17:268–277.
13. Mulderink T, Gitelman D, Mesulam M-M, Parrish T. On the use of caffeine as a contrast booster for BOLD fMRI studies. NeuroImage 2002; 15:37–44.
14. Classen J, Knorr U, Werhahn K. Multimodal output mapping of human central motor representation on different spatial scales. J Physiol 1998; 512:163–179.
15. Perrine K, Uysal S, Dogali M, Devinsky O. Functional mapping of memory and other nonlinguistic cognitive abilities in adults. In: Devinsky O, Beric A, Dogali M, eds. Electrical and Magnetic Stimulation of the Brain and Spinal Cord. New York: Raven Press, 1993:165–177.
16. Cohen L, Brasil-Neto J, Pascual-Leone A, Hallet M. Plasticity of cortical motor output organization following deafferentation, cerebral lesions, and skill acquisition. In: Devinsky O, Beric A, Dogali M, eds. Electrical and Magnetic Stimulation of the Brain and Spinal Cord. New York: Raven Press, 1993:187–200.
17. Karl A, Birbaumer N, Lutzenberger W, Cohen LG, Flor H. Reorganization of motor and somatosensory cortex in upper extremity amputees with phantom limb pain. J Neurosci 2001; 21:3609–3618.
18. Roux F, Boulanouar K, Ibarrola D, Tremoulet M, Chollet F, Berry I. Functional MRI and intraoperative brain mapping to evaluate brain plasticity in patients with brain tumours and hemiparesis. J Neurol Neurosurg Psychiatry 2000; 69:453–463.
19. Cohen L, Ziemann U, Chen R, Classen J, Hallett M, Gerlott C, Butefisch C. Studies of neuroplasticity with transcranial magnetic stimulation. J Clin Neurophysiol 1998; 4:305–324.
20. Boroojerdi B, Ziemann U, Chen R, Butefisch C, Cohen L. Mechanisms underlying human motor system plasticity. Muscle Nerve 2001; 24:602–613.
21. Chen R, Corwell B, Yaseen Z, Hallett M, Cohen L. Mechanisms of cortical reorganization in lower-limb amputees. J Neurosci 1998; 18:3443–3450.
22. Weber M, Eisen A. Magnetic stimulation of the central and peripheral nervous systems. Muscle Nerve 2002; 25:160–175.
23. Kosslyn S, Pascual-Leone A, Felician O, Camposano S, Keenan J, Thompson W, Ganis G, Sukel K, Alpert N. The role of area 17 in visual imagery: Convergent evidence from PET and rTMS. Science 1999; 284:167–170.
24. Chen R, Gerloff C, Classen J, Wassermann E, Hallett M, Cohen L. Safety of different inter-train intervals for repetitive transcranial magnetic stimulation and recomendations for safe ranges of stimulation parameters. EEG Clin Neurophysiol 1997; 105:415–421.
25. Walsh V, Cowey A. Transcranial magnetic stimulation and cognitive neuroscience. Nat Rev/Neurosci 2000; 1:73–79.
26. Flitman S, Grafman J, Wassermann E, Cooper V, O'Grady J, Pascual-Leone A, Hallet M. Linguistic processing during repetitive transcranial magnetic stimulation. Neurology 1998; 50:175–181.
27. Hilgetag C, Theoret H, Pascual-Leone A. Enhanced visual spatial attention ipsilateral to rTMS-induced 'virtual lesions' of human parietal cortex. Nat Neurosci 2001; 4:953–957.
28. Boroojerdi B, Phipps B, Kopylev L, Wharton C, LG C, Grafman J. Enhancing analogic reasoning with rTMS over the left prefrontal cortex. Neurology 2001; 56:526–528.
29. Rossini P, Pauri F. Neuromagnetic integrated methods tracking human brain mechanisms of sensorimotor areas 'plastic' reorganisation. Brain Res Rev 2000; 33:131–154.
30. Rossini P, Caltagirone C, Castriota-Scanderberg A, Cicihelli P, Del Gratta C, Demartin M. Hand motor cortical area reorganization in stroke: A study with fMRI, MEG and TCS maps. NeuroReport 1998; 9:2141–2146.
31. Flor H, Braun C, Elbert T, Birbaumer N. Extensive reorganization of primary somatosensory cortex in

chronic back pain patients. Neurosci Lett 1997; 224: 5–8.

32. Wikstrom H, Roine R, Aronen H, Salonen O, Sinkkonen J, Ilmoniemi R, Huttunen J. Specific changes in somatosensory evoked magnetic fields during recovery from sensorimotor stroke. Ann Neurol 2000; 47:353–360.

33. Fuchs A, Jirsa V, Kelso J. Theory of the relation between human brain activity (MEG) and hand movements. NeuroImage 2000; 11:359–369.

34. Crease R. Biomedicine in the age of imaging. Science 1993; 261:554–561.

35. Green J, Bialy Y, Sora E. High-resolution EEG in poststroke hemiparesis can identify ipsilateral generators during motor tasks. Stroke 1999; 30:2659–2665.

36. Nuwer M. Assessment of digital EEG, quantitative EEG, and EEG brain mapping. Report of the American Academy of Neurology. Neurology 1997; 49:277–292.

36a. Kaipio M-L, Cheour M, Ceponiene R, Ohman J, Alku P, Naatanen R. Increased distractability in closed head injury as revealed by event-related potentials. NeuroReport 2000; 11:1463–1468.

37. Cameron K, Yashar S, Wilson C, Fried I. Human hippocampal neurons predict how well word pairs will be remembered. Neuron 2001; 30:289–298.

38. Krelman G, Koch C, Fried I. Imagery neurons in the human brain. Nature 2000; 408:357–361.

39. Haglund M, Ojemann G, Hochman D. Optical imaging of epileptiform and functional activity in human cerebral cortex. Nature 1992; 358:668–671.

40. MacVicar B. Mapping neuronal activity by imaging intrinsic optical signals. The Neuroscientist 1997; 3:381–388.

41. Wang G, Tanaka K, Tanifuji M. Optical imaging of functional organization in the monkey inferotemporal cortex. Science 1996; 272:1665–1668.

42. Cannestra A, Pouratian N, Bookheimer S, Martin N, Becker D, Toga A. Temporal spatial differences observed by functional MRI and human intraoperative optical imaging. Cereb Cortex 2001; 11:773–782.

43. Cannestra A, Bookheimer S, Pouratian N, O'Farrell A, Sicotte N, Toga A. Temporal and topographical characterization of language cortices using intraoperative optical intrinsic signals. NeuroImage 2000; 12:41–54.

44. Cannestra A, Black K, Martin N, Cloughesy T, Woods R, Toga A. Topographical and temporal specificity of human intraoperative optical intrinsic signals. NeuroReport 1998; 9:2557–2563.

44a. Fallgatter A, Strik W. Right frontal activation during the continuous performance test assessed with near-infrared spectroscopy in healthy subjects. Neurosci Lett 1997; 223:89–92.

45. Sakatani K, Xie Y, Lichty W, Li S, Zuo H. Language-activated cerebral blood oxygenation and hemodynamic changes of the left prefrontal cortex in poststroke aphasic patients. Stroke 1998; 29:1299–1304.

46. Kleinschmidt A, Obrig H, Requardt M, Meerboldt K-D, Dirnagl U, Villringer A, Frahm J. Simultaneous recording of cerebral blood oxygenation changes during human brain activation by magnetic resonance imaging and near-infrared spectroscopy. J Cereb Blood Flow Metab 1996; 16:817–826.

47. Miyai I, Tanabe H, Sase I, Eda H, Oda I, Konishi I, Tusunazawa Y, Suzuki T, Yanagida T, Kubota K. Cortical mapping of gait in humans: A near-infrared spectroscopic topography study. NeuroImage 2001; 14:1186–1192.

48. Saitou H, Yanagi H, Hara S, Tsuchiya S, Tomura S. Cerebral blood volume and oxygenation among poststroke hemiplegic patients: Effects of 13 rehabilitation tasks measured by near-infrared spectroscopy. Arch Phys Med Rehabil 2000; 81:1348–1356.

49. Prichard J, Rosen B. Functional study of the brain by NMR. J Cereb Blood Flow Metab 1994; 14:365–372.

50. Reddy H, Narayanan S, Matthews P, Hoge R, Pike G, Duquette P. Relating axonal injury to functional recovery in MS. Neurology 2000; 54:236–239.

51. Garnett M, Blamire A, Corkill R, Cadoux-Hudson K, Rajagopalan B, Styles P. Early proton magnetic resonance spectroscopy in normal-appearing brain correlates with outcome in patients following traumatic brain injury. Brain 2000; 123:2046–2054.

52. Kamada K, Saguer M, Moller M, Wicklow K, Katenhauser M, Kober H, Vieth J. Functional and metabolic analysis of cerebral ischemia using magnetoencephalography and proton magnetic resonance spectroscopy. Ann Neurol 1997; 42:554–563.

53. Silvestrini M, Cupino LM, Placidi F, Diomedi M, Benardi G. Bilateral hemispheric activation in the early recovery of motor function after stroke. Stroke 1998; 29:1305–1310.

54. Silvestrini M, Troisi E, Matteis M, Razzano C, Caltagirone C. Correlations of flow velocity changes during mental activity and recovery from aphasia in ischemic stroke. Neurology 1998; 50:191–195.

55. Frackowiak R. Functional mapping of verbal memory and language. Trends Neurosci 1994; 17:109–115.

56. Friston K. Imaging neuroscience: principles or maps. Proc Natl Acad Sci USA 1998; 95:796–802.

57. Wittenberg G, Bastian A, Dromerick A, Thach W, Powers W. Mirror movements complicate interpretation of cerebral activation changes during recovery from subcortical infarction. Neurorehabil Neural Repair 2000; 14:213–221.

57a. Mattay VS, Fera F, Tessitore A, Hariri A, Das S, Callicott J, Weinberger DR. Neurophysiological correlates of age-related changes in human motor function. Neurology 2002; 58:630–635.

57b. Smith MJ, Adams LF, Schmidt P, Rubinow D, Wasserman E. Effects of ovarian hormones on human cortical excitability. Ann Neurol 2002; 51:599–603.

58. Rademacher J, Burgel U, Geyer S, Schormann T, Freund H-J, Zilles K. Variability and asymmetry in the human precentral motor system: A cytoarchitectonic and myeloarchitectonic brain mapping study. Brain 2001; 124:2232–2258.

59. Decety J. Can motor imagery be used as a form of therapy? J NIH Res 1995; 7:47–48.

60. Friston K, Price C, Fletcher P, Moore C, Frackowiak R, Dolan R. The trouble with cognitive subtraction. NeuroImage 1996; 4:97–104.

61. Sartori G, Umilta C. How to avoid the fallacies of cognitive subtraction in brain imaging. Brain Lang 2000; 74:191–212.

62. Gusnard D, Raichle M. Searching for a baseline: Functional imaging and the resting human brain. Nat Rev Neurosci 2001; 2:685–694.

63. Marchal G, Serrati C, Baron J, Rioux P, Petit-Taboue M, Viader F, de la Sayette V, Le Doze F,Lochon P, Derlon J, Orgogozo J. PET imaging of cerebral perfusion and oxygen consumption in acute ischaemic stroke: Relation to outcome. Lancet 1993; 341:925–927.

64. Kushner M, Reivich M, Fieschi C, Silver F, Chawluk J, Rosen M, Greenberg J, Burke A, Alavi A. Metabolic and clinical correlates of acute ischemic infarction. Neurology 1987; 37:1103–1110.

65. Heiss W-D, Emunds H-G, Herbolz K. Cerebral glucose metabolism as a predictor of rehabilitation after ischemic stroke. Stroke 1993; 24:1784–1788.

66. Giubilei F, Lenzi G, DiPiero V, Pozzilli C, Pantano P, Bastianello S, Argentino C, Fieschi C. Predictive value of brain perfusion single-photon emission computed tomography in acute ischemic stroke. Stroke 1990; 21:895–900.

67. Davis S, Chua M, Lichtenstein M, Rossiter SC, Binns D, Hopper JL. Cerebral hypoperfusion in stroke prognosis and brain recovery. Stroke 1993; 24:1691–1696.

68. Pantano P, Formisano R, Ricci M, Di Piero V, Sabatini V, Di Poti B, Rossi R, Bozzao L, Lenzi GL. Motor recovery after stroke. Brain 1996; 119:1849–1857.

69. Miyai I, Blau A, Reding M, Volpe B. Patients with stroke confined to basal ganglia have diminished response to rehabilitation efforts. Neurology 1997; 48:95–101.

70. Weiller C, Chollet F, Friston K, Wise R, Frackowiak R. Functional reorganization of the brain in recovery from striatocapsular infarction in man. Ann Neurol 1992; 31:463–472.

70a. Graziano M, Taylor C, Moore T. Complex movements evoked by microstimulation of precentral cortex. Neuron 2002; 34:841–851.

71. Kwan L, Reed B, Eberling J, Schuff N, Tanabe J, Jagust W. Effects of subcortical cerebral infarction on cortical glucose metabolism and cognitive function. Arch Neurol 1999; 56:809–814.

72. Reed B, Mungas D, Weiner M, Jagust W. Memory failure has different mechanisms in subcortical stroke and Alzheimer's disease. Neurology 2000; 48: 275–284.

73. Silverman D, Small G, Chang C, Lu C, Cummings JL, Phelps M. Positron emission tomography in evaluation of dementia. JAMA 2001; 286:2120–2127.

74. Fendrich R, Wessinger C, Gazzaniga M. Technical notes: Sources of blindsight. Science 1993; 261:493–495.

75. Escudero J, Sancho J, Bautista D, Escudero M, Lopez-Trigo J. Prognostic value of motor evoked potential obtained by transcranial magnetic stimulation on motor function recovery in patients with acute ischemic stroke. Stroke 1998; 29:1854–1859.

76. Heald A, Bates D, Cartlidge N, French JM, Miller S. Longitudinal study of central motor conduction time following stroke: 2. Central motor conduction measured within 73 h after stroke as a predictor of functional outcome at 12 months. Brain 1993; 116: 1371–1385.

77. Mills K. Magnetic brain stimulation: A tool to explore the action of the motor cortex on single human spinal motoneurones. Trends Neurosci 1991; 14:401–405.

78. Seitz R, Azari N, Knorr U, Binkofski F, Herzog H, Freund H-J. The role of diaschisis in stroke recovery. Stroke 1999; 30:1844–1850.

79. Binkofski F, Seitz R, Arnold S, Classen J, Benecke R, Freund H-J. Thalamic metabolism and corticospinal tract integrity determine motor recovery in stroke. Ann Neurol 1996; 39:460–470.

80. Iglesias S, Marchal G, Rioux P, Beaudouin V, Hauttement JL, Baron JC. Do changes in oxygen metabolism in the unaffected cerebral hemisphere underlie early neurological recovery after stroke? A positron emission tomography study. Stroke 1996; 27:1192–1199.

81. Remy P, Zilbovicius M, Cesaro P. Primary somatosensory cortex activation is not altered in patients with ventroposterior thalamic lesions. Stroke 1999; 30:2651–2658.

82. Kaas J, Ebner F. Intrathalamic connections: A new way to modulate cortical plasticity? Nat Neurosci 1998; 1:341–342.

83. Bowler J, Wade J, Jones B, Nijran K, Jewkes RF, Cuming R, Steiner TJ. Contribution of diaschisis to the clinical deficit in human cerebral infarction. Stroke 1995; 26:1000–1006.

84. Mimura M, Kato M, Sano Y, Kojima T, Naeser M, Kashima H. Prospective and retrospective studies of recovery in aphasia. Brain 1998; 121:2083–2094.

85. Bergsneider M, Hovda D, Shalmon E, Kelly D, Vespa P, Martin N, Phelps M, McArthur D, Caron M, Kraus J, Becker D. Cerebral hyperglycolysis following severe traumatic brain injury in humans: A positron emission tomography study. J Neurosurg 1997; 86:241–251.

86. Bergsneider M, Hovda D, McArthur D, Etchepare M, Huang S, Sehati N, Satz P, Phelps M, Becker D. Metabolic recovery following human traumatic brain injury based on FDG-PET: Time course and relationship to neurological disability. J Head Trauma Rehabil 2001; 16:135–148.

87. Oder W, Goldenberg G, Spatt J, Podreka J, Binder H, Deeke L. Behavioural and psychological sequelae of severe closed head injury and regional cerebral blood flow: A SPECT study. J Neurol Neurosurg Psychiatry 1992; 55:475–480.

88. Laatsch L, Pavel D, Jobe T, Lin Q, Quintana J-C. Incorporation of SPECT imaging in a cognitive rehabilitation therapy programme. Brain Inj 1999; 13:555–570.

89. Fontaine A, Bazin B, Mangin J-F. Metabolic correlates of poor outcome in severe closed head injury: A high resolution FDG-PET study. Neurology 1994; 44(Suppl 2):A175.

90. Fontaine A, Azouvi P, Remy P, Bussel B, Samson Y. Functional anatomy of neuropsychological deficits after severe traumatic brain injury. Neurology 1999; 53:1963–1968.

91. Kampfl A, Schmutzhard E, Franz G, Pfausler G, Haring H-P, Ulmer H, Felber S, Golaszewski S, Aichner F. Prediction of recovery from post-vegetative state with cerebral magnetic resonance imaging. Lancet 1998; 351:1763–1767.

92. Laureys S, Goldman S, Phillips C, Van Bogaert P, Aerts J, Luxen A, Franck G, Maquet P. Impaired effective cortical connectivity in vegetative state: Preliminary investigation using PET. NeuroImage 1999; 9:377–382.

92a. Schiff N, Ribary U, Moreno DR, Beattie B, Kroneberg E, Blasberg R, Plum F. Residual cerebral activity and behavioural fragments can remain in the persistently vegetative brain. Brain 2002; 125:1210–1234.

93. Fridman E, Hanakawa T, Wu C-Y, Cohen L. Involvement of the premotor cortex in motor recovery after stroke. Neurology 2002; 58(suppl 3); A30–A31.

94. Karni A, Meyer G, Jezzard P, Adams M, Turner R, Ungerleider S. Functional MRI evidence for adult motor cortex plasticity during motor skill learning. Nature 1995; 377:155–158.

95. Karni A, Meyer G, Hipolito C, Jezzard P, Adams M. The acquisition of skilled motor performance: Fast and slow experience-driven changes in primary motor cortex. Proc Natl Acad Sci USA 1998; 95:861–868.

95a. Small SL, Hlustik P, Noll D, Genovese C, Solodkin A. Cerebellar hemisphere activation ipsilateral to the paretic hand correlates with functional recovery after stroke. Brain 2002; 125:1544–1557.

96. Cramer S, Finklestein S, Schaechter J, Bush G, Rosen B. Activation of distinct motor cortex regions during ipsilateral and contralateral finger movements. J Neurophysiol 1999; 981:383–387.

96a. Calautti C, Leroy F, Guincestre J-Y, Marie R-M, Baron J-C. Sequential activation brain mapping after subcortical stroke: changes in hemispheric balance and recovery. NeuroReport 2001; 12:3883–3886.

96b. Feydy A, Carlier R, Roby-Brami A, Bussel B, Maier M. Longitudinal study of motor recovery after stroke. Stroke 2002; 33:1610–1617.

97. Weiller C, Juptner M, Fellows S, Rijntjes M, Leonhardt G, Kiebel S, Müeller S, Diener C, Thilmann AF. Brain representation of active and passive movements. NeuroImage 1996; 4:105–110.

98. Alary F, Doyon B, Loubinoux I. Event-related potentials elicited by passive movements in humans: Characterization, source analysis, and comparison to fMRI. NeuroImage 1998; 8:377–390.

99. Picard N, Strick P. Motor areas of the medial wall: A review of their location and functional activation. Cereb Cortex 1996; 6:342–353.

100. Cramer S, Nelles G, Schaechter J, Kaplan J, Finklestein S, Rosen B. A functional MRI study of three motor tasks in the evaluation of sroke recovery. Neurorehabil Neural Repair 2001; 15:1–8.

101. Staines W, McIlroy W, Graham S, Black S. Bilateral movement enhances ipsilateral cortical activity in acute stroke: A pilot functional MRI study. Neurology 2001; 56:401–404.

102. Mudie M, Matyas T. Can simultaneous bilateral movement involve the undamaged hemisphere in reconstruction of neural networks damaged by stroke? Disabil Rehabil 2000; 22:23–37.

103. Calautti C, Leroy F, Guincestre J-Y, Baron J-C. Dynamics of motor network overactivation after striatocapsular stroke. Stroke 2001; 32:2534–2542.

104. Mima T, Sadato N, Yazawa S. Brain structures related to active and passive finger movements. Brain 1999; 122:1989–1997.

105. Loubinoux I, Carel C, Alary F, Boulanouar K, Rascol O, Chollet F. Within-session and between-session reproducibility of cerebral sensorimotor activation: A test-retest effect evidenced with functional MRI. J Cereb Blood Flow Metab 2001; 21:592–607.

106. Carel C, Loubinoux I, Boulanouar K, Manelfe C, Rascol O, Celsis P, Chollet F. Neural substrate for the effects of passive training on sensorimotor cortical representation: A study with functional MRI in healthy subjects. J Cereb Blood Flow Metabol 2000; 20:478–484.

107. Nelles G, Spiekrammann G, Jueptner M, Leonhardt G, Diener H. Evolution of functional reorganization in hemiplegic stroke: A serial positron emission tomographic activation study. Ann Neurol 1999; 46:901–909.

108. Weiller C. Imaging recovery from stroke. Exp Brain Res 1998; 123:13–17.

109. Netz J, Lammers T, Homberg V. Reorganization of motor output in the non-affected hemisphere after stroke. Brain 1997; 120:1579–1586.

110. Marshall R, Perera G, Lazar R, Krakauer J, Constantine R, DeLaPaz R. Evolution of cortical activation during recovery from corticospinal tract infarction. Stroke 2000; 31:656–661.

111. Weiller C, Ramsay S, Wise R, Frackowiak R. Individual patterns of functional reorganization in the human cerebral cortex after capsular infarction. Ann Neurol 1993; 33:181–189.

112. Alagona G, Delvaux V, Gerard P, DePasqua V, Pennisi G, Delwaide P, Nicoleti F, de Noordhout AM. Ipsilateral motor responses to focal transcranial magnetic stimulation in healthy and acute stroke patients. Stroke 2001; 32:1304–1309.

113. Chiappa K, Cros D, Kiers L, Triggs W, Clouston P, Fang J. Crossed inhibition in the human motor system. J Clin Neurophysiol 1995; 12:82–96.

114. Bruce I, Siu L. Electromyographic activity in a distant muscle during simple voluntary movements: An unexpected hand-eye linkage. Electromyogr Clin Neurophysiol 1998; 38:405–409.

115. Brodal A. Self-observations and neuroanatomical considerations after a stroke. Brain 1973; 96:675–694.

116. Colebatch J, Gandevia S. The distribution of muscular weakness in upper motor neuron lesions affecting the arm. Brain 1989; 112:749–763.

117. Prigatano G, Wong J. Speed of finger tapping and goal attainment after unilateral cerebral vascular accident. Arch Phys Med Rehabil 1997; 78:847–852.

118. Cramer S, Nelles G, Benson R, Kaplan J, Parker R, Rosen B. A functional MRI study of subjects recovered from hemiparetic stroke. Stroke 1997; 28:2518–27.

119. Cao Y, D'Olhaberriague L, Vikingstad E, Levine S, Welch K. Pilot study of functional MRI to assess cerebral activation of motor function after poststroke hemiparesis. Stroke 1998; 29:112–122.

120. Pineiro R, Pendlebury S, Johansen-Berg H, Matthews P. Functional MRI detects posterior shifts in primary sensorimotor cortex activation after stroke: Evidence of local adaptive reorganization? Stroke 2001; 32:1134–1139.

121. Blood K, Perlman S, Bailliet R. Visual cortex hyperactivity during arm movements in brain injured individuals: Evidence of compensatory shifts in functional neural systems. J Neuro Rehabil 1991; 5: 211–217.

122. Johansen-Berg H, Christensen V, Woolrich M, Matthews P. Attention to touch modulates activity in both primary and secondary somatosensory areas. NeuroReport 2000; 11:1237–1241.

123. Sanes J, Schieber M. Orderly somatotopy in primary motor cortex: Does it exist? NeuroImage 2001; 13:968–974.

124. Harris J, Petersen R, Diamond M. The cortical distribution of sensory memories. Neuron 2001; 30: 315–318.

125. Buchel C, Coull J, Friston K. The predictive value of changes in effective connectivity for human learning. Science 1999; 283:1538–1541.

126. Chugani H, Shewmon D, Peacock W, Mazziotta J, Shields WD, Phelps ME. Surgical treatment of intractable neonatal-onset seizures: the role of PET. Neurology 1988; 38:1178–1188.

127. Sabatini U, Toni D, Pantano P, Brughitta G, Pandovani A, Bozzao L, Lenzi GL. Motor recovery after early brain damage. Stroke 1994; 25:514–517.

128. Chugani H, Phelps M, Mazziotta J. Positron emission tomography study of human brain functional development. Ann Neurol 1987; 22:487–497.

129. Benecke R, Meyer B, Freund H. Reorganisation of the descending motor pathways in patients after hemispherectomy and severe hemispheric lesions demonstrated by magnetic brain stimulation. Exp Brain Res 1991; 83:419–426.

130. Palmer E, Ashby P, Hajek V. Ipsilateral fast corticospinal pathways do not account for recovery in stroke. Ann Neurol 1992; 32:519–525.

131. Carr L, Harrison L, Evans A, Stephans J. Patterns of central motor reorganization in hemiplegic cerebral palsy. Brain 1993; 116:1223–1247.

132. Thickbroom G, Byrnes M, Archer S, Nagarajan L, Mastaglia F. Differences in sensory and motor cortical organization following brain injury early in life. Ann Neurol 2001; 49:320–327.

133. Topka H, Cohen L, Cole R, Hallett M. Reorganization of corticospinal pathways following spinal cord injury. Neurology 1991; 41:1276–1283.

134. Bruehlmeier M, Dietz V, Leenders K, Roelcke U, Missimer J, Curt A. How does the human brain deal with a spinal cord injury? Euro J Neurosci 1998; 10:3918–3922.

135. Green J, Sora E, Bialy Y, Ricamato A, Thatcher R. Cortical motor reorganization after paraplegia. Neurology 1999; 53:736–743.

136. Mikulis D, Jurkiewicz M, McIlroy W, Staines W, Rickards L, Kalsi-Ryan S, Crawley AP, Fehlings MG, Verrier MC. Adaptation in the motor cortex following cervical spinal cord injury. Neurology 2002; 58:794–801.

137. McAllister T, Saykin A, Flashman L, Sparling M, Johnson SC, Yanofsky N. Brain activation during working memory 1 month after mild traumatic brain injury. Neurology 1999; 53:1300–1308.

138. Christodoulou C, DeLuca J, Richer J, Madigan N. Functional magnetic resonance imaging of working memory after traumatic brain injury. J Neurol Neurosurg Psychiatry 2001; 70:161–168.

139. Bookheimer S, Strojwas M, Cohen M, Saunders A, Pericak-Vance M, Mazziota J, Small G. Patterns of brain activation in people at risk for Alzheimer's disease. New Engl J Med 2000; 343:450–456.

140. Lombardi W, Andreason P, Sirocco K, Rio D, Gross R, Umhau J, Hammer D. Wisconsin Card Sorting Test performance following head injury: Dorsolateral fronto-striatal circuit activity predicts perseveration. J Clin Experi Neuropsychol 1999; 21:2–16.

141. Duncan J, Owen A. Common regions of the human frontal lobe recruited by diverse cognitive demands. Trends Neurosci 2000; 23:475–483.

142. Brewer J, Zhao Z, Desmond J, Glover G, Gabrieli J. Making memories: Brain activity that predicts how well visual experience will be remembered. Science 1998; 281:1185–1187.

143. Breiter H, Aharon I, Kahneman D, Dale A, Shizgal P. Functional imaging of neural responses to expectancy and experience of monetary gains and losses. Neuron 2001; 30:619–639.

144. Damasio A, Grabowski T, Bechara A, Damasio H, Ponto L, Parvizi J, Hichwa R. Subcortical and cortical brain activity during the feeling of self-generated emotions. Nat Neurosci 2000; 3:1049–1056.

145. Henson R, Shallice T, Dolan R. Neuroimaging evidence for dissociable forms of repetition priming. Science 2000; 287:1269–1272.

146. Waxman S. Acquired channelopathies in nerve injury and MS. Ann Neurol 2001; 56:1621–1627.

147. Lee M, Reddy H, Johansen-Berg H, Pendlebury S, Jenkinson M, Smith S, Palace J, Matthews P. The motor cortex shows adaptive functional changes to brain injury from multiple sclerosis. Ann Neurol 2000; 47:606–613.

148. Filippi M, Rocca M, Falini A, Caputo D, Ghezzi A, Colombo B, Scotti G, Comi G. Correlations between structural CNS damage and functional MRI changes in primary progressive MS. NeuroImage 2002; 15:537–546.

148a. Pantano P, Iannetti GD, Caramia F, Mainero C, Lenzi GL. Cortical motor reorganization after a single clinical attack of multiple sclerosis. Brain 2002; 125:1607–1615.

148b. Staffen W, Mair A, Zauner H, Unterrainer J, Niederhofer H, Ladurner. Cognitive function and fMRI in patients with multiple sclerosis. Brain 2002; 125:1275–1282.

149. Reddy H, De Stefano N, Mortilla M, Federico A, Matthews P. Functional reorganization of motor cortex increases with greater axonal injury from CADASIL. Stroke 2002; 33:502–508.

150. Filippi M, Rocca M, Columbo B, Falini A, Codella M, Scotti G, Comi G. Functional magnetic resonance imaging correlates of fatigue in multiple sclerosis. NeuroImage 2002; 15:559–567.

151. Garraghty P, Kaas J. Functional reorganization in adult monkey thalamus after peripheral nerve injury. NeuroReport 1991; 2:747–750.

152. Pons T, Garraghty P, Ommaya A, Mishkin M. Massive cortical reorganization after sensory deafferentation in adult macaques. Science 1991; 252: 1857–1860.

153. Kaas J, Florence S, Jain N. Reorganization of sensory systems of primates after injury. The Neuroscientist 1997; 3:123–130.

154. Jones E, Pons T. Thalamic and brainstem contributions to large-scale plasticity of primate somatosensory cortex. Science 1998; 282:1121–1125.

155. Roricht S, Meyer B-U, Niehaus L, Brandt S. Long-term reorganization of motor cortex outputs after arm amputation. Neurology 1999; 53:106–111.

156. Weder B, Herzog H, Seitz R, Nebeling B, Kleinschmidt A, Huang Y. Tactile exploration of shape after subcortical ischaemic infarction studied with PET. Brain 1994; 117:593–605.

157. Liepert J, Bauder H, Miltner W, Taub E, Weiller C. Treatment-induced cortical reorganization after stroke in humans. Stroke 2000; 31:1210–1216.

158. Liepert J, Miltner W, Bauder H, Sommer M, Dettmers C, Taub E, Weiller C. Motor cortex plasticity during constraint-induced movement therapy in stroke patients. Neurosci Lett 1998; 250:5–8.

159. Nelles G, Jentzen W, Jueptner M, Muller S, Diener H. Arm training induced brain plasticity in stroke studies with serial positron emission tomography. NeuroImage 2001; 13:1146–1154.

159a. Carey JA, Kimberley T, Lewis S, Averbach E, Dorsey L, Rundquist P, Ugurbil K. Analysis of fMRI and finger tracking training in subjects with chronic stroke. Brain 2002; 125:773–788.

160. Levy C, Nichols D, Schmalbrock P, Keller P, Chakeres D. Functional MRI evidence of cortical reorganization in upper-limb stroke hemiplegia treated with constraint-induced movement therapy. Am J Phys Med Rehabil 2001; 80:4–12.

161. Dobkin B, Sullivan K. Sensorimotor cortex plasticity and locomotor and motor control gains induced by body weight-supported treadmill training after stroke. Neurorehabil Neural Repair 2001; 15:258.

162. Dobkin B, Davis B, Bookheimer S. Functional magnetic resonance imaging assesses plasticity in locomotor networks. Neurology 2000; 54(suppl 3):A8.

163. Dobkin B. Spinal and supraspinal plasticity after incomplete spinal cord injury: Correlations between functional magnetic resonance imaging and engaged locomotor networks. In: Seil F, ed. Progress in Brain Research. Vol. 128. Amsterdam: Elsevier, 2000:99–111.

163a. Conforto A, Kaelin-Lang A, Cohen LG. Increase in hand muscle strength of stroke patients after somatosensory stimulation. Ann Neurol 2002; 51:122–125.

163b. Fraser C, Power M, Hamdy S, Rothwell J, Hobday D. Driving plasticity in human adult motor cortex is associated with improved motor function after brain injury. Neuron 2002; 34:831–840.

164. Price C. The anatomy of language: Contributions from functional neuroimaging. J Anat 2000; 197:335–359.

165. Heiss W-D, Kessler J, Karbe H, Fink G, Pawlik G. Cerebral glucose metabolism as a predictor of recovery from aphasia in ischemic stroke. Arch Neurol 1993; 50:958–964.

166. Heiss W-D, Kessler J, Thiel A, Ghaemi M, Karbe H. Differential capacity of left and right hemispheric areas for compensation of poststroke aphasia. Ann Neurol 1999; 45:430–438.

167. Weiller C, Isensee C, Rijntjes M, Huber W, Woods R, Diener IIC. Recovery from Wernicke's aphasia: A positron emission tomographic study. Ann Neurol 1995; 37:723–732.

167a. Leff A, Crinion J, Scott S, Turkheimer F, Howard D, Wise R. A physiological change in the homotopic cortex following left posterior temporal lobe infarction. Ann Neurol 2002; 51:553–558.

168. Gabrieli J, Poldrack R, Desmond J. The role of left prefrontal cortex in language and memory. Proc Natl Acad Sci USA 1998; 95:906–913.

169. Cao Y, Vikingstad E, George K. Cortical language activation in stroke patients recovering from aphasia with functional MRI. Stroke 1999; 30:2331–2340.

170. Rosen H, Petersen S, Linenweber B, Snyder A, Dromerick A, Corbetta M. Neural correlates of recovery from aphasia after damage to left inferior frontal cortex. Neurology 2000; 55:1883–1894.

171. Thulborn K, Carpenter P, Just M. Plasticity of language-related brain function during recovery from stroke. Stroke 1999; 30:749–754.

172. Musso M, Weiller C, Kiebel S. Training-induced brain plasticity in aphasia. Brain 1999; 122:1781–1790.

173. Crinion J, Lambdon-Ralph M, Warburton L, Howard D, Wise R. Cortical regions involved in recovery of speech comprehension following left temporal lobe infarction. Neurology 2002; 58(suppl):in press.

174. Binder J, Rao S, Hammeke T, Frost J, Bandettini P, Bobholz J, Frost J, Myklebust B. Lateralized human brain language systems demonstrated by task subtraction functional magnetic resonance imaging. Arch Neurol 1995; 52:593–601.

175. Garavan H, Kelley D, Rosen A, Rao S, Stein E. Practice-related functional activation changes in a working memory task. Microsc Res Tech 2000; 51:54–63.

176. McIntosh A, Rajah M, Lobaugh N. Interactions of prefrontal cortex in relation awareness in sensory learning. Science 1999; 284:1531–1533.

177. Pizzamiglio L, Perani D, Cappa S, Vallar G, Paolucci S, Frazio F. Recovery of neglect after right hemisphere damage. Arch Neurol 1998; 55:561–568.

178. de Frockert J, Rees G, Frith C, Lavie N. The role of working memory in visual selective attention. Science 2001; 291:1803–1806.

179. Kujala T, Alho K, Naatanen R. Cross-modal reorganization of human cortical functions. Trends Neurosci 2000; 23:115–120.

180. Cohen L, Celnik P, Leone A, Corwell B, Faiz L, Hallet M. Functional relevance of cross-modal plasticity in blind humans. Nature 1997; 389:180–183.

181. Pascual-Leone A, Wassermann E, Sadato N, Hallett M. The role of reading activity on the modulation of motor cortical outputs to the reading hand in Braille readers. Ann Neurol 1995; 38:910–915.

182. Lee D, Lee J, Oh S, Kim S-K, Kim J-W, Chung JK, Lee MC, Kim CS. Cross-modal plasticity and cochlear transplants. Nature 2001; 409:149–150.

183. Crisostomo E, Duncan P, Propst M, Dawson D, Davis J. Evidence that amphetamine with physical therapy promotes recovery of motor function in stroke patients. Ann Neurol 1988; 23:94–97.

184. Dam M, Tonin P, De Boni A, Pizzolato G, Casson S, Ermani M, Freo U, Piron L, Battistin L. Effects of fluoxetine and maprotiline on functional recovery in poststroke hemiplegic patients undergoing rehabilitation therapy. Stroke 1996; 27:1211–1214.

185. Walker-Batson D, Smith P, Curtis S, Unwin H, Greenlee R. Amphetamine paired with physical therapy accelerates motor recovery after stroke. Stroke 1995; 26:2254–2259.

186. Grade C, Redford B, Chrostowski J, Toussaint L, Blackwell B. Methylphenidate in early poststroke recovery: A double-blind, placebo-controlled study. Arch Phys Med Rehabil 1998; 79:1047–1050.

187. Walker-Batson D, Unwin H, Curtis S. Use of amphetamine in the treatment of aphasia. Restor Neurology Neurosci 1992; 4:47–50.

188. McDowell S, Whyte J, D'Esposito M. Differential effect of a dopaminergic agonist on prefrontal func-

tion in traumatic brain injury patients. Brain 1998; 121:1155–1164.

189. Goldstein L. Potential effects of common drugs on stroke recovery. Arch Neurol 1998; 55:454–456.

190. Mann J, Malone K, Diehl D, Perel J, Nichols T, Mintun M. Positron emission tomographic imaging of serotonin activation effects on prefrontal cortex in healthy volunteers. J Cereb Blood Flow Metab 1996; 16:418–426.

191. Davidson R, Putnam K, Larson C. Dysfunction in the neural circuitry of emotion regulation-a possible prelude to violence. Science 2000; 289:591–594.

192. Loubinoux I, Boulanouar K, Ranjeva J-P, Carei C, Rascol O, Chollet F. Cerebral functional magnetic resonance imaging activation modulated by a single dose of the monamine neurotransmission enhancers fluoxetine and fenozolone during hand sensorimotor tasks. J Cereb Blood Flow Metab 1999; 19:1365–1375.

193. Loubinoux I, Pariente J, Carel C, Rascol O, Manelfe C, Chollet F. Motor output and dexterity are enhanced after a single dose of serotonin reuptake inhibitor: A double-blind, placebo-controlled, multidose fMRI study in healthy subjects. Neurology 2001; 56(suppl):A254.

194. Hasbroucq T, Rihet P, Blin O, Possamai C-A. Serotonin and human information processing: fluvoxamine can improve reaction time performance. Neurosci Lett 1997; 229:204–208.

195. Pariente J, Loubinoux I, Carel C, Albucher J, Rascol O, Chollet F. Fluoxetine modulates motor performance and cerebral activation of patients recovering from stroke. Ann Neurol 2001; 50:718–729.

196. Mattay V, Berman K, Ostrem J, Esposito G, Van Horn J, Bigelow L, Weinberger D. Dextroamphetamine enhances "neural network-specific" physiological signals: A positron-emission tomography rCBF study. J Neurosci 1996; 16:4816–22.

197. Mattay V, Callicott J, Bertolino A, Heaton I, Frank J, Coppola R, Berman K, Goldberg T, Weinberger D. Effects of dextroamphetamine on cognitive performance and cortical activation. NeuroImage 2000; 12:268–275.

198. Strafella A, Paus T, Barrett J, Dagher A. Repetitive transcranial magnetic stimulation of the human prefrontal cortex induces dopamine release in the caudate nucleus. J Neurosci 2001; 21:RC157 (1–4).

199. Kessler J, Thiel A, Karbe H, Heiss W. Piracetam improves activated blood flow and facilitates rehabilitation of poststroke aphasic patients. Stroke 2000; 31:2112–2116.

200. Ziemann U, Chen R, Cohen L, Hallett M. Dextromethorphan decreases the excitability of the human motor cortex. Neurology 1998; 51:1320–1324.

201. Kuhl D, Koeppe R, Minoshima S, Snyder S, Ficaro E, Kilbourne M. In vivo mapping of cerebral acetylcholinesterase activity in aging and Alzheimer's disease. Neurology 1999; 52:691–699.

202. Pfefferbaum A, Desmond J, Galloway C, Menon V, Glover G, Sullivan E. Reorganization of frontal systems used by alcoholics for spatial working memory: An fMRI study. NeuroImage 2001; 14:7–20.

203. Mazziotta J, Toga A, Frackowiak R. Brain Mapping: The Methods. New York: Academic Press, 1996.

204. Moonen C, Bandettini P. Functional MRI. Berlin: Springer-Verlag, 1999.

205. Friston K. Experimental design and statistical methods. In: Mazziotta J, Toga A, Frackowiak R, eds. Brain Mapping: The Disorders: Academic Press, 2000:33–56.

206. Smith E, Jonides J. Storage and executive processes in the frontal lobes. Science 1999; 283:1657–1661.

207. Owen A. The role of the lateral frontal cortex in mnemonic processing: The contribution of functional neuroimaging. Exp Brain Res 2000; 133:33–43.

208. Worsley K, Liao C, Aston J, Petre V, Duncan H, Morales F, Evans AC. A general statistical analysis for fMRI data. NeuroImage 2002; 15:1–15.

209. Poldrack R. Imaging brain plasticity: Conceptual and methodological issues-a theoretical review. NeuroImage 2000; 12:1–13.

210. Nudo R, Wise B, SiFuentes F, Milliken G. Neural substrates for the effects of rehabilitative training on motor recovery after ischemic infarct. Science 1996; 272:1791–1794.

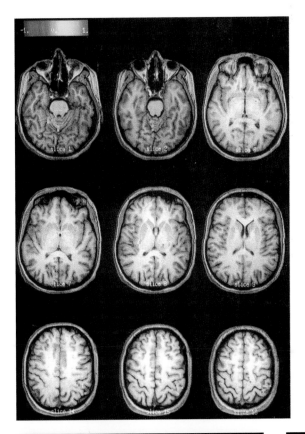

Color Figure 1–8. A functional magnetic resonance imaging study of repetitive flexion and extension of the fingers of the right hand reveals correlated activations in the contralateral primary sensorimotor cortex, supplementary motor area, putamen, and thalamus, and in the ipsilateral putamen and cerebellum. The inferior parietal sensorimotor coordinating regions are bilaterally activated. Activated pixels correspond to a cluster of more than 3 contiguous pixels that have an autocorrelation coefficient of −1 (blue) to +1 (red). Source: Lehericy et al., 1998,[210] with permission.

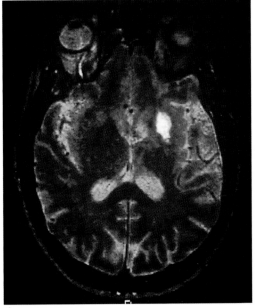

A

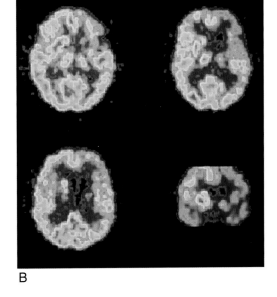

B

Color Figure 2–2. (A) T$_2$-weighted magnetic resonance imaging (MRI) scan shows an infarction of the left caudate and anterior limb of the internal capsule from a patient who suffered an occlusion of the recurrent artery of Heubner. The thalamus and cortex appear normal. His residual impairment included difficulty learning novel information, poor working memory, and a self-described daunting difficulty in thinking creatively. (B) A positron emission tomography (PET) scan shows the regional metabolic activity for 2-deoxyglu-cose. White and red colors represent the highest level of metabolic activity. The top two axial cuts show hypometabolism within the injured left striatum and uninjured, but connected thalamus and dorsolateral frontal lobe. The bottom right coronal cut also shows the marked asymmetry in transsynaptic activity between the normal right and abnormal left subcortical gray matter and frontal cortex. The diaschisis and hypometabolism is within the frontal-subcortical circuit.

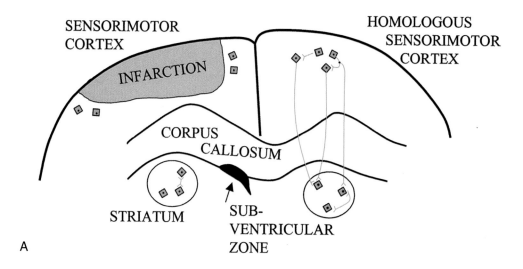

A

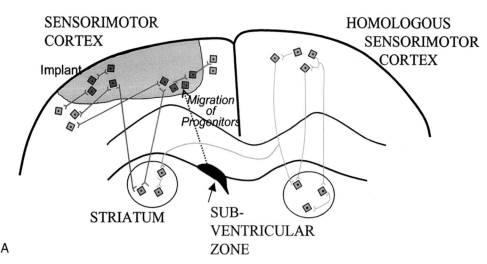

A

Color Figure 2–5. Potential mechanisms for neural repair after stroke are depicted in a rat model. (*A*) The infarction damages the pyramidal cells of the sensorimotor cortex for the forelimb representation and the ipsilateral corticostriatal projections. These projections are shown in the homologous contralateral cortex. Intrinsic responses such as dendritic proliferation between neurons (orange) in the homologous cortex may follow. (*B*) Endogenous precursor cells (red) from the subventricular zone that ordinarily migrate to the olfactory bulb may be incited to proliferate, differentiate, and migrate to the perinfarct tissue. The neuroblasts form local corticocortical circuits and projection circuits to the striatum with uninjured neurons (red and orange neurons). Another circuit is shown, formed by exogenous stem cells or neural precursors (blue) that were expanded *ex vivo* and implanted into the margins of the infarct. Rostrocaudal corticocortical circuits (red and orange neurons) may restore association pathways for sensorimotor and cognitive functions. The projection fibers from the implant to the striatum may improve sensorimotor control. In addition, corticostriatal projection fibers from the uninvolved cortex (orange neurons) produce axon collaterals that cross the corpus callosum in response to synchronous electrical and molecular signals for regenerative genes. Signals in the milieu of the denervated striatum, perhaps neurotrophins or axon guidance molecules, lead these collaterals to synapse in the striatum of the infarcted hemisphere.

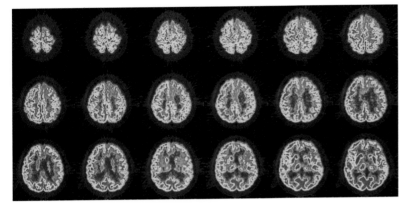

Color Figure 3-3. Resting positron emission tomograph (left hemisphere on reader's right) using fluorodeoxyglucose from a previously high functioning patient who had a stroke in the left anterior and dorsal thalamus 3 months earlier associated with hypertension. The family was told that the stroke was a minor one and he could return to ordinary activities. From left to right and top to bottom, the axial slices go from higher to lower levels of the cerebrum. Metabolism is scaled as highest (red) to lower (yellow), then green, then blue (cerebrospinal fluid). Asymmetric hypometabolism is seen in the left hemisphere in posterior frontal cortex (high cuts) and the dorsolateral and frontal cortex on lower cuts (second and third rows). The bottom row reveals diminished activity in the left thalamus and basal ganglia (last 4 cuts on the right).

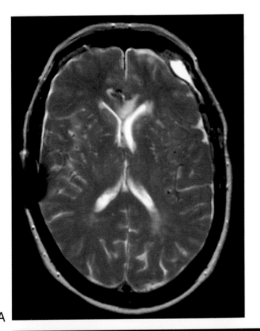

Color Figure 3–4. (*A*) Axial view of magnetic resonance imaging study shows the anterior midline infarction that accompanied a subarachnoid hemorrhage from an anterior communicating aneurysm. The lesion damaged the inferior aspect of the corpus callosum and undercut the septal region, which receives input from the ventral tegmental tract and sends projections to the hippocampus. (*B*) Six months after the stroke, a positron emission tomography scan using ^{18}fluorodeoxyglucose was performed at rest. Hypometabolism is found in the bilateral frontal lobes, but especially affects frontal–subcortical circuits on the left more than the right that include the dorsolateral prefrontal cortex, thalamus, and basal ganglia, best appreciated on the images at the bottom row to the right.

A

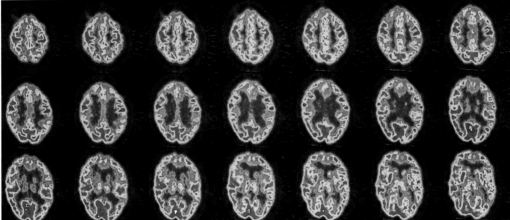

B

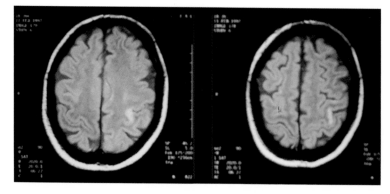

Color Figure 3–5. Serial functional magnetic resonance imaging (fMRI) study of recovery of hand grasping. (*A*) An infarct in the primary motor cortex has high T$_2$ weighted signal near the hand sulcal notch. (*B*) The subject lightly squeezed a sponge ball for 30 seconds at 0.5 Hz alternating with 30 seconds of rest during the fMRI activation. Four serial studies are shown. Functional MRI reveals an evolution of changes in the representations for this action as motor control improves (see Experimental Case Study 3–2). Arrow points to the hand notch representation.

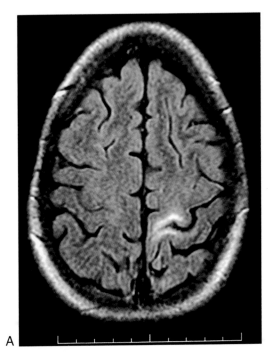

A

Color Figure 3–7. (*A*) The magnetic resonance study using a FLAIR sequence reveals a lesion of the U-fibers under the primary motor cortex in the leg/trunk representation. A young woman presented with weakness of the right leg brought on by prolonged bicycling. She had subtle weakness of the iliopsoas and gluteal muscles on examination. Immediately after performing 20 jumping jacks, however, paresis in all muscles of the right leg and subtle paresis of the right shoulder girdle occurred, lasting less than 2 minutes. Laboratory studies and a subsequent bout of left leg paresthesias established the diagnosis of multiple sclerosis. This reversible fatigability with repetitive movements suggests impaired central conduction of spared or partially spared fibers that cannot keep up with activity-dependent demand. (*B*) This series of functional magnetic resonance imaging studies reveals activation of the wrist and the low trunk/hip representations that surround the affected cortical mantle. The cortex above the plaque could not be activated by a wrist or back motor task. This finding may be related to deafferentation of the motoneurons or neuronal dysfunction from the proximal axon injury by the plaque. A relatively larger activation than expected for a wrist and low paraspinal muscle movement at just 0.5 Hz suggests reorganization of peri-plaque motor representations. Arrows point to the plaque and area medial to it for the back muscles.

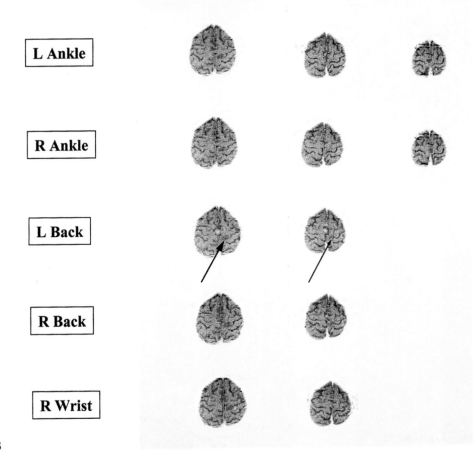

B

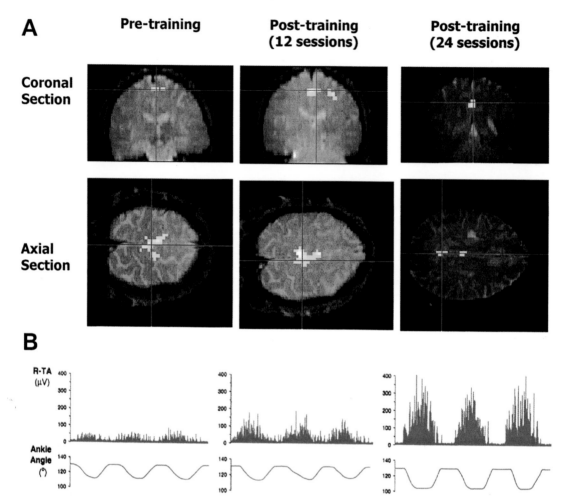

Color Figure 3–8. Pre-training: Six months after a left subcortical infarct, the patient walked slowly over ground, usually caught the toe at initial leg swing, and showed asymmetrical stance and swing times. A functional magnetic resonance imaging (fMRI) study of voluntary ankle dorsifexion at 0.5 Hz for 30 seconds was compared to rest. The fMRI studies were analyzed by SPM. In addition, significantly activated pixels ($p < 0.01$) were located in a region-of-interest analysis of primary somatosensory cortex/primary motor cortex (S1M1) and supplementary motor area (SMA). (*A*) A rather diffuse activation was initially present in bilateral SMA and prefrontal cortex with a modest activation in contralateral S1M1. (*B*) Raw rectified electromyographic (EMG) activity of the affected tibialis anterior tested for the same movement revealed low-amplitude bursts. Post-training after 12 sessions of body weight-supported treadmill training at 1.8–2.2 mph: (*A*) Activations converge more into the bilateral SMA. (*B*) Walking velocity increased by 40% and kinematics during stepping improved. Electromyographic burst amplitude increased, but the off-period remained abnormal. Post-training after 24 sessions at treadmill speeds up to 2.5 mph: (*A*) Activations are highest in contralateral S1M1 and SMA and similar in distribution to healthy subjects. (*B*) Walking velocity further improved 15% and foot clearance, stride length, and symmetry of stance and swing times for the legs was near normal. Electromyographic bursts are higher in amplitude and have clear on and off times, suggesting better motor control of the tibialis anterior and ankle dorsiflexion.

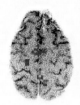 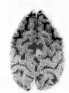

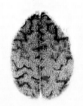 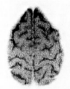 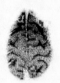

Color Figure 3–9. Functional magnetic resonance imaging activation study of 20° of voluntary repetitive ankle dorsiflexion at 0.5 HZ in a healthy volunteer before and 3 hours after a single dose of fluoxetine, 10 mg. Activity became more focused in primary sensorimotor cortex in the leg representation and in SMA. This suggests greater synaptic efficacy, perhaps associated with greater sensory drive, given the persistent parietal activity. The drug could also have raised the excitability of these regions at rest, so that foot movements caused less relative increase in activation. Three control subjects showed the same changes, whether the serotonergic agent was given for a first or second study.

Right Foot Dorsiflexion

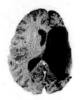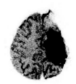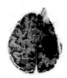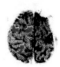

Left Foot Dorsiflexion

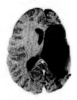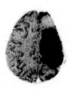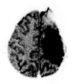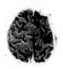

Color Figure 12–3. Functional magnetic resonance imaging (BOLD technique) with region-of-interest analysis reveals differences in the recruitment pattern during ankle dorsifexion of the right (top) and left (bottom) ankles in a youngster who suffered a perinatal stroke in a left middle cerebral artery distribution causing a congenital right hemiparesis. Refractory seizures led to a partial hemispherectomy at 10 years of age. She was able to walk with minimal paresis and selectively dorsiflex the affected ankle. At age 11, dorsiflexion of the right foot at 0.5 Hz activated the contralesional sensory cortex, supplementary motor area, and precentral frontal cortex, along with spared ipsilesional cingulate cortex and SMA. Dorsiflexion of the unaffected left foot elicited typical primary sensorimotor, parietal, and SMA activity, and no cingulate activation. The study suggests bilateral contributions to motor control for the right foot and greater input from spared cingulate motor cortex than normally found on the side of the lesion.

Chapter 4

Neurostimulators and Neuroprostheses

Along with the generation of axons and neurons to aid neurorecovery, the first quarter of the 21st century will see the creation of interfaces that allow neurons to drive or be driven by computers and micromachines (Table 4–1). Such human-machine interfaces may reduce impairments and disabilities. At a minimum, they will lessen handicaps by making the environment more negotiable.

Several neuroprostheses are available for purchase. They employ electrical stimulation of nerves and motor points in muscle to permit grasping with a plegic hand or to empty a neurogenic bladder. Simple neurorobotic devices have been created for quadriplegic subjects. Patterns of cerebral electrical activity extracted by a computer interfaces with levers or cursors to produce movements, words, and environmental controls. Brain-derived signals may soon command neuroprostheses. The cochlear implant restores hearing for people with acquired deafness. Visual prostheses that stimulate visual cortex are becoming feasible.

Computational power in inexpensive computers has grown so great that neurorobotic and neuroprosthetic devices may eventually manage complex tasks, most likely when stimulation sequences and intensities come to be guided by sensory feedback.[1] Miniaturization is also progressing quickly. Microelectromechanical systems (MEMS) such as pressure sensors, accelerometers, optical switches, actuators, pumps, gears, and pulleys that fit on a grain of rice or ride a red blood cell are improving manufactured goods and health-care items. The MEMS and even tinier nanoelectronic devices now analyze bodily fluids and measure skin pressure or blood pressure after implantation. These sensors, analyzers, and motors may soon become integrated into neurorobotic and neuroprosthetic stimulation and feedback devices that can be implanted within a cortical or subcortical neuronal assembly or along a central or peripheral nerve. Nanodevices may read and pulse neurons with electrical and chemical signals, drugs, neurotransmitters, or trophic agents. Neurons that form a circuit with semiconductor chips[2] may further integrate MEMS devices with the nervous system. Such cyborg-like modules of silicon neurons could partially patch a disconnection in a cortical or spinal circuit.

Improvements in CNS and PNS signal processing, in the size, cost, and functionality of implanted sensors and stimulators, in online functional and chemical imaging, in targeted drug delivery, in tissue engineering, and in

Table 4–1. **Bionic Approaches for Movement**

Interface Approach	Likely Consumers	Types of Actuators
Brain-machine	Mechanical assist for paralyzed persons	Motors to control robotic arm
Brain-computer	Communication for paralyzed persons	Computer screen to move a cursor
Peripheral-machine	Amputees or persons with weakness and intact central nervous system	Motors for prosthetic hand
Hybrid brain-machine	Complete spinal cord injury	Brain control of *FreeHand* device
Computer-brain	Parkinson's disease	Muscles

Source: adapted from W. Craelius, 2002.[66]

fiber-optic approaches to stimulation and sensing may allow clinicians the opportunity to partially substitute for impaired sensation, movement, and some cognitive processes using a biologic and microelectronic tool kit. Up until now, painstaking research and development has gone into less exotic neurostimulators and neuroprostheses. Bionics, however, is on the threshold of creating devices that find and decipher the neural signals that express cognitive control over important movements from within their residual pathways.

PERIPHERAL NERVOUS SYSTEM DEVICES

Functional Neuromuscular Stimulation

The term functional neuromuscular stimulation (FNS) will be used to describe devices that produce functional movements of paralyzed muscles to lessen disability. Functional electrical stimulation (FES) is a term often used interchangeably. I will apply it, however, to describe electrical stimulation devices that were designed primarily to increase muscle volume and strength or to decrease hypertonicity, but not to directly affect self-care skills. A diaphragmatic pacing system, then, would fall under the category of FNS. Functional neuromuscular stimulation devices have faced a difficult road in reaching consumers.[3] Once a device is available, commercialization faces struggles with regulatory agencies over safety and efficacy, as well as with liability issues, cost-benefit analyses, and production costs for items that may have a very limited market.

GENERAL DESIGN FEATURES

Electrical stimulation produces an all-or-nothing depolarization of axons and their terminal branches in muscle. Fast, fatigable motor units are recruited first. The motor point is the most common site for direct electrical stimulation. From here, a mix of fast and slow muscle fibers are recruited as current spreads from an electrode. Functional neuromuscular stimulation requires an intact motor unit. If anterior horn cells have been destroyed, roots torn or avulsed, or peripheral nerves severed, electrical stimulation fails. The nerves and motor points affected by complete brachial plexopathies, central cord injuries, and conus/cauda equina trauma cannot be activated.

The amount of current delivered to a given region determines the success of muscle contraction. The current produced by a stimulator at a surface or implanted electrode is adjusted by its pulse waveform, usually a square wave, and especially by its amplitude and duration. Frequency adjustments of pulse cycles per second aim for a tetanic contraction, which occurs at 15 Hz–30 Hz. When magnetic stimulators are used, coil shape and placement, the magnetic gradient, and pulse duration manipulate the current. High rates of stimulation and a larger duty cycle, which is the ratio of time that the stimulator is on compared to off, produce neuromuscular fatigue. The main contraindications to stimulation include pacemakers, high susceptibility to cardiac arrhythmias, and autonomic instability, along with severe bone demineralization or wounds in the region induced to contract. Implanted electrodes and stimulators that are placed under the skin become a contraindication for imaging studies by MRI and can lead to complications such as bacteremia in people with prosthetic heart valves.

Portable FNS systems powered by batteries allow consumers to learn how to time the onset and offset of the desired muscle contraction and movement. The trainer sets the stimulus parameters through trial and error and practice with the subject. On–off switches of many varieties are positioned wherever most accessible for the subject. A hand-held button, heel switch, or joint position sensor may, for example, trigger movements during walking. A shoulder movement, wrist angular transducer, and voice activation switch have worked for stimulation of the upper extremity. The switch connects to the stimulator with its programmed microprocessors. The microprocessors control the firing parameters of each channel and activate an electrode wired to a muscle. From 4 to 16 muscles of an extremity are modulated, firing in various combinations of timed contractions. Sensory feedback to create a closed loop FNS system is a research and development goal.[4] Real time data on changing joint torques and positions, acceleration of the limb, cutaneous pressure at the fingertips, and other parameters will increase the functionality of FNS systems.

Short-term or intermittent stimulation sessions employ surface electrodes with low impedances placed over muscles. Long-term stimulation for daily use is most practical using electrodes implanted near each muscle's motor point with connecting wires that run under the skin to the stimulator. Implanted electrodes are designed for easy placement, immobility once in the contracting muscle, minor tissue responses to prevent infection and scarring, and durability. Electrodes designed for injection by a hypodermic needle under fluoroscopy must be quite thin and have barbs to keep them in place. Surgically implanted electrodes can be thicker and more durable and placed in the muscle or sewn onto the epimysium. A wireless, injectable electrode called the *BION* was released in 2000 to evaluate its utility in clincial applications (Advanced Bionics Corp, Sylmar, CA; A.E. Mann Foundation for Scientific Research, Santa Clarita, CA).[5] The ceramic case is approximately 2.5 mm wide and 15 mm long. It includes an antenna that allows it to receive and transmit data by radiofrequency telemetry. Thus, a *BION* can be designed to provide sensory feedback from stretch or local forces for example. A magnetic stimulator must be close by to trigger each *BION*.

SYSTEMS FOR THE UPPER EXTREMITY

The first commercial neuroprosthesis for hand grasping with implanted electrodes is the $35,000 *FreeHand* system (NeuroControl Corp., Cleveland, OH).[6] Most users have a cervical SCI with residual ability to flex the elbow and extend the wrist, but cannot use their hands. An external shoulder position transducer activates an external programmable control unit. The unit is wired to a subcutaneously implanted receiver/stimulator with eight channels. The outlets are wired to epimysial electrodes sutured onto the adductor pollicus, extensor pollicis longus, abductor digitorum brevis, extensor digitorm communis, and flexor digitorum superficialis muscles and, sometimes, other groups such as flexor digitorum profundus and flexor pollicus longus for a stronger palmar or lateral prehension grasp. The receiver/stimulator is placed on the chest near the opposite shoulder.

FreeHand users are pretrained to produce a tenodesis grasp by wrist dorsiflexion. Proportional control of grasp arises from the external transducer. The subject chooses either a lateral pinch to hold small objects or a palmar grip for larger items. A quick jerk of the shoulder locks that position and another quick jerk unlocks and releases the grip. The system is programmed in 1 day using varible levels of electrical stimulation at each electrode. The system appears to be biologically and electrically safe over several years of follow-up, with less than 2% rate of infection or electrode failure. A survey of 34 users found that 88% felt the neuroprosthesis had a positive impact and improved their activities of daily living.[7] Only 5 patients reported not using the device almost daily.

A lighter control unit or implanted module, more channels, sensory feedback within a closed-loop system, activation of more proximal muscles such as the deltoid, supraspinatus, pectoralis, and biceps[8] or the triceps, forearm pronator and supinator, and intrinsic hand muscles,[9] an integrated bimanual system for quadriplegic patients, and telemetrically controlled direct nerve or muscle microstimulators like the *BION*[10] may be added in the future to make *FreeHand*-like devices even more acceptable to patients and to further increase functional capabilities. Kilgore, Peckham and colleagues at Case Western Reserve have successfully implanted a joint angle transducer and a myoelectric signal sensor that provides feedback to a FreeHand-type system. The commercial viability of the *FreeHand* device, however, is uncertain.

The first commercial surface electrode-driven device for grasping is the Handmaster (NESS Ltd. Ra'anana, Israel), which has found some use in quadriplegic patients with at least C-5 intact and in hemiplegic patients with poor hand function.[11] Electrodes attached to a molded forearm orthosis that reaches across the wrist stimulates the wrist and finger flexors and extensors in synchrony. The external control unit operates from a button managed by the subject for the level of output that allows grasp, holding, or release. Uncontrolled trials of patients with a chronically hemiplegic hand showed a decrease in hypertonicity with up to 3 hours of daily stimulation for several months. A 5-week uncontrolled trial assessed subjects before and after 5 weeks of supervised home stimulation performed as they carried out a set of tasks (G. Alon, University of Maryland). The 75 patients could voluntarily flex and extend the elbow and wrist 20° and at least slightly extend the second and third digits, so they were much like subjects who have been studied in trials of constraint-induced movement therapy. A mean of 60 hours of upper extremity practice plus stimulation led to post-test improvements in functional skills such as the nine-hole peg test and led to gains similar to those of other mass practice paradigms. A randomized trial that includes a specified training paradigm for intentional movement-associated electrical stimulation for acute or chronic patients with impaired hand function is needed.

SYSTEMS FOR STANDING AND WALKING

Peroneal nerve stimulation to enable ankle dorsiflexion has a long anecdotal history as an adjunct to step training in hemiplegic subjects. The stimulus can be evoked by a hand switch, by a heel switch, or a more sophisticated tilt sensor called the *Walk-Aide* (Neuromotion Inc., Edmonton, Canada). Many systems from laboratories in Europe, Asia, and the United States have demonstrated that four electrodes per leg can allow paraplegic people who have good trunk control to maintain standing.

The only commercial device to assist stepping, the Parastep System (Sigmedics, North-field, IL), uses six surface electrodes to stimulate the gait cycle as subjects hold on to a rolling walker.[12] Stimulation of the quadriceps muscles and push off with the arms permits standing up. Constant stimulation maintains standing. A step button on the walker stops quadriceps firing as one leg starts its swing phase and activates a triple flexion response by peroneal nerve stimulation. The patient releases the button after the hip flexes and switches on the quadriceps stimulator for stance. The other leg is then stimulated to aid swing. The hip does not go into extension and the knee often is in full extension (the ground reaction vector is anterior to it) to passively maintain stance. This slow step-like gait does not reproduce the sensory inputs that ordinarily drive walking (see Chapter 1, under Central Pattern Generation). Users generally step approximately 150 feet before resting. The FNS device also allows standing to be incorporated into some daily activities.

Devices with 16 to 48 implanted electrodes also permit stepping over ground. These FNS systems mostly assist hip flexion for swing and knee extension for stance. The media hype since the 1980s about their potential has not led to a commercially viable product in North America or Europe. Systems for standing for patients with paraplegia[13] and for step training in hemiplegic subjects[14] show promise in work going on at neuroengineering sites such as the Cleveland FES Center at Case Western Reserve University and its Veterans Administration affilliate. Successful FNS for walking requires continuous problem solving by an experienced physical therapist who can match the abilities of the patient and the FNS system to the kinematic, kinetic, and temporal features of the gait cycle.[15] Aside from the complexities of electrode construction and instrumentation, the composition and control of the sequential firing train that produces a safe, nonrobotic-looking gait pattern over flat and uneven ground pose ongoing challenges.

The intuition and trial-and-error approach of physical therapists, engineers, and physicians is at least as important as the functionality of a FNS system for training stepping in paraplegic patients and augmenting ambulation for patients who have some motor control. Careful studies will determine whether FNS enhances locomotor recovery beyond the time of use of a device in patients who have some lower extremity motor control. External stimulation may not lead to motor learning or induce cortical adaptations unless the intervention is provided within a learning paradigm. If some aspects of the gait cycle improve during FNS, producing more normal locomotor-associated sensory inputs to the cord and brain during locomotion and allowing intense task-specific practice, then fMRI studies may be able to demonstrate resulting neuroplasticity in sensorimotor regions.

SYSTEMS FOR BOWEL AND BLADDER

Functional neuromuscular stimulation has been successful in patients who have upper motor neuron spinal lesions from trauma, multiple sclerosis, and other causes of a fixed myelopathy.[16] Electrical stimulation has been tried within the lower cord, pudendal nerve, and bladder detrusor. The best results involve stimulation of the ventral sacral roots from S-2 to S-4, usually after a dorsal rhizotomy to reduce bladder hyperrreflexia.[17] Rhizotomy can, however, reduce sexual responsiveness, especially in women with spinal cord lesions.[18] The devices may also improve bowel evacuation and produce a penile erection. A commercial device, the $25,000 *Vocare Bladder Stimulator* (NeuroControl Inc, Cleveland, OH), includes electrodes placed after a T-12 to L-1 laminectomy as cuffs over the sacral roots in the intradural or epidural surrounds. The electrodes are wired to a subcutaneous radio-frequency receiving coil coupled to an external stimulator. Pulsed electrical stimuli, usually at approximately 24 Hz, activate the detrusor more slowly than the striated muscle of the external sphincter. The bladder pressure rises and sphincter pressure falls after a series of pulses, emptying the bladder in spurts.

Telemetric stimulation of S-2 using an implanted stimulator has shown promise in restoring continence and voiding on command after SCI.[19] Magnetic stimulation of the abdomen, which spreads to the sacral nerves, has been used in a similar fashion for bladder and bowel emptying.[20] Single sacral root electrical stimulation can reduce urge incontinence.[21] No FNS system for micturition has proven useful for people with lower motor neuron lesions following, for example, a conus/cauda equina SCI. Patients with this lesion may benefit from electrodes placed within the bladder wall, but the wires are subject to movement and difficult to arrange for effective stimulation in the absence of preganglionic parasympathetic innervation.

FUNCTIONAL ELECTRICAL STIMULATION

Many muscle-stimulating devices have been developed to increase muscle mass or aerobic conditioning, to inhibit hypertonicity, to reduce shoulder subluxation, and to interact with a form of biofeedback to try to improve motor control.[22,23] These interventions are discussed in Chapters 5 and 9. A commercial bicycle ergometer called the *ERGYS* (Therapeutic Technologies, Inc., Tampa FL) uses surface electrodes over the bilateral quadriceps, hamstrings, and gluteal muscles to sequentially activate leg forces on the pedals. As muscle strength increases, contractions are made against greater ergometer resistance. Chapter 10 reviews the purported benefits of this exercise for paraplegic people.

PHOTONICS

A fiber-optic system could stimulate, inhibit, and modulate spinal and peripheral neural tissue. Light impulses have been developed to target the release of chemically caged neurotransmitters and drugs. Fiber-optic sensors can detect chemicals in their milieu. Such sensors provide a source of feedback signals that may be incorporated for monitoring the effects of a pharmacologic or specific neural repair intervention.

Nerve Cuffs

Direct stimulation and recording from nerve roots and peripheral nerves may improve the functionality of systems for hand use, walking, sensory feedback, micturition, ventilation via the diaphragm, pain control, cranial nerve sensorimotor activities, and neural repair. At least four types of nerve cuffs are in development.[24] At least one commercial nerve cuff is available for experimental use in animal models and subjects (NeuroStream Technologies Inc., Burnaby, BC, Canada). Positive demonstrations of a closed loop system that reads sensory feedback from heel contact to toe-off during the

quired from EEG field potentials over the surface of the scalp, dura, or subdural regions or from the spike potentials of small clusters of neurons picked up by microelectrode arrays from motor cortex or cognitive planning regions such as parietal mirror neurons or supplementary motor cortex. A variety of brain signals have been employed.[41] The signals are digitized and processed by a variety of algorithms to extract specific features, such as the amplitude of an evoked potential or a specific rhythm from sensorimotor cortex or the firing rate of cortical spikes. These signals reflect CNS function before the action or thought occurs, so they imbue the user's intent. A translation algorithm takes the particular electrophysiologic features chosen to give simple commands to a device, such as a word processor, virtual keyboard, Web site, an upper extremity neuroprosthesis, or to a *thought translation device*.[39]

An ideal brain–computer interface would have an open architecture for self-learning of multisensory inputs and outputs, employ noninvasive recordings, be portable and cosmetically acceptable, quickly allow a trainer to determine if the patient can achieve a good enough performance to benefit, readily allow training to achieve and maintain performance, manage a range of devices for everyday use, pay attention to the social environment and factors that may affect the user's motivation, and lend itself to testable hypotheses for clinical research.

Little is known about the ability of patients who have a progressive disease such as ALS to be able to maintain a particular physiologic activity that can be processed. Much more research is needed to optimize training paradigms. At the second international meeting of Brain–Computer Interfaces for Communication and Control Group in 2002, a dozen working devices were described, including models for general purpose systems such as the BCI 2000, a collaboration from Wolpaw, Birbaumer, Pfurtscheller and colleagues,[41] and systems from Guger Technologies (Graz, Austria) and Brainware (Rome, Italy). Systems range from two to four surface electrodes with telemetry capability to 64 electrodes imbedded in a cap wired to amplifiers and processors to silicon-based implantable microelectrode arrays that can stimulate and record from a region the size of a dime and deliver drugs (www.eecs.umich.edu/NELab).

FIELD POTENTIALS

If a subject can move the eyes to lighted targets such as letters, a brain-computer interface can translate the visual evoked response by the photic drive into a yes/no or on/off action. If no eye movement or EMG activity is available to a subject, slow cortical potentials, P300 evoked potentials, and mu and beta rhythms have been studied for their signaling efficacy.[40]

The P300 appears over the parietal cortex when an unexpected or significant auditory, visual, or sensory stimulus occurs. The basis for use of an evoked response potential is that the component measured such as the peak after 300 ms represents a specific activity of the brain invoked to serve a specific processing function. The amplitude of the P300 does have a proportional relationship to the probability that an item seen is the oddball for each type of task. With little or no training, the user watches a six by six matrix of rows and columns that contain the letter or word of interest flash every 125 ms. The user counts the times the symbol to be communicated is flashed. About five symbols per minute can be discerned, but responses may habituate and make the brain–computer interface less reliable.

The idling activity over primary sensorimotor cortex includes a variety of 8–12 Hz mu and 18–26 Hz beta rhythms. Movement and preparation for movement decreases these rhythms, called event-related desynchronization, especially contralaterally. Relaxation after a movement increases the rhythm, called event-related synchronization. With considerable training, subjects can learn to increase the amplitude of mu over the left vertex by, for example, imagining movement of the right hand, and decrease the amplitude by, for example, imagining movement of the left foot. The basis for these changes appears to be the enhanced attention given to the focus coupled to inhibition of attention to other stimuli (surround inhibition), modulated by thalamocortical and different portions of reticular nucleus cells that correspond to distinct sensory modules, such as the hand and foot.[40a] Normal and quadriplegic subjects who were trained to vary the amplitude or synchronization of their mu and beta EEG activity learned to use this electrical output to control the vertical and horizontal direction of movement of a computer cursor.[41,42] With operant conditioning, patients learn to signal about five letters a minute. Greater information processing of a responsive rhythm improves the capacity of interfaces for movement-related and thought-related controllers. Subjects tend to reach a level of accuracy for up and down cursor movements of 65%–80%. Errors in target selection are associated with a positive potential over the vertex, which could be used to cancel the previous choice. Specific imagined movements and combinations of movements may be translatable into still better control algorithms.

Slow cortical potentials are low voltage EEG signals found over the vertex that evolve over less than 10 seconds. Movement induces a negative potential and positive potentials accompany reduced cortical activity. The subject operantly learns to move a cursor toward a target such as a letter or icon at the bottom of a screen by inducing a more positive slow or more negative slow potential.[43] Activation of the cortical attentional-motor network during the negative potential and best performance correlate with activation by fMRI in the basal ganglia and deactivation in the supplementary motor area.[41] Activations occur as well in the dorsolateral prefrontal cortex and primary sensorimotor cortex. One of the clinical applications of this approach enabled a patient with amyotrophic lateral sclerosis to select items such as words and pictograms on a computer screen.[44] Practice often requires approximately 1000 trials over 15 or more sessions to achieve an accuracy of better than 65%.

Normal and quadriplegic subjects who were trained to vary the amplitude or synchronization of their mu and beta EEG activity learned to use this electrical output to control the vertical and horizontal direction of movement of a computer cursor.[41,42] With practice, patients learn to signal approximately five letters a minute. Greater information processing of a responsive rhythm improves the capacity of interfaces for movement-related and thought-related controllers. A patient can be trained to incorporate the cortical rhythm associated with imagining a movement to control a cursor.[43] One of the more remarkable clinical applications of a device uses cortical slow potentials to enable a patient with amyotrophic lateral sclerosis to select items such as words and pictograms on a computer screen.[44]

Extracted EEG signals allow subjects to perform simple tasks slowly. The strategy is safe and relatively inexpensive, but primarily applicable to the person who lacks all movement. Training of ill, fatigued, and less than highly motivated subjects limits success. The instructor must pay attention to how practice and feedback are provided. Thought translation is more exotic and less practical than simpler solutions for the quadriparetic person. A lighted pointer moved by even slight head motion or a muscle that the patient twitches enough to activate a microswitch will work much faster when interfaced to an interactive computer program for typing, selecting items on a screen, and controlling the nearby environment.

NEURONAL SPIKE POTENTIALS

Cortically implanted and subdural electrodes sense focal brain activity. The ability of neuroscientists to record from 50 to over 100 neurons at a time and analyze what aspects of movement or vision or other properties the cells are tuned to has given neuroprosthesis and neurorobotic researchers an opportunity to aim for smart, real-time brain controllers (Fig. 4–1). Many technological problems to safe, longstanding wire implants and signal processing have been overcome in the past few years.[45] Further innovations will be needed to produce a practical and highly efficacious neuroprosthetic command signal. Some interesting examples of successes are relevant to rehabilitation.

Signals recorded from 25 to 50 neurons of the motor cortex in the forelimb representation of a rat were used to control a robotic lever.[38] The animal first trained to depress the lever to get a drop of water. Within several days, the processed signals that arose from the monitored cortical neurons were used by the investigators to depress the lever, before the rat's forearm did so. The lever, then, became a real-time neurorobotic device. Chapin and colleagues extended this work to primates.[38] Arrays of 16 to 32 microwires were implanted into the bilateral dorsal premotor, primary motor, and posterior parietal cortices. Two monkeys trained at two tasks while they were being recorded. They moved a manipulandum left or right to a visual cue and made 3-dimensional hand movements to reach for a treat at one of four places on a tray. By modeling parameters from the neuronal assemblies associated with the upper extremity movements needed to accomplish each task, the investigators showed that firing patterns from the neurons could be transformed to control prosthetic limb movements. The control of complex movements still needs to be demonstrated. To date, neural recordings from one implanted electrode in the motor cortex of a paralyzed subject did come to control the movement of a cursor on a computer screen.[46]

Another brain-machine interface is even more remarkable in its simplicity for the thought-control of movements.[47] A microarray of 100 electrodes was inplanted into M1 of monkeys to record from 7 to 30 neurons. The investigators created a filter method that weighted the sum of neural firing to mathematically translate the output to accurately reflect the trajectory of the monkey's hand as it moved a cursor to reach stationary targets on a screen. The neuronal firing data were built into a model for movement with decoding filters based on 1–2 minutes of recordings from M1. Several adjustments corrected the alogorithm. Little training was required before the monkey was facile in being able to use its own neural activity-based signal to carry out the tracking task without moving its arm. Thus, rapid learning and sensory feedback were

quickly reflected in the output of the M1 neurons and the model of neural control was easily adjusted to offer an effective decoder for a brain-machine interface.

Another group of investigators recorded from 18 neurons in the hand region of M1 as monkeys tracked a moving object on a screen with visual feedback with the hand actually reaching into space and with just the recorded neurons controlling a cursor.[47a] A mathematical algorithm tracked changes in cortical tuning properties during this and related tasks for fast and slow brain-controlled movements. The tuning parameters of the neurons changed when switching from the hand-controlled to brain-controlled tasks, consistent with notions about how learning induces activity-dependent plasticity (see Chapter 1). Remarkably, almost every neuron within a microelectrode array contributes some aspect of the intended movement, suggestive of a locally distributed network within a single map of the workspace of the hand around the body.[47b] With practice, the neurons can be trained to make a range of 3-dimensional movements with the accuracy and speed of normal arm movements and maintain this control. Thus, by using control algorithms for changes in what neurons are tuned to during mental practice, a neuroprosthesis or other brain-machine interface ought to serve robust functions for a paralyzed person who can learn with modest effort.

Strategies for the cortical control of a neuroprosthesis or robotic device will take advan-

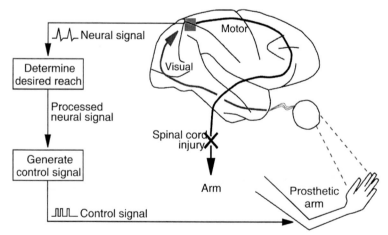

Figure 4–1. General design for a neuroprosthesis that takes neuronal signals associated with the thought of a movement, processes this electrical activity to generate a control signal, and moves the plegic arm using a system of functional neuromuscular electrical stimulation.

tage of the distributed network for motor control, allowing perhaps just one or two sites to control devices. Representational plasticity for movements that results from practice at a task will also strengthen the control of the recorded assembly for that movement over time. Other regions of the brain, such as those with mirror neurons that are active during both the observation and imitation of a movement, may rapidly acquire firing patterns that the prosthesis uses to control new movements. In a sense, then, the neuroprosthesis will be self-learning, rewarded by behavioral success, and potentially modulated by pharmacologic interventions. As technical limitations lessen and mathematical encoding of neural signals improves, the activity of assemblies of cells may be used to specify more complex multijoint and bilateral movements, a trajectory for reaching, or a signal for the end point of a movement.

Intracranially implanted neuroprostheses composed of microchips seem potentially feasible given the plasticity of the CNS. Although still far from a reality, multichip modules that incorporate the nonlinear dynamics and adaptive properties of neurons and neural networks[48] are being designed to communicate with uninjured surrounding cortical tissue by conforming to the cytoarchitecture of the environs. The brain and silicon module may adapt to each other for tasks represented by this integrated network. Neurons may even be a component of a chip.[2]

Sensory Prostheses

Auditory prostheses are a reality. The cochlear implant has restored speech discrimination to thousands of people. At least seven commercial varieties are available. A microphone by the external ear picks up acoustic signals, converts sound into electric signals, and delivers them to the electronic signal processor. Signals are transmitted to an electrode array implanted into the scala tympani of the cochlea, into the auditory nerve, or near target neurons. Despite what may seem a rather crude stimulation system of fewer than 25 electrodes, practice and cortical plasticity lead to reasonable speech discrimination, but usually less ability to appreciate music.

Visual prostheses are a work in progress. Several designs for a visual prosthesis have been offered, depending on the location of the cause of blindness. A retinal prosthesis can make use of the selective survival of inner layer retinal cells for people with macular degeneration or retinitis pigmentosa by directly stimulating them, bypassing damaged photoreceptors. With complete retinal or optic nerve damage, the stimulation must include the occipital visual cortex. One approach captures images with a camera and a stimulating device activates an implanted microarray. The density of the array and just what properties it signals determines the size of the visualized pixels.[49] As the number increases, especially beyond a matrix of pixels that is approximately eight by eight, visual acuity improves enough to make out coarse features.

As noted in Chapter 3, functional imaging reveals that the auditory cortex may be limited in its ability to use information from a cochlear implant if the brain has had no prior auditory experience. If a visual neuroprosthesis becomes available for people with longstanding or congenital blindness, the prior experience of visual cortex may alter its effectiveness. For example, new visual inputs to visual and visual association cortices may have to compete with auditory or finger sensory inputs (from reading Braille). The potential plasticity of these systems may be evaluated with fMRI or PET activation paradigms.

ROBOTIC AIDS

Robots that may help disabled people are likely to be programmed for a select number of task-specific actions, such as delivering items from one place to another or assisting mobility.[50] Available machines programmed to travel down a corridor by sensing the location of the walls are too crude to help patients with neurologic impairments. Researchers in this field, however, suggest that robotic technology will lead to more complex capabilities induced by autonomous learning during real-world interactions with objects (www.yobotics.com/).[51] A number of countries have funded research on robotic devices for specific tasks, such as finding land mines, moving items, and surveying the environs. Biomimetic robots are built to mimic the innate sensorimotor behaviors of the not-so-smart American lobster, for example (see www.neurotechnology.neu.edu). This water robot was engineered by observing the movements of the lobster under many circumstances and recreating its actions with an electronic system that parallels the lobster's nervous system. Electronic command neurons, coordinating neurons, central pattern generators, and sensory feedback allow software to manage a remarkably modest number of circuits to mimic all locomotor activities. Such neurocreations may extend the reach of the disabled.

Intelligent wheelchairs and lightweight exoskeletons with sensors and tiny actuators worn under clothes and powered without leaden battery packs could also serve a robotic function. An ankle-foot orthosis, for example, is a passive device that is not as compliant as an ankle, does not adapt over time to the changing needs of its user, and cannot reproduce biologic behaviors. The U.S. armed forces have funded research for the development of tiny joint actuators built into exoskeletons that aim to enable a soldier to leap over walls and run at great speeds. These exoskeletons may find their greatest benefit in helping the mobility and self-care activities of the disabled. For rehabilitation at present, the most successful robotic efforts have been simple devices designed to enhance the retraining of movement. The International Conference on Rehabilitation Robotics (ICORR) presents biannual updates on robotic devices that replace or augment diminished physical and cognitive capabilities.

Upper Extremity

The *MIT-MANUS* is a robot control system with 2° of freedom that moves, guides, and can perturb elbow and shoulder movements on a flat surface.[52] The subject's forearm and hand are attached to the robotic arm. Subjects practice by trying to move their hands to targets shown on a screen. They get visual feedback regarding the positions of their hands in relation to the target. The robot's impedance controller allows a patient to make smooth movements as the robot passively or actively assists the arm as needed. A randomized clinical trial of patients with a hemiparetic arm carried out 2 weeks after a stroke showed greater gains in proximal arm strength for the robotic-treated group compared to the control group.[53] The

motor score on the Functional Independence Measure was also higher, but the tests of self-care were not specifically carried out with the affected upper extremity. Subjects assigned to the robotic received a total of 25 hours of activity for the affected arm. Those assigned to the control group had considerably less specific proximal arm therapy of any kind, so an intensity of practice effect, rather than a motor learning paradigm, may have accounted for the differences in outcomes. The investigators aim to develop an additional robotic component that incorporates arm motion with 3° of freedom and robotic manipulation of wrist and hand movements.

The Mirror Image Motion Enabler (*MIME*) is an upper extremity robotic device offering 6° of freedom.[54] Robot-assisted movements can be made passively toward a predetermined target, with assistance after the patient triggers the initial force of movement to a target, with viscous resistance from the robot, and bimanually so that the affected arm is a slave to a controller device on the unaffected arm. Hemiparetic subjects can practice preprogramed reaching movements in multiple planes with an assist from the robotic arm or can carry out bilateral shoulder and elbow movements with the affected arm following the kinematics of the unaffected arm. A 6-axis sensor measures the forces and torques between the robot and the hemiparetic arm. A trial with 27 hemiparetic patients compared *MIME* robotic therapy to neurodevelopmental therapy each for 24 1-hour sessions over 2 months.[55] Thus, an attempt was made to control for intensity of therapy, but large differences in the amount of arm movement practice are still likely. The group assigned to the robotic arm had greater gains in strength and reach at 2 months and did better on ADLs at 6 months.

The Assisted Rehabilitation and Measurement (ARM) Guide offers 3° of freedom to assist forward reaching in the typical workspace of the arm.[56] The patient initiates reaching and the Guide completes a smooth trajectory through the full range of available passive motion. A control group with hemiparesis that practices free reaching shows similar gains as the ARM group if the number of movements practiced is equal. A European group developed a robotic with 3° of freedom called the *Haptic Master* that integrates reaching exercises with a virtual environment. A wheel-steering device created by the SEAT project in Palo Alto records the force exerted by each hand and encourages more selective control by the hemiparetic arm. Combinations of devices have also been proposed, such as bilateral ARM Guides with *MIME* control software. A device with these characteristics could measure torques and the coordination of reaching to targets, as well as allow for studies of the efficacy of unilateral and bimanual practice.

The usual goal for these robotic devices is to help the subject complete a goal-directed movement within the ordinary workspace of the arm, to let subjects practice without the constant attention of a therapist, and to measure changes in forces and trajectories along with behaviors. Studies to date do not reveal whether repeated attempts at movement or the assistance offered by a robotic device is most critical to any gain in range or proximal strength. Such gains are not necessarily associated with improved functional use of the arm. The hand has been most difficult to robotize. Without training for wrist and finger extension and several types of grasp or pinch, these devices will have limited value for patients with moderate to severe impairments. Safety, cost, machine feedback that best induces learning and neuroplasticity, posttraining generalization to real-world tasks, the design of clinical trials to test interventions built around a robot assist, and the need for ongoing engineering expertise to modify the devices must be addressed.

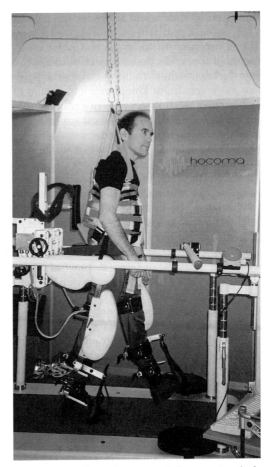

Figure 4–2. The Lokomat exoskeleton assists body weight-supported treadmill stepping without on-line sensory feedback.

Lower Extremity

Spurred on by reports of the efficacy of treadmill training with partial body weight support and of task-specific, mass practice, investigators in North America, Europe, and Japan have designed robotic systems to assist walking on a treadmill. A few exoskeletal devices are works in progress to fully control stepping in place on a treadmill. The initial version of the Lokomat (Hocoma, Switzerland) includes four rotary ball screw joints driven by DC motors that allow hip and knee flexion and extension.[57] The exoskeleton is adjustable for different leg shank lengths and hip widths (Fig. 4–2). The motors are programmed to take the legs through typical stance and swing cycles. A parallelogram mechanism that moves vertically, counterbalanced by a gas spring, supports the weight of the exoskeleton. The torques across each hip and knee are adjusted by a computer to allow a patient to use the exoskeleton as a partial assist for stepping. The next goal is to permit partial robotic assistance with torque feedback controls. The so-called *Autoambulator*, built by the HealthSouth healthcare group, includes a pair of rotating arms that assist treadmill stepping and monitor joint torques. No reports have been published regarding this device. An electromechanical *gait trainer* is on the verge of commercial availability.[58,59] Patients place one foot on each of two long foot plates connected to a crank system driven by motors. The foot plates move in an ellipsoid pattern. The gear system also controls a harness worn by the patient to allow vertical displacement during stepping. The system responds to the torques

27. Clark K, Naritoku D, Smith D, Browning R, Jensen R. Enhanced recognition memory following vagus nerve stimulation in human subjects. Nat Neurosci 1999; 2:94–98.

27a. Talwar S, Xu S, Hawley E, Weiss S, Moxon K, Chapin JK. Rat navigation guided by remote control. Nature 2002; 417:37–38.

28. Katayama Y, Fukaya C, Yamamoto T. Poststroke pain control by chronic motor cortex stimulation: Neurological characteristics predicting a favorable response. J Neurosurg 1998; 89:585–591.

29. Pinter M, Gerstenbrand F, Dimitrijevic M. Epidural electrical stimulation of posterior structures of the human lumbosacral cord: 3. Control of spasticity. Spinal Cord 2000; 38:524–531.

30. Dimitrijevic M, Gerasimenko Y, Pinter M. Evidence for a spinal central pattern generator in humans. Ann NY Acad Sci 1998; 860:360–376.

31. Herman R, He J, D'Luzansky S, Willis W, Dilli S. Spinal cord stimulation facilitates functional walking in a chronic incomplete spinal cord injured. Spinal Cord 2002; 40:65–68.

32. Tresch M, Saltiel P, Bizzi E. The construction of movement by the spinal cord. Nat Neurosci 1999; 2: 162–167.

33. Mushahwar V, Horch K. Selective activation and graded recruitment of functional muscle groups through spinal cord stimulation. Ann NY Acad Sci 1998; 860:531–535.

34. Tresch M, Bizzi E. Responses to spinal microstimulation in the chronically spinalized rat and their relationship to spinal systems activated by low threshold cutaneous stimulation. Exp Brain Res 1999; 129:401–416.

35. Kargo W, Giszter S. Rapid correction of aimed movements by summation of force-field primitives. J Neurosci 2000; 20:409–426.

36. Barbeau H, McCrea D, O'Donovan M, Rossignol S, Grill W, Lemay M. Tapping into spinal circuits to restore motor function. Brain Res Rev 1999; 30:27–51.

37. Barinaga M. Turning thoughts into actions. Science 1999; 286:888–890.

38. Chapin J, Moxon K, Markowitz R. Real-time control of a robot arm using simultaneously recorded neurons in the motor cortex. Nat Neurosci 1999; 2:664–670.

39. Kubler A, Neumann N, Kaiser J, Kotchoubey B, Hinterberger T, Birbaumer N. Brain-computer communication: self-regulation of slow cortical potentials for verbal communication. Arch Phys Med Rehabil 2001; 82:1533–1539.

40. Farwell L, Donchin E. Talking off the top of your head: Toward a mental prosthesis utilizing event-related brain potentials. Electroencephalogr Clin Neurophysiol 1988; 70:512–523.

40a. Suffczynski P, Kalitzin S, Pfurtscheller G, Lopes da Silva F. Computational model of thalamo-cortical networks. Int J Psychophysiol 2001; 43:25–40.

41. Wolpaw JR, Birbaumer N, McFarland D, Pfurtscheller G, Vaughan TM. Brain-computer interfaces for communication and control. Clin Neurophysiol 2002; 113:767–791.

42. Miner L, McFarland D, Wolpaw J. Answering questions with an electroencephalogram-based brain-computer interface. Arch Phys Med Rehabil 1998; 79: 1029–1033.

43. McFarland D, Miner L, Vaughan T, Wolpaw J. Mu and beta rhythm topographies during motor imagery and actual movements. Brain Topogr 2000; 12:177–186.

44. Birbaumer N, Ghanayim N, Hintergerger T, Iversen I, Flor H, Kotchoubey B, Kübler A, Perelmouter J, Taub E. A spelling device for the paralysed. Nature 1999; 398:297–298.

45. Moxon K, Morizio J, Chapin J, Nicolelis M, Wolf P. Designing a brain-machine interface for neuroprosthetic control. In: Chapin J, Moxon K, eds. Neural Prostheses for Restoration of Sensory and Motor Function. Boca Ratan: CRC Press, 2001:179–219.

46. Kennedy P, Bakay R, Moore M. Direct control of a computer from the human nervous system. IEEE Trans Rehabil Eng 2000; 8:198–202.

47. Serruya M, Hatsopoulos N, Paninski L, Fellows M, Donoghue J. Instant neural control of a movement signal. Nature 2002; 416:141–142.

47a. Taylor DM, Helms Tillery S, Schwartz AB. Direct cortical control of 3D neuroprosthetic devices. Science 2002; 296:1829–1832.

47b. Graziano M, Taylor C, Moore T. Complex movements evoked by microstimulation of precentral cortex. Neuron 2002; 38:841–851.

48. Tsai H, Tai J, Sheu B, Tanguay A, Berger T. Design of a scalable and programmable hippocampal neural network multi-chip module. Soc Neurosci Abstr 1999; 25:902.

49. Normann R, Maynard E, Rousche P, Warren D. A neural interface for a cortical vision prosthesis. Vision Res 1999; 39:2577–2587.

50. Regalbuto M, Krouskop T, Cheatham J. Toward a practical robotic aid system for people with severe physical disabilities. J Rehabil Res Dev 1992; 29:19–26.

51. Weng J, McClelland J, Pentland A, Sporns O, Stockman IS, M, Thelen E. Autonomous mental development by robots and animals. Science 2001; 291:599–600.

52. Krebs H, Volpe B, Aisen M, Hogan N. Increasing productivity and quality of care: Robot-aided neurorehabilitation. J Rehab Res Dev 2000; 37:639–652.

53. Volpe B, Krebs H, Hogan N, Edelstein L, Diels C, Aisen M. A novel approach to stroke rehabilitation: Robot-aided sensorimotor stimulation. Neurology 2000; 54:1938–1944.

54. Burgar C, Lum P, Shor P, Van der Loos M. Development of robots for rehabilitation therapy: the Palo Alto VA/Stanford experience. J Rehab Res Dev 2000; 37:663–73.

55. Lum P, Burgar C, Majimundar M, Van der Loos M. Robot-assisted movement training compared to conventional therapy techniques for the rehabilitation of upper limb motor function following stroke. Arch Phys Med Rehabil 2002; 83:952–959.

56. Reinkensmeyer D, Kahn L, Averbuch M, McKenna-Cole A, Schmit B, Rymer Z. Understanding and treating arm movement impairment after chronic brain injury: Progress with the ARM guide. J Rehab Res Dev 2000; 37:653–662.

57. Colombo G, Joerg M, Schreier R, Dietz V. Treadmill training of paraplegic patients using a robotic orthosis. J Rehab Res Dev 2000; 37:693–700.

58. Hesse S, Uhlenbrock D. A mechanized gait trainer for restoration of gait. J Rehabil Res Dev 2000; 37: 701–708.

59. Hesse S, Werner C, Uhlenbrock D, Frankenberg S, Bardeleben A, Brandl-Hesse B. An electromechanical gait trainer for restoration of gait in hemiparetic stroke patients. Neurorehabil Neural Repair 2001; 15:39–50.

60. Taga G, Yamaguchi Y, Shimizu H. Self-organized control of bipedal locomotion by neural oscillators in unpredictable environment. Biol Cybern 1991; 65:147–159.

61. Burns R, Crislip D. Using telerehabilitation to support assistive technology. Assist Technol 1998; 10:126–133.

62. Reinkensmeyer D, Lum P, Winters J. Emerging technologies for improving access to movement therapy following neurologic injury. In: Winters J, Robinson C, Simpson R, Vanderheiden G, eds. Emerging and Accessible Telecommunications, Information and Healthcare Technologies: IEEE Press, 2002.

63. Jack D, Boian R, Merians A, Tremaine M, Brurdea G, et al. Virtual reality-enhanced stroke rehabilitation. IEEE Trans Neural Syst Rehabil Eng 2001; 9:308–318.

64. Holden M, Todorov E, Callaban J, Bizzi E. Virtual environment training improves motor performance in two patients with stroke: case report. Neurol Rep 1999; 23:57–67.

65. Kurzweil R. Merging human and machine. Comput Graph World 2000; 23:24–27.

66. Craelius W. The bionic man: restoring mobility. Science 2002; 295:1018–1021.

PART II

COMMON PRACTICES
ACROSS DISORDERS

Chapter 5

The Rehabilitation Team

The goals of neurologic rehabilitation, to help patients become as functional as possible across interacting impairments, disabilities, and personal needs, require a team of professionals who partner in inpatient and outpatient settings. I will refer to the team of rehabilitation specialists, such as nurses, physical therapists, physicians, and others, as rehabilitation clinicians or *rehabilitationists*, to best convey their equality at the patient's bedside. Together, they practice the experiential art and science of the possible.

Rehabilitationists provide what many programs call intensive and comprehensive neurologic rehabilitation. These loosely defined designations mean something different in every program of inpatient or outpatient care. Intensive does not imply a particular intensity of practice. Intensive may mean that a patient is assigned to 3 hours a day with therapists. In reality, the patient may actively participate in therapy for considerably less time. Comprehensive may mean that most disciplines are represented, not that their activities aim to restore a broad range of functions. To the patient, comprehensive care may mean satisfying all health-related needs.

Inpatient and outpatient therapy are constrained by the costs of care. The duration and intensity of rehabilitation is also constrained by the ability of a therapist or a team to articulate the value of continuing to work on an aspect of disability and to offer an evidence-based practice to enhance gains. The length of inpatient rehabilitation stays has been declining in the United States since 1985. This trend may continue with the institution of a Prospective Payment System under Medicare and Medicaid (www.access.gpo.gov/nara/index.html) based upon the diagnosis, subscores of the Functional Independence Measure (FIM), and a minor adjustment for comorbid conditions. The opportunities to offer patients therapy beyond limited compensatory skills for basic activities of daily living (ADLs) depends upon research that demonstrates evidence-based interventions.

THE TEAM APPROACH

The team approach takes many forms. In a *multidisciplinary* model, each member with specialty training treats particular disabilities. In an *interdisciplinary* model, roles blend. An

Table 5–1. Sample Patient Satisfaction Questions for Inpatient Rehabilitation Answered on a Likert Scale

1. Did your progress meet your expectations?
2. Did you meet your goals?
3. Did the program prepare you to return home?
4. Did the program enable you to take better care of yourself and train the family in your care?
5. Did you interact well with your therapists, nurses, physicians?
6. Did the nurses respond in reasonable time to your needs?
7. Did your doctor answer your medical questions?
8. Do you understand how to use your medicines?
9. Was the discharge planning satisfactory?
10. Did you learn to use the equipment ordered by your therapists?
11. Do you understand your home and outpatient therapy schedule and goals?
12. Would you recommend this program to others who need rehabilitation?

physician, in 1887, to start a neurologic rehabilitation clinic. He had his ataxic patients, many with tabes dorsalis, practice upper extremity coordination and walking tasks and incorporated parallel bars into gait training. His methods gained adherents in the United States[9] and led to the first hospital gymnasium at the Salpétrière in Paris, the most famous neurology department of its day. The French named the process rééducation fonctionelle in 1893. Hirschberg, a French neurologist, published the first book about applying Frenkel's methods to patients with hemiplegia in 1912, 10 years after Frenkel had published his text, *Treatment of Tabetic Ataxia by Means of Systematic Exercise* (Blackiston's Sons Co., Philadelphia). Physiatrists evolved from the need for a rehabilitation discipline after World War II and drew on methods for the management of victims of spinal cord injury and polio. Thus, from their roots in syphilis, polio, and war-related trauma, neurologists and physiatrists are most likely to participate with an inpatient team.

Responsibilities

Physicians are especially responsible for anticipating and managing the medical complications and rehabilitation needs of their patients (see Chapter 8). In addition, physicians who specialize in neurologic rehabilitation educate patients and families about the consequences and overall prognosis and management of the nervous system disease and of new disabilities.

Physicians should explain to both patient and primary care doctor the indications for medications, measures for secondary prevention of complications, management of risk factors for recurrence or exacerbation of the disease, and the type and duration of rehabilitative interventions. In a study of disagreements between physicians and patients about their encounters, the discrepancies were greatest when, in the patient's opinion, the physician paid little attention to psychosocial issues or drew a quick conclusion about the problem without helping the patient understand the basis for the decision.[10] The rehabilitation specialist is also in the best position to articulate the impact of disability to employers and government agencies so that patients can obtain equipment, services, and pertinent disability reports.[11]

Rehabilitation physicians tend to be the facilitators of the team, especially on an inpatient service. Here, the physician leads a weekly team conference that reviews the progress of the patient in reaching the functional goals that will permit a discharge to the home. To do this well, the physician must help build the team's infrastructure and understand the practices of its disciplines. The conference allows the team to share notes and thoughts about each patient and to solve lingering problems. A physician leader articulates, mobilizes, and persuades the patient, family, and team of therapists toward goals that they come to share. The team conference is a good time to review imaging studies that are pertinent to the patient's impairments and to teach, for example, about nervous system anatomy and physiology, the effects of medications, and motor and neurobehavioral disorders. Team meetings and journal clubs may be used to discuss new and relevant research articles that are pertinent to patient care.

Interventions

The physician's history, examination, and review of laboratory and neuroimaging studies are critical to the team's formulation of how impairments will affect rehabilitation potential. For example, the recorded history must include details about the patient's premorbid functional activities, physical fitness, mood, and lifestyle. These elements will impact rehabilitation care and goal-setting. The examination must explore the patient's attention, memory, ability to learn, judgement, language, behavior, mood, and executive functions. Strength is assessed and recorded in terms of graded manual muscle testing, functional movements, and fatigability with repetitive muscle contractions. Although neuroimaging studies cannot themselves predict impairments and prognosis, tests such as computerized tomography (CT) and magnetic resonance imaging (MRI) offer useful insights. For example, profound dysphagia may not have been expected in a patient with a recent lacunar infarct in the left internal capsule. An MRI scan that reveals an old, silent lacuna in the right basis pontis, however, offers insight into the cause of a pseudobulbar palsy and alters the prognosis.

The clinician superimposes the specific contributions of neurologic, musculoskeletal, cardiopulmonary, and other impairments on a map of the patient's functional abilities and disabilities. For example, does spasticity or palpably tender musculoligamentous tissue cause pain or limit movement? Does a medication or episodic orthostatic hypotension lessen attention span and endurance for exercise? Is hyponatremia or anemia having negative clinical consequences? Does a muscle group show increased paresis with a few repetitive contractions against resistance, suggesting central or peripheral mechanisms of fatigability that may impede repeated use of a limb? Are cognitive problems related only to the cerebral injury, or does a metabolic abnormality, a medication or, in an older person, an underlying dementia

augment the findings? The evaluation also emphasizes the patient's premorbid experience with pain and disability and the present degree of disability. By teasing out the patient's prior level of competence in physical, mental, and psychosocial functioning in light of new impairments and disability, the physician can put perspective on the mutual goals of patient, family and the rehabilitation team.

During inpatient care, the physician explores the small personal matters that mean much to patients. These issues include interference with sleep. For example, do medications or blood draws taken too early in the morning or late in the evening awaken the patient? Is insomnia associated with anxiety or depression, a noisy roommate, and pain at rest or with certain movements? Sleep deprivation may thwart rehabilitation efforts by preventing the consolidation of skills learning and experience-dependent gains in the performance of motor and perceptual procedural memory tasks.[12] Other daily discussions may center on the regularity of bowel movements, symptoms that point to a urinary tract infection, phlebitis or aspiration, as well as caloric and fluid intake, short-term therapy goals, how the patient and family are coping with unexpected burdens, and plans for discharge and outpatient care. The physician also reinforces the therapeutic approaches made by the team at its weekly conferences. During daily rounds, the physician encourages patients to spend more time out of bed, reiterates specific exercises for improving endurance, motor control, and skills that can be performed alone or with family, and reexamines patients for changes in impairments and gains in functional activities. The physician must explain the value of new medications and frequently reassess the need for drugs still taken. Families and people with neurologic diseases are quick to check for experimental and alternative treatments on the Internet and in articles. The physician needs to put animal research results, ongoing clinical trials, uncontrolled use of substances that include much hype by the seller, and alternative medicine approaches into perspective.

A responsible clinician never ignores or underestimates the meaning of a patient's symptoms or a family's concerns. Nor does the compulsive clinician ever disregard the insights of the rest of the team. A modest decline in attention span or exercise tolerance noted by the speech therapist or occupational therapist may mean, for example, incipient sepsis, a new metabolic complication, or side effects of a medication. A few minutes of assessment and explanation prevents lost opportunities to uncover unrecognized problems and misunderstandings. Vigilance is necessary in regard to identifying inpatient and outpatient medical and disability-related complications and for the pursuit of opportunities to improve the function and quality of life of patients.

During outpatient care, physicians must develop their skills at counseling about matters such as exercise[13] and specific directions about home practice paradigms for motor and cognitive retraining. I make it a point to review the details of how the patient is practicing to improve the functional use of an affected upper extremity, language and memory skills, and socialization. I observe for any irregularities in gait that require fine tuning and practice (see Chapter 6). I reiterate how task-specific practice may alter the brain's representations for these activities and improve the patient's abilities, even years after the initial neurologic illness. For patients with chronic diseases that progress, practice is perhaps even more important, since it may spur gradual neural reorganization to maintain function (see Chapter 3).

The rehabilitation physician works with the patient's primary care physician to monitor for medical complications and any decline in functioning. A follow-up by 1 month after inpatient discharge and at 3 and 6 months for disabled patients will allow adjustments in the formal and informal rehabilitation program, changes in assistive devices and braces, and ascertainment of community resources over the time that most patients make their fastest improvements.

With a background in general medicine, neuromedicine, neuroscience, mechanisms of plasticity, and scientific experimentation, rehabilitation physicians should serve as clinician-scientists. The physician can encourage therapists to weigh, formulate, and test strategies. Drawing upon current literature and by collaboration with basic and clinical researchers, the neurologic rehabilitation specialist assesses and develops interventions. During ward rounds and team meetings, a good leader amiably questions whether particular practices of the team reflect the best means of restoration for a patient. As much as is feasible, the physician should insist on definable interventions. If one approach is not working, a different approach can then be defined and tested. Reproducible measures of success, such as changes in the time needed to eat a meal or walk 50 feet, help label success beyond nonparametirc tools that are used to define levels of independence (see Chapter 7). Access to a good database drawn from the literature, the institution's prior cases, and national studies such as the Uniform Data System For Medical Rehabilitation[14] helps put features of the recovery of impairments and disabilities into perspective. This information stimulates collective deliberations that may build a consensus toward alternative solutions and the design of a single-case study or larger clinical trial. Newly shared knowledge gives the team a greater sense of competence and gets all rethinking what they do. Clinical research energizes the team.

NURSES

Responsibilities

Inpatient rehabilitation nurses monitor the vexing medical complications that accompany neurologic disease and immobility. Nurses initiate passive range of motion of paretic limbs, follow through on preventative measures for deep vein thrombosis, and turn an immobile patient every 2 hours, along with other measures to prevent pressure ulcers over bony prominences. They protect patients from being pulled across the bed, which can shear the skin, and work out ways to prevent incontinence so that moisture does not macerate the skin. Nurses also educate ancillary hospital personnel who might tug and sublux a paretic shoulder. Other responsibilities include assessments for sleep disorders such as apneic spells, respiratory function, swallowing, nutrition, and bowel and bladder function; training in self-catheterization, care of skin and self-medication; education about disease and personal matters such as sexuality; and practice in self-care skills outside the formal therapy setting. Nurses check supine and sitting or standing blood pressure and pulse rate when indicated and can teach hypertensive patients and their families how do use a digital blood pressure cuff for home monitoring. Diabetics are taught about diet, exercise, medications, and glucose self-monitoring techniques. A nurse practitioner can be a great asset to the physician and team on a busy inpatient service, especially in a university hospital, where patients tend to have complex medical illnesses and needs.

Interventions

Nurses are on the front line, where they must help balance between what a patient can reasonably do alone and the assistance a patient requires. They have to be attuned to fluctuations in the stamina and alertness of their patients that may affect taking fluids and performing ADLs. By observing the patient and family in less structured activities, away from the formal therapy provided by other team members, nurses provide unique insight into physical and emotional functioning. Nurses are also in an ideal position to get patients to comply with lifestyle changes for disease prevention. Nurses should be armed with information and hand-out materials regarding primary and secondary disease prevention. Along with the physician, psychologist, and social worker, they can initiate discussions about drug abuse with young patients on a TBI or SCI unit. For new medication that will be used after hospital discharge, nurses can develop cues and rituals with the patient and caregiver that reinforce compliance.[15] Rehabilitation nurse specialists and nurse practitioners are playing greater roles in managing medical, social, and case management issues for inpatients and outpatients. The Association of Rehabilitation Nurses has excellent resources for continuing education (www.rehabnurse.org).

PHYSICAL THERAPISTS

Responsibilities

Physical therapists or physiotherapists (PTs) contribute especially to the rehabilitation of disabilities associated with bed mobility, transfers to a chair or toilet, stance, and ambulation. Their assessments emphasize measures of voluntary movement, sensory appreciation, range of motion, strength, balance, fatigability, mobility and gait, and functional status. The clinician's goals for neurologic rehabilitation aim toward compensatory strategies for carrying out ADLs, such as the use of a wheelchair, as well as interventions to lessen specific impairments when time allows. Therapists play a primary role in managing musculoskeletal and radicular pain, contractures, spasticity, and deconditioning.

Like other rehabilitationists, PTs have increasingly sought strategies to improve the accuracy and reproducibility of clinical evaluations and their applications.[16] Some of the common approaches to movement-related problems are listed in Table 5–2. Two broad categories of exercise programs, therapeutic exercise and the so-called neurophysiologic and neurodevelopmental approaches, have received the most attention in the past. Newer concepts related to neuroplasticity, motor control, and how motor skills are learned are merging with these.[17] An evolving systems theory of motor control has been suggested as a framework for structuring clinical practices in PT.[18] This approach views movement as resulting from the dynamic interplay between multiple CNS, peripheral, and biomechanical systems that organize around a behavioral goal that is

Table 5–2. **Practices in Physical and Occupational Therapy**

Therapeutic exercise and reeducation	Massed practice
Neurofacilitation techniques	Biofeedback
Proprioceptive neuromuscular facilitation	Virtual environment training
Bobath	Musculoskeletal techniques
Brunnstrom	Electromyogram-triggered neuromuscular
Rood	stimulation
Motor skills learning	Orthotics and assistive devices
Task-oriented practice	
Forced use	

constrained by the environment. Shumway-Cook and Woollacott emphasize this mindset in describing task-oriented approaches to quantify and manage the functional skills and impairments that impede performance. Chapter 1 describes the framework for understanding theories regarding motor control and Chapter 2 discusses how extrinsic manipulations alter neruoplasticity.

Success in retraining during rehabilitation depends on diverse variables that include the characteristics of a task, changing contexts and environments when performing a task, psychological reinforcements, motivation, attention, memory for carry-over of what is taught, environmental distractions, anxiety, sleep deprivation, and family support. All can influence how, for example, motor and cognitive programs are built, shaped, and refined as the patient acquires a new skill. The daily practices of most neurologic PTs reveal an eclectic, problem-oriented approach.

Interventions for Skilled Action

COMPENSATORY EXERCISE AND REEDUCATION

Muscle reeducation evolved primarily for the management of polio, but these programs of exercise of muscle were considered less useful for rehabilitating patients with upper motor neuron syndromes. Traditional exercise programs emphasize repetitive passive and active joint-by-joint exercises and resistance exercises in anatomical planes to optimize strength and range of motion.[19] The approach aims to prevent the complications of immobilization, such as contractures, muscle atrophy, and spasticity. Therapists train residual motor skills, often of the uninvolved side, to compensate for impairments. The acquisition of self-care and mobility skills often takes precedence over the quality of movement, so long as patients are safe. Upper and lower extremity orthotics and assistive devices tend to be used early in therapy to speed functional compensation.

When needed, therapists also employ breathing and general conditioning exercises and energy conservation techniques, particularly to reduce the energy cost of a pathological gait.[20] Strengthening and conditioning are achievable within the context of almost any

neurologic disease.[21] These interventions are important to maintain functional activities in aging patients, maintain cardiorespiratory fitness, and prevent complications related to disuse or to overuse of weak muscles.

Muscle Strengthening

The schools of neurofacilitation generally frown upon attempts to strengthen muscles that are hypertonic (see next section). The concern is that this leads to heightened spasticity and diminished motor control. Strengthening exercises, however, may be underutilized by therapists who are aiming only for compensatory gains in function or for more precise motor control.[22] Some studies support the value of strengthening exercises to improve mobility in patients with upper motor neuron lesions.[23,24] Strengthening also improves movements that are *speed-sensitive*, in that they have strict timing requirements and require forces of varying intensity.[25]

Excessive resistance exercise that reinforces a flexor synergy at, for example, the biceps may have a negative impact. Daily repeated arm curls against high resistance by a patient who has poor elbow extension could potentially enhance elbow flexor tone and shoulder adduction to the point of driving the fist of the dystonic hemiparetic arm up into the patient's neck and jaw. A variety of experimental studies, however, suggest that hemiparetic subjects can increase force output when pushing against higher loads, such as when pedaling to gain muscular force output, without any worsening of motor control.[26–28] Bicycle pedaling movements tend to put greater demands on the stronger leg, but the reciporocal movements allow force output by the weaker leg and probably lessen any chance of inducing excessive postexercise hypertonicity. Use of the large leg muscles by pedaling against resistance even at only 20 cycles per minute or by walking on a treadmill also improves cardiovascular fitness in patients who have at least fair motor control.[29,30]

NEUROFACILITATION APPROACHES

Many schools have developed what their proponents call neurophysiologic approaches. Techniques are based mostly on interpretations of Sherrington's neurophysiologic studies in the early 20th century. In addition, these approaches were first formulated from the founding advocate's observations of children with cerebral palsy and adults with hemiplegic stroke. The approaches involve hands-on interaction between the therapist and the patient. The interventions utilize sensory stimuli and reflexes to facilitate or inhibit muscle tone and patterns of movement. Therapy aims to elicit individual and whole limb muscle movements, but schools vary in whether they try to initially elicit mass flexor or extensor patterns of movement called synergies. Therapists may try to activate or suppress a stretch reflex, the asymmmetric and symmetric tonic neck reflexes, the tonic labyrinthine reflex, and withdrawal and extensor reflexes. They use stimuli that include muscle or tendon vibration, joint compression, skin stroking, and other sensory inputs that elicit reflexive movement and positive and negative supporting reactions.

Neurodevelopmental Techniques

Most schools have emphasized a progression in the sequence of therapies reminiscent of the neurodevelopmental evolution from reflexive to more complex movements. Neurodevelopmental techniques (NDT) call for reproducing the developmental sequence shown by infants as they evolve motor control. Based on hands-on experience with children with cerebral palsy, practitioners believe that normal movement requires normal postural responses, that abnormal motor behaviors are compensatory, and that the quality of motor experiences helps train subjects for normal movement. Practitioners emphasize normal postural alignment prior to any movement. Mobility activities proceed in a developmental pattern from rolling onto the side with arm and leg flexion on the same side, to extension of the neck and legs while prone, to lying prone while supported by the elbows, and then to static and weight-shifting movements while crawling on all four extremities. These mat activities are followed by sitting, standing, and, finally, walking. Different schools vary in their attempts to activate or mimimize reflexive movements and to train functional movements during ordinary physical activities.

One of the potential problems with NDT is the delay of standing and walking until the patient has achieved relative control of proximal and distal muscles. This delay in weight-bearing could lead to complications such as deep vein thrombosis in acute stroke patients.[31] It could also delay the recovery of stepping, if one believes that a task-oriented therapy for ambulation is most likely to provide the sensory feedback and learning stimuli that can modulate neural assemblies and step generators at several levels of the neuraxis.

Proprioceptive Neuromuscular Facilitation

This empiric technique, initiated by Kabat and Knott, arose in part from observing smooth, coordinated, diagonal and spiral movements in athletes at the peak of their physical efforts.[32] Proprioceptive neuromuscular facilitation (PNF) facilitates mass movement patterns against resistance in a spiral or diagonal motion during flexion and extension. It is based on the belief that since anterior horn cells for synergistic muscles are near each other, an appropriate level of resistance will bring about changes in muscle tone by overflow to these motoneurons. The therapist utilizes proprioceptive sensory stimuli and brain stem reflexes to facilitate the desired movement and inhibit unwanted movements. For example, the therapist places the upper extremity in extension, abduction, and internal rotation. While the subject's arm is rotated and extended from the side, it is moved into flexion, adduction, and external rotation. Specific techniques include repeated quick stretch, contraction, contraction-relaxation, and rhythmic stabilization in which the patient tries to hold the arm still as resistance is applied by the therapist in an opposite direction. Proprioceptive neuromuscular facilitation stretching techniques call for an isometric contraction of the muscle under stretch, such as the hamstrings, followed by a concentric contraction of the opposing quadriceps muscle during stretch of the hamstrings, designated as contract-relax agonist-contract (CRAC). This sequence is thought to alter the responses of muscle spindles in a way that increases the maximum range of motion; stimulation may increase in force produced by each muscle as well.[33] Numerous specific exercise patterns are described by the practitioners of PNF. Similar spiral and diagonal movement patterns are later used for functional activities and walking. Proprioceptive neuromuscular facilitation has been applied to diseases of the motor unit as well.

Bobath

This NDT approach popularized by the Bobaths aims to give patients control of abnormal patterns of posture and movement associated with spasticity by inhibiting pathological reflexes.[34] In this theory, abnormal motor tone and primitive postural reactions are the key factors that interfere with proper motor functioning. Abnormal movements provide abnormal sensory feedback, which reinforces limited, nonselective, abnormal movement. Methods continue to evolve.[35] Therapists use reflex inhibitory patterns to reduce tone and abnormal postures and they stimulate advanced postural reactions to enhance motor recovery. They use pressure or support on key proximal limb or trunk points to inhibit or facilitate movement. They avoid inducing associated reactions in a muscle group away from the body part that is active and overflow movements within the same limb. Bobath therapists especially avoid provoking mass flexor shoulder, elbow, and wrist synergies of the arm, as well as extensor knee and plantarflexor ankle synergistic movements of the leg. For example, the hemiplegic patient with flexor spasticity of an arm that rides up during walking is trained to bend forward in a chair with the arm hanging down. The subject moves and swings the affected arm and then swings both arms. The subject slowly sits upright with the neck flexed while the arm hangs, then raises the head and stands. When the elbow starts to flex again, the patient repeats these steps.

Strengthening exercises are generally not used by Bobath therapists. During the early stages of recovery, weight bearing, postural responses, and selective movements are emphasized. Ankle-foot orthoses are discouraged, because braces are believed to facilitate abnormal tone. Bobath's approach is the most popular form of NDT used for the rehabilitation of patients with hemiplegia. Indeed, it has become synonymous with the term NDT. A survey of United Kingdom physiotherapsits found the Bobath approach preferred by 67% of senior physiotherapists.[36] Approximately 30% prefer an eclectic approach. The Bobath therapists said they delay task-related therapies if the patient does not have normal tone and cannot use normal patterns of movement, although they are not opposed to using walking aides and orthotics if these conditions were met. These beliefs, however, are not backed by data from clinical trials or by information drawn from current theories regarding motor learning and practice-induced skills learning and associated neuroplasticity.

Johnstone's technique[37] has similarities to Bobath's in its developmental approach, but adds a pressure splint around the affected arm or leg. The inflatable splint provides even pressure across joints and allows weight bearing, for example, on the arm through the extended wrist. This technique is said to increase sensory input and decrease hypertonicity, according to the detailed description for therapy provided by this British therapist.

Brunnstrom

Brunnstrom's training procedures facilitate synergies by using cutaneous and proprioceptive sensations and tonic neck and labyrinthine reflexes.[38] In contrast to Bobath's approach, this technique initially promotes associated reactions, mass movement synergies, primitive postural reactions, and strengthening exercises. Specific techniques are recommended for each of the 6 stages of recovery that emerge: (1) flaccidity, (2) limb synergies with onset of spasticity, (3) increased spasticity and some voluntary control of synergies, (4) control of movement out of synergy, (5) selective over synergistic movement, and (6) near normal control. These stages of recovery have been used as both descriptors and, inappropriately, as outcome measures in some studies. In clinical practice, Brunnstrom's approach is mostly restricted to patients who have persistent hypotonia and hemiplegia.

Rood

Margaret Rood's approach emphasizes the use of specific sensory stimuli to facilitate tonic and then phasic muscle contractions.[39] High threshold receptors are thought to increase tonic responses and low threshold receptors activate phasic ones. Sensory stimuli include fast brushing, light touch, stroking, icing, stretching, tapping, applying pressure and resistance, and truncal rocking and rolling. The response to cutaneous and other sensory inputs is used to facilitate developmental patterns and then purposeful movement. One common technique is light brushing of the lips to facilitate both flexion of the hemiplegic arm and a hand-to-mouth pattern of movement. Rood's approach was never formalized as thoroughly as other NDT strategies.

Efficacy of Neurofacilitation Techniques

The approaches of the pioneering schools of physical therapy were derived from clinical observations that drew upon narrow assumptions about motor control. Techniques use normal movement as their point of reference, view the nervous system as a hierarchal organization that can be approached at the level of reflex activity, and see recovery from brain and spinal injury following a predictable sequence similar to infant development. None of these assumptions can be taken as correct. For example, techniques for shifting weight onto the affected hemiparetic leg prior to stepping has been a maxim of developmental approaches. Joint compression is considered to increase proprioceptive and cutaneous stimuli, affect tone, and help train the leg to participate in postural tasks. One study, however, suggested that loading only accentuates the extensor synergy of the lower leg muscles, rather than facilitating normal postural responses.[40] Kinematic studies of the recovery of upper extremity movement for reaching also refute the developmental notion that movement within a synergistic pattern of flexion or extension of a whole limb precedes more selective movements outside of the synergy.[41] Indeed, some synergistic movements can be eliminated simply by changing the context of the elicited movement. For example, the influential study of motor recovery after hemiplegia by Twitchell,[42] from which the Brunnstrom technique derives its stages, is often quoted as the evidence for specific stages of recovery of the upper extremity. Was Twitchell correct? He claimed that flexion of the elbow and shoulder precede movements in extension. When the paretic arm is supported to allow free movements of the forearm in a horizontal plane just below shoulder level, however, flexion and extension of the elbow and shoulder often can be brought out independently. Many patients have extension of the elbow that comes in earlier and better than flexion.[43] The potential for

recovery of some motor control must take into account the context of a movement, from what position it begins, the patient's goal, the ways in which movement toward the goal is reinforced, and other perhaps less visible issues.

The NDT schools disagree over the use of resisted muscle activity, compensatory movements, and overflow or associated reactions. Bobath teaches that these increase abnormal movements, whereas Kabat encourages resistance exercises, and Brunnstrom uses associated reactions early in treatment. At least one Brunnstrom technique for eliciting associated reactions has received some support.[44] In the hemiplegic patient, resisting hip movements by the nonparetic leg increased the magnitude of the torque in an opposite direction in the paretic hip group. This approach may both strengthen and improve the motor control of hip movements, particularly if resistance is applied to the normal leg during gait training and during treadmill training with body weight support.

Some of the neurophysiologic principles used by the schools appear reasonable. Predictable motor responses are elicited by reflex reactions, by vibration to stimulate a muscle contraction,[45] by cutaneous stimulation to facilitate a voluntary contraction,[46] and by upper extremity weight-bearing through the extended elbow and heel of the hand to normalize corticospinal facilitation of motoneuronal excitability.[47] Any carry-over of responses into functional or volitional movement begins to stretch the imagination, however. Consider the tonic neck reflexes after a brain injury. Turning the head to the hemiplegic side can facilitate the triceps, whereas turning toward the unaffected side may induce flexion and abduction of the paretic shoulder. Neck extension can facilitate extension of the affected arm and flexion of the leg. Neck flexion may produce flexion of the arms and extension of the legs. Bilateral responses are most remarkable after diffuse TBI and incomplete cervical SCI. These reflexes can be used to position patients and alter tone on a mat or in a chair. Manipulation of the reflexes has not been shown to enhance the recovery or quality of movement and functional use of the limbs, however. The attention the schools place on the use of sensory inputs to elicit and reinforce certain movements (see Chapter 1) still has an important place in any style of PT. Some of the other specific hands-on methods of the schools of therapy may produce a positive outcome, even if some of the theory is suspect.

The better-designed studies that have compared these approaches have been carried out in patients with stroke (see Chapter 9). No advantages were demonstrated for one technique over another. A meta-analysis of 37 pediatric subjects, mostly with cerebral palsy, suggested a small positive treatment effect from NDT alone or combined with another approach, compared to other approaches.[48] All of those trials have serious methodologic flaws.

Studies of the efficacy of particular schools of therapy have used outcome measures that emphasize independence in ADLs and not an outcome directly related to the primary focus of their techniques of physiotherapy, which is motor performance and patterns of movement.[49] Outcome measures probably need to be more appropriately linked to the type and purpose of the intervention to demonstrate differences between approaches, if any exist. Also, treatment can be efficacious for its intended proximal purpose, but not necessarily contribute to the goal of functional gains.

Studies of efficacy should concentrate on the best well-defined practice for an important goal that may, in theory, be modulated by the intervention. For example, instead of trying to assess an effect of the Bobath method on a standard test of mobility and self-care skills, the research design could assess an aspect of movement of the affected upper extremity that is treated by the method. Then, a change in impairment can be correlated with an increase in functional use of the arm that requires the movement pattern. A study of one school over another is probably not feasible or worthwhile, if the search is for the best physiotherapy that will optimally improve ADLs and mobility. The methods of the schools are not likely to be reproducible in a reliable way for clinical research and their philosophies are too far from any scientific underpinning to justify an exclusive emphasis of one over another.

Evidence from many studies of neuroplasticity (see Chapters 1 and 3) suggests that therapy structured around learning new sensorimotor relationships in the wake of altered motor control will be more effective than methods that aim to foster a developmental sequence. The approach of task-oriented motor learning attempts to put this notion into practice.

TASK-ORIENTED TRAINING

An evolving approach to therapy combines several theories of motor control and principles of motor learning. *Motor control* subsumes studies of the neural, physical, and behavioral aspects of movement. *Motor learning* includes studies of the acquisition of skilled movements as a consequence of practice, drawn mostly from work in animal and human experimental psychology. The approach, task-oriented training, includes many models of motor control, including pattern generation, relationships between kinematic variables and functional movements, representational plasticity induced by practice, and the interdependency and reciprocity of neuronal networks and the distributed control of a movement throughout these systems (see Chapter 1).

Task-oriented motor learning emphasizes visual, verbal, and other sensory feedback to achieve task-specific movements, in contrast to neurophysiologic techniques that rely on cutaneous, proprioceptive, and other sensory stimuli to elicit facilitation and inhibition of movement patterns. The therapist does not necessarily seek to shape normal movement in the patient. For any particular task, the motor control model stresses methods to solve a motor problem, rather than strategies to relearn a normal pattern of movement. Therapists use cognitive and sensory feedback to train the patient with an impaired nervous system to accomplish a relevant task in any of a variety of ways, but not necessarily by striving to train the patient in a particular pattern of muscle activation. The goal becomes error detection, which the PT uses to help patients correct themselves during the practice of reaching, standing up, or moving in a variety of environmental conditions. This approach for physical, occupational, or speech therapy offers a script for the roles of problem solving, sensory experience, sensorimotor integration, motivation, and reward, all of which are encoded within the ordinary workings of neural assemblies and their connections.

The task-oriented approach assumes that success after practice under one condition does not necessarily transfer to another related task.

For example, in one study, weight-shift training in hemiparetic patients while standing improved the symmetry of weight bearing and balance in stance, but the gains did not improve lower extremity symmetry during walking.[50] This finding is consistent with motor learning concepts. Practice at hitting a golf ball is not likely to improve a baseball player's batting average any more than a static therapy can train a patient to perform a dynamic activity. For gait, a task-specific physical therapy has to include stepping at reasonably normal speeds, not weight shifting alone. A program of early locomotor training made possible by body weight-supported treadmill stepping fits into this conceptual model.[51]

The task-oriented approach for training cognitive and motor skills requires formalized techniques that everyone on the rehabilitation team employs. In rehabilitation settings, little attention has been paid to whether or not typical training procedures—not what is taught but how it is taught—optimize gains in cognitive skills, motor functions, and self-care and community activities. The essence of therapy for any disability, indeed, for acquiring any novel motor skill, is *practice*. What must be reconsidered, however, is that a practice session can have a powerful, but only temporary effect. A positive effect on performance during a training session may not lead to long-term learning. The goal of practice should be a permanent effect. A learned behavior must carry over when practice conditions and cues are no longer provided to the patient.

Therapists employ practice procedures and reinforcements, using a task-oriented approach, to increase the speed or quality of a patient's performance during training. The physical or occupational therapist may assist the subject to approximate a movement toward its final goal by providing partial assistance. Positioning is often critical for better performance of a motor task. Restraint of the trunk during reaching, for example, may improve the range of movement of the arm by limiting abnormal, compensatory muscle recruitment of the trunk and shoulder girdle.[52] Therapists may change the demands of a task in terms of speed, accuracy, and timing. Sensory substitution is often allowed in an effort to solve a motor problem. For balance, visual fixation may counteract vestibular dysfunction or loss of proprioception.

An important rehabilitative outcome is to have patients practice in a way that enhances post training performance and to transfer training to related tasks under differing conditions in the patient's environment. At first, it may seem counterintuitive that any training procedure that speeds the rate of improvement or results in a more effective performance during therapy would do anything other than enhance learning and subsequent long-term performance. Research on the processes that lead to learning in normal subjects, however, suggests that retention and the ability to generalize may depend heavily on the type of practice used, regardless of the learner's immediate success during the acquisition phase.[53]

MOTOR LEARNING APPROACHES

Motor learning depends upon the interactions of pathways for sensation, cognition, and skilled movement within the context of real-world environments. Motor learning can arise from procedural or declarative learning (see Chapter 1). In the former, practice leads to improved performance for a particular activity, without awareness of the rules that led to the gains. Patients with stroke and with TBI often have preserved procedural learning abilities.[54] In declarative learning, knowledge is consciously recallable. Nonassociative and especially associative learning often play a role in relearning during rehabilitation. A verbal cue given during the swing phase of walking made in concert with a physical assist for foot placement may come to be associated, so that the verbal cue alone is adequate. This *classical conditioning* response is most effective during tasks with cues that are meaningful to the patient. *Operant conditioning* is a trial and error approach in which a rewarded behavior tends to be selected by the subject over alternative behaviors. Biofeedback relies on this type of learning.

What are some of the variables that a rehabilitation team may manipulate to get permanent rather than simply transitory effects during a therapy session? In normal subjects, variations in a few standard training conditions may slow the rate of improvement or lower performance at the end of the acquisition phase, but may enhance posttraining performance.[55,56]

Blocked and Random Practice

Blocked practice, the mass repetition of a drill, improves performance during the phase of acquisition. Random schedules of practice, in which several motor or verbal tasks are given so that the same task is not practiced on successive trials and repetition of any one task is widely spaced, will degrade success during acquisition. The term *contextual interference* describes distractors involved when a subject carries out more than one activity within a training session. In normal subjects, random schedules of practice enhance retention over the long run and can improve performance in contexts other than those evident during training.[57] This finding suggests that random practice adds difficulty for the learner during acquisition, but prevents superficial rehearsal. Unlike blocked practice, it forces the learner to design or retrieve a different strategy for each trial. Practice at performing a task along a single dimension, such as tossing beanbags into a basket at one distance or walking only on a smooth flat surface, produces better accuracy during acquisition than variable practice, in which a person tosses bags at different distances or walks on a variety of surfaces. Variable practice, however, seems to force a change in behavior from trial to trial that improves performance on tests of long-term retention of the motor skill and generalizes the skill to other settings.[55] Variable practice, then, strengthens the processes or rules between the outcome of a goal-directed movement and the parameters for that movement, such as postural adjustments, the sequence of movements, firing rates of agonist and antagonist muscles, and error-detection.

How much practice is needed to master a new skill? A strong relationship exists between performance and the time spent on deliberate practice.[58] For example, by age 20 years, the best professional musicians have practiced for more than 10,000 hours, nearly twice as much as less accomplished groups of expert musicians and 8000 hours more than amateur musicians of the same age. Deliberate practice is sustained for 3 to 5 hours every day for years in elite performers. Only approximately 50 hours of training is typically needed to achieve effortless performance of everyday activities such as learning to drive a car. Even this amount of practice at a particular activity is unlikely to be achieved during rehabilitation for

at least 1 month after onset of a neurologic illness.

Feedback

Feedback has been provided during training by several means. Verbal or visual information can be related to the activity itself, called *knowledge of performance*, or to the consequences of the action, called *knowledge of results*. Concurrent performance feedback includes hand-over-hand assistance to reach an object or to guide the hand with verbal cues. Knowledge of results offers feedback at the end of the attempted movement, providing a verbal cue about how to better approach the task on the next attempt. Any schedule of feedback that is frequent and accurate and immediately modifies what the learner does will increase learning during the acquisition phase. Retention in normal subjects was better for learning a complex arm movement, however, when subjects received feedback after every 15 trials compared to after every trial.[59] In a name-learning experiment in which subjects received feedback about correctness either 100% of the time or had feedback gradually withdrawn over the first few trials to 50%, learning was similar during the acquisition phase, but it was better in the 50% group as the retention interval increased.[60] Schmidt and Winstein suggested that very frequent feedback may interfere with information processing, response-induced kinesthetic feedback, effective error detection, or the evolution of a stabilized cognitive and motor representation that helps to sustain performance on later tests of retention.

Motor Learning After Brain Injury

In people without a brain injury, then, repetitious practice with minimal rest and no contextual interference between sessions, along with continuous guidance or frequent feedback, may improve performance during the training session. The improvement, however, tends not to carry over to a later time as well as when practice involves a random ordering of tasks and less frequent external reinforcement. Brain-injured patients undergoing rehabilitation may respond differently to variations in practice and feedback than normal subjects. Subjects with frontal-subcortical damage after TBI, for example, often do less well in dual tasks that divide their attention.[61] For mentally re-tarded subjects, block practice was superior to random practice.[62] Subjects with Alzheimer's disease who trained in a beanbag tossing task learned as well as older healthy controls under the condition of constant practice, but the subjects performed worse with blocked practice and considerably worse with random practice.[63] The impaired subjects were also less able than the controls to transfer the skill to tossing horseshoes. A group of subjects with an acquired amnestic disorder from trauma, encephalitis, or stroke were trained in strategies that lessened the likelihood that they would make mistakes while learning new information or a new skill. This *errorless practice* led to enhanced learning and reduced forgetting, compared to trial-and-error learning strategies.[64] Thus, at least in patients with poor episodic memory who cannot remember enough to eliminate their mistakes during training trials, errorless learning may be superior to random practice and errorful learning techniques. Other variables such as the age of a patient and the novelty of a motor task may also lessen the differences between types of practice and levels of feedback.[65] Clinical trials of errorless practice compared to errorful practice for learning motor skills, for behavioral modification, and for cognitive problems such as hemi-inattention are needed in patients with cerebral lesions who have mild to moderate impairment in working memory, memory consolidation, or memory retrieval.

Two well-designed trials offer insight into learning paradigms. Subjects with a chronic hemiparetic stroke improved as much as an age-matched healthy control group in the acquisition and retention of an upper extremity task.[66] The 40 subjects had left or right hemispheric strokes. They grasped a joy stick with the unaffected hand and used elbow movements to try to quickly reproduce a sinusoidal line that appeared on a screen. Visual feedback was provided that compared their drawing to the graphic stimulus after a trial. Feedback after every trial did not lead to different outcomes when compared to feedback on an average of 67% of the trials. Despite cognitive impairments in the stroke group, procedural learning, then, was intact.

In 24 subjects with chronic stroke, random practice of functional activities using the hemiparetic left or right arm for reaching and grasp-ing items led to better retention over time compared to blocked practice.[67] Despite the contextual interference of intermixing other tasks such as pointing and touching during learning in the random-practice group, both groups acquired their learning within the same number of trials. Thus, random practice did not impede the rate of gains, and still increased retention. Patients whose brain injury involves the hippocampus, cerebellum, or basal ganglia may not learn as quickly or fully as the subjects involved in these two studies of motor learning, however (see Chapter 1).

Studies are still needed that enter subjects in the first several weeks after stroke or head injury and that provide as much practice as may be needed to show differences in acquisition and retention for contextual learning compared to errorless practice. In addition, the types of learning that can be transferred from one hand to the other, such as the timing of a movement rather than the forces exerted,[68] and the value of bimanual task training under various practice conditions[69,70] need further assessment in patients. The overall evidence suggests, however, that drill-sergeant therapists who try to stamp in retention with blocked practice and constant attention to the details of performance need to reconsider their approach to training. If a task requires minimal variations under constant conditions, say relearning to use a toothbrush to brush the teeth, it is probably best trained with little variation. Practice designed to promote active involvement of subjects in solving the demands of goal-directed actions, however, ought to take a more open approach.

Training Techniques

One of the first formalized physical therapy techniques to draw upon the literature of motor learning marks the transition from the neurophysiologic to a task-oriented approach by therapists.[71,72] Carr and Shepherd offered a model of therapy that trains functional actions in a task-specific and context-specific manner. Patients practice the action to be learned with many repetitions to strengthen muscles and to optimize learning of the target action. Their use of learning principles was initially less well developed. Physiotherapists and other rehabilitationists are, however, developing interventional strategies around these notions of task-oriented therapies.[66,67,73–76] A growing variety of clinical trials confirm that greater intensity of task-oriented practice for walking or dextrous use of the upper extremity leads to significantly better functional outcomes for that task compared to nonspecific training.[77,78]

Constraint-induced movement therapy can be considered a corollary to the task-oriented motor learning concept, with an emphasis on massed practice. The technique has shown promise in hemiparetic patients who had at least 20° of wrist extension and 10° of finger extension. The strategy calls for forced use of the affected upper extremity and may include gradual *shaping* of a variety of functional movements to overcome what is theorized as learned nonuse of the limb.[79] Learned nonuse may derive from unsuccessful early attempts to use the affected limb after a stroke or, in studies of monkeys, after deafferentation of the upper extremity.[80] The failure in attempts to use an arm may lead to behavioral suppression and masks any subsequent ability of the limb. Positive reinforcement comes from successful use of the unaffected arm, which leads to the permanent compensatory behavior of nonuse of the paretic hand. Restraining the normal arm and engaging the affected one in the practice of functional tasks improved the strength, frequency, and quality of its daily use in a small 2-week trial.[81] The addition of a shaping paradigm of reinforcement to elicit functional movements appeared to have a longer lasting effect than did conditioned response training in only one study,[79] but did not improve outcomes or was not necessary for success in others.[69,82–84] In shaping with forced use, the patient receives feedback during the steps it takes to improve from a rudimentary early training response, such as slow extension of the elbow, through a more complex response, such as using the proximal arm to push a shuffleboard puck to a target. The notion of shaping, drawn from the psychology literature, has been rather vague when applied to rehabilitation efforts and its relevance to motor learning is yet to be demonstrated.

As discussed earlier, therapy structured around learning new sensorimotor relationships in the wake of altered motor control seems more likely to be effective than methods that only foster a developmental sequence. Constraint-induced movement therapy protocols have not, to date, defined a specific style of feedback. A large randomized clinical trial called EXCITE is in progress in the United States to test the efficacy of constraint-induced movement therapy from 3 to 9 months after a stroke. The trial is not testing a definable shaping or reinforcement protocol. A positive trial of body weight-supported treadmill training for stroke,[85] an ongoing trial of this approach for acute spinal cord injury,[51,86] and a successful treatment for certain types of aphasia[87] also employed forms of task-specific, massed practice with elements of constraint.

Some potential practical limitations of a task-oriented model deserve mention. The therapist must assess and design interventions that work through a wide range of sensorimotor and cognitive limitations encountered during tasks. The patient must be able to absorb information about goals and reinforcements. Training for tasks should occur across many natural or simulated settings. Changing the context of the task allows the patient to develop better problem-solving skills, serves as a better reinforcer, and leads to greater generalizability when the patient attempts a similar task in another setting. Such practice takes considerable time and must be shown to be a cost-effective approach. Task-oriented techniques, then, challenge the creativity of the therapist, as well as the residual cognitive skills of the brain-injured patient.

Paradigms must be defined and tested with controlled trials to find optimal schedules for practice and for feedback during rehabilitative training. The type, frequency, intensity, and delay in providing knowledge of results or knowledge of performance require more systematic study. The practice variables that affect the learning of movements that subserve motor functions in normal subjects may differ among individual patients who suffer from the spectrum of brain injuries. For the physical therapist, speech pathologist, and occupational therapist, however, any information about variations of verbal and kinesthetic feedback that may optimize their efforts would be invaluable. From the point of view of neuroplasticity, sensorimotor cortical representations and other signs of reorganization are most likely to accompany rewarded, goal-directed, task-specific practice (see Chapters 1 and 3). One type of training paradigm may be more effective than another, however, in engaging and remodeling cortical representations. Activation studies with functional MRI or PET may help predict whether or not a particular learning paradigm will incorporate the neural networks that must be included to optimize the acquisition of a skill or behavior.

MENTAL PRACTICE

As noted in Chapters 1 and 3, the processes underlying the perception of human actions are biologically complementary to the production of those movements. Imagining an action in the mind's eye evokes the representations involved in learning and retrieving that movement. Elite athletes such as platform divers and gymnasts rehearse through imagery in the moments preceding their performance. Although not all patients with a brain injury may be able to do this when cognition is impaired, mental practice can be encouraged for specific skills during training.

BIOFEEDBACK

Biofeedback (BFB) includes a variety of instrumented techniques that make subjects aware of physiologic information with the goal of learning to regulate the monitored function. In the neurologic rehabilitation setting, BFB has been used primarily to improve postural balance and motor performance. Feedback can be derived from changes in the center of gravity, changes in joint angles, and other physiologic signals. The nervous system ordinarily interacts with environmental signals as people move. Movement paced by music or by a metronome is a relative form of BFB and a potentially valuable tool for therapists.[88] Movement on a beat adds automaticity to repetitive actions. Subjects who were instructed to repeatedly flex a finger between two beats, for example, had a less stable pattern of coordination and movement frequency than when the subjects were instructed to make an extension movement on the beat.[89]

Electromyographic Biofeedback

Electromyographic (EMG) BFB to improve upper and lower extremity muscle activity, to decrease cocontraction of muscles, and to increase functional movements has been tried across many diseases, including stroke, SCI, TBI, multiple sclerosis, neuropathies, and cerebral palsy.[90] For the most part, support for this approach derives more from the enthusiasm of a case series than from controlled studies. A meta-analysis of 79 studies of EMG BFB for lower extremity function revealed a likely increase in ankle dorsiflexor strength compared to conventional therapy in ambulators when started 3 or more months poststroke.[91] Stride length and walking speed were not clearly improved. A meta-analysis of the intervention for upper extremity gains showed no effect compared to conventional therapies.[92] The poor design of most clinical trials limits any conclusions about efficacy, but the evidence does not favor the general use of EMG BFB.

The link between surface EMG changes during BFB and motor control is not simple, so the rationale for using the technique has inherent scientific limitations. Electromyographic activity and isometric muscle force in normal subjects have a rather linear relationship. A proportional effect is not necessarily present in spastic or paretic muscle, where great variability exists in the ease of recruitment of motor units. Other confounding relationships between muscle activity and function include the velocity of movement, the muscle length when a contraction is initiated, the duration of contraction, the instructions given to peform a movement, the intent of the movement, the spontaneous strategy used, and the resulting kinematics. For example, in a study of the recovery of reaching, the peak velocity of the required movement increased and the time to reach toward a target decreased, without any associated increase in the force or any change in the level of surface EMG activity in the muscles activated during the task.[41] Electromyographic BFB, then, could not contibute to gains in motor control in this setting.

Electromyographic BFB is often conceptualized as a means to help the patient learn motor control. Many of the studies that employed the technique for the upper extremity suggest that it can improve performance during training, but not necessarily when visual or auditory guidance ceases. In a single training session of pursuit tracking movements in 16 hemiparetic subjects, continuous EMG BFB from the spastic elbow flexors did not improve tracking any more than in the control group. Indeed, the intervention negatively affected the transfer of gains in speed and accuracy when the BFB was discontinued.[93] These findings raise the issue

tional therapist presents activities in a way that elicits the retention and transfer of particular skills for use in a functional setting.[106] For example, in one study, upper extremity reaching by subjects with spasticity after TBI improved the arm's range of motion significantly more after game playing than after rote exercise.[107] In another study, limb kinematics improved in normal and hemiparetic subjects when training included purposeful goals with objects of interest.[108] Thus, practice in object-related tasks, rather than simple repetition of reaching and grasping items that bear no significance to a person, may provide more concrete sensory information and offer rewards that motivate performance. Instructions to patients ought to direct attention toward the task's items and goals. More studies will determine how these practice and training factors generalize to functional activities and to patients with varieties of cognitive dysfunction, such as hemi-inattention.

Neurofacilitory handling and positioning techniques are still used by occupational therapists to provide cues for postural alignment during functional movement activities. The ability to learn postural adjustments from these cues may improve with active planning, initiation, execution, and termination of sequential movements that include changes in posture through open-ended tasks and random practice on several tasks in the same training session.[75] Testing approaches to skills training is especially appropriate for the primary goal of the occupational therapist, which is to help patients become competent problem solvers across a variety of functional tasks and in different performance contexts.

SENSORY RE-EDUCATION

Studies of cortical and thalamic representational plasticity provide a theoretical basis for techniques of sensory re-education after stroke.[109,110] Somatosensory cortical maps undergo rapid modulation that depends on task-specific sensory processing (see Chapter 1). Tonic sensory flow may be as important for movements requiring corticospinal control as sensory feedback.[111,112] If some afferent pathways and somatosensory cortical areas are intact, then neuronal receptive fields that had not been excited by sensory inputs prior to an injury may be trained to appreciate inputs from the arm and hand. Rehabilitation goals include the following:

1. Improve the appreciation of spatial and temporal patterns of skin contact as the fingers move over the edges, surfaces, and textures of objects
2. Identify and manipulate objects
3. Improve precision movements
4. Adjust grip forces
5. Prevent nonuse of the partially deafferented hand
6. Enhance daily manual activities

Sucessful sensory retraining was demonstrated in the 1930s when monkeys were trained to discriminate manipulated objects by shape, texture, and weight and then relearned these distinctions after a parietal lobe ablation.[113] Few studies have provided more than anecdotal or single-case examples of this recovery in man after stroke, but sensory retraining techniques have potential efficacy.[114-116] Dystonia of the hand that develops in people who make repetitive task-specific movements is associated with abnormal sensory processing (Chapter 1) and has been treated by techniques of sensory retraining. Affected patients have been taught to make the sensory discriminations needed to read braille or received multimodel retraining designed to activate BA 3a and 3b with proprioceptive and muscle afferent inputs or somatosensory inputs, respectively. Each approach has had moderate success in lessening the impact of dystonia on handwriting and similar activities.[116a]

ORTHOTICS

Upper extremity orthoses are frequently used for patients with upper and lower motor neuron impairments. The devices stabilize or stretch a joint in a chosen position, prevent contractures, assist the function of nearby muscles that may otherwise be at a biomechanical disadvantage, provide an attachment for an assistive device such as a cup, and, perhaps, reduce hypertonicity. Static orthoses allow no motion of the primary joint. Dynamic orthoses allow some controlled movements by employing elastic, wire, or powered levers that compensate for weakness or an imbalance in the strength of synergist and antagonist muscles. Devices for prehension are usually driven by finger or wrist movements.

Shoulder slings and resting hand splints may improve function, lessen tone, and limit contractures and pain, but the supporting data are scanty.[117] These orthotics will protect a paretic shoulder from painful subluxation and a dangling misplaced hand from being bruised. Dorsal and volar resting splints that extend up the forearm and across the wrist have been found in some small studies to reduce tone in adults and children.[118,119] A dorsal splint that provides a Bobath reflex-inhibiting pattern, as well as a splint that partially supinates the forearm and abducts the thumb and fingers, may be effective.[120] Therapists have used an inflatable splint around the whole forearm and hand with fingers in abduction to produce a similar inhibitory effect per the Johnstone approach, although the technique was not efficacious as a resting splint in one trial.[121] The daily amount of wear, length of time of use, and lasting effect after removal vary considerably in these studies. Thus, the choice of a splint often depends more on personal experience. Measuring cost-effectiveness is difficult.

The hemicuff and Bobath slings are often used to reduce shoulder subluxation as a prophylactic measure to avoid pain. Adjustable fabric shoulder straps pull the cloth cuff around the elbow and forearm and lift the humerus toward the glenoid fossa. The Bobath sling raises the humeral head via a foam rubber roll under the axilla. Other than serving as a warning not to yank the patient's arm, these slings have not been shown to prevent a painful shoulder.

ADAPTIVE AIDS

Adaptive aids are assistive devices that extend capabilities for home, work, and leisure. Recent designs for items from wheelchairs to utensils create a positive, even a sporty and aesthetically pleasing character. Clever industrial designs, lightweight materials, computers, and electronics offer a growing list of ways to diminish disabilities and handicaps. Computer and software manufacturers, including Apple and IBM, have development programs for people with special needs. Cellular phones and hand-held messaging and Internet devices give relatively immobile people powerful links for communicating with significant others and business associates and enlarge their safety net. Table 5–3 lists

Table 5–3. **Adaptive Aids for Daily Living**

Feeding
    Utensil: thickened or palm handle; cuff holder
    Dish: scoop; food guard; suction holder
    Cup: no spill covers; holders; straws
    Finger foods
Bathing
    Shower seat, transfer bench
    Washing: mit, long handle scrub brush, hose
    Safety: grab bars; tub rails
Dressing
    Velcro closures: shoes, pants
    Button hook, zipper pull
    Low closet rods
    Long handle comb, hair brush
Toileting
    Toilet safety rails; raised seat
    Commode
Mobility
    Prefabricated ramps
    Stair lifts
    Wheelchairs
    Transfer devices and ceiling-mounted track lifts
    Automobile and van: lifts, hand controls, specialty designs

Communication
    Cellular phone, hand-held Internet device
    Universal infrared transmitter controller
Computer Workstation
    Slip-on typing aid
    Environmental controls
    Communication: spoken words; voice synthesis; voice recognition for printing
    Interface adaptations: keyboard, microswitch, voice activation
Miscellaneous
    One-handed jar opener
    Door knob extension
    Book holder, page turner
    Holder for cutting with loop scissor or knife
    Long-reach jaw grabbers
    Standing frames
Sports and Hobbies
    Needle holder for one-handed knitting
    Action Life Glove: double tunnel loops hold pool cue, fishing rod, gym equipment
    Strong Arm fishing rod holder

some especially functional, off-the-shelf items. Other simple or highly engineered items can contribute to independent living.

A wide variety of portable communication devices are available commercially for the patient who cannot speak and has little or no limb movement. Some software can "learn" to predict the next word and list words and word endings often chosen by the user. These packages include speech synthesizers. Portable computers can be controlled with small one-handed keyboards or microswitches that move a cursor with a flicker of the user's residual motion, even if that is only a twitch of the frontalis muscle. Patients can operate on-screen keyboards with a mouse under ultrasonic or infrared head control, by blowing into a straw, and by voice recognition. With additional interfaces, these controls can access telephones, lights, alarms, intercoms, and other home and work electronic equipment. These devices are of particular value to the patient with quadriparesis from SCI, ALS, or stroke. Head controllers that allow a quadriplegic patient to control the pointer or mouse cursor of a computer with slight head movements allow such people to work productively. Most systems work by proportional gain of neck movements (*HeadMaster Plus*, Prentke Romich Corp, Wooster OH; *Tracker 2000*, Madentec Ltd, Edmonton, Canada). Organizations such as RESNA and the U.S. Veterans Administration, funding agencies such as the U.S. Department of Ed-

ucation, and groups such as the Applied Science & Engineering Laboratories at the University of Delaware's A.I. DuPont Institute regularly publish evaluations of computer devices and software for communication.

More remarkable tools for the disabled include robotic manipulators, mobile robots, manipulations of a virtual reality environment, and neuroprostheses (see Chapter 4). Interfaces that can convert a muscle or eye movement or a cerebral biosignal into a control signal for a computer are available (e.g., BioControl Systems, Inc., Palo Alto, CA). As aids become more sophisticated, designers and manufacturers will have to consider the varied needs of the disabled person, otherwise clever products in search of a use will result.

WHEELCHAIRS

Over 2 million people in the United States use wheelchairs. The first reliable folding manual wheelchair was designed by Everest and Jennings in 1939 and commercial battery-run wheelchairs did not appear until the 1950s. Although the technology allowed such devices to have been developed much sooner, even the inventors called their wheelchairs invalid chairs, suggesting that anyone who needed a wheelchair was not independent or bright enough to maneuver one. Many health plans seem to review the need for a disabled person to have a lightweight, well-fitted wheelchair with the same attitude.

Table 5–4. **Wheelchair Prescription Parameters**

Frame	Leg and footrest
Material	Height; adjustment from edge of seat
Weight	Fixed, removable, swing-away; straps
Seat	Wheels
Height, width, depth, angle	Materials—alloys, plastic
Sling or cushioned; inserts	Tires—width, tread; pneumatic or solid
Cushion—elastic foam,viscoelastic foam, air or	Angulation
viscous fluid filled, alternating pressure	Handrims
Back	Front casters
Height; fixed or reclining; head rest	Brakes—locking, backsliding
Flexible, custom molded; foam or gel inserts	Anti-tip bars
Arms	Power supply; control system
Height—fixed or adjustable	
Fixed, removable, swing-away	
Arm troughs; clear plastic lap board;	
power controls	

Chairs range from the depot type that others push, lightweight ones for self-propelling, ultra lightweight chairs for highly active people, and sports chairs for rapid mobility and turns on a tennis or basketball court. In general, an ultra lightweight wheelchair is more durable and adjustable than a lightweight chair for active people.

Wheelchair prescriptions must take into account many factors, particularly for the highly mobile paraplegic person or for the quadriparetic person who needs an electric wheelchair system.[122] A prescription specifies the dimensions and components listed in Table 5–4. Many models of different weights and materials are available from vendors. Wheelchair clinics in rehabilitation facilities bring in representatives of manufacturers to match the patient's needs. Considerations include safety, comfort, trunk and thigh support, skin and pressure point protection, type of transfers into the chair, ease of propulsion, transportability, use for recreation or on uneven terrain, special accommodations for work, control systems, barriers such as narrow doorways, and anticipation about changes related to progression of impairments. For example, the hemiplegic patient may require a seat set low enough to allow one leg to help propel the chair. An active young person will develop wheelchair skills over time that require fewer safety features, allow the wheel axle to set forward for greater maneuverabilty, and improve pushrim biomechanics. Training in best biomechanics for wheelchair use and in strength and endurance exercises may help reduce injuries. Some studies estimate that two-thirds of manual users suffer arm pain and many develop compression neuropathies.[123]

Seat cushions vary in their stability, pressure distribution, thermal conduction, weight, and shear characteristics. Cushions help support the low back as well as protect the skin. Ideally, each cushion would include pressure mapping technology and self-adjust to prevent pressure sores and provide optimal sitting comfort and stability. Available seats carry trade-offs. A ROHO air cushion ought to equalize pressure by its interconnected flexible air chambers, but does not have as stable a base as the Jay2 viscous fluid and foam base. Cut-out foam cushions redistribute pressure but may put pressure on areas other than the buttocks. Dynamic cushions with air cylinders are expensive and of uncertain reliability.

A powered wheelchair run by a joystick, sip-and-puff, chin, or voice-command controller may be ideal for a quadriparetic patient who has cerebral palsy or a cervical cord injury, but would be hazardous for a patient with hemi-inattention or poor judgment. Electric powered wheelchairs have electromechanical brakes that release when power is applied to the motors. Controller software has greatly improved safety and drivability by matching the program to a person's abilities. Sensors that avoid obstacles and tracking technology that can preprogram a chair's path are available, but not used much yet. Hybrid wheelchairs (Yamaha) are becoming available. Pushing on the rim activates an electric hub motor for a boost, especially up hills. The *IBOT* (Johnson and Johnson; ≈$22,000) adds a new dimension to mobility. This remarkable vehicle includes gyroscopes for balance, has a 4-wheel rotating base to maneuver over curbs, stands the user upright, and ascends and descends stairs.

Motorized scooters with 3 or 4 wheels are convenient for community mobility for patients who are limited to home ambulation. Some paraparetic patients, particularly those with multiple sclerosis or diseases of the motor unit such as postpolio, find that scooters allow them efficient mobility. Patients must be able to transfer easily and have good trunk and upper extremity motor control. Some lightweight scooters can be taken apart in 3 pieces. A portable phone in the home and a cellular phone for the community provide great convenience and measures of safety to the patient who is confined to a wheelchair or scooter. Ongoing studies in ergonomics, engineering, computerized safety and control devices, and materials for seating systems, wheels, and frames should continue to refine the wheelchair.

SPEECH AND LANGUAGE THERAPISTS

At least 1 in 3 early survivors of an acute stroke or serious traumatic brain injury has dysarthric speech or aphasia. The dementias, brain tumors, meningoencephalitides, and other neurologic diseases also affect language. The prevalence of aphasia is uncertain, but given the frequency of all of these entities, an annual incidence of 200,000 cases in the United States seems likely. Articulatory disorders and oropharyngeal dysphagia are even more common, in both acute and chronic or degenerative neu-rologic diseases. Speech therapists generally take the lead in assessing and managing these problems. Because neurogenic dysphagia has significant medical consequences, its assess-ment and management is covered in Chapter 8.

Responsibilities

DYSARTHRIA

Dysarthria arises from injury to the neural path-ways for articulation, the shaping of sounds within the mouth. Laryngeal activity, respiratory movements, and articulatory activity are hierar-chically controlled by multiple brain stem nu-clei, as well as pyramidal and extrapyramidal pathways, and mediofrontal regions for volun-tary control of initiation and suppression of vo-cal utterances.[124] Weakness, slowness, and in-coordination can be appreciated in a patient's phonation, respiratory support for speech, res-onance, and prosody. Therapists will also char-acterize the patient's vocal quality, pitch, and loudness, particularly for sounds made with the vocal cords abducted (voiceless sounds such as "f" and "s") or adducted and vibrating (voiced sounds such as "v" and "z"). Laryngoscopy and pulmonary function tests such as the forced ex-piratory volume can help localize associated im-pairments. Acoustic analysis provides an objec-tive measure of the dysphonic voice and can guide therapy.[125]

A few syndromes are common. Bilateral cerebral lesions produce a pseudobulbar palsy with spastic dysarthia. This effortful articula-tion is hyponasal, harsh, and strained. The flac-cid dysarthia from lower motor neuron and mo-tor unit dysfunction is characterized by breathy short phrases and hypernasal, imprecise artic-ulation. Other categories include the monoto-nous, soft rushes of a Parkinson's hypokinetic dysarthia, the distortions associated with dys-tonias, and the dysrhythmic pitch and prosody of an ataxic dysarthia.

APHASIA

The speech and language therapist must de-termine whether a patient has a disorder of lan-guage and, if so, the way this interacts with overall cognitive function. Formal and informal testing leads to a classification of the problem.

Many formal tests of the components of speech and language have come into common use by therapists and for clinical studies. Table 7–5 lists some of the well-standardized testing tools.

Table 5–5 lists the most common clini-coanatomic classification of the aphasias. From 20% to 50% of aphasic patients do not easily fit into a classic category. Many patients have partial features of a syndrome or have mixed syndromes. Some studies have found so little correlation between the traditional aphasia subtype classification and anatomical localiza-tion that they question its utility.[126] Other in-vestigators found that problems in repetition, mutism, fluency, and verbal comprehension did adhere to the classic clinical-anatomic clas-sification of aphasia.[127] As locations on a map of brain and language, this schematic is highly simplified. For example, Broca's aphasia in-volves several regions of the left hemisphere in addition to the frontal operculum and usually evolves from incomplete recovery of a more se-vere aphasia.[128] Damage only within Broca's area causes transient mutism or a disorder of articulation. The presence or absence of the pathways for the activational, semantic, motor planning, and articulatory aspects of language determines the kind of function that follows this anterior injury. Most importantly, the lan-guage tasks used to classify aphasia in Table 5–5 have not been connected to neurobiologi-cally identified processes. The classifications have heuristic value, but may not hold up as knowledge of large-scale cortical networks in-creases (see Chapter 1).

Cortical stimulation studies in people un-dergoing craniotomies and functional neu-roimaging studies reveal specialized language sites with separable linguistic functions and other sites with overlapping functions. For ex-ample, lexical processing is more diffusely rep-resented compared to morpheme-syntactic processing.[129–132] The left temporal lobe en-codes word meanings, but sentence compre-hension is highly distributed. Lesions confined to a handful of specific sites tend to predict particular disorders.[127,133] For example, (1) in-jury to the anterior superior temporal gyrus dis-rupts sentence comprehension, especially of grammar; (2) injury of the posterior superior temporal gyrus affects echoic verbal memory, producing Wernicke's aphasia; (3) damage to the posterior temporal lobe and underlying

Table 5–5. **Traditional Aphasia Syndromes**

Type	Expression	Comprehension	Repetition	Brodmann Area Injured	Adjunct Therapy
Broca's	Effortful, nonfluent, agrammatic Anomia: Proper and common nouns Proper nouns	Mostly intact	Impaired; best for nouns and action verbs	44,45; +/− nearby 6, 8,9,10,46, subcortex 20,21 38	MIT; VCIU; manual signing; HELPSS; RET; MIPT; bromocriptine
Wernicke's	Melodic, fluent, phoneme and word choice errors	Impaired; reading better	Impaired	22; +/− 37,39,40	SLAC
Global	Nonfluent; expletives facial and intonation expression	Poor; best for personally relevant material	Absent	Above Combined	VAT; symbols; computerized systems
Conduction	Fluent; letter and word substitutions	Mostly intact	Poor for sentences and multisyllabic words	40,41,42 subinsula	PACE
Transcortical Motor	Decreased fluency	Mostly intact	Mostly intact	Anterior/ superior to Broca's	Bromocriptine
Sensory	Fluent; substitutions	Impaired	Mostly intact	Posterior/ inferior to Wernicke's	
Subcortical Basal Ganglia	Transient mutism; decreased fluency or dysarthria	Mildly impaired	Intact or mildly impaired	Caudate head, anterior limb of internal capsule	
Thalamus	Fluent; neologisms	Mildly impaired	Intact	Antero-lateral	
Right hemisphere	Impaired prosody and organization of a narrative	Impaired recognition of emotional tone	Impaired attention	Parallels with Broca & Wernicke areas	

MIT, melodic intonation therapy; VCIU, voluntary control of involuntary utterance; HELPSS, Helm-elicited language program for syntax stimulation; RET, response elaboration training; MIPT, multiple input phoneme therapy; SLAC, sentence level auditory comprehension; VAT, visual action therapy; PACE, promoting aphasics' communicative effectiveness.

white matter disrupts the lexical-semantic network and produces poor naming skills even with priming and choice, especially if the middle temporal gyrus is involved; (4) a lesion in the superior arcuate fasciculus prevents information in language cortex from reaching the motoric controls for speech, often causing recurrent utterances; and (5) damage to the insula within the superior tip of the precentral gyrus causes at least a transient apraxia of speech.

Certain aphasic disorders are highly associated with particular lesions. For example, (1) mutism involves fronto-putaminal lesions; (2) repetition deficits involve lesions of the external capsule and posterior internal capsule; (3) phonemic paraphasia involves damage to the external capsule that extends to the posterior temporal lobe or internal capsule; and (4) perseveration involves a lesion of the caudate nucleus. For rehabilitation therapy, the broadly defined features used to classify patients in Table 5–5 often do not address in enough detail the underlying disturbances of aphasic language. Thus, traditional pigeonholes for classification may not direct treatment optimally.

Interventions for Dysarthria and Aphasia

DYSARTHRIA

Therapies aim to improve the patient's speech intelligibility, volume, and fluidity by means of exercises for affected structures. Patients may be trained to slow their articulation, use shorter sentences, maximize breath support, extend the jaw's motion, and purposefully place the tongue or exaggerate articulatory movements. A modest Valsalva exercise may increase adduction of the vocal folds. By increasing vocal cord adduction and respiratory support for speech, patients with extrapyramidal disorders often improve their intelligibility (Lee Silverman Voice Treatment).[134] Relaxation techniques may lessen the strained vocal quality in patients with a pseudobulbar palsy. Behavioral retraining methods include pacing vocalizations by an external cue, using delayed auditory feedback by speaking into an echoic device, and use of a *Speech Enhancer* (Electronic Speech Enhancement, St. Louis) that amplifies the voice and clarifies dysarthric speech.

Surface electromyographic electrodes placed over the anterior cervical strap muscles can provide feedback about laryngeal elevation.

Some patients benefit from oral prosthetic devices when weakness of muscles around the velopharyngeal port impairs resonance. A palatal lift may help both spastic and flaccid dysarthric patients. So-called pressure consonants such as *t*, *s*, and *p* sounds may improve with a lift in place. For very soft or monotone speech, a portable amplifier can reestablish functional communication. Apraxia of oromotor function, which refers to the inability to carry out volitional movements with the articulators, is managed by methods that overlap those used to treat dysarthia.

APHASIA

Treatment for aphasia is based on the clinical evaluation of the patient's cognitive and linguistic assets and deficits. The therapy plan is fine tuned by standardized language and neuropsychologic tests, knowledge of the cortical and subcortical structures damaged, and the ongoing response to specific therapies. The patient's casual interactions with the family and rehabilitation team often broaden the analysis of the patient's linguistic and nonlinguistic strengths and weaknesses for communication. The speech therapist must assist the team, as well as the patient, to understand the processes and strategies that the patient will employ to communicate. Successful treatment approaches depend on the profile of impaired and spared abilities and build upon the patient's residual problem-solving strategies and memory. The therapist manages aspects of behavioral compensation, substitutive reorganization, and psychosocial responses to disability. Language therapists usually employ an idiosyncratic combination of techniques. Approaches to children with aphasia may differ considerably from therapy for adults, not only in regard to development, but also in relation to the greater plasticity shown in studies of children.[135] Aphasia therapy, in general, is efficacious after stroke,[136] which is discussed further in Chapter 9.

General Strategies

Speech therapists attempt to circumvent, deblock, or help the patient compensate for defective language behaviors. For patients with impaired expression and comprehension of language, the therapist's first challenge is to quickly obtain reliable verbal or gestural "yes–no" responses. Otherwise, aphasic patients may feel isolated, even angry and frustrated, and may withdraw from those around them. Initial treatments for aphasia often deal with tasks that relate to self-care, the immediate environment, and emotionally positive experiences. As specific syndromes of impairments evolve during assessment and treatment, a variety of specific techniques can be applied. One note of caution. Some patients become upset and withdraw from therapists and family or friends whom they perceive to be talking down to them. Nothing turns them away from therapy more than seemingly irrelevant, simple, repetitive tasks. The inpatient and outpatient rehabilitation team and family help the aphasic person most when they show patience and use consistent techniques to aid expression and comprehension.

Different models of conceptualizing language lead to variations in the approaches that may be taken.[137] Models include (1) modality-specific, (2) linguistic, (3) language module processing, (4) minor hemisphere mediation, (5) functional communication, and (6) hybrid therapy approaches. Each therapy task in each of these models has its rationale, drawn from small group studies of normal and impaired subjects. Without greater knowledge of the cognitive architecture of language, however, these models will have limited success for aphasia therapy.[138] Future models may combine information about processing single words, sentences, and discourse with the memory substrates needed for these forms of visual and auditory communication and with their physiologic and anatomic substrates drawn from functional anatomic imaging with PET, fMRI, and other tools (see Chapter 3).

Within any of the conceptual models, a patient can be diagnosed with multiple language processing impairments, instead of a specific syndrome of aphasia. The aim of the neurolinguistic assessment of aphasia is to specify types of representations or units of language, such as simple words, word formation, sentences, and discourse, that are abnormally processed during speech, auditory comprehension, reading, and writing.[139,140] For each unit, the therapist ascertains how the disturbance affects linguistic forms, such as phonemes, syntactic structures, and semantic meanings. Some of these distinctions are made by a speech therapist's traditional evaluation. For example, the therapist assesses differences in the ability to express or understand words that are familiar or novel, regular or irregular, and concrete or abstract. A traditional analysis often is not as detailed as a neurolinguistic one. Perhaps greater clarification of the nature of the patient's impairments will produce additional therapeutic strategies,[141,142] ones that sift through the real architecture of language processing.

The most common intervention takes a *stimulation-facilitation* approach. Therapists employ visual and verbal cueing techniques that include picture-matching and sentence-completion tasks, along with frequent repetition and positive reinforcement as the patient approaches the desired responses (Table 5–6). One major goal is to activate connections be-

Table 5–6. **Traditional Aphasia Therapy Tasks**

Body part identification	Contextual cueing
Word discrimination	Phonemic and semantic word retrieval strategies
Word to picture matching	Priming for responses
Yes–no response reliability	Melodic stimulation
Auditory processing at the phrase, then sentence level	Graphic tasks–tracing, copying, word completions
Word, phrase, then sentence level reading	Calculations
Gestural expression and pointing	Pragmatic linguistic and nonlinguistic conversational skills
Oral-motor imitation	Psychosocial supports
Phoneme, then word repetition	
Verbal cueing for words and sentence completion	

tween related words and meanings and to prime subjects to do this faster and more spontaneously. Some preliminary studies suggest that priming techniques (see Chapters 1 and 11) may improve certain language functions. Priming, a phenomenon present even in amnestic patients, relies on cues and prompts to drive recall of information previously provided to the subject. Patients with poor comprehension of spoken words may respond to auditory priming to complete a task, even though the patients do not comprehend the studied items.[143] Auditory perceptual priming may, then, depend upon access to a presemantic (knowledge about the world) auditory word-form system. Few well-designed studies, however, have been published of word–word and sentence–word priming paradigms in aphasic patients.[144] Such *semantic priming* may not be preserved in some aphasic patients, since it involves a network that includes the left inferior prefrontal cortex. Of interest, when semantic priming is intact, cortical regions that had been engaged when a word was first seen are relatively deactivated when the word reappears, which is consistent with the decrease in reaction time induced by prior exposure.[145] The pathway for processing has been greased.

Related techniques that expose aphasic patients to target items also improve their performance via implicit or nonconscious memory. Implicit reading strategies help a person with an acquired alexia read. A task that requires alexic patients to name a written word tends to produce a letter-by-letter reading strategy.[146] When instructed to make a lexical decision or semantic judgement about rapidly presented words, some patients are able to switch to a whole-word reading strategy.

The intensity and specificity of practice may be most important in testing for advantages of conceptual models for therapy. Several studies have examined this issue. One well-designed clinical trial employed a picture card game in which a group of aphasic patients were prompted to request and provide a card of depicted objects in their hand. The results suggest that behaviorally relevant mass practice for at least 3 hours a day for 10 days that also constrained the use of nonverbal communication and reinforced appropriate responses within a group setting could improve comprehension and naming skills over less intensive and formalized therapy.[87] Researchers continue to ex-

amine how each parameter of a retraining program built upon any of these models may improve outcomes, including manipulations of the frequency and duration of a specific treatment approach, the use of blocked practice or contextual interference, the type and frequency of reinforcement with knowledge of performance and results, the advantages of group versus individual therapy, and the use of a professional therapist or trained helper.

Therapies for Specific Syndromes

A handful of techniques have been designed and evaluated for specific aphasia syndromes and neurolinguistic impairments.[139,147,148] The evidence for efficacy of these structured approaches to difficulties in expression and comprehension rests on small group and case studies. Table 5–5 lists the most thoroughly evaluated adjunct techniques that include a well-documented procedure for the intervention. These approaches often overlap. For example, for several approaches, the clinician controls perseverative utterances by holding up a hand and instructing the desperate patient to watch and listen, but not try to speak. Then, the patient watches the clinician's mouth pronounce a word as the clinician taps on the patient's arm to help define the start and end of the word. The clinician repeats this approach a half-dozen times before allowing the patient to attempt the word.

Melodic intonation therapy (MIT) is one of the few interventions that can be defined and applied consistently enough to make it applicable for research.[149] In MIT, therapists and patients melodically intone multisyllabic words and commonly used short phrases while the therapist taps the patient's left hand to mark each syllable.[150] Words are produced with an exaggerated prosody that includes high and low pitches at short and longer durations. Gradually, the continuous voicing and tapping is withdrawn. Melodic intonation therapy works best in Broca's aphasics with sparse or stereotyped nonsense speech and good auditory comprehension. Short-term, qualitative benefits have been shown for this demanding approach. Melodic intonation therapy can also lead to gains in patients with a severe apraxia of speech. A PET study showed that word repetition during MIT compared to repetition without the sounds of MIT caused a decrease in cerebral blood flow in the right hemisphere's homologue region for Wernicke's area and increased flow to the left hemisphere, especially in Broca's area and adjacent prefrontal cortex.[151] Melodic intonation therapy, then, induces a systematic change in how the acoustic features of spoken and perceived speech are engaged by the brain after a left hemispheric stroke. Intensive practice in the approach may help to reactivate the left prefrontal region in relation to improved expression. As described in Chapter 3, functional imaging studies suggest that greater recovery in aphasics occurs when peri-injury language areas are activated, rather than when nondominant homoguous cortical regions are engaged.

When a single sound, word, or phrase overwhelms any other attempted output, the voluntary control of involuntary utterance (VCIU) program can help the patient gain control over perseverative intrusions.[152]

The agrammatism of Broca's aphasia has been treated with the Helm-elicited language program for syntax stimulation (HELPSS),[153] which uses a series of drawings that picture common activities. The therapist provides a brief verbal description that ends with a question about the story and contains a target sentence. After the patient responds with the target words, the patient is asked to complete the story without benefit of having heard the target sentence. Each probe seeks a target response that requires an increasingly more difficult syntactic construction.

Some patients with little or only stereotyped output, even with impaired comprehension, have responded to multiple input phoneme therapy (MIPT).[154] The theory behind the approach is that markedly apractic-aphasic patients who produce only stereotypies are caught in a verbal motor loop. Once an utterance is made, the loop strengthens and each attempt at volitional speech elicits the loop. Multiple input phoneme therapy is a 22-step hierarchic program that builds from an analysis of phonemes produced by the patient. The therapist controls the patient's struggle to articulate, then elicits a target phoneme to build consonant blends, multisyllabic words, and eventually sentence production.

Response elaboration training (RET) shapes and chains the responses patients give to their descriptions of familiar activities in line drawings.[155] The technique reinforces informational content, rather than linguistic form.

Some mute or nonfluent aphasics can acquire a limited but useful repertoire of gestures, such as those drawn from *American Indian sign language*.[156] Sign language requires left hemisphere language areas.

Attempts to improve comprehension for patients with global and Wernicke's aphasia take many forms. The sentence level auditory comprehension (SLAC) program trains patients to discriminate consonant-vowel-consonant words that are the same or differ by only one phoneme (e.g. bill, pill, fill).[157] Patients then try to associate the word sounds with the written word and later try to identify the target word embedded in a sentence. Gains in some patients have generalized to improved scores on the Token Test for comprehension. The SLAC program[141] calls upon the neurolinguist's understanding of phonemic, syntactic, and lexical deviations.

For global aphasics, nonverbal communication with pantomime through a technique called visual action therapy (VAT) may decrease limb apraxia and improve auditory comprehension.[158] Patients are taught to use hand gestures with real items, then gestures without the items. Programmed instruction has been combined with operant conditioning for the global aphasic patient, but the efficacy was limited.[159] Another technique, called promoting aphasics' communicative effectiveness (PACE), emphasizes the ideas that need to be conveyed in face-to-face interactions during real bouts of communication with nontherapists, rather than linguistic accuracy.[160] This experiential technique aims to develop any modality that can be used to transmit a message, such as limited speech, limb or facial gestures, and drawing. Success with VAT and PACE suggests that the left hemisphere has a linguistic, rather than a general symbolic specialization for the components of language. The dominant hemisphere produces sign and spoken language, whereas both hemispheres are capable of producing the nonlinguistic gestures of pantomime.[161] Pointing to pictured objects with the proximal right arm may improve simultaneous vocal naming after a stroke, perhaps by activating attention in the dominant hemisphere.[162]

Pragmatics refers to the use of language in a social context. Along with the attentional, memory, and other cognitive problems of patient's with TBI, pragmatic communication is often impaired.[163] The communication abili-

and tennis possible. The same holds for snow skiing.[177,178] Over 200 local, national and international organizations have developed rules and equipment for at least 75 sports and recreational activities that take into account a range of functional abilities.[21] The United States Adaptive Recreation Center in Bear Lake, CA (www.usarc.org) is one of many services to provide information and training in sports activities. Self-esteem and problem-solving skills may grow as a disabled person learns a martial art or engages in outdoor experiential educational pursuits such as traversing a ropes course 30 feet above the ground.

More research is needed to design exercise and recreational programs for younger and older people with neurologic diseases. These studies should assess both useful and possibly injurious effects. Outcome measures may include medical morbidity such as pressure sores, blood pressure, and lipid levels, endurance for instrumental ADLs, leisure-time physical activity, and quality of life, with follow up through mid and late life. Sports and exercise activities could easily be incorporated into subacute and chronic neurologic rehabilitation programs to enhance and maintain functional recovery and to build self-esteem.

OTHER TEAM MEMBERS

The rehabilitation team looks to many other professionals, including case managers who act as ombudsmen for patients, nutritionists, vocational counselors, bioengineers, orthotists, and, increasingly, clinical researchers and statisticians. The ethicist may become an even more valued member. Ethical dilemmas are bound to increase as society sets limits on whom receives what treatment and for what amount of time. Will inpatient units no longer accept elderly inpatients who are not candidates for cardiopulmonary resuscitation? Will inpatient units no longer provide rehabilitation if it is less expensive for patients to remain disabled? Will rehabilitationists be able to carry out research to improve outcomes and then apply group studies of cost-effective interventions to the individual patient?

Staying current within their areas of expertise has become an increasingly challenging task for the team. Computerized publication services or regular down-loading from library databases can make updating more efficient. Scores of basic science, applied science, general clinical, and specialized clinical journals and books contain information relevant to those who practice neurologic rehabilitation. This depth of intellectual activity offers a view of the expanding boundaries of the disciplines and knowledge that are relevant to neurologic rehabilitation.

SUMMARY

An interdisciplinary team approach to issues of medical care, mobility, self-care and community skills, cognition and language, and psychosocial needs by physicians, nurses, therapists, social workers, psychologists, and others embodies what is peculiar and remarkable about the culture of a neurologic rehabilitation service. This culture concerns itself as much with the experience of illness and disability of the patient and family as with the details of a particular disease. Each team member bears key responsibilities for the team and each brings a point of view about the basis and style for assessments and interventions.

Most physical and cognitive interventions require practice carried out in a learning paradigm that, ultimately, modulates neural networks. Consideration must be given to the goal of an intervention, the intensity and duration of treatment, and the schema of practice. Every approach to therapy is open to challenge. Every challenge deserves thought on how to better understand and manage a behavioral phenomenon and its neural correlates. Rehabilitationists must continue to prove whether specific approaches to particular impairments and disabilities are better than other therapies. The settings for these clinical experiments include inpatient rehabilitation, initial outpatient therapy after an acute illness, chronic care, and office follow-ups in which a clinician identifies a persistent problem, say slow community ambulation, and provides a brief pulse of therapy to achieve a particular aim, say walking speed greater than 1.8 mph. The interdisciplinary team owes itself continuing education about theories and studies in each of its fields that reach conferences and publications. This intellectual vigor will help everyone best manage the consequences of brain and spinal dysfunction in patients with impairments and disabilities.

REFERENCES

1. Charon R. Narrative medicine. JAMA 2001; 286:1897–1902.
2. Dobkin B. Brain Matters: Stories of a Neurologist and His Patients. New York: Crown Publishers, 1986.
3. Haas J, Mackenzie C. The role of ethics in rehabilitation medicine. Am J Phys Med Rehabil 1993; 72:48–51.
4. Pound P, Gompertz P, Ebrahim S. Patients' satisfaction with stroke services. Clin Rehabil 1994; 8:7–17.
5. Keith R. The comprehensive treatment team in rehabilitation. Arch Phys Med Rehabil 1991; 72:269–274.
6. Kalra L. The influence of stroke unit rehabilitation on functional recovery from stroke. Stroke 1994; 25:821–825.
7. Kramer A, Steiner J, Schlenker R, Eilertsen TB, Hrincevich CA, Tropea DA, Ahmad LA. Outcomes and costs after hip fracture and stroke: A comparison of rehabilitation settings. JAMA 1997; 277:396–404.
8. Duncan P, Horner R, Reker D, Samsa G, Hoenig H. Adherence to postacute rehabilitation guidelines is associated with functional recovery in stroke. Stroke 2002; 33:167–178.
9. Bettman B. Frenkel's treatment of ataxia by means of exercise. JAMA 1897; 28:5–8.
10. Rohrbaugh M, Rogers J. What did the doctor do? When physicians and patients disagree. Arch Fam Med 1994; 3:125–129.
11. Salan S. What makes a good disability evaluation report? The Neurologist 1998; 4:269–276.
12. Stickgold R, James L, Hobson A. Visual discrimination learning requires sleep after training. Nat Neurosci 2000; 3:1237–1238.
13. Group. Activity Counseling Trial. Effects of physical activity counseling in primary care: The Activity Counseling Trial. JAMA 2001; 286:677–687.
14. Granger C, Hamilton B. The Uniform Data System for Medical Rehabilitation report of first admissions for 1992. Am J Phys Med Rehabil 1994; 73:51–55.
15. Cramer J. Identifying and improving compliance patterns: A composite plan for health care providers. In: Cramer J, Spilker B, eds. Patient Compliance in Medical Practice and Clinical Trials. New York: Raven Press, 1991:387–392.
16. Mitchell R. The quality of evaluation in physical therapy. Crit Rev Phys Rehabil Med 1992; 4:61–77.
17. Lister M. Contemporary Management of Motor Control Problems: Proceedings of the II Step Conference. Alexandria, VA: Foundation for Physical Therapy, 1991:278.
18. Shumway-Cook A, Woollacott M. Motor Control. Philadelphia: Lippincott Williams & Wilkins, 2001.
19. Basmajian J, Wolf S. Therapeutic Exercise. Baltimore: Williams & Wilkins, 1990:460.
20. Waters R, Yakura J. The energy expenditure of normal and pathological gait. Crit Rev in Phys Rehabil Med 1989; 1:183–209.
21. Dobkin B. Exercise fitness and sports for individuals with neurologic disability. In: Gordon S, Gonzalez-Mestre X, Garrett W, eds. Sports and Exercise in Midlife. Rosemont, IL: American Academy of Orthopedic Surgeons, 1993:235–252.
22. Miller G, Light K. Strength training in spastic hemiparesis: Should it be avoided? Neurorehabilitation 1997; 9:17–28.
23. Bohannon R. Relevance of muscle strength to gait performance in patients with neurologic disability. J Neuro Rehabil 1989; 3:97–100.
24. Inuba M, Edberg E, Montgomery J, Gillis K. Effectiveness of functional training, active exercise and resistive exercise for patients with hemiplegia. Phys Ther 1973; 53:28–35.
25. Corcos D. Strategies underlying the control of disordered movement. Phys Ther 1991; 71:25–32.
26. Benecke R, Conrad B, Meinck H, Hohne J. Electromyographic analysis of bicycling on an ergometer for evaluation of spasticity of lower limbs in man. In: Desmedt J, ed. Motor Control Mechanisms in Health and Disease. New York: Raven Press, 1983.
27. Brown D, Kautz S, Dairaghi C. Muscle activity adapts to anti-gravity posture during pedalling in persons with post-stroke hemiplegia. Brain 1997; 120:825–837.
28. Brown D, Kautz S. Increased workload enhances force output during pedaling exercise in persons with poststroke hemiplegia. Stroke 1998; 29:598–606.
29. Potempa K, Lopez M, Braun L, Szidon JP, Fogg L, Tincknell T. Physiological outcomes of aerobic exercise training in hemiparetic stroke. Stroke 1995; 26:101–105.
30. Macko R, Smith G, Dobrovolny C, Sorkin J, Goldberg A, Silver K. Treadmill training improves fitness reserve in chronic stroke patients. Arch Phys Med Rehabil 2001; 82:879–884.
31. Bromfield E, Reding M. Relative risk of deep vein thrombosis or pulmonary embolism post stroke based on ambulatory status. J Neurol Rehab 1988; 2:51–57.
32. Voss D, Ionta M, Myers B. Proprioceptive Neuromuscular Facilitation. Philadelphia: Harper & Row, 1985:370.
33. Liebesman J, Cafarelli E. Physiology of range of motion in human joints: A critical review. Crit Rev Phys Rehabil Med 1994; 6:131–160.
34. Bobath B. Adult Hemiplegia. Oxford: Heinemann, 1990:190.
35. Valvano J, Long T. Neurodevelopmental treatment: A review of the writings of the Bobaths. Pediatr Phys Ther 1991:125–129.
36. Lennon S, Baxter D, Ashburn A. Physiotherapy based on the Bobath concept in stroke rehabilitation: A survey within the UK. Disabil Rehabil 2001; 23:254–262.
37. Johnstone M. Restoration of Motor Function in the Stroke Patient. London: Churchill Livingstone, 1978:187.
38. Brunnstrom S. Movement Therapy in Hemiplegia. Philadelphia: Harper & Row, 1970:190.
39. Stockmeyer S. An interpretation of the approach of Rood to the treatment of neuromuscular dysfunction. Am J Phys Med 1967; 46:900–956.
40. Dickstein R, Edmondstone M, Stivens K. Therapeutic weight shift in hemiparetic patients: Surface electromyographic activity of lower extremity muscles during postural tasks. J Neurol Rehabil 1990; 4:17–25.
41. Trombly C. Observations of improvement of reaching in five subjects with left hemiparesis. J Neurol Neurosurg Psychiatry 1993; 56:40–45.

42. Twitchell T. The restoration of motor function following hemiplegia in man. Brain 1951; 74:443–480.
43. Wing A, Lough S, Turton A, Fraser C, Jenner JR. Recovery of elbow function in voluntary positioning of the hand following hemiplegia due to stroke. J Neurol Neurosurg Psychiatry 1990; 53:126–134.
44. Gauthier J, Bourbonnais D, Filiatrault J, Gravel D, Arsenault AB. Characterization of contralateral torques during static hip efforts in healthy subjects and subjects with hemiparesis. Brain 1992; 115: 1193–1207.
45. Hagbarth K-E, Eklund G. The effects of muscle vibration in spasticity, rigidity, and cerebellar disorders. J Neurol Neurosurg Psychiat 1968; 31:207–213.
46. Matyas T, Galea M, Spicer S. Facilitation of the maximum voluntary contraction in hemiplegia by concomitant cutaneous stimulation. Am J Phys Med 1986; 65:125–134.
47. Brouwer B, Ambury P. Upper extremity weight-bearing effect on corticospinal excitability following stroke. Arch Phys Med Rehabil 1994; 75:861–866.
48. Ottenbacher K, Biocca R, DeCremer O, Gevelinger M, Jedlovec KB, Johnson MB. Quantitative analysis of the effectiveness of pediatric therapy. Phys Ther 1986; 66:1095–1101.
49. Ashburn A, Partridge C, De Souza L. Physiotherapy in the rehabilitation of stroke: A review. Clin Rehabil 1993; 7:337–345.
50. Winstein C, Gardner E, McNeal D. Standing balance training: Effect on balance and locomotion in hemiparetic adults. Arch Phys Med Rehabil 1989; 70:755–762.
51. Dobkin B. Overview of treadmill locomotor training with partial body weight support: A neurophysiologically sound approach whose time has come for randomized clinical trials. Neurorehabilitation and Neural Repair 1999; 13:157–165.
52. Michaelsen S, Luta A, Roby-Brami A, Levin M. Effect of trunk restraint on the recovery of reaching movements in hemiparetic patients. Stroke 2001; 32:1875–1883.
53. Schmidt R, Wrisberg G. Motor Learning and Performance. Champaign, IL: Human Kinetics, 2000.
54. Pohl P, McDowd J, Filion D, Richards L, Stiers W. Implicit learning of a perceptual-motor skill after stroke. Phys Ther 2001; 81:1780–1789.
55. Schmidt R. Motor learning principles for physical therapy. In: Lister M, ed. Contemporary Management of Motor Control Problems. Alexandria, VA: Foundation for Physical Therapy, 1991:49–63.
56. Winstein C. Knowledge of results and motor learning—Implications for physical therapy. Phys Ther 1991; 71:140–149.
57. Wulf C, Schmidt R. Variability in practice: Facilitation in retention and transfer through schema formation or context effects? J Mot Behav 1988; 20: 133–149.
58. Ericcson K, Lehmann A. Expert and exceptional performance: Evidence on maximal adaptations on task constraints. Ann Rev Psychol 1996; 47:273–305.
59. Schmidt R, Lange C, Young D. Optimizing summary knowledge of results for skill learning. Hum Move Sci 1990; 9:325–348.
60. Winstein C, Schmidt R. Reduced frequency of knowledge of results enhances motor skill learning. J Exp Psychol 1990; 16:677–691.
61. Leclercq M, Couillet J, Azouvi P, Marlier N, Martin Y, Strypstein E, Rousseaux M. Dual task performance after severe diffuse traumatic brain injury or vascular prefrontal damage. J Clin Exp Neuropsychol 2000; 22:339–350.
62. Heitman R, Gilley W. Effects of blocked versus random practice by mentally retarded subjects on learning a novel skill. Percept Mot Skills 1989; 69:443–447.
63. Dick M, Hsieh S, Dick-Muehlke C, Davis D, Cotman C. The variability of practice hypothesis in motor learning: Does it apply to Alzheimer's disease? Brain Cogn 2000; 44:470–489.
64. Wilson B, Baddeley A, Evans J, Shiel A. Errorless learning in the rehabilitation of memory impaired people. Neuropsychol Rehabil 1994; 4:307–326.
65. Magill R, Hall K. A review of the contextual interference effect in motor skill acquisition. Hum Move Sci 1990; 9:241–289.
66. Winstein C, Merians A, Sullivan K. Motor learning after unilateral brain damage. Neuropsychologia 1999; 37:975–987.
67. Hanlon R. Motor learning following unilateral stroke. Arch Phys Med Rehabil 1996; 77:811–815.
68. Teixeira L. Timing and force components in bilateral transfer of learning. Brain Cogn 2000; 44:455–469.
69. van der Lee J, Wagenaar R, Lankhorst G, Vogelaar T, Deville W, Bouter L. Forced use of the upper extremity in chronic stroke patients: Results from a single-blind randomized clinical trial. Stroke 1999; 30:2369–2375.
70. Andres F, Mima T, Schulman A. Functional coupling of human cortical sensorimotor areas during bimanual skill acquisition. Brain 1999; 122:855–870.
71. Carr J, Shepherd R. A Motor Relearning Programme for Stroke. London: W Heinemann, 1987.
72. Carr J, Shepherd R. Neurological Rehabilitation: Optimizing Motor Performance. Oxford: Butterworth Heinemann, 1998.
73. Dean C, Shepherd R. Task-related training improves performance of seated reaching tasks after stroke. Stroke 1997; 28:722–728.
74. Pohl P, Winstein C. Practice effects on the less-affected upper extremity after stroke. Arch Phys Med Rehabil 1999; 80:668–675.
75. Sabari J. Motor learning concepts applied to activity-based intervention with adults with hemiplegia. Am J Occup Ther 1991; 45:523–530.
76. Yaguez L, Nagel D, Hoffman H. A mental route to motor learning: improving trajectorial kinematics through imagery training. Behav Brain Res 1998; 90:95–106.
77. Kwakkel G, Wagenaar R, Koelman T, Lankhorst G, Koetsier J. Effects of intensity of rehabilitation after stroke: A research synthesis. Stroke 1997; 28: 1550–1556.
78. Kwakkel G, Wagenaar R, Twisk J, Lankhorst G, Koetsier J. Intensity of leg and arm training after primary middle cerebral artery stroke: A randomised trial. Lancet 1999; 354:191–196.
79. Taub E, Crago J, Burgio L, Groomes TE, Cook EW 3rd, DeLuca SC, Miller NE. An operant approach to rehabilitation medicine: Overcoming learned nonuse by shaping. J Exp Anal Behav 1994; 61:287–318.
80. Knapp H, Taub E, Berman A. Movements in monkeys with deafferented limbs. Exp Neurol 1963; 7:305–315.

81. Taub E, Miller N, Novack T, Cook EW 3rd, Fleming WC, Nepomuceno CS, Connell JS, Crago JE. Technique to improve chronic motor deficit after stroke. Arch Phys Med Rehabil 1993; 74:347–354.

82. Liepert J, Bauder H, Miltner W, Taub E, Weiller C. Treatment-induced cortical reorganization after stroke in humans. Stroke 2000; 31:1210–1216.

83. Dromerick A, Edwards D, Hahn M. Does the application of constraint-induced movement therapy during acute rehabilitation reduce arm impairment after ischemic stroke? Stroke 2000; 31:2984–2988.

84. Taub E, Wolf S. Constraint induced movement techniques to facilitate upper extremity use in stroke patients. Top Stroke Rehabil 1997; 3:38–61.

85. Visintin M, Barbeau H, Korner-Bitensky N, Mayo N. A new approach to retrain gait in stroke patients through body weight support and treadmill stimulation. Stroke 1998; 29:1122–1128.

86. Dobkin B, Apple D, Barbeau H, Saulino M, Fugate L, Scott M. Randomized trial of body weight-supported treadmill training after acute spinal cord injury. Neurorehabil Neural Repair 1999; 13:50.

87. Pulvermuller F, Neininger B, Elbert T, Mohr B, Rockstroh B, Koebbel P, Taub E. Constraint-induced therapy of chronic aphasia after stroke. Stroke 2001; 32:1621–1626.

88. Thaut M, Kenyon G, Schauer M, McIntosh G. The connection between rhythmicity and brain function. IEEE Eng Med Biol 1999; March/April:101–108.

89. Fuchs A, Jirsa V, Kelso J. Issues in the coordination of human brain activity and motor behavior. Neuroimage 2000; 11:375–377.

90. Basmajian J. Biofeedback for neuromuscular rehabilitation. Crit Rev Phys Rehabil Med 1989; 1:37–58.

91. Moreland J, Thomson M, Fuoco A. Electromyographic biofeedback to improve lower extremity function after stroke: A meta-analysis. Arch Phys Med Rehabil 1998; 79:134–140.

92. Moreland J, Thomson M. Efficacy of electromyographic biofeedback compared with conventional physical therapy for upper-extremity function in patients following stroke: A research overview and meta-analysis. Phys Ther 1994; 74:534–543.

93. Bate P, Matyas T. Negative transfer of training following brief practice of elbow tracking movements with electromyographic feedback from spastic antagonists. Arch Phys Med Rehabil 1992; 73:1050–1058.

94. Cauraugh J, Light K, Kim S, Thigpen M, Behrman A. Chronic motor dysfunction after stroke: Recovering wrist and finger extension by electromyography-triggered neuromuscular stimulation. Stroke 2000; 31:1360–1364.

94a. Cauraugh J, Kim S. Two coupled motor recovery protocols are better than one. Stroke 2002; 33:1589–1594.

95. Todorov E, Shadmehr R, Bizzi E. Augmented feedback presented in a virtual environment accelerates learning of a difficult motor task. J Mot Behav 1997; 29:147–158.

96. Jack D, Merians A, Adamovich S, Tremaine M, Poizner H. A virtual reality-based exercise program for stroke rehabilitation, ASSETS 2000, Arlington, Va, 2000. Fourth ACM SIGCAPH Conference on Assistive Technologies.

97. Holden M, Todorov E, Callaban J, Bizzi E. Virtual environment training improves motor performance in two patients with stroke: Case report. Neurol Rep 1999; 23:57–67.

98. Riva G, Bolzoni M, Carella F, Rovetta A, Galimberti C, Griffin MJ, Lewis CH, Luongo R, Mardegan P, Melis L, Molinari-Tosatti L, Poerschmann C, Rushton S, Selis C, Wann J. Virtual reality environments for psycho-neuro-physiological assessment and rehabilitation. In: Westwood J, Hoffman H, Stredney D, Weghorst S, eds. Medicine Meets Virtual Reality: IOS Press, 1998:34–45.

99. Grealy M, Johnson D, Rushion S. Improving cognitive function after brain injury: the use of exercise and virtual reality. Arch Phys Med Rehabil 1999; 80:661–667.

100. Katz N, Marcus S, Weiss P. Purposeful activity in physical rehabilitation. Crit Rev Phys Rehabil Med 1994; 6:199–218.

101. Trombly C. Occupational Therapy for Physical Dysfunction. Baltimore: Williams & Wilkins, 1995.

102. Soderback I, Ekholm J. Occupational therapy in brain damage rehabilitation. Crit Rev Phys Rehabil Med 1993; 5:315–355.

102a. Liberman RP, Wallace C, Blackwell G, Kopelowicz A, Vaccaro J, Mintz J. Skills training versus psychosocial occupational therapy for persons with persistent schizophrenia. Am J Psychiatry 1998; 155:1087–1091.

103. Newell K, Valvano J. Therapeutic intervention as a constraint in learning and relearning movement skills. Scand J Occup Ther 1998; 5:51–57.

104. Mathiowetz V, Haugen J. Motor behavior research: Implications for therapeutic approaches to central nervous system dysfunction. Am J Occup Ther 1994; 48:733–745.

105. Poole J. Application of motor learning principles in occupational therapy. Am J Occup Ther 1991; 45:531–539.

106. Jarus T. Motor learning and occupational therapy: The organization of practice. Am J Occup Ther 1994; 48:810–816.

107. Sietsema J, Nelson D, Mulder R, Mervau-Scheidel D, White BE. The use of a game to promote arm reach in persons with traumatic brain injury. Am J Occup Ther 1993; 47:19–24.

108. Wu C-Y, Trombly C, Lin K-C, Tickle-Degnen l. A kinematic study of contextual effects on reaching performance in persons with and without stroke: Influences of object availability. Arch Phys Med Rehabil 2000; 81:95–101.

109. Recanzone G, Merzenich M, Jenkins W, Grajski K, Dinse H. Topographic reorganization of the hand representation in cortical area 3b of owl monkeys trained in a frequency-discrimination task. J Neurophysiol 1992; 67:1031–1056.

110. Godde B, Stauffenberg B, Spengler F, Dinse H. Tactile coactivation-induced changes in spatial discrimination performance. Neuroscience 2000; 20:1597–1604.

111. Braun C, Heinz U, Schweizer R, Wiech K, Bribaumer N, Topka H. Dynamic organization of the somatosensory cortex induced by motor activity. Brain 2001; 124:2259–2267.

112. Rossi S, Pasqualetti P, Tecchio F, Sabato A, Rossini P. Modulation of corticospinal output to human hand muscles following deprivation of sensory feedback. NeuroImage 1998; 8:163–175.

113. Ruch T, Fulton J, German W. Sensory discrimination in monkey, chimpanzee and man after lesions of the parietal lobe. Arch Neurol Psychiatry 1938; 39:914–918.

114. Dannenbaum R, Dykes R. Sensory loss in the hand after sensory stroke: Therapeutic rationale. Arch Phys Med Rehabil 1988; 69:833–839.

115. Carey L, Matyas T, Oke L. Sensory loss in stroke patients: Effective training of tactile and proprioceptive discrimination. Arch Phys Med Rehabil 1993; 74:602–611.

116. Yekutiel M, Guttman E. A controlled trial of the retraining of the sensory function of the hand in stroke patients. J Neurol Neurosurg Psychiatry 1993; 56:241–244.

116a. Zevner K, Bara-Jimenez W, Noguchi P, Goldstein S, Dambrosia J, Hallett M. Sensory training for patients with focal hand dystonia. Ann Neurol 2002; 51:593–598.

117. Naganuma G, Billingsley F. The use of hand splints with the neurologically involved child. Crit Rev Phys Rehabil Med 1990; 2:87–100.

118. McPherson J, Kreimeyer D, Aalderks M, Gallagher T. A comparison of dorsal and volar resting hand splints in the reduction of hypertonus. Am J Occup Ther 1982; 36:664–670.

119. Exner C, Bondere B. Comparative effects of three hand splints on bilateral hand use, grasp and arm-hand posture in hemiplegic children. Occup Ther J Res 1983; 3:75–81.

120. Casey C, Kratz E. Soft splinting with neoprene: the thumb abduction supinator splint. Am J Occup Ther 1988; 42:395–399.

121. Poole J, Whitney S, Hangeland N, Baker C. The effectiveness of inflatable pressure splints on motor function in stroke patients. Occup Ther J Res 1990; 10:360–366.

122. Giannini M. Choosing A Wheelchair System. J Rehabil Res Dev 1990; Clinical supplement #2:1–118.

123. Rodgers M, Keyser R, Rasch E, Gorman P, Russell P. Influence of training on biomechanics of wheelchair propulsion. J Rehabil Res Dev 2001; 38:505–511.

124. Jurgens U. Neural pathways underlying vocal control. Neurosci Biobehav Rev 2002; 26:235–258.

125. Kempler D. Speech pathology: Evaluation and treatment of speech, language, cognitive, and swallowing disorders. In: Meyerhoff W, Rice D, eds. Otolaryngology—Head and Neck Surgery. Philadelphia: WB Saunders, 1992:128–151.

126. Willmes K, Poeck K. To what extent can aphasic syndromes be localized? Brain 1993; 116:1527–1540.

127. Kreisler A, Godefroy O, Delmaire C, Debachy B, Leclercq M, Pruvo JP, Leys D. The anatomy of aphasia revisited. Neurology 2000; 54:1117–1123.

128. Mohr J, Pessin M, Finkelstein S, Funkenstein HH, Duncan GW, Davis KR. Broca's aphasia: Pathologic and clinical findings. Neurology 1978; 28:311–324.

129. Bhatnagar S, Mandybur G, Buckingham H, Andy O. Language representation in the human brain: Evidence from cortical mapping. Brain Lang 2000; 74:238–259.

130. Damasio H, Grabowski TJ, Tranel D, Ponto LLB, Hichwa RD, Damasio AR. Neural correlates of naming actions and of naming spatial relations. NeuroImage 2001; 13:1053–1064.

131. Dhond R, Buckner R, Dale A, Marinkovic K, Halgren E. Spatiotemporal maps of brain activity underlying word generation and their modification during repetition priming. J Neurosci 2001; 21: 3564–3571.

132. Wise R, Scott S, Blank S, Mummery C, Murphy K, Warburton E. Separate neural subsystems within 'Wernicke's area.' Brain 2001; 124:83–95.

133. Dronkers N, Refern B, Knight R. The neural architecture of language disorders. In: Gazzaniga M, ed. The New Cognitive Neurosciences. Boston: MIT Press, 2000:949–958.

134. Ramig L. Voice therapy for neurologic disease. Curr Opin Otolaryngol Head Neck Surg 1995; 3:174–182.

135. Bates E, Reilly M, Wulfeck B, Dronkers N, Opie M, Fenson J, Kriz S, Jeffries R, Miller L, Herbst K. Differential effects of unilateral lesions on language production in children and adults. Brain Lang 2001; 79:223–265.

136. Robey R. A meta-analysis of clinical outcomes in the treatment of aphasia. J Speech Lang Hear Res 1998; 41:172–187.

137. Horner J, Loverso F, Gonzalez Rothi L. Models of aphasia treatment. In: Chapey R, ed. Language Intervention Strategies in Adult Aphasia. Baltimore: Williams & Wilkins, 1994:135–145.

138. Blumstein S, Milberg W. Neural systems and language processing: Toward a synthetic approach. Brain Lang 2000; 71:26–29.

139. Caplan D. Toward a psycholinguistic approach to acquired neurogenic language disorders. Am J Speech Lang Path 1993; 2:59–83.

140. Pinango M. Semantic operations in aphasic comprehension: Implications for the cortical organization of language. Brain Lang 2001; 79:297–308.

141. Byung S. Sentence processing deficits: Theory and therapy. Cogn Neuropsychol 1988; 5:629–676.

142. Mitchum C. Traditional and contemporary views of aphasia: Implications for clinical management. Top Stroke Rehabil 1994; 1:14–36.

143. Schacter D, McGlynn S, Milberg W, Church B. Spared priming despite impaired comprehension: Implicit memory in a case of word meaning deafness. Neuropsychol 1993; 7:107–118.

144. Bates E, Marangolo P, Pizzamiglio L. Linguistic and nonlinguistic priming in aphasia. Brain Lang 2001; 76:62–69.

145. Wagner A, Koutstaal W, Maril A, Schacter D, Buckner R. Task-specific repetition priming in left inferior prefrontal cortex. Cereb Cortex 2000; 10: 1176–1184.

146. Coslett H, Saffran E, Greenbaum S, Schwartz H. Reading in pure alexia: The effect of strategy. Brain 1993; 116:21–37.

147. LaPointe L. Aphasia and Related Neurogenic Language Disorders. New York: Thieme Medical Publishers, 1990.

148. Helm-Estabrooks N, Albert M. Manual of Aphasia Therapy. Austin, TX: Pro-Ed, 1991.

149. Benson D, Dobkin B, Rothi L, Helm-Estabrooks N, Kertesz A. Assessment: Melodic intonation therapy. Neurology 1994; 44:566–568.

150. Helm-Estabrooks N, Nicholas M, Morgan A. Melodic Intonation Therapy Program. San Antonio: Special Press, 1989.

151. Belin P, Van Eeckhout P, Zilbovicius M, Remy P,

Francois C, Guillaume S, Chain F, Rancurel G, Samson Y. Recovery from nonfluent aphasia after melodic intonation therapy: A PET study. Neurology 1996; 47:1504–1511.

152. Helm N, Barresi B. Voluntary control of involuntary utterances. In: Brookshire R, ed. Clinical Aphasiology. Minneapolis: BRK Publishers, 1980:308–315.

153. Helm-Estabrooks N, Ramsberger G. Treatment of agrammatism in long-term Broca's aphasia. Br J Disord Commun 1986; 21:39–45.

154. Stevens E. Efficacy of multiple input phoneme therapy in the treatment of severe expressive aphasia and apraxia of speech. Phys Med Rehabil: State of the Art Reviews 1989; 3:194–199.

155. Kearns K. Broca's aphasia. In: LaPointe L, ed. Aphasia and Related Neurogenic Language Disorders. New York: Thieme, 1990.

156. Guilford A, Scheurele J, Sherik P. Manual communication skills in aphasia. Arch Phys Med Rehabil 1982; 63:601–604.

157. Naeser M, Haas G, Mazurski P, Laughlin S. Sentence level auditory comprehension treatment program for aphasic adults. Arch Phys Med Rehabil 1986; 67:393–399.

158. Helm-Estabrooks N, Fitzpatrick P, Barresi B. Visual Action therapy for global aphasia. J Speech Hear Disord 1982; 47:385–389.

159. Lincoln N, Pickersgill M. The effectiveness of programmed instruction with operant training in the language rehabilitation of severely aphasic patients. Behav Psychotherapy 1984; 12:237–248.

160. Davis G, Wilcox M. Adult Aphasia Rehabilitation: Applied Pragmatics. San Diego: College-Hill Press, 1985.

161. Corina D, Vaid J, Bellugi U. The linguistic basis of left hemisphere specialization. Science 1992; 255:1258–1260.

162. Hanlon R, Brown J. Enhancement of naming in nonfluent aphasia through gesture. Brain Lang 1990; 38:298–314.

163. Bara B, Cutica I, Tirassa M. Neuropragmatics: Extralinguistic communication after closed head injury. Brain Lang 2001; 77:72–94.

164. Prutting C, Kirchner D. A clinical appraisal of the pragmatic aspects of language. J Speech Hear Disord 1987; 52:105–119.

165. Johannsen-Horback H, Cegla B, Mager U. Treatment of chronic global aphasia with a nonverbal communication system. Brain Lang 1985; 24:74–82.

166. Steele R, Kleczewska M, Carlson G, Weinrich M. Computers in the rehabilitation of chronic, severe aphasia: C-VIC cross modal studies. Aphasiology 1992; 6:185–194.

167. Aftonomos L, Steele R, Wertz R. Promoting recovery in chronic aphasia with an interactive technology. Arch Phys Med Rehabil 1997; 78:841–6.

168. Deloche G, Ferrand I, Dordain M, et al. Confrontation naming rehabilitation in aphasics: A computerised written technique. Neuropsycholog Rehabil 1992; 2:117–124.

169. Weinrich M, Boser K, McCall D, Bishop V. Training agrammatic subjects on passive sentences: Implications for syntactic deficit theories. Brain Lang 2001; 76:45–61.

170. Sarno M, Sarno J, Diller L. The effect of hyperbaric oxygen on communication function in adults with aphasia secondary to stroke. J Speech Hear Res 1972; 15:42–48.

171. Huber W, Willmes K, Poeck K, Van Vleymen B, Deberdt W. Piracetam as an adjuvant to language therapy for aphasia: A randomized double-blind placebo-controlled pilot study. Arch Phys Med Rehabil 1997; 78:245–250.

172. Walker-Batson D, Curtis S, Natarajan R, Ford J, Dronkers N, Salmeron E, Lai J, Unwin D, Feeney D. A double-blind placebo-controlled study of the use of amphetamine in the treatment of aphasia. Stroke 2001; 32:2093–2098.

173. Livneh H, Antonak R. Psychosocial reactions to disability: A review and critique of the literature. Crit Rev Phys Rehabil Med 1994; 6:1–100.

174. Lazarus R, Folkman S. Stress, Appraisal & Coping. New York: Springer Publishing, 1984.

175. Cohen S, Syme S. Social Support and Health. New York: Academic Press, 1985.

176. Shepard R. Benefit of sport and physical activity for the disabled: Implications for the individual and for society. Scand J Rehabil Med 1991; 23:233–241.

177. Laskowski E. Snow skiing for the physically disabled. Mayo Clin Proc 1991; 66:160–172.

178. Cooper R. Wheelchair racing sports science: A review. J Rehabil Res Dev 1990; 27:295–312.

Chapter 6

Approaches for Walking

Ambulation is often the highest immediate rehabilitative priority for patients following a stroke, the Guillain-Barre syndrome, and brain or spinal cord injury. Patients with progressive diseases such as multiple sclerosis, Parkinson's disease, and myopathies, as well as the elderly who develop proximal weakness and imbalance associated with deconditioning, arthritic pain, contractures or a spinal stenosis aim for continued independent walking, in part to lessen the burden of care they may pose for significant others.

The neurorehabilitation team may not place as high a value on ambulation as the patient and family does. The goal of treatment may be safe and energy-efficient mobility, which could mean using a wheelchair or incorporating assistive devices to walk short distances in the home. Most disabled patients reach the same

conclusion. The specific means of safe and independent mobility does not correlate with health-related quality of life.

For the assessment of ambulation, the physical therapist, physician, and orthotist rely on an observational analysis of the gait pattern combined with measures of strength, sensation, balance, and muscle tone. Trial-and-error interventions and, sometimes, a formal gait analysis, help formulate the treatment approaches and the prognosis for gains in walking over time. This chapter bridges portions of the preceding and next chapter by describing assessments of the most common gait deviations, routine and newer therapeutic interventions, and outcome measures.

NORMAL GAIT

The network mechanisms for postural and locomotor control managed by cortical, subcortical, and spinal processing modules, described in Chapter 1, must be kept in mind when considering normal and abnormal gait (see Fig. 1–1). Walking and carrying out tasks while standing require a remarkable level of sensorimotor integration, cognition, and procedural learning.

Observational and quantitative methods that evaluate human locomotion assess the cyclical movements that occur between successive contacts with the heel of the same foot. From heel strike to heel strike, the best form of visual analysis of the gait cycle divides walking into the stance and swing phases of one of the legs, shown in Figure 6–1. The clinician notes single-limb and double-limb support times, shown in Figure 6–2, looking for asymmetries

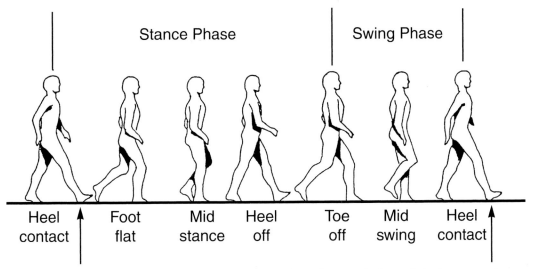

Figure 6–1. Changing positions of the legs during the phases of a single gait cycle from right heel contact to the next right heel contact.

between the legs in duration of stance. Some of the more easily observed joint angles made by the trunk, pelvis, hip, knee, and ankle during the stance and swing phases are described in Table 6–1. Figure 6–3 collates the simultaneous temporal relationships between the muscles that burst, the level of limb loading, and the joint angles at the hip, knee, and ankle during each subphase of a normal stance and swing cycle at the casual walking speed of 2.5 mph. By observing the key movements in Table 6–1 and extrapolating from Figure 6–3, the clinician can usually determine what a patient needs to practice and whether a brace is likely to be of help.

During the normal gait cycle, each activated muscle fires briefly. Muscles act either as a shock absorber for deceleration, through a lengthening or eccentric contraction, or as an accelerator, by a shortening or concentric contraction. These contractions permit fine control of forward progression during stepping and maintain a stable upright posture. Properly timed changes in the joint angles at the hip, knee, and ankle help minimize the energy expended as ambulators shift their center of gravity. For the stance and swing phases of the step cycle, these changes include:

1. Early in the stance phase, the knee flexes approximately 15°.

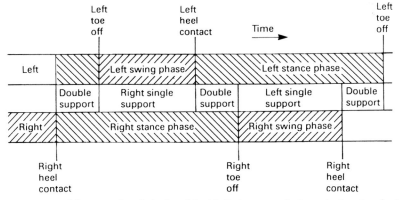

Figure 6–2. Average temporal features of single-limb and double-limb support during a single gait cycle. Approximately 60% of the cycle is in stance during walking at the casual speed of 2.5 mph.

Table 6–1. **Readily Observable Components of a Gait Cycle**

STANCE PHASE	
Pelvis	Lateral and horizontal shift to the stance leg
Hip	Extension
Knee	Flexion upon loading
	Extension at mid stance
	Flexion at foot push off
Ankle	Dorsiflexion at heel contact, then plantarflexion with a propulsive rocker motion of the foot
	Dorsiflexion as the lower leg moves over the foot
	Plantarflexion for push off

SWING PHASE	
Pelvis	Drops at toe off, then rotates forward
Hip	Flexion to "shorten" the leg
Knee	Flexion to "shorten" the leg, then extension just before heel contact
Ankle	Dorsiflexion for heel strike

2. During the first part of stance, controlled plantarflexion allows the transfer of weight from the heel to the flat foot. The heel-strike to foot-flat to push-off action of the foot is a forward rocker motion that maintains forward momentum. The plantarflexors normally perform 80% of the positive work of gait.

3. The knee flexes approximately 30°–40° near the end of stance.

4. The hip extends approximately 10° late in stance with an eccentric contraction of the iliopsoas muscle.

5. The pelvis is displaced toward the stance limb.

6. The combination of hip extension and unloading of the leg that starts the swing phase and loading the opposite leg that is in mid stance provide the most important sensory inputs to the spinal cord for the stance to swing transition.

7. In the swing phase, the pelvis rotates, so that the swinging hip moves forward faster than the hip that is in stance.

8. The pelvis tilts down on the side of the swinging hip, under the control of the opposite hip abductors.

9. The hamstrings contract eccentrically to slow the lower leg's momentum and to terminate the swing phase.

10. The thoracolumbar paraspinal muscles help control the trunk. People with low back pain often experience pain at heel strike or as the swing phase is initiated, because these muscles contract.

Healthy elderly people walk more slowly and have a shorter stride length than young adults. Table 6–2 shows the modest declines reported for casual and maximum walking speeds as people age. Walking speed over a short distance serves as an overall marker for the quality of the gait pattern. Table 6–3 provides a conversion table for the more frequently used measurement units of walking speed. Hemiplegia, paraplegia, disorders of the motor unit, extrapyramidal disorders, the ataxias, and hydrocephalus all cause changes in the temporal and kinematic variables of the gait cycle.

NEUROLOGIC GAIT DEVIATIONS

The Rancho Los Amigos charting system provides one of several available systematic observational methods for gait analysis.[1,2] The approach incorporates 32 of the most common gait deviations that can affect the trunk, pelvis, hip, knee, ankle, foot and toes during swing and stance. The more commonly observed deviations are listed in Table 6–4 for the stance phase and in Table 6–5 for swing.[1,3] These deviations from normal are best interpreted by referring to the joint angle, muscle on and off activity, and ground reaction forces detailed in Figure 6–3.

Observational methods for measuring the outcomes of rehabilitative interventions are probably reliable only in the hands of experienced clinicians.[4] Also, data from normal walkers are not necessarily appropriate for comparing and correcting characteristics of a patient's hemiplegic gait. Patients should be trained, however, with the template of Figure 6–3 in mind so that optimal facilitation of gait through sensory feedback is achieved.

Hemiparetic Gait

After an upper motoneuron injury, myriad combinations of problems can interfere with

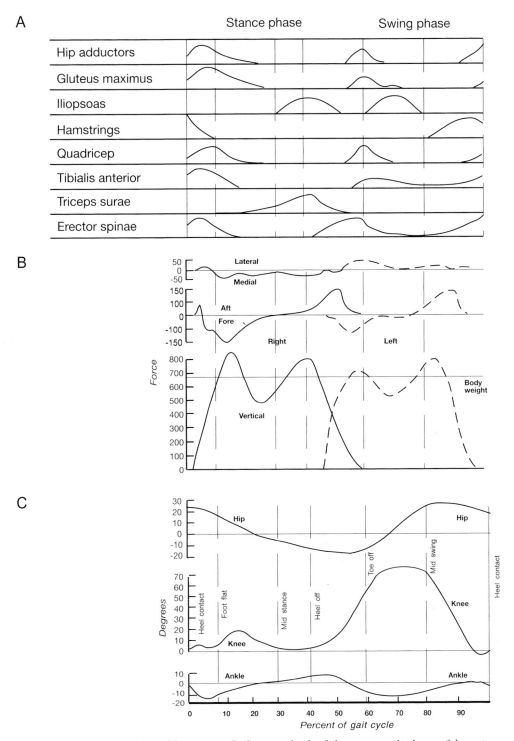

Figure 6–3. (*Top*) Linear envelopes of the timing and relative amplitude of electromyographic bursts of the major muscle groups from heel contact to heel contact. (*Middle*) Kinetic study of the lateral, fore-aft, and vertical components of the ground reaction force in newtons, for the right foot (solid line) and the left foot (dashed). (*Bottom*) Kinematic study of the average joint angles made at the hip (flexion is a positive angle), knee (flexion positive), and ankle (dorsiflexion positive). Walking speed is 2.5 mph.

Table 6–2. **Average Walking Speeds for Short Distances in Healthy Men and Women**

Decade	20s	30s	40s	50s	60s	70s
CASUAL (meters/minute)						
Men	84	88	88	84	82	80
Women	84	85	84	84	78	76
MAXIMUM (meters/minute)						
Men	152	147	148	124	116	125
Women	148	150	127	120	106	105

Source: Adapted from Bohannon, 1997[64]

the gait pattern. These deficits include weakness, impaired activation of muscles, coactivation of muscle groups, hypertonicity, leg length asymmetries of more than approximately 1 inch, laxity of ligaments, joint and soft tissue stiffness, contractures, and pain. Therapists make their adjustments to deviations that occur during the six most easily separable events of the gait cycle (Fig. 6–1), as described in the following paragraphs.

GAIT DEVIATIONS

Figure 6–4 shows the kinematics of the hemiplegic leg during a step cycle.

1. *Initial contact with heel strike:* Normally, work at the knee flexors is mostly eccentric during weight acceptance in stance. This lengthening muscle contraction prevents hyperextension of the knee. The tibialis anterior contracts eccentrically the foot to the ground to touch, rather than to

slap. The patient with hemiplegia may lose heel strike and the heel-to-forefoot rocker action that increases the length of a step and adds forward propulsion. Instead, the patient may land flat-footed or on the forefoot, due to poor ankle dorsiflexion and knee extension. Poor dorsiflexion can arise from a heel cord contracture, from sustained or early activation of the antagonist muscle group, the triceps surae, and from a synergistic pattern that prevents the combination of hip flexion, ankle dorsiflexion, and knee extension.

2. *Foot flat or load acceptance:* Normally, rapid passive plantarflexion is restrained by the tibialis anterior and toe extensor muscles, and by flexion of the knee, which occurs when the tibia moves forward faster than the thigh. These actions prevent the vertical force at load acceptance from rapidly building up at impact. The initial rocker action at the ankle and foot

Table 6–3. **Measurement Units to Quickly Convert the Range of Common Walking Speeds**

cm/second	meters/minute	feet/second	km/hour	mph
5	3	0.16	0.18	0.11
10	6	0.33	0.36	0.22
20	12	0.66	0.66	0.45
30	18	0.98	1.08	0.67
45	27	1.48	1.62	1.01
100	60	3.28	3.60	2.24
125	76	4.10	4.50	2.80

Table 6–4. Stance Phase: Observational Analysis of Common Hemiparetic Gait Deviations

Deviations	Etiology	Consequences
Hip adduction	Increased adductor activity Inadequate strength of abductors	Narrow base of support Loss of balance
Contralateral pelvic drop	Weakness or inadequate control of hip abductors	Decreased stance stability
Inadequate hip extension	Inadequate quadriceps Hip flexion contracture Increased activity of hip flexors Excessive knee flexion posture	Increased energy demand Decreased forward progression and velocity
Inadequate knee extension	Inadequate quadriceps strength/control Knee flexion contracture Increased hamstring or gastrocnemius activity Inadequate hip extension or excessive dorsiflexion	Increased energy demand Decreased stance time Decreased forward progression and velocity
Knee extensor thrust	Inadequate quadriceps control Increased quadriceps or plantarflexion activity Ankle instability Plantar flexion contracture	Loss of loading response at knee Decreased forward progression and velocity Joint pain
Excessive plantar flexion	Increased plantar flexion activity Inadequate plantar flexion strength/control Plantar flexion contracture	Decreased forward progression and velocity Compensatory postures Increased energy demand Shortened stance time
Excessive dorsiflexion	Accommodation for knee flexion contracture Plantar flexion paresis	Stance instability Decreased stance time Compensatory hip and knee flexion requiring increased energy Decreased forward progression/velocity
No heel off	Inadequate plantar flexion strength/control Restricted ankle or metatarsal motion	Decreased pre-swing knee flexion Decreased forward progression/velocity
Excess varus	Increased invertor muscle activity	Unstable base of support Decreased forward progression/velocity
Clawed toes	Increased toe flexor muscle activity or weak intrinsic foot muscles Exaggerated compensation for poor balance Toe flexion contracture	Pain from skin pressure and weight bearing on toes Decreased forward progression/velocity

also reduces this impact. In the hemiplegic patient who immediately loads the forefoot, the tibia is forced back and the knee is thrust into extension, thereby impeding forward momentum. The foot may rotate in varus onto its lateral aspect

and becomes an unstable weight-bearing surface. The quadriceps may give way so the knee buckles or the knee may hyperextend and snap back.

3. *Midstance:* At this point, the leg in swing passes the stance leg and the feet come

Table 6–5. Swing Phase: Observational Analysis of Common Hemiparetic Gait Deviations

Deviations	Etiology	Consequences
Impaired hip flexion	Increased extensor activity at knee and ankle Inadequate control of hip flexors	Decreased forward progression and velocity Shortened step length Increased energy demand
Impaired knee flexion	Inadequate pre-swing knee flexion Increased knee extensor activity Contracture Hamstring paresis	Toe drag at initial swing
Inadequate knee extension at end of swing	Knee flexion contracture Flexor synergy or withdrawal prevents knee extension during hip flexion Increased knee flexor activity	Shortened step length Decreased forward progression and velocity
Hip adduction	Increased adductor activity Excessive flexor or extensor synergy	Swing limb abuts stance limb or unsafely narrows base of support Decreased forward progression
Excessive plantar flexion at mid to end swing	Inadequate dorsiflexion strength Contracture Increased plantar flexor activity or extensor synergy	Toe drag Initial contact with foot flat or toes first Loss of loading response at ankle

next to each other. The body slows its forward velocity as it progresses over the stance leg. The trunk is at its highest point, creating the potential energy of height, and is displaced to a maximum toward the stance leg. The hip extends. The quadriceps muscles stop contracting and the soleus contracts to slow the forward motion of the tibia. The ground reaction force moves forward along the foot as the ankle rotates from approximately 15° of plantarflexion to 10° of dorsiflexion. The gluteus muscles contract on the opposite side to maintain pelvic alignment. In the hemiplegic patient, the inability to dorsiflex the ankle about 5° may hyperextend the knee or lean the trunk forward. This deviation slows momentum and causes a shorter step by the opposite leg. If the soleus contraction is inadequate, the quadriceps muscles continue to fire to compensate for the dorsiflexed ankle. If the quadriceps cannot compensate, the patient must avoid early stance phase knee flexion and maintain the knee extension that was initiated during the swing phase. The leg, then, is stiff.

4. *Terminal stance or heel off:* This phase occurs just before heel contact by the opposite leg. The trunk loses vertical height and the iliopsoas muscle contracts eccentrically to resist the hip as the leg extends from the hip. The knee peaks in its extension and begins to flex and the gastrocnemius joins the soleus contraction to oppose dorsiflexion. In the patient with hemiplegia, contractures or spastic clawing of the toes may prevent weight from advancing to the forefoot. Weight bearing on flexed toes is also painful and increases hypertonicity. In addition, the opposite pelvis may drop from impaired hip abductor muscle activity.

5. *Toe off and initial swing:* Stance ends and swing begins at the end of the second double-limb support phase. Gravity, the rectus femoris, and hip adductor muscles flex the hip. The rectus femoris also controls knee flexion by an eccentric contraction. Muscles that act across the ankle stabilize the foot as the triceps surae muscles contract. The ground reaction force rapidly dissipates through the metatarsal heads. Work at the ankle is

mostly concentric and is highest at push-off. The hemiplegic patient often misses this phase because of sustained knee extension from excessive quadriceps activity or as compensation for poor calf control. Patients also compensate for toe drag by circumducting the leg or by vaulting off or leaning toward the normal leg.

6. *Midswing:* The swing phase involves approximately 40% of the normal gait cycle. The timing of midswing corresponds to midstance for the other leg. Swing has an initial acceleration at the hip powered by the iliopsoas and other flexor muscles and a deceleration phase controlled by contraction of the hamstrings group. The knee flexes like a pendulum, driven by hip flexion. At the end of swing, the hamstrings prevent knee hyperextension. The toe clears the ground by less than 3 cm as a result of contraction of the tibialis anterior muscle, which places the ankle in a neutral position, and from shortening the leg as the knee flexes. The hemiplegic patient often cannot flex at the hip and ankle while extending the knee. The leg becomes functionally too long. Hip hiking powered by the paraspinal and abdominal muscles is one energy-taxing compensatory strategy when the hamstrings are weak. The knee may extend prematurely, so the leg is too long near the end of swing. Circumduction, vaulting off the foot of the stance leg, and excessive hip and knee flexion from a prominent footdrop are other gait deviations that act as compensatory techniques.

In summary, the hemiplegic gait is prone to:
1. A shorter step length with the unaffected leg
2. Longer stance duration, mostly from longer double-limb support time with shorter time on the paretic leg
3. Shorter duration of swing
4. Greater flexion at the hip during midstance, which, by moving the center of mass forward, is associated with an increased knee extensor moment
5. Decreased lateral shift to the paretic side during single-limb support
6. Less knee flexion and ankle dorsiflexion during swing, compensated by circumduction of the affected leg

WALKING SPEED

Casual walking speed in hemiplegic gait is about half of the walking speed of age-matched normal subjects. Mean ranges for gait speed in several studies of recovery from hemiplegic stroke have been as low as 25 to 50 cm/second,[5] compared to the 130 cm/second (2.9 mph or 50 feet in 12 seconds)[6] for the elderly listed in Table 6–2. A prospective observational study of 185 patients admitted for inpatient rehabilitation found a change in walking velocity from a median of 45 cm/second on admission to 55 cm/second at discharge.[7] Speed is a good reflection of the overall gait pattern. Because speed is determined by cadence and step length, one approach to increasing speed for hemiparetic patients is to decrease the longer double-limb support time and single-limb support time of the unaffected leg.[8] The single-limb stance time on the affected leg may be abnormal in relation to the decreased proportion of time spent in stance, but the actual time may be near normal, from approximately 0.3 to 0.5 seconds.

Although patients with hemiplegia experience no increase in the rate of energy expenditure, mostly because they walk so slowly, the energy demand on them is higher because it takes longer to cover a given distance.[9] The distance walked by the patient in increments of 3 minutes may be considerably less than by a normal subject. Thus, rehabilitation interventions for ambulation ought to aim not only for independent walking for 150 feet, which is the ceiling criteria used by the Barthel Index and Functional Independence Measure (see Chapter 7). Interventions should also aim to improve walking speed.

The probability of being referred for inpatient rehabilitation within 10 days of a stroke is very high for patients who walk <30 cm/second and low for those who walk >60 cm/second.[10] Once patients reach a threshold velocity of 40 cm/second for home ambulation,[11] therapy ought to aim for faster walking speeds and for more energy efficient distances traveled to permit unlimited community activities. Community ambulation usually takes a walking velocity of 60 to 80 cm/second[11] or walking at over 1.5 mph.

Paraparetic Gait

The observational gait of patients with spastic paraparesis reveals a variety of compensatory mechanisms to achieve locomotion. The deviations noted for hemiplegic gait apply to both lower extremities. Hip and knee flexion can be prominent in swing and stance, especially in patients with a cervical central cord syndrome. The gait may look like the stepping pattern of a child with spastic diplegia from cerebral palsy. Heel contact may be absent, replaced by a plantarflexed or flat-footed initial floor contact. Excess plantar flexion in early stance prevents the ankle from dorsiflexing into a position where the plantarflexors can contribute to forward impulse by an active push-off.[12] Poor proprioception at a knee and ankle joint also contributes to pathologic gait deviations.

Electromyographic (EMG) analysis often shows a prolonged duration of EMG activation with premature recruitment and delayed relaxation compared with healthy persons.[13] The EMG bursts tend to be flat with decreased or absent peaks. The rectus femoris and gastrocnemius muscles show reduced activity over the whole step cycle, whereas the tibialis anterior may show increased activity during early swing. Prolonged bursts can accompany passive muscle lengthening.

Gait with Peripheral Neuropathy

Injury to even a single nerve may cause considerable deviations and secondary compensations in gait. For example, paralysis of the tibialis anterior muscle decreases walking velocity by several mechanisms. Step length decreases, mostly on the nonparalyzed side. On the paralyzed side, one may find a decrease in ankle dorsiflexion moment at the end of stance, a decrease in vertical ground reaction force, a decrease in weight transfer to the forward part of the foot, a decrease in knee extensor range and torque in the stance phase, an increase in ankle dorsiflexion range in stance, and increased energy cost.[14] A peroneal palsy causes yet greater changes. Step length decreases on the nonparalyzed side. On the paralyzed side, vertical forces on push-off decrease, the knee extensor moment with stance decreases, the plantar flexion moment with early stance decreases, and the dorsiflexion moment with late stance decreases. Ankle inversion occurs at heel strike. To achieve foot clearance, hip and knee flexion must increase during swing.[15]

Gait with Poliomyelitis

Anterior trunk flexion with knee hyperextension is a common compensation for severe quadriceps weakness from polio. This paresis can cause degenerative disease of the knee joints. Weakness of other muscle groups, such as the paraspinals and hip and ankle movers, yield a variety of gait deviations and compensatory strategies. Severely affected patients require bracing the ankles and knees.

QUANTITATIVE GAIT ANALYSIS

Biomechanics, kinesiology, electrophysiology, and computer modeling have contributed to research into the mechanisms and evaluation of normal and pathologic gait. Quantitative methods of gait analysis draw from these disciplines. Studies reveal information about normal[16] and abnormal[17] motor control and can lead to therapeutic interventions and to assessments that monitor change reliably. Some of the practical techniques for gait analysis are listed in Table 6–6. Quantitative clinical stud-

Table 6–6. Techniques for Gait Analysis

TIME-DISTANCE VARIABLES
Footswitch stride analyzer
Footprint analysis
Conductive or pressure-sensitive walkway
KINEMATICS
Electrogoniometers
Computerized video analysis with joint markers
Electromagnetic field motion analysis
DYNAMIC ELECTROMYOGRAPHY
Surface and fine wire electrodes
KINETICS
Force plate in walkway or treadmill
Piezoelectric and load cell force transducers in shoes
METABOLIC ENERGY EXPENDITURE
Oxygen consumption by respirometry

ies for neurologic diseases are usually reserved for children who have cerebral palsy who may undergo an invasive intervention such as a tendon lengthening or a dorsal rhizotomy, as well as for orthopedic procedures that include a tendon lengthening or transposition, and sometimes to determine which muscle groups should be silenced with an injection of botulinum toxin or phenol.

Temporal Measures

The least complicated and expensive instrumented techniques use footswitches under the heel, under the heads of the first and fifth metatarsal, and under the great toe. While in contact with the ground, each small transducer's circuit closes and produces a voltage signal on a strip chart or computer. From this signal, temporal and distance measures are obtained, including speed, cadence (step frequency), stride length (the distance between two consecutive heel strikes by the same foot), step length (the distance between left and right heel strikes), and the percent of the gait cycle spent in single-limb (swing phase) and double-limb (stance phase) support. Retest reliability is good, but random and systematic errors and the inherent variability of overground velocity can make serial measures difficult to interpret.[18]

Footswitch techniques reveal asymmetries between the limbs, such as documenting the frequent finding of a reduced stance time on a hemiparetic leg. These techniques can measure improvement in the symmetry of the swing phase and in the stance-to-swing ratio that is associated with motor recovery after stroke.[19] They cannot, alone, assess deviations in the gait pattern or compensatory strategies.

Kinematics

Whole limb motion can be recorded with electrogoniometers placed across each joint. Movement in one plane or, for more sophisticated devices, in three planes, produces a change in resistance and a recordable voltage that reveals the change in joint angles. Motion-analysis systems increasingly use front and side cameras that videotape the movements of accurately placed reflective markers or light-emitting

diodes.[20] By a variety of techniques, the data are digitized to make a moving stick figure. Changes in the angles of one or more joints can be derived across the gait cycle. Fiber-optic systems that embed wires in a pair of trousers and electromagnetic field techniques are yet more sophisticated means to evaluate kinematics.

Figure 6–3C shows the sagittal plane kinematics of the hip, knee, and ankle during a normal step cycle. Figure 6–4 shows the joint angles of a 70-year-old man with a left hemiparesis caused by a right internal capsule infarction who walks with a cane at his preferred cadence without an ankle-foot orthosis. Hip, knee, and ankle flexion are much less than in a healthy person. On a coronal view, one would appreciate a modest amount of leg circumduction, used by the patient to help clear the foot. Plots of one joint angle versus another during the step cycle provide a more dynamic view of gait deviations.[21]

Electromyography

Electromyography (EMG) recordings during gait reveal the onset, duration, and amplitude of muscle bursts in relation to the step cycle (Figure 6–3A). Dedicated recording and signal processing systems have defined EMG patterns in relation to footswitch signals.[22] Surface and fine wire electrodes can be attached to cable or to telemetry systems. The raw EMG signal is usually processed by full wave rectification, which reflects the absolute value of the signal's amplitude. Further low pass filtering gives a linear envelope or moving average signal, as depicted in Figure 6–3.

Recordings show when the muscle is active or changes its activity, but tell nothing about strength, voluntary control, or whether the muscle contraction is concentric or eccentric. Muscle timing errors during gait have been defined as premature, prolonged, continuous, curtailed, delayed, absent, and out of phase.[20] This categorization provides information related to motor control and has led to strategies such as tendon releases and transfers. In pathologic gaits, individual patients can be compared over time in regard to the timing of bursts among groups. Amplitude changes in paretic muscles that are reassessed at different times, however, are difficult to interpret, unless nor-

estimated by comparing the heart rate before and after 3 minutes of walking.[25] Over a wide range of walking speeds, normal children and those with cerebral palsy also show a linear relationship between heart rate and oxygen uptake.[26]

APPROACHES TO RETRAINING AMBULATION

One of the foremost goals of the hemiparetic or paraparetic patient is to achieve independent ambulation. Patients who require more than minimal assistance to walk a short distance, 10 to 15 feet, by the end of their acute hospitalization have the most common disability that leads to transfer to an inpatient rehabilitation program. The physical therapist develops strategies to improve ambulation, but the entire team reinforces techniques for head and trunk control, sitting and standing balance, transfers, and a safe and energy-efficient reciprocal pattern for gait. The most appropriate targets for gait interventions are still uncertain. Most work has centered upon balance, weight-bearing, leg symmetry in swing and stance times, normalizing strength, and improving motor control.[27]

Conventional Training

Pregait training often includes neurophysiologic and neurodevelopmental techniques to elicit movements and develop sitting and standing balance (see Chapter 5). Mat activities include rolling or rotating at the hip to elicit flexion, as well as supine bridging, kneeling and half-kneeling. No data are available to determine whether or not this approach is worth the time and effort compared to immediately finding a technique that helps the patient stand and train in stepping. Most therapists will work to elicit selective muscle contractions and to strengthen muscle groups using resistance exercises and functional exercises, such as sitting on a large ball and repeated sit-to-stand movements. Another goal is to increase the range of motion of shortened muscles and stiff joints.

Gait training conventionally begins once the patient has adequate endurance and stability to stand in the parallel bars or at a hemibar. The therapist often must block the knee and help

control the paretic trunk and leg. Some therapists will use bracing at this point to enable weight bearing, but this approach raises the hair of therapists who abide by the Bobath school.

The therapist concentrates on the most prominent deviations from normal during the gait cycle. Isolated component movements of the step cycle may be practiced, such as weight-shifting and limb-loading. In addition, the therapy team may intervene to diminish hypertonicity with inhibitory exercises and try out various assistive devices such as walkers and canes. An ankle-foot orthosis may be necessary to gain safe control of the ankle and knee. Occasionally, functional electrical stimulation is employed to elicit ankle dorsiflexion or a quadriceps muscle contraction for knee control. Therapists often have to improvise to enable patients to work around premorbid medical conditions such as painful arthritis in the knees to enable ambulation (Fig. 6–5).

Outpatient therapy tends to concentrate on improving stride length, swing and stance symmetry of the legs, speed, stair climbing, balance on uneven ground, and confidence in moving about in the community. Therapists continue to provide physical and verbal cues to correct the pattern of gait. Energy consumption is higher with a limp than with a normal gait pattern and rises faster with an increase in speed. The therapist helps the patient find a functional compromise between speed, safety, and energy demand. The need for bracing and assistive devices tends to change over the first 6 months after a stroke and over a longer period for paraparetic patients. Antispasticity medications for walking-induced symptoms and signs of hypertonicity such as clonus and spasms are rarely needed during the inpatient care of patients with a first stroke, but may be worth trying in patients with chronic upper motoneuron lesions.

Physicians may follow patients for months or years after formal therapy ends. Each visit is an opportunity to reevaluate the gait pattern and offer adjustments to be practiced. I often draw upon several notions to improve walking skills and help establish practice parameters for patients and caregivers to follow. The first is the apparent benefit of using rhythmic proprioceptive signals to help engrain stepping during BWSTT and the enhancements in gait symmetry that also accompany rhythmic auditory

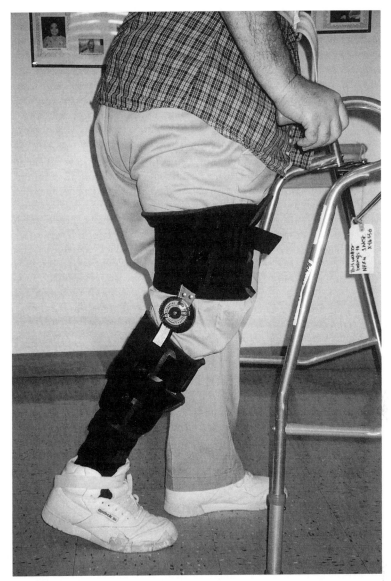

Figure 6–5. Improvisation is essential during the rehabilitation of patients who have premorbid impairments that interfere with therapy goals. This patient had a stroke causing right hemiparesis and impaired ambulation. As motor control improved, his chronic knee pain and atrophy of the quadriceps from degenerative joint disease continued to limit ambulation. A flexible knee brace and frontwheel walker enabled him to more easily load the knee in the stance phase of gait and he immediately became independent in ambulation.

signals for stepping.[28,29] The second is the critical effect on the gait cycle in animal and human studies of loading the stance leg at the moment of onset of initiating swing of the opposite leg (Chapters 1 and 2). If asymmetries between the legs in either stance or swing times are apparent, one can instruct the patient to load the stance leg as if pushing through the floor, much the way a ballerina en pointe works. At the moment of that extra sense of loading, the patient initiates swing with the opposite leg. Alternating load-and-swing then helps engrain the rhythm of stepping. The physician can also reinforce the need to get at least 10° of hip extension at the end of the stance phase and the aim for heel strike at the initiation of stance, rather than landing with a flat foot. In addition, I encourage the patient to keep a log that I can review that shows the incremental gains in distance and time spent walking each day, parameters we have agreed are feasible, for the purposes of locomotor practice and to build endurance.

Task-Oriented Training

This approach includes muscle strengthening, strategies that meet the requirements of walking such as training on a treadmill, and practice under varied conditions on different surfaces and at greater walking speeds (see Chapter 5). Task-specific therapy for gait, including treadmill training, shows promise for improving the quality and speed of overground ambulation and enhancing fitness and strength compared to conventional training.[5,30–32]

BODY WEIGHT–SUPPORTED TREADMILL TRAINING

With the aim of developing a task-oriented approach to the retraining of walking that could be instituted as soon as possible after onset of a stroke or spinal cord injury, clinical investigators have developed training protocols drawn from basic studies of the sensorimotor mechanisms that drive locomotion (see Chapter 1).[33–35] The approach can be called body weight–supported treadmill training (BWSTT). Upright posture is controlled by placing the patient in a modified mountain climbing harness attached to an overhead lift. The patient is suspended over a treadmill belt and bears whatever amount of weight on the legs that prevents the knees from buckling and enables the therapists to assist the legs to step. A variety of stepping parameters have been juggled by trainers, systematically or subconsciously, such as the levels of weight support and treadmill speeds, the duration of weight support, the number and duration of training sessions, and methods to optimize the kinematics, kinetics, timing of muscle bursts, and temporal features of the step cycle.[34] The approach allows physical therapists to do hands-on therapy under conditions they can control and vary within the learning paradigm they choose. Potential advantages and disadvantages are shown in Table 6–7.

Several groups of investigators have studied paraparetic patients who had minimal sensori-

motor function in the legs. With BWSTT, some patients achieved independent treadmill walking and became able to step overground.[36–38] Only quasi-experimental studies of patients with spinal cord injury, however, have been carried out using BWSTT. A randomized clinical trial of patients with acute, incomplete SCI will be completed in 2004.[34]

The largest randomized clinical trial of BWSTT in stroke subjects to date was carried out by Visintin and colleagues.[39] This trial showed that treadmill training alone was less successful than treadmill training with partial body weight support, especially for patients who initially walked very slowly (see Chapter 9). Thus, the trial sought out any advantage of the addition of weight support to treadmill walking and did not compare a task-oriented therapy to a conventional approach for locomotor rehabilitation. Small trials of BWSTT have been carried out in patients with Parkinson's disease,[40] multiple sclerosis, and cerebral palsy[41] with favorable reports of at least short-term gains.

As noted in Chapter 1, sensory inputs from the lower extremities[42–45] during step training with BWSTT are appreciated by the locomotor region of the cord, and to a varying degree can be appreciated by the efference copy system of the cerebellum[46] and higher motor centers.[47] Such inputs would likely resculpt cortical and subcortical movement representations for locomotion (Fig. 3–8). For physical therapists, the use of BWSTT offers a neurophysiologically sound approach, but the actual requirements for assisting the legs of patients to optimize segmental sensory inputs and maximize the motor control available to patients, as well as the best use of parameters such as treadmill speeds and levels of weight support, are still being defined and tested.[34,48–50] As this technique evolves, additional locomotor approaches are being added, including functional electrical stimulation,[51,52] dorsal lumbar epidural cord stimulation,[53] robotic assists,[54] and attempts at pharmacologic augmentation of stepping[55] and of motor learning.[56,57]

Assistive Devices

Assistive devices include a wide variety of braces, canes, and walkers. Randomized trials of the utility of common assistive devices or

Table 6–7. **Rationales for and Against Body Weight-Supported Treadmill Training**

TRAINING ADVANTAGES

Initiates step training and upright posture as early as possible after onset of disability

Therapists can readily optimize kinematics, kinetics, and temporal parameters of walking

Allows practice at normal walking velocities

Encourages exercise to increase fitness, prevent disuse leg muscle atrophy, and lessen chance for deep vein thrombosis

Provides task-oriented mass practice under varying conditions of limb loading and walking speed to augment motor learning

Allows immediate and delayed feedback for reinforcement of motor learning; subject uses a mirror for visual feedback

Readily accommodates add-on experiments, e.g., functional electrical stimulation

May induce activity-dependent plasticity

    Afferent inputs modulate spinal and supraspinal activity

    Practice reorganizes spared pathways and sensorimotor representations

    Repetitive sensory inputs facilitate long-term potentiation, spinal neurotrophin release, and neurotransmitter modulation at spinal and supraspinal levels (see Chapter 2)

TRAINING DISADVANTAGES

Lengthy experiential training of physical therapists; must learn how to provide minimum physical assistance, learn best hand-hold locations, visualize ongoing kinematics, and cue patients

Physically demanding on therapists

Costly over short run; requires 2–3 trainers, lift system, treadmill, and space; may require a robotic stepper device

No consensus methodology yet for training

May seem antithetical to Bobath and neurodevelopmental approaches

Definitive randomized clinical trials to show efficacy still in progress

---

comparisons between devices have not been reported.

ORTHOTICS

Lower extremity bracing systems are employed to improve stability during stance, to clear the foot during swing, to position the foot at heel contact, to increase step length, to conserve energy during walking, and to compensate for impaired motor control, weakness, and joint deformities. As a result of shortened inpatient stays, ankle-foot orthoses (AFOs) tend to be fitted during inpatient rehabilitation programs to help enable ambulation in patients with a central or peripheral lesion. Indications for an AFO include inadequate dorsiflexion for initial heel contact and primarily for toe clearance during midswing, excessive hip-hiking during swing, medial-lateral subtalar instability during stance, tibial instability during stance, uncontrolled foot placement caused by sensory loss, and after an operative heel cord lengthening. The typical patient with an upper motoneuron lesion who needs an AFO for safe community ambulation has impaired proprioception at the ankle and knee, little or no voluntary control of the ankle movers, and no synergistic dorsiflexion of the ankle during the swing phase. The typical patient with a neuropathy who needs an AFO has diabetes mellitus, poor sensation over the sole of the foot and some decrease in proprioception, as well as weakness of all the ankle movers.

Hemiparetic patients who recover little ankle movement, whose foot tends to turn over during gait, or who lack enough knee control to prevent it from snapping back usually can be managed with a polypropylene AFO that is fitted to the patient's needs. Studies confirm the clinical impression that energy demands,[9] gait speed, and the gait pattern can be improved with an AFO.[58] Patients with stroke who require an AFO for a drop foot or spastic equinus or equinus-varus foot are more impaired in motor function, balance, and in the ability to walk and climb stairs at admission and discharge from inpatient rehabilitation than patients who do not need an AFO.[59] From 20% to 25% of patients on an inpatient service will be sent home with an AFO.

A comparison of wearing and not wearing an AFO during gait analysis of hemiparetic subjects reveals that the AFO improves toe clearance by decreasing plantar flexion, improves pivoting over the affected ankle, may increase knee and hip flexion, diminishes EMG activity in the tibialis anterior, increases quadriceps muscle activity during initial stance and midstance as the leg is being loaded, and may decrease premature or excessive gastrocnemius activity in terminal swing.[60] For hemiplegic pa-

tients, an AFO in 5° of dorsiflexion increases walking speed, increases the duration of heel-strike and midstance, and improves the knee flexion moment in midstance.[58] An AFO for hemiparetic patients should increase step length and swing time, and improve stance time for the affected leg. The orthotic may increase walking speed. By aiding toe clearance, the risk of falls decreases.

Many patients are concerned that an AFO will reduce the likelihood of improving ankle movement. In patients with a drop foot from peripheral causes and in healthy subjects, an AFO initially decreases mean EMG by 7% and 20% in early stance, respectively, but after 6 weeks of use, total EMG activity did not differ from initial levels.[61] Thus, wearing an AFO may not particularly limit gains for ankle dorsiflexion during gait training and everyday walking. Stepping practice without an AFO, however, at least during BWSTT, may decrease cutaneous and proprioceptive inputs associated with the gait cycle that contribute

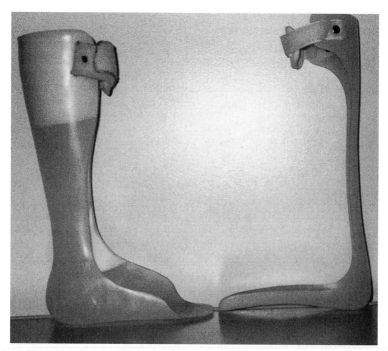

Figure 6–6. Solid ankle, thermoplastic, molded ankle-foot orthoses (AFOs) that fit into a shoe. (*A*) This lightweight, cosmetically acceptable design can help control the motion of the ankle in the sagittal plane, aiding heel strike and toe clearance and limiting knee flexion or extension depending upon the angle that the ankle joint is set. Greater stability for varus and valgus control is achieved by extending the mediolateral flanges at the distal leg and around the foot and by using straps with Velcro closures across the front of the ankle. (*B*) This leaf-spring variation in design offers little mediolateral control, but permits flexibility at the ankle during the phases of stance, while preventing foot drop during swing.

to the sensory cues for the reorganization of stepping.

Observation of the gait pattern is usually enough to determine the need for a trial with an orthosis. Often, clinicians can judge the likelihood that the device will control the ankle and knee if they can manually stabilize the affected leg when the patient stands and bears weight on it. The physical therapist and orthotist, through trial and error, determine the best fit, strapping system, and flexibility of AFO that benefits the patient most.

Most patients with hemiparesis, paraparesis, or a neuropathy can be managed with a thermoplastic orthosis (Fig. 6–6). The lateral flanges can be extended for varus and valgus control of the ankle. Padding helps protect the skin. Clinicians must monitor for signs of pressure over the skin, especially over the malleoli. Velcro straps allow one-handed closure of the brace and can help hold the heel in place. The straps may also pinch the skin, however. In patients with greater spasticity, the plastic can be extended toward the forefoot and higher up the tibia. A pad or plastic ridge under the distal metatarsals can reduce clawing of the toes. These polymer AFOs should easily fit into a shoe secured by laces or Velcro straps. Shoewear will influence the alignment of the orthotic. If the knee buckles during stance, angling the AFO in slight plantarflexion will extend the knee earlier. Dorsiflexing the AFO will decrease knee hyperextension and help prevent the snapping back that causes instability and pain in early stance and midstance.

The Valens caliper is primarily used in Germany and Switzerland and is comparable to a rigid thermoplastic AFO. The caliper includes a rigid upright medial bar and a calf band, an outside T-strap to correct a varus position, and an ankle stop that allows a chosen amount of dorsiflexion or plantarflexion.[60] The apparatus attaches to a firm shoe. For patients with profound sensorimotor impairment, a double upright metal brace may be indicated, but a well-constructed AFO will usually suffice. A metal double-upright brace offers greater rigidity for mediolateral ankle instability and allows more versatility in adjustments for the amount of plantar and dorsiflexion that may change over time. Double-upright braces, however, tend to be expensive, heavy, and cosmetically unappealing to patients. They are rarely indicated after a stroke.

An articulated AFO with a posterior stop (Fig. 6–7) prevents plantarflexion caused by hypertonicity. In addition, it permits dorsiflexion and makes standing up easier because of the give at the ankle. As the patient regains greater leg control, the AFO can be remodeled by cutting away the medial and lateral flanges or tibial portion to give the AFO greater flexibility.

Lightweight plastic knee-ankle-foot orthoses (KAFO) with locking metal knee joints can assist patients who have a profound polyneuropathy, muscular dystrophy, myelomeningocele, and spinal cord injury. Exoskeletal systems with wire cables that link flexion of one hip to extension of the opposite hip for patients with paraplegia are described in Chapter 10.

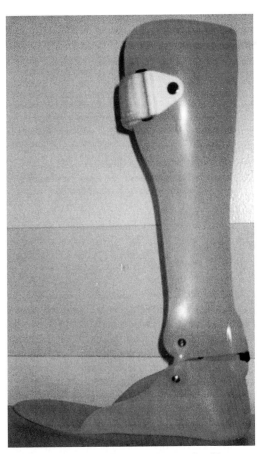

Figure 6–7. Plastic ankle-foot orthosis with ankle articulation provides mediolateral stability and allows less superimposed control of the ankle as the patient's motor control improves. The articulation permits the tibia to flex over the foot upon standing up.

CANES AND WALKERS

These devices improve stability by providing a lever arm that handles a modest force and generates a moment to assist the hip abductors. In addition, the devices reduce loading on the knee and share the body's weight between the leg and device. The metabolic energy expenditure of various forms of assisted gait varies with the device, with the impairment, with the patient's cardiovascular status, and especially with upper limb strength.[62] The pattern of gait with and without a cane usually does not differ in relation to symmetry of stance and swing times and EMG activity of the affected leg.[63]

Walking aids fall into several categories, although many models exist for each. Clinicians can obtain some sense of what may help most by walking beside and slightly behind the patient while gently holding onto a safety belt around the patient's waist. The physician can also let patients use his or her forearms as a sort of walker to appreciate the amount of force exerted by their arms. Placing a hand under the patient's grip on a cane or walker also provides a sense of how much weight the patient needs to transfer to the device.

Rolling walkers allow a step-through gait pattern, whereas a pick-up walker tends to foster a slower step-to pattern and interferes with the automaticity of the gait cycle. Walkers with four large wheels are least likely to dampen forward momentum for stepping. Walkers can be rigged with seats, baskets, horns, and racing stripes. For patients with ataxia, heavy walkers with brakes and wheels are best. For patients with Parkinson's disease, a four-wheel rolling walker with brakes and a resistive stop against the back wheels may prevent a rapid festinating gait, without interfering with forward momentum. Users need to be trained to stand upright and not place their center of mass too forward.

Single-point canes offer the narrowest base of support and vary in whether forces are distributed directly beneath or in front of the tip. Quadcanes and hemiwalkers offer a wider base for stability, but may rock if the prongs are not all in contact with the floor. Forearm or Lofstrand crutches are excellent for unloading the legs and for balance, but they may cause strain on the hands, wrists or elbows. They are reserved for patients with paraparesis caused by poliomyelitis, a low thoracic spinal cord injury, or a conus/cauda equina injury. A cane held opposite the paretic leg helps to keep the pelvis level during stance on the weak leg. The cane should swing forward with the involved limb and should bear most weight during stance on that leg. Hand grips are usually set at a height that allows approximately 20°–30° of elbow flexion. A single-point cane should hold less than 20% of a person's weight. Therapists and family may need to reinforce how to properly use an assistive device, especially for patients with cognitive impairment.

SUMMARY

A careful visual analysis of the stance and swing phases of the gait cycle aids the rehabilitation of walking. The clinician uses a mental picture of optimal patterns of muscle firing, kinematics, and kinetics, as well as the temporal features of ambulation, to make suggestions to patients about improving the stance and swing phases of gait. Walking velocity, cadence, and leg symmetries in stride length and swing and stance times are useful for serial comparisons of the effectiveness of physical and drug therapies for ambulation. Quantitative laboratory studies of the gait cycle are rarely needed for clinical care, except perhaps preoperatively for surgical interventions to improve stepping and for drug injections for dysfunctional muscle firing.

At every outpatient visit, the clinician ought to review the gait pattern with the patient and make explicit recommendations about modest adjustments that the patient can then practice. Disabled patients need encouragement to attempt to walk faster and farther.

The best approaches to the retraining of ambulation have yet to be defined. Research continues into the optimal use of task-oriented training procedures, interventions that aim to optimize the sensory inputs associated with locomotion such as BWSTT, and other accessory approaches such as functional electrical stimulation, pharmacologic therapies combined with training, and more functionally adaptable assistive devices. The best approaches will, however, always require motivation and practice.

REFERENCES

1. Gillis K. Observational gait analysis. In: Scully R, Barnes M, eds. Physical Therapy. Philadelphia: JB Lippincott, 1989:670–695.

2. Rancho Professional Staff Association. Normal and Pathological Gait Syllabus. Downey, CA: Rancho Los Amigos Hospital, 1981.

3. Lehmann J, de Lateur B, Price R. Biomechanics of abnormal gait. Phys Med Rehabil Clin N Am 1992; 3:125–138.

4. Krebs D, Edelstein J, Fishman S. Reliability of observational kinematic gait analysis. Phys Ther 1985; 65:1027–1034.

5. Richards C, Malouin F, Wood-Dauphinee S, Williams JI, Bouchard JP, Brunet D. Task-specific physical therapy for optimization of gait recovery in acute stroke patients. Arch Phys Med Rehabil 1993; 74:612–620.

6. Reuben D, Siu A. An objective measure of physical function of elderly outpatients. J Am Geriatr Soc 1990; 38:1105–1112.

7. Baer G, Smith M. The recovery of walking ability and subclassification of stroke. Physiother Res Int 2001; 6:135–144.

8. Goldie P, Matyas T, Evans O. Gait after stroke: initial deficit and changes in temporal patterns for each gait phase. Arch Phys Med Rehabil 2001; 82:1057–1065.

9. Waters R, Yakura J. The energy expenditure of normal and pathological gait. Crit Rev Phys Rehabil Med 1989; 1:183–209.

10. Salbach N, Mayo N, Higgins J, Ahmed S, Finch L, Richards C. Responsiveness and predictability of gait speed and other disability measures in acute stroke. Arch Phys Med Rehabil 2001; 82:1204–1212.

11. Perry J, Garrett M, Gromley J, Mulroy S. Classification of walking handicap in the stroke population. Stroke 1995; 26:982–989.

12. Winter D. Energy generation and absorption at the ankle and knee during fast, natural, and slow cadences. Clin Orthop Rel Res 1983; 175:147–154.

13. Conrad B, Benecke R, Meinck H. Gait disturbances in paraspastic patients. In: Delwaide P, Young R, eds. Clinical Neurophysiology in Spasticity. Amsterdam: Elsevier, 1985:155–174.

14. Lehmann J, Condon S, deLateur B, Smith J. Gait abnormalities in tibial nerve paralysis. Arch Phys Med Rehabil 1985; 66:80–85.

15. Lehmann J, Condon S, deLateur B, Price R. Gait abnormalities in peroneal nerve paralysis and their corrections by orthoses. Arch Phys Med Rehabil 1986; 67:380–86.

16. Winter D. The Biomechanics and Motor Control of Human Gait. Waterloo, Ontario: Waterloo University Press, 1987.

17. Perry J. Gait Analysis. Thorofare, NJ: Slack, Inc., 1992.

18. Hill K, Goldie P, Baker P, Greenwood K. Retest reliability of the temporal and distance characteristics of hemiplegic gait using a footswitch system. Arch Phys Med Rehabil 1994; 75:577–583.

19. Brandstater M, deBruin H, Gowland C, Clark B. Hemiplegic gait: Analysis of temporal variables. Arch Phys Med Rehabil 1983; 64:583–587.

20. Harris G, Wertsch J. Procedures for gait analysis. Arch Phys Med Rehabil 1994; 75:216–225.

21. Winstein C, Garfinkel A. Qualitative dynamics of disordered human locomotion: A preliminary study. J Mot Behav 1989; 21:373–391.

22. Perry J, Bontrager E, Bogey R, Gronley JK, Barnes LA. The Rancho EMG analyzer: A computerized system for gait analysis. J Biomed Eng 1993; 15:487–496.

23. Knutsson E, Richards C. Different types of disturbed motor control in gait of hemiparetic patients. Brain 1979; 102:405–430.

24. Lamontagne A, Malouin F, Richards C. Locomotor-specific measure of spasticity of plantarflexor muscles after stroke. Arch Phys Med Rehabil 2001; 82:1696–1704.

25. Waters R, Hislop H, Perry J, Antonelli D. Energetics: Application to the study and management of locomotor disabilities. Orthop Clin North Am 1978; 9:351–377.

26. Rose J, Gamble J, Burgos A, Medeiros J, Haskell WL. Energy expenditure index of walking for normal children and for children with cerebral palsy. Dev Med Child Neurol 1990; 32:333–340.

27. Bohannon R. Gait performance of hemiparetic stroke patients: Selected variables. Arch Phys Med Rehabil 1987; 68:777–781.

28. McIntosh G, Thaut M, Rice R, Prassas S. Rhythmic facilitation of gait kinematics in stroke patients. J Neurol Rehabil 1995; 9:131.

29. Thaut M, Kenyon G, Schauer M, McIntosh G. The connection between rhythmicity and brain function. IEEE Eng Med Biol 1999; March/April:101–108.

30. Malouin F, Potvin M, Prevost J, Richards C, Wood-Dauphinee S. Use of an intensive task-oriented gait training program in a series of patients with acute cerebrovascular accidents. Phys Ther 1992; 72:781–793.

31. Dean C, Richards C, Malouin F. Task-related circuit training improves performance of locomotor tasks in chronic stroke: A randomized, controlled pilot trial. Arch Phys Med Rehabil 2000; 81:409–417.

32. Smith G, Silver K, Goldberg A, Macko R. "Task-oriented" exercise improves hamstring strength and spastic reflexes in chronic stroke patients. Stroke 1999; 30:2112–2118.

33. Dobkin B. Neurologic rehabilitation: Neural substrates for the effects of rehabilitative training. Neurol Network Comment 1997; 1:121–126.

34. Dobkin B. Overview of treadmill locomotor training with partial body weight support: A neurophysiologically sound approach whose time has come for randomized clinical trials. Neurorehabil Neural Repair 1999; 13:157–165.

35. Barbeau H, Norman K, Fung J, Visintin M, Ladouceur M. Does neurorehabilitation play a role in the recovery of walking in neurological populations? Ann N Y Acad Sci 1998; 860:377–382.

36. Dietz V, Wirz M, Curt A, Colombo G. Locomotor patterns in paraplegic patients: training effects and recovery of spinal cord function. Spinal Cord 1998; 36:380–390.

37. Wernig A, Nanassy A, Miller S. Maintenance of locomotor abilities following Laufband (treadmill) therapy in para- and tetraplegic persons: Follow-up studies. Spinal Cord 1998; 36:744–749.

38. Barbeau H, Ladouceur M, Norman K, Pepin A, Leroux A. Walking after spinal cord injury: Evaluation, treatment and functional recovery. Arch Phys Med Rehabil 1999; 80:225–235.

39. Visintin M, Barbeau H, Korner-Bitensky N, Mayo N. A new approach to retrain gait in stroke patients through body weight support and treadmill stimulation. Stroke 1998; 29:1122–1128.

40. Miyai I, Fujimoto Y, Ueda Y, Yamamoto H, Nozaki S, Saito T, Kang J. Treadmill training with body weight

support: Its effect on Parkinson's disease. Arch Phys Med Rehabil 2000; 81:849–852.

41. Schindl M, Forstner C, Kern H, Hesse S. Treadmill training with partial body weight support in nonambulatory patients with cerebral palsy. Arch Phys Med Rehabil 2000; 81:301–306.

42. Pearson K, Misiaszek J, Fouad K. Enhancement and resetting of locomotor activity by muscle afferents. Ann N Y Acad Sci 1998; 860:203–215.

43. Van Wezel B, Ottenhoff F, Duysens J. Dynamic control of location-specific information in tactile cutaneous reflexes from the foot during human walking. J Neurosci 1997; 17:3804–3814.

44. Nielsen J, Petersen N, Fedirchuk B. Evidence suggesting a transcortical pathway from cutaneous foot afferents to tibialis anterior motoneurones in man. J Physiol 1997; 501:473–484.

45. Duysens J, Pearson K. From cat to man: Basic aspects of locomotion relevant to motor rehabilitation of SCI. NeuroRehabil 1998; 10:107–118.

46. Jueptner M, Weiller C. A review of differences between basal ganglia and cerebellar control of movements as revealed by functional imaging studies. Brain 1998; 121:1437–1449.

47. Muir G, Steeves J. Sensorimotor stimulation to improve locomotor recovery after spinal cord injury. Trends Neurosci 1997; 20:72–77.

48. Field-Fote E. Spinal cord control of movement: implications for locomotion rehabilitation following spinal cord injury. Phys Ther 2000; 80:477–484.

49. Behrman A, Harkema S. Locomotion training after human spinal cord injury: a series of case studies. Phys Ther 2000; 80:688–700.

50. Harkema S, Dobkin B, Edgerton V. Pattern generators in locomotion: Implications for recovery of walking after spinal cord injury. Top Spinal Cord Inj Rehabil 2000; 6:82–96.

51. Daly J, Ruff R. Electrically induced recovery of gait components for older patients with chronic stroke. Am J Phys Med Rehabil 2000; 79:349–360.

52. Wieler M, Stein R, Ladouceur M, Whittaker M, Barbeau H. Multicenter evaluation of electrical stimulation systems for walking. Arch Phys Med Rehabil 1999; 80:495–500.

53. Herman R, He J, D'Luzansky S, Willis W, Dilli S. Spinal cord stimulation facilitates functional walking in a chronic incomplete spinal cord injured. Spinal Cord 2002; 40:65–68.

54. Colombo G, Joerg M, Schreier R, Dietz V. Treadmill training of paraplegic patients using a robotic orthosis. J Rehab Res Dev 2000; 37:693–700.

55. Fung J, Stewart J, Barbeau H. The combined effects of clonidine and cyproheptadine with interactive training on the modulation of locomotion in spinal cord injured subjects. J Neurol Sci 1990; 100:85–93.

56. Dobkin B. Driving cognitive and motor gains with rehabilitation after brain and spinal cord injury. Curr Opin Neurol 1998; 11:639–641.

57. Dobkin B. Neurorehabilitation: Greater plasticity through chemicals and practice. Neurol Network Commen 1998; 2:171–174.

58. Lehmann J, Condon S, Price R, deLateur B. Gait abnormalities in hemiplegia: Their correction by ankle-foot orthoses. Arch Phys Med Rehabil 1987; 68:763–71.

59. Teasell R, McRae M, Foley N, Bhardwaj A. Physical and functional correlations of ankle-foot orthosis use in the rehabilitation of stroke patients. Arch Phys Med Rehabil 2001; 82:1047–1049.

60. Hesse S, Werner C, Matthias K. Non-velocity-related effects of a rigid double-stopped ankle-foot orthosis on gait and lower limb muscle activity of hemiparetic subjects with an equinovarus deformity. Stroke 1999; 30:1855–1861.

61. Geboers J, Drost M, Spaans F, Kuipers H, Seelen H. Immediate and long-term effects of ankle-foot orthosis on muscle activity during walking. Arch Phys Med Rehabil 2002; 83:240–245.

62. Deathe A, Hayes K, Winter D. The biomechanics of canes, crutches, and walkers. Crit Rev Phys Rehabil Med 1993; 5:15–29.

63. Hesse S, Jahnke M, Schaffrin A, Luecke D, Reiter F, Konrad M. Immediate effects of therapeutic facilitation on the gait of hemiparetic patients as compared with walking with and without a cane. Electroencephalogr Clin Neurophysiol 1998; 109:515–522.

64. Bohannon R. Comfortable and maximum walking speed of adults agd 20 to 79 years: Reference values and determinants. Age Ageing 1997; 26:15–19.

Chapter 7

Assessment and Outcome Measures for Clinical Trials

Is our approach to therapy for an individual patient's specific disability better than another approach? This question fuels scientific, social, ethical, economic, and political facets of the practices of neurologic rehabilitation. At a time when public health initiatives tend to defer to the marketplace and to consumer choice, disabled people need evidence about rehabilitation practices, not slick advertisements and untestable claims. Measured outcomes in comparison studies must be interpreted in relation to their statistical significance and clinical importance.

A national research agenda in the United States, called *Healthy People 2010*,[1] described 110 health objectives for people with disabilities. Measures of disability and interventions for disability lag well behind those objectives.[2] The time has come for rehabilitationists to hush their complaints about those who may be perceived as regulating or interfering with the care of patients, such as case managers, insurers, and government agencies. Instead, each member of the rehabilitation team, university research programs, and health care organizations should commit resources to test specific interventions and settings for care. Those who practice neurologic rehabilitation and those who pay for rehabilitation are obligated to demonstrate just which approaches produce the best of possible outcomes, so that all stakeholders can define what ought to be provided to patients.

Research on the effectiveness and appropriateness of medical interventions has increasingly affected the practices of health professionals. Outcomes research, which examines the end results of health services, includes the study of the experiences, preferences, and values of patients.[3] The goal of this field is to create a compendium of scientific evidence about the best decisions that can be made by

271

providers and patients. To study the best ways to lessen impairments, disabilities, and handicaps in patients with neurologic diseases, rehabilitationists need reliable and valid measurement instruments that are sensitive to important changes. Those who pay for health care, along with the rehabilitation team, also require meaningful measures gathered for internal program evaluations, individual patient monitoring, quality assurance, quality improvement, and for determination of the cost-effectiveness of procedures.

No ideal scales and measuring tools exist for neurologic rehabilitation, so researchers and practitioners must interpolate from what a tool purports to offer and how best to make use of it.[4] Clinical researchers around the world have made progress in the conceptualization and measurement of physical and cognitive impairments, of disabilities mostly related to *activities of daily living* (ADLs), of handicap, and of the domains of health-related *quality of life* (QOL). The World Health Organization introduced a revision of its conceptual framework of disability in its International Classification of Functioning and Disability (ICIDH-2). The new classification, available on the WHO web site (www.who.int/icidh/), examines activities that disabled people can and cannot do and whether people actually perform and participate in these activities. The dimensions of the WHO classification also include personal and environmental factors that affect functioning. The emphasis on activities, participation, and contextual factors interacting with impairments and disabilities may influence the design of new tools.

This chapter examines some of the existing measurement tools most successfully employed for neurologic diseases across levels of impairment, disability, and QOL. Measurement tools will sit idly in a file cabinet, however, without good ideas that need testing. A tool becomes useful when a research protocol specifies an outcome assessment relevant to the rehabilitation intervention and measured by the instrument. Well-defined interventions and solid assessment and outcome measures point to clear answers about efficacy only when deployed within a well-designed clinical trial. This chapter also introduces some of the experimental designs and statistical methods suited for trials of rehabilitation interventions. The need for creative designs for clinical trials becomes es-

pecially cogent as rehabilitationists begin to test biologic and neuroprosthetic therapies.

PRINCIPLES OF MEASUREMENT

The choice of tools for assessments and outcomes and the choice of statistical methods to assess tools requires a general grasp of measurement principles.

Types of Measurements

Nominal measures classify items into categories that have no particular ordered relationship to one another. Only the number of subjects, for example, who fall within a group are counted, such as males and females or subjects with strokes who have either a left hemiplegia versus right hemiplegia versus no weakness.

With an *interval* scale, the numerical differences between measured points are interpretable. The distance, for example, between a joint angle of 10° and 18° is the same as the difference between 25° and 33°. Quantification requires instrumentation. Measures that use an interval scale with magnitude and an absolute zero, such as the force exerted by a concentric muscle contraction in newton-meters or the time in seconds to walk 50 meters, are also *ratio* scales. Temperature is not a ratio scale, because, for example, 38°C is not twice as hot as 19°C, although it is 19°C warmer.

Ordinal scales measure magnitude by a predetermined order among possible responses in a classification, but do not possess equal intervals and may not have an absolute zero. Most rehabilitation measures have magnitude, but do not possess equal intervals or an absolute zero. These ordinal scales can be viewed as having numerically ordered *ranks*. The British Medical Council scale for strength—from 0 equals no movement to 5 equals full resistance—is an ordinal one, as are any of the functional assessment scales where zero means dependent, 1 means physical assistance is needed, and 2 means independence. These consecutive grades are not linear, however. A gain from 0 to 1 is not the equivalent of a gain from 1 to 2. Separate items on scales like the Functional Independence Measure and Barthel Index can be summed, so that higher scores indicate greater independence. A change from a score on the Barthel Index from 30 to 60 may come to be correlated with the capacity to live at home after a stroke, but rehabilitation has not made the patient twice as independent.

Methods of analysis developed for interval or ratio measures can, however, be applied to ordinal data that approximate, for example, a continuous underlying measure of functionality. In addition, hierarchical ordinal scales for a specific function, such as mobility, that are set up in their order of difficulty (for example, wheelchair transfers, wheelchair mobility, room ambulation, stair climbing, community ambulation) can be given a coefficient of scalability and reproducibility using the Guttman scaling procedure.

The *Rasch analysis* is a sophisticated approach for transforming ordinal data into interval data to create a more linear measure in scales used for functional assessment.[5] The underlying concept is that each item or test has a certain level of difficulty. Each person has a certain level of ability. Success and failure rates on test items are a function of both parameters. Data items are positioned along the measurement continuum according to how difficult they are for patients. Patients are positioned by their ability to perform the items. In this model, the log odds of an individual item, which are the successes of the patient on an item divided by the failures of the patient on the same item, are equal to the independence of the patient, which is the log of successes minus the log of failures. An iterative procedure using a Rasch analysis software program computes estimates of item difficulty, associated errors of measurement, and each item's fit into the measurement model. An estimate of each item's difficulty, expressed in logits, locates each item on a continuous and additive scale, so that a change of, 3 points on the scale has equal value at any level. New ordinal scales may need to be designed to take full advantage of Rasch analysis.

Reliability and Validity

For research and clinical applications, measurement tools must be reliable and valid. *Reliability* is the extent to which the measure yields the same score when no true change in what is measured has occurred. Reliability, or consistency, is not unlike a measure's signal-to-noise ratio, taking into account random errors, inherent biases, and systemic errors. *Validity* is the degree to which a measure reflects what it is meant to measure. A measure may always yield the same score for a patient, but it may not be a measure of its intended purpose. Validity may also describe the range of interpretations that are appropriate to place upon a score. What does a score mean within the confines of a particular study? Reliability and validity are never all or nothing attributes.

Reliability measures take several forms. *Interrater reliability* needs to be demonstrated for measures that require a rating by someone other than the patient. The statistics most commonly used to indicate reliability include Pearson correlations, Kappa correlations, and the intraclass correlation coefficient. The intraclass correlation addresses specifically the degree to which scores from the same rater are more similar to one another than they are to scores from other raters. For example, a very good standard interobserver agreement for measures of a group is 0.70 and for an individual is 0.90, using the Kappa statistic for nominal and ordinal data. A Kappa of <0.40 indicates poor agreement.

Test–retest reliability compares measures at two points in time, close enough so that no true change should have occurred. For functional assessments, the fewer the steps in a scale, the higher the level of agreement, but sensitivity to change and the ability to discriminate between two populations tend to fall. Reliability of scales with many items is often assessed by Cronbach's reliability coefficient, which measures internal consistency of the items. This analysis detects the relatedness of items that can be correctly added together. A score of >0.80 is excellent and a score of <0.70 suggests an inadequate level of internal consistency.

An assessment measure becomes validated by an accumulation of analyses of validity. *Content validity* may be decided subjectively by a panel of experts who suggest whether items and their measure are appropriate and cover the domain of interest. Choices must be made about which items are most commmon and important to the population being studied. This *face validity*, the logic of a measure, is especially important. The clinician, not the statistician, draws from knowledge and experience to determine what is relevant and practical about a scale. In rehabilitation, one must especially consider whether or not an instrument is valid

Table 7–2. **Standard Tools to Measure Neurologic Impairments**

CONSCIOUSNESS	SENSORIMOTOR SCALES
Glasgow Coma Scale	Modified Ashworth Scale of spasticity
Rancho Los Amigos Level of Cognitive Function	Fugl-Meyer Assessment of Motor Performance
Coma Recovery Scale[16]	Motor Assessment Scale
Galveston Orientation and Amnesia Test	Motricity Index
	Berg Balance Scale
COGNITION	Action Research Arm Test
	Wolf Motor Function Test
General	Grip strength
Wechsler Adult Intelligence Scale-III (verbal and performance IQ)	National Institutes of Health Stroke Scale
Raven's Progressive Matrices (nonverbal test)	Scandinavian Stroke Scale
Mini-Mental State Examination	Kurtzke Functional System and Expanded Disability Status Scale for multiple sclerosis
Neurobehavioral Cognitive Status Examination	United Parkinson's Disease Rating Scale
Halstead-Reitan	ASIA Neurological and Functional Classification for SCI
Memory, Learning	Tufts Quantitative Neuromuscular Examination
Wechsler Memory Scale	
Rivermead Behavioral Memory Test	**TIMED PERFORMANCE**
Selective Reminding Test	
Rey Auditory Verbal Learning Test	Timed self-care tasks
California Verbal Learning Test	Physical Performance Test
Benton Visual Retention Test	Tufts Assessment of Motor Performance
Rey-Osterieth visual learning complex	Timed walk for 10 meters or 50 feet
	Distance walked in 2 or 6 minutes
Attention/Concentration/Set Shifting/Processing Speed	Modified Emory Functional Ambulation Profile
Trail-Making Test A and B	Reaction times for a visuomotor task
Digit Span	Purdue Grooved Pegboard
Paced Auditory Serial Addition Test	9-Hole Peg Test
	Finger tapping
Perception	
Hooper Visual Organization Test	**INSTRUMENTED EVALUATIONS**
Line Bisection	
Cancellation Test for visual neglect	Gait analysis
	Step counter
Executive Functions	Heart rate monitor
Wisconsin Card Sorting Test	Strength: dynamometry
Stroop Color and Word Test	Balance: center of pressure on force plate
Porteus Maze	Range of motion: goniometry
Rey Complex Figure Copy and Recall Test	Electromagnetic limb tracking devices
	Metabolic energy expenditure
	Instrumented neurologic examination

ASIA, American Spinal Injury Association; SCI, spinal cord injury.

For a specific neurologic disease or range of impairments, a battery of core tests can describe patient populations across facilities and provide some common measures across interventional studies, especially in stroke and brain injury. For example, the Consortium to Establish a Registry for Alzheimer's Disease (CERAD) combined nine standard tests to monitor the course of patients with this dementia.[20] Across institutions, the test battery was found to be re-

Table 7–3. **Glasgow Coma Scale**

Examiner's Test	Patient's Response	Assigned Score	
Eye opening	Spontaneous speech	Opens eyes on own	4
	Pain	Opens eyes when asked in a loud voice	3
	Pain	Opens eyes to pressure	2
	Pain	Does not open eyes	1
Best motor response	Commands	Follows simple commands	6
	Pain	Pulls examiner's hand away to pressure	5
	Pain	Pulls a part of body away with pressure	4
	Pain	Decorticate posturing	3
	Pain	Decerebrate posturing	2
	Pain	No motor response to pressure	1
Verbal response	Pain	Converses and states where he is, who he is, the month and year	5
	Speech	Confused or disoriented	4
	Speech	Talks so examiner can understand, but makes no sense	3
	Speech	Makes sounds, not understood	2
	Speech	Makes no noise	1

liable, sensitive to change, and easily administered. Validity has been supported by clinical–pathological correlations. The 17 American rehabilitation programs that comprise the Traumatic Brain Injury Model systems project have used 15 standard tests prior to inpatient discharge.[21] Tests of language function are often included in batteries (see Chapter 5), including the Token Test for the ability to follow spoken directions and generation of a list of words starting with a specified letter, such as the FAS test.

The *Mini-Mental State Examination* (MMSE) is perhaps the most frequently employed cognitive screening test, but it has limited sensitivity in detecting language dysfunction[22] and usually cannot detect the cognitive basis for disability in the neurorehabilitation population.

Table 7–4. **Galveston Orientation and Amnesia Test**

1. What is your name? (2) _____ When were you born? (4) _____ Where do you live? (4) _____
2. Where are you now? (5) city _____ (5) hospital_____ (unnecessary to state name of hospital)
3. On what date were you admitted to this hospital? (5) _____ How did you get here? (5) _____
4. What is the first event you can remember <u>after</u> the injury? (5) _____
   Can you describe in detail (e.g., date, time, companions) the first event you can recall <u>after</u> injury? (5) _____
5. Can you describe the last event you recall <u>before</u> the injury? (5) _____
   Can you describe in detail (e.g., date, time, companions) the first event you can recall <u>before</u> the injury? (5) _____
6. What time is it now? _____ (-1 for each $1/2$ hour removed from correct time to maximum of -5)
7. What day of the week is it? _____ (-1 for each day removed from correct one)
8. What day of the month is it? _____ (-1 for each day removed from correct date to maximum of -5)
9. What is the month? _____ (-5 for each month removed from correct one to maximum of -15)
10. What is the year? _____ (-10 for each year removed from correct one to maximum of -30)
Total Score (100 − total error points) _____

The MMSE has had its greatest impact on detecting a decline over time in people with Alzheimer's disease. Scoring needs to be considered within educational and age-adjusted norms.[23,24]

The *Neurobehavioral Cognitive Status Examination* (NCSE) includes 10 scales and is more sensitive to cognitive impairments than the MMSE.[25] The NCSE uses a graded series of tasks within domains such as orientation, attention, constructions, memory, language including comprehension, naming and repetition, abstractions, and social judgment. Scores have correlated with stroke rehabilitation outcomes on the Barthel Index.[26] Other batteries of frequently used and lesser known tests that extract greater information about a patient include an assessment for impairment in sensorimotor integration,[27] perceptual function,[28] and a variety of attempts to develop disease-specific test batteries, especially for stroke and cerebral trauma.

The PASAT finds its most extensive use in studies of TBI and in the MSFC. An examiner's own version of the PASAT can be carried out at the bedside to obtain a sense of processing speed for auditory information and mental flexibility, as well as the ability to perform calculations. The patient is instructed to listen to a random string of digits from 1 to 9 presented every 2 to 3 seconds and to add the last digit spoken to the preceding one. For example:

stimulus	2	7	4	3	...
response	—	9	11	7	...

The MSFC employs 60 sums in its alternate forms of the PASAT.

A new generation of cognitive tests may evolve from tasks that aim to activate regions of the brain during functional neuroimaging procedures. For example, the *N-back* test performed during fMRI may reveal different levels of working memory capacity in subjects who perform the test equally well (see Chapter 3). Another potential innovation will be to define measures of the so-called *theory of mind* capacity. This approach to cognition requires subjects to model the mental states of others. Theory of mind may produce probes of perceptions, attitudes, opinions, intentions about acting, and other attributions about oneself and others.[29] These measures would be especially valuable for studies of patients with TBI.

Speech and Language

Tests for aphasia may evaluate many aspects of speech and language, such as grammar, syntax, word finding, naming, auditory comprehension, reading, writing, articulation, presence of paraphasic errors, and other modalities (Table 7–5). The lengthier and rather inclusive batteries include the *Boston Diagnostic Aphasia Examination* (BDAE) and the Porch Index. These tests take from 1 to 3 hours to complete. The Western Aphasia Battery includes many of the tasks in the BDAE but is shorter and perhaps easier for the physician to understand, because it parallels a typical bedside test of language. The Token Test, with its large and small circles and squares of 4 colors, picks up more subtle impairments in comprehension and prepositional language. Tools for assessing functional communication usually require approximately a 15-minute examination. For example, the American Speech-Language-Hearing Association recommended its 43-item rating scale that includes social communication, expressing daily needs, and the ability to plan.[30]

Table 7–5. Diagnostic Tests for Aphasia

GENERAL SKILLS
Porch Index of Communicative Ability
Boston Diagnostic Aphasia Examination
Neurosensory Center Comprehensive Examination for Aphasia
Western Aphasia Battery
Aachen Aphasia Test (German)
Milan Aphasia Test (Italian)

FUNCTIONAL COMMUNICATION
Communication Abilities in Daily Living
Functional Communication Profile
Functional Assessment of Communication Skills (American Speech-Language, Hearing Association)

SPECIALIZED
Revised Token Test
Boston Naming Test
Boston Assessment of Severe Aphasia
Aphasia Severity Rating Scale
Rating Scale Profile of Speech Characteristics

Sensorimotor Impairment Scales

STRENGTH

Strength is most commonly measured by the 5 grades of the British Medical Council Scale. This scale is least sensitive to change at grade 4, which describes movement against less than full resistance. This scale may be incorporated into other scales for a specific muscle group innervated by a particular root level, as in the American Spinal Injury Association Motor Score (see Chapter 10). Hand-held dynamometry can be performed at most muscles in a sensitive and reliable way,[31,32] but limb positioning and rater experience are critical. Many devices measure grip and pinch strength, although the reproducibility and validity of these tests are often unclear.[33] Grip strength, tested by a Jamar dynamometer with the elbow extended, is used to monitor diseases of the motor unit and correlates with overall strength in the elderly. The Tufts Quantitative Neuromuscular Examination[34] battery uses an inexpensive, nonportable strain gauge to quantitate maximal voluntary isometric contraction of many muscles, along with pulmonary function tests that reflect strength. This system has been successfully used in longitudinal studies and in a randomized trial with ciliary neurotrophic factor in patients with amyotrophic lateral sclerosis.

The most objective, reliable, and sensitive, but expensive and cumbersome, instruments are the commercially available isokinetic dynamometers. These computerized devices measure torque throughout range of motion as the limb moves at a constant velocity. Their programs provide data on the pattern of force generation, on the effect of speed on the development of force, on the work performed, and on fatigability.[35] Eccentric and concentric contractions can be evaluated. Hand-held computerized dynamometry for finger pinch, hand squeeze, and finger tapping produces continuous data and may be of value during functional imaging studies.[36] Computerized dynamometry also serves as a measure of spasticity.

SPASTICITY

A number of clinical examination (Table 7–6) and instrumented (Table 7–7) measures of spasticity have been developed that are meant

Table 7–6. **Clinical Measures of Spasticity**

MODIFIED ASHWORTH SCORE[38]

0	No increase in muscle tone
1	Slight increase in tone, producing a catch and release or minimal resistance at the end of range when the joint is moved in flexion or extension
2	Slight increase in tone, manifested by a catch followed by minimal resistance through the remainder of range of motion, but the joint is still easily moved
3	More marked increase in tone through most of the range of motion, but the joint is still easily ranged
4	Considerable increase in tone, and passive movement difficult
5	Affected joint rigid in flexion or extension

SPASM SCORE[257]

0	No spasms
1	Mild spasms induced by stimulation
2	Spasms fewer than 1 per hour
3	More than 1 per hour
4	More than 10 per hour

Sources: Bohannon and Smith, 1987[38]; Meythaler et al., 1992.[257]

to reveal the effects of interventions on tone and provide insight into mechanisms (see Chapter 2).

Clinical Scales

The history of how and when hypertonicity interferes with a patient's activities is the most useful way to determine whether or not an intervention is needed. Bouts of clonus and flexor and extensor spasms during ambulation, driving, wheelchair push-up pressure releases, transfers, reclining, bed mobility, sleep, sexual function, and during self-care activities can be counted over the course of a day or week. A self-rating visual analogue scale that allows patients to grade themselves may give insight into diurnal variations or activity-dependent spasms. The patient bisects a 10 cm line scaled as *no spasticty* on the far left and *most imaginable spasticity* on the far right. This approach correlates with the Modified Ashworth Scale.[37]

The Modified Ashworth Scale[38] has good in-

Table 7–7. **Clinical Techniques to Measure Spasticity**

MECHANICAL METHODS

Pendulum drop with relaxation index

Manual stretch with EMG response

Dynamometry with ramp, sinusoidal, or random
movements

    Controlled displacement with torque or EMG
    response

    Controlled torque with displacement or EMG
    response

NEUROPHYSIOLOGIC METHODS

H-reflex

    H_{max}/M_{max}

    H suppression by vibration

    H recovery after conditioning stimulus train

    Audiospinal modulated H-reflex[258]

Dynamic integrated EMG recruitment periods

    Bicycle ergometry[259]

    Treadmill walking

Joint probability density amplitudes

Kinematic gait studies with angle-angle plots

EMG, electromyographic; H, Hoffman.

terrater reliability and reproducibility if done under the same conditions, such as similar positioning of the patient. No universal technique is employed, despite its frequent use in clinical trials. The scale attempts to quantify the resistance to passive range of motion across a single joint. The Ashworth has been a primary outcome measure for clinical trials of drug interventions with injections of botulinum toxin, oral tizanidine, and intrathecal baclofen, as well as for surgical interventions such as dorsal rhizotomy. No direct relationship, however, exists between changes in the Ashworth score and improvements or declines in functional activities. The Tone Assessment Scale is one of many attempts to improve upon the information gained by the Ashworth Scale by asessing tone in different postures, but adds little information and no greater interrater reliability compared to the Ashworth.[39]

Associated reactions are another potential, if rather gross measure of an aspect of spasticity. An involuntary movement of the spastic limb can often be elicited by a forceful movement in another part of the body. With standing up,

for example, the hemiparetic arm may flex. These movements can be counted or the change in angle of a joint measured.[40]

Electrophysiologic Techniques

The Hoffman's reflex (H-reflex) has been used in clinical settings.[41,42] The amplitude of the H response compared to the motor (M) response (H_{max}/M_{max} ratio) measures the excitability of the soleus motoneurons that respond to supramaximal stimulation of the sciatic nerve. Tested at rest, the ratio tends to increase with spasticity, but studies have not shown it to correlate with the intensity of spasticity. The ratio and H-reflex amplitude increase significantly approximately 3 months after a clinically complete spinal cord injury.[43] The hyperactive H-reflex was not consistently modulated during ambulation in spastic paretic subjects, unlike normal subjects, so its usefulness as a measure of reflex abnormality may be limited.[44] The gain of the H-reflex in some spastic patients may already be so high that the response cannot rise with stimulation.

The $H_{max\ vibration}/H_{max\ control}$ decreases with spasticity. This ratio measures the inhibition of the soleus monosynaptic reflex by vibration at 100 Hz over the Achilles tendon. The decrement is caused by presynaptic inhibition of Ia fibers exerted through interneurons that make GABAergic connections with the terminal arborizations of Ia fibers. Spasticity is also associated with brief facilitation of the H-reflex recovery curve, rather than the normal suppression, after it is conditioned by a train of four 300 Hz shocks applied to the posterior tibial nerve at the ankle. This presumably reflects the hyperexcitability of motoneurons. Several of these electrophysiologic tests were used in spastic patients in an attempt to detect and best treat the predominant pathophysiology underlying their hypertonicity and hyperreflexia.[45] Diazepam, and to some degree tizanidine, increased vibratory inhibition of the H-reflex. Baclofen facilitated the H-reflex recovery curve. The drugs did not affect the H_{max}/M_{max} ratio.

Biomechanical Techniques

Biomechanical techniques evaluate changes in the phasic and tonic reflex activity of the muscles across a joint.

For the Wartenberg pendulum or *drop* test, the subject is supine or propped up 45° with the legs dangling over the edge of a table. The tester lifts a relaxed leg to the horizontal and releases it so the leg swings by gravity alone. With quadriceps and hamstrings spasticity, the initial swing from full extension usually will not reach the vertical, whereas a healthy person's leg will flex beyond that to approximately 70°. The maximum angular velocity, knee angle in flexion, and number of swings tend to decrease with hypertonicity. Commercially available isokinetic exercise equipment, an electrogoniometer that records the changing knee joint angle, or a computerized video for studying leg kinematics can be used to make this reproducible, although perhaps theoretically flawed, measure of hypertonicity.[46] The drop test provided more detailed and observer-independent measurements than the Ashworth score in studies of chronic hemiplegia after stroke[47] and in patients with multiple sclerosis,[48] and correlated with the Ashworth score in a study of tizanidine in spastic paraparetic subjects with SCI.[49] The antispasticity effects of clonidine, cyproheptadine, and baclofen were revealed by a video motion analysis of the pendulum test in patients with spastic SCI.[50]

Devices such as dynamometers can quantitate the torque or amount of force elicited by motorically moving the elbow, wrist, knee, or ankle over a particular angle at a specified velocity. Dynamometry quantitates the threshold angle at which the torque or EMG starts to increase in an initially passive muscle. This approach measures an aspect of muscle tone by the resistance (usually the eccentric torque) produced with passive isokinetic movement of e.g., the knee in different displacements. Although this emulates what the clinician tests qualitatively, results from different laboratories are often inconsistent. Differences may be related to idiosyncrasies in equipment and technique, the joint tested, and the patient population studied. For example, biomechanical evidence has been used to support the opposing hypotheses that spastic hypertonia at the elbow results primarily from:

1. A decrease in stretch reflex threshold and preserved reflex gain, implying that the motoneurons activated at smaller joint angles and lower angular velocities start out more depolarized;[51] and

2. A pathological increase in stretch reflex gain, implying that the response is mediated by a late polysynaptic pathway, probably from muscle spindle afferents;[52] and

3. Responses that differ under passive and active movements; for example, with active flexion, a change is more apparent in reflex gain than in reflex threshold, but a change in the mechanical properties of the muscle is also important.[53]

Studies of stretch-evoked EMG and torque signals do distinguish healthy subjects from patients with marked hypertonicity, such as subjects with complete SCI.[54] The meaning of differences in these measures across subjects who have hypertonicity and of differences in the effects of interventions such as medication for spasticity on passive isokinetic movements is moot.

Several measurement strategies were compared in a study of 10 chronically hemiplegic patients.[47] The Ashworth and Fugl-Meyer scores correlated with torque and EMG measurements during ramp-and-hold angular displacements about the elbow and with a pendulum test of the affected leg. The results were reproducible over several weeks. The H/M ratio showed a wide intrasubject variation and did not correlate with the clinical picture. Correlations among these methods point more to their fair reliability than to the validity of the measures as biologic or clinical markers for functionally important conditions.

Electromyographic and Kinematic Methods

Abnormal coactivation of antagonist muscle groups, as well as inappropriate timing of muscle activity, may interfere with walking in patients with an upper motor neuron (UMN) syndrome. A formal gait analysis (see Chapter 6) with surface EMG and kinematic studies can quantify dynamic muscle and joint relationships. Task-specific studies of spasticity and disordered motor control are more likely to shed light on the clinical measurement and implications of the UMN syndrome for rehabilitation than measures made by passive movements at single joints to ascertain an Ashworth score or an H-reflex in a supine patient.

Gait analysis by Richards and colleagues shows that in patients with spasticity after a hemiparetic stroke, the EMG bursts arise from an abnormal muscle-lengthening, velocity-sensitive activation pattern during stance, rather than the usual length-dependent activation pattern of the nonparetic leg.[55] This abnormal response to muscle stretch may serve as a dynamic, locomotor-based measure of spasticity. The measure is task-specific in that muscle-lengthening velocity during swing did not cause an abnormal response, muscle strength did not correlate with the measure, and the presence of ankle clonus and passive resistance on the Ashworth Scale did correlate.

For another gait measure, the EMG from each muscle from initial foot contact with the floor to the next ipsilateral foot contact is integrated and normalized to 100% of the step cycle. The patient's EMG data are then divided into windows that identify when each muscle is active or not active compared to the timing of the activity of normal controls. An index is defined as the ratio of integrated EMG area in ordinarily "off" windows to that in the "on" windows. If the timing of muscle activity in a patient is similar to that of normal subjects, the index is a small fraction. For patients with significant spasticity or disordered motor control, muscles are on when they would be off in controls, so the ratio is greater than one.[56] The analysis provides a dynamic within-step quantification of inappropriate activity with respect to the step cycle for each muscle studied. Drawbacks include the complexity of obtaining the data and performing the analysis, getting measures on normals and patients walking at about the same speed, and taking into account the great variation in the EMG bursts of normals and spastic patients during ambulation.

Quantitative measures of spasticity or of disordered motor control that are sensitive to functionally important actions of the arm and leg need further development for a clinical setting. Single-joint movements are of less importance to rehabilitationists than are dynamic multijoint, movement-evoked responses of the motor system.

MOTOR PERFORMANCE

Several reliable and valid measures of sensorimotor impairment are a bridge to tests of disability. These tests assess the performance of the affected limbs within the context of the motor components of ADLs. The Fugl-Meyer Assessment of Physical Performance,[57] devel-

oped for the evaluation of hemiplegic stroke, is a bit cumbersome to perform, but may be the most employed impairment tool for clinical practice and research in stroke. This index scores defined actions at each limb joint based on whether they are accomplished by selective muscular contractions or by an abnormal synergistic pattern. Thus, an isolated biceps contraction with resistance is scored as better than the same resistance produced by a flexor synergy response by the arm. This distinction is important in measuring a change in motor control in patients with upper motor neuron impairment. The upper extremity and lower extremity motor function score components (maximum of 66 and 34, respectively) can be converted into percentages of the total possible score for that extremity to compare changes in percent recovery over time.[58] Total motor scores can help stratify patients for outcome studies in stroke (0–35, severe; 36–55, moderately severe; 56–79, moderate; and >79, mild).[59,60] Table 7–8 shows the scoring system for the lower extremity.

The Motricity Index[61] for arm and leg function has been used in several outcome studies of stroke (see Chapter 9), but should be valid for any upper motor neuron disease. Weighted scores are given for levels of ability for a thumb and forefinger pinch and for power at the elbow flexors, shoulder abductors, hip and ankle flexors, and knee extensors. The Motor Assessment Scale captures eight motor functions on a 7-point ordinal scale, such as supine to sitting and sitting to standing and a measure of muscle tone, and tends to correlate with the Fugl-Meyer Scale.[62] The Modified Motor Assessment Scale uses a 6-point scoring system.[63] Scores correlate with the Barthel Index after stroke.[64]

Manual Tests

Many tests have been designed specifically to assess the sensorimotor function and coordination of the upper extremity, especially for patients with hemiparetic stroke. The Action Research Arm Test includes 19 items scored on a 4-point ordinal scale, but the sum score from 0 to 57 is usually treated as an interval scale.[65] Subjects are graded by the quality of grasp, grip, and pincer movements using small items and for larger hand movements. The test can be timed to better differentiate a score of 2

Table 7–8. Fugel-Meyer Scale for Leg Movement and Sensation and Balance

Area	Test	Scoring Criteria	Maximum Possible Score	Attained Score
Lower Extremity (supine)	I. Reflex activity-tested in supine position Achilles _____ Patellar _____	0-No reflex activity 2-Reflex activity	4	
	II. A. Flexor Synergy Hip flexion _____ Knee flexion _____ Ankle dorsiflexion _____	0-Can not be performed 1-Partial motion 2-Full motion	6	
	B. Extensor synergy (motion is resisted) Hip extension _____ Adduction _____ Knee extension _____ Ankle plantar flexion ____	0-No motion 1-Weak motion 2-Almost full strength compared to normal		
Sitting (knees free of chair)	III. Movement combining synergies A. Knee flexion beyond 90° ___	0-No active motion 1-From slightly extended position knee can be flexed, but not beyond 90° 2-Knee flexion beyond 90°		
	B. Ankle dorsiflexion _____	0-No active flexion 1-Incomplete active flexion 2-Normal dorsiflexion	4	
Standing	IV. Moving out of Synergy (hip at 0°) A. Knee flexion _____	0-Knee cannot flex without hip flexion 1-Knee begins flexion without hip flexion but does not reach 90°, or hip flexes during motion 2-Full motion as described		
	B. Ankle dorsiflexion _____	0-No active motion 1-Partial motion 2-Full motion	4	
Sitting	V. Normal reflexes Knee flexors _____ Patellar _____ Achilles _____	0-2 or 3 are markedly hyperactive 1-1 reflex is hyperactive, or 2 reflexesare lively 2-No more than 1 reflex lively	2	
Supine	VI. Coordination/speed—heel to opposite knee (5 repetitions in rapid succession) A. Tremor _____	0-Marked tremor 1-Slight trmor 2-No tremor		

Continued on following page

=

Table 7–8.—*continued*

Area	Test	Scoring Criteria	Maximum Possible Score	Attained Score
	B. Dysmetria _____	0-Pronounced or unsystematic 1-Slight of systematic 2-No dysmetria		
	C. Speed _____	0-6 seconds slower than unaffected side 1-2–5 seconds slower 2-Less than 2 seconds difference	6	
		Total lower extremity score for patient		___
Sensation				
Upper and Lower Extremities	I. Light touch a. Upper arm _____ b. Palm of hand _____ c. Thigh d. Sole of foot _____	0-Anesthesia 1-Hyperesthesia/dysesthesia 2-Normal _____	8	
	II. Proprioception a. Shoulder b. Elbow c. Wrist d. Thumb e. Hip f. Knee g. Ankle h. Toe	0-No sensation 1-Three quarters of answers are correct, but considerable difference in sensation compared with unaffected side 2-All answers are correct, little or no difference	16	

(performed abnormally) and 3 (movement performed normally). The test takes less than 10 minutes.

The Wolf Motor Function Test includes 15 timed tasks that are rated on a 6-point functional ability scale.[66] The test has high reliability for testing rehabilitation interventions for the upper extremity such as constraint-induced movement therapy. It takes from 30 to 40 minutes to complete. Such tests require a careful set up of items, seating with the subject's back against a chair, and clear instructions. The Test Evaluant les Membres superieurs des Personnes Agees (TEMPA) includes 9 unilateral and bimanual tasks related to upper extremity ADLs.[67] Each task is timed and given a functional rating. Examples include opening a jar and spooning coffee grains into a cup, placing coins into a slot, and tying a scarf around the neck. The test correlates with the Action Research Arm Test for subjects who can offer resistance in most upper extremity muscle groups.

Hand dexterity can be tested with the Jebsen-Taylor Test of Hand Function, the 9-Hole Peg Test, the Purdue Pegboard Test, or the Box and Block Test. These involve lifting and placing small items. Although many other instruments to measure hand function and upper extremity tasks exist, most were designed for patients with arthritis or for recovery after hand surgery. Tests of upper extremity function for patients undergoing neurorehabilitation need finer calibration to reflect a hierarchy of impairments in motor control and of levels of disability.

Disease-Specific Scales

Many other ordinal and quantitative tests of sensorimotor and oculobulbar function are in common use or have been instrumented.[68,69] Disease-specific ordinal measures with good reliability include the NIHSS for stroke,[70] the Kurtzke Expanded Disability Status Scale (EDSS) for multiple sclerosis,[71] and most portions of the United Parkinson's Disease Rating Scale.[72] The Canadian Neurological Stroke Scale, Scandinavian Stroke Scale (SSS), and NIHSS use different grading schemes for strength, sensation, language, alertness, visual fields, gaze, and neglect, but serve as reliable and valid measures of impairment for patients with acute and chronic stroke. The scales are not readily interconverted, however.[73] The SSS correlates well with the Barthel Index in patients with acute stroke followed through rehabilitation.[74,75] The NIHSS performed 7 days after a stroke forecasts both good recovery and severe disability at 3 months.[76] The NIHSS also defined the severity of impairment observed during inpatient stroke rehabilitation.[77] The Orpington Prognostic Scale (Table 7–9) is a bit easier to use compared to the NIHSS and may be modestly better as a predictor of ADLs at 3–6 months following a mild to moderate stroke.[78] A modified NIHSS may offer greater reliability than the NIHSS, at least for acute stroke studies.[79] These scales of stroke impairment underestimate functional outcomes for disability and psychosocial functioning.[80]

Instrumented Scales

Instrumented approaches have been attempted for multiple sclerosis[81] and Parkinson's disease,[72] but highly quantitative approaches to tremor, coordination, balance, and reaction times, among other tasks, have not found a niche in outcome studies. Mechanical goniometry is adequate for static range of motion measures in neurologic diseases, but electrogoniometers are required for dynamic studies, particularly in gait analysis. Methods for the analysis of gait patterns are reviewed in Chapter 6. When the question is how much walking is carried out by a disabled person, computerized data can be obtained from a foot switch, a pedometer set to stride length, or a more sophisticated accelerometer attached to the leg.[82]

Fiber-optic technology and software programming, initially applied to make the DataGlove[83] and a suit for whole-body virtual reality experiments, offer methodologies to assess limb positions during complex movements

Table 7–9. **The Orpington Prognostic Score**

Clinical Impairment	Score
ARM STRENGTH (MEDICAL RESEARCH COUNCIL GRADE)	
5	0.0
4	0.4
3	0.8
1–2	1.2
0	1.6
PROPRIOCEPTION (EYES CLOSED)	
Locates affected thumb	
Accurately	0.0
Slight difficulty	0.4
Finds thumb via arm	0.8
Unable	1.2
BALANCE	
Walks 10 feet without help	0.0
Maintains stance	0.4
Maintains sitting position	0.8
No sitting balance	1.2
COGNITION (1 POINT FOR EACH CORRECT ANSWER)	
Age of patient	
Time to nearest hour	
Name of hospital	
Month	
Years of World War II	
Name of U.S. President	
Year	
Date of birth	
Count backwards from 20	
Recall address given at start of testing	
Mental Test Score	
10	0.0
8–9	0.4
5–7	0.8
0–4	1.2

The total score is the sum of 1.6 plus the motor, proprioception, balance, and cognition subscores.

across joints and in three dimensions. Electromagnetic motion tracking devices (Polhemus, Vermont) on a limb can display real-time movements on a computer screen as a task is carried out in a virtual coordinate frame of reference using 3-dimensional graphics (see Chapter 5). With proper software, the accuracy, trajectory, speed, reaction time and other parameters of movement can be measured. This approach holds great promise for the measurement of otherwise elusive parameters.

TIMED TASKS

Direct observation of a patient's physical functioning requires more staff time, training, and effort than a self-report or proxy report by a family member. Direct observation built upon a set of rules for how the task should be completed provides generally a more objective serial measure, however. From the point of view of measurement, a timed performance task is even more attractive. Timed self-care tasks, the time needed to walk a particular distance in the range of 25 to 300 feet, and the distance walked within a given time, usually ranging from 2 to 6 minutes, all potentially add to the reproducibility and sensitivity to change of repeated measures. Tests of walking endurance such as the distance covered in a 2-minute walk are reliable indicators and can be more sensitive to change during stroke rehabilitation than the walking subscore of the Functional Independence Measure or speed of ambulation over 50 feet.[63,84] The Rivermead Mobility Index, a questionnaire about mobility, was found in one study to be as reliable and valid as a 1-meter timed walk and 2-minute walking distance test in patients receiving rehabilitation for a variety of neurologic diagnoses.[85]

The time it takes to perform a task may reflect disability. Timed motor tasks are considered generally as measures of impairment, if the scale is not about level of dependence and if a factor analysis done on subjects who carry out the tasks reveals loading on specified impairments. Distinctions can blur. For example, the test with Standard Practical Equipment uses four levels of dependence to grade 12 observed household tasks, such as inserting an electrical plug into a socket and using a key to unlock a lock.[86] The factors that explained most of the variance of the 12 tasks were mobility and balance, cognition, and coordination and hand function. If the well-defined lock-opening task were timed, it would not be any less a measure of impairment of upper extremity sensorimotor function and dexterity than, say, the

timed Purdue Grooved Pegboard or the 9-Hole Peg Test.[87]

The Physical Performance Test (PPT)[88] was devised as a quick screen of the elderly to measure common domains of function, including upper body strength and dexterity, mobility, and stamina in tasks that simulated ADLs (Table 7–10). Although its set of tasks and the range of scores derived from reliability and validity studies would not likely apply to severely impaired rehabilitation inpatients, we have found the PPT to be useful in an outpatient clinic. Further development of similar quantitative approaches would aid decision-making regarding whether a patient is becoming more or less impaired or functional. For example, if an outpatient with a stroke takes longer to walk 50 feet and to climb steps by serial testing, and if no medical complication accounts for the decline, the physician may order a brief pulse of physical therapy.

The Tufts Assessment of Motor Performance (TAMP)[89] was designed for the neurologically impaired, with the notion that any functional activity requires at least several distinct gross and fine motor performance capabilities. The TAMP defines 32 motor tasks that encompass the domains of mobility, ADLs, and physical aspects of communication. It goes beyond any other impairment or disability instrument by creating five measures to evaluate each task: time to completion, a 5-point scale of assistance needed, dichotomous scales to indicate the normality of the approach used and to rate the normality of specific gross and fine movements, and a 3-point proficiency scale to rate movement control and accuracy of the task. A factor analysis of these measurement dimensions reduced the large set of variables to seven factors that included tasks associated with mat mobility, dynamic balance, ambulation, working fasteners, gross and fine manipulation, grasp and release, and typing.[90] Although the TAMP, as it exists, is daunting, continued psychometric analyses could eliminate redundant items, determine unidimensional variables, identify how motor performances change after an impairment and during rehabilitation, and establish the most sensitive measures of change. This methodology is no different from the challenge posed in the construction of meaningful measures of disability and QOL.[6]

Table 7–10. **The Physical Performance Test**

Task	Time	Scoring	Score
1. Write the sentence, (whales live in the blue ocean)	____seconds	≤10 seconds = 4 10.5–15 seconds = 3 15.5–20 seconds = 2 >20 seconds = 1 Unable = 0	____
2. Simulate eating	____seconds	≤10 seconds = 4 10.5–15 seconds = 3 15.5–20 seconds = 2 >20 seconds = 1 Unable = 0	____
3. Lift a book and put it on a shelf	____seconds	≤2 seconds = 4 2.5–4 seconds = 3 4.5–6 seconds = 2 >6 seconds = 1 Unable = 0	____
4. Put on and remove a jacket	____seconds	≤10 seconds = 4 10.5–15 seconds = 3 15.5–20 seconds = 2 >20 seconds = 1 Unable = 0	____
5. Pick up penny from floor	____seconds	<2 seconds = 4 2.5–4 seconds = 3 4.5–6 seconds = 2 >6 seconds = 1 Unable = 0	____
6. Turn 360°	Discontinuous steps Continuous steps Unsteady (grabs, staggers) Steady	0 2 0 2	____
7. Walk 50 feet	____seconds	≤15 seconds = 4 15.5–20 seconds = 3 20.5–25 seconds = 2 >25 seconds = 1 Unable = 0	____
8. Climb one flight of stairs	____seconds	<5 seconds = 4 5.5–10 seconds = 3 10.5–15 seconds = 2 >15 seconds = 1 Unable = 0	____
9. Climb stairs	Number of flights of stairs up and down (maximum 4)	____	
Total Score (maximum 36 for 9–item, 28 for 7–item)		____ 9-item ____ 7-item	

BALANCE

Measures of balance and mobility can be acquired with and without instrumentation. Elderly subjects have been graded on getting up and sitting down in a chair, withstanding a nudge to the sternum, reaching up and bending over, standing with head turning and eyes closed, and by observing the initiation of ambulation and the patient's step height, step symmetry, path deviation, and turning.[91] The timed Up And Go test scores the risk of falling and the time taken to rise from an arm chair, walk 3 meters, turn, and walk back and sit down.[92] Balance and mobility interact with other measures. For example, walking speed and symmetry of the swing phase of gait in hemiplegics correlates with the Brunnstrom stage of motor recovery and the Fugl-Meyer score.[93] Gait velocity, cadence, degree of independence, and appearance show significant correlations with muscle strength of the hemiparetic lower extremity.[94] Self-selected walking velocity and maximal speed are cumulative quality scores of the patient's ability and confidence in walking.

Balance has been measured by ordinal scales (0 = unable to stand with feet apart, to 6 = able to stand on one leg for 60 seconds), by timed efforts,[95] by balance beam walking, and by the distance along a yard stick that a patient can reach while sitting or standing in place.[96] Testing single-limb balance has limited usefulness in many neurologically impaired patients, especially inpatients.

The Berg Balance Scale includes 14 tasks scored on a 5-point ordinal scale and has excellent reliability and validity mostly in stroke studies.[97] Subjects move through a series of everyday but increasingly difficult positions, from sitting to single limb stance, that diminish the base of leg support. The test examines truncal support as well, so it includes several measures that may be affected by an intervention to enhance mobility. It takes 15 minutes to carry out.

Instrumented techniques include standing on a force plate to measure sway, to measure the ability to maintain the body's center of gravity or center of pressure, and to assess the symmetry of weight bearing on each leg.[98,99] Other measures of balance include kinematic analysis during attempts at maintaining balance, the pattern and latencies of leg muscle EMG responses after perturbing a standing patient, and computerized moving platform posturography. Dynamic posturography has been somewhat useful in detecting elderly patients at risk for falls[100] and for evaluating vestibular disorders.[101] The technique includes recording changes in the center of gravity in standing subjects during small, brief rotational and translational movements of a force plate and to combinations of visual and somatosensory inputs. The reliability of this method and its validity for other neurologic impairments is uncertain.

BEHAVIORAL MEASURES

Behavioral Modification

The rehabilitation team often seeks to alter a patient's behavior. One approach targets a behavior over time and monitors change with an interval measure (Table 7–11).[102] This approach has been called Goal Attainment Scaling when the outcome measure is a 5-point scale ranging from −2 (much less than expected) to 0 (expected level) to +2 (much better than expected).[103] The outcome measures may also be more specific. For example, a male patient with a frontotemporoparietal infarction and hemi-inattention to his left hemispace is instructed to shave his entire face with an electric razor in front of a mirror. The therapist records the number of verbal cues required to remind him that he is not yet finished whenever he stops. In addition, the therapist tallies the number of times he discontinues the task, the amount of facial area shaved after a given time, and the total time to completion with cues as needed. The targeted behavior is monitored daily during morning self-care activities.

In another variation, the therapist sets the goal of no choking during six feedings in a day for a dysphagic patient who coughs if liquids are swallowed quickly. The patient must remember to limit intake to one sip at a time with a straw and to properly position the head before each swallow. The number of times that the correct technique is used independently for the first dozen swallows is graphed over each of the six feedings. The graph also serves as visual feedback for the subject.

Table 7–11. A Strategy for Measuring Change in Behaviors

1. Specify a discrete target behavior and associated conditions.
2. Define an observable or measurable action that operationalizes the behavior.
3. Sample the behavior by a chosen measure, e.g., frequency or duration of the behavior in a given time.
4. Score subject on the measure 3 times before the intervention, at specified times while on the intervention, and after completing the intervention.

This measurement approach to assess behavioral changes over time has been employed especially in patients with TBI who show aberrant behaviors, such as agitation, poor impulse control, or poor listening skills. Rewards, such as tokens that can be used to buy candy or musical recordings, may reinforce appropriate behaviors when tied to better behavior. A behavioral approach lends itself to single-case study designs for testing an intervention. If the behavioral measurement is to be used across patients or to evaluate an intervention for statistical purposes, the investigator must assess for interrater reliability and use one of the graphing techniques described in the section on clinical trials in this chapter.

Neurobehavioral Scales

The Neuropsychiatric Inventory (NPI)[104] was developed to assess psychopathology in people with Alzheimer's disease. It also has great potential for studies of TBI, stroke, and other diseases that affect the frontal and temporal lobes. The NPI includes 10 neurobehavioral and 2 neurovegetative domains. An informed caregiver responds yes or no to the presence of symptoms for each domain and rates their frequency, severity, and the distress they cause the caregiver.

The Neurobehavioral Rating Scale, most often used in patients with TBI, is a structured interview with a formal mental status examination. It includes 27 variables that can be grouped as loading on the four factors shown in Table 7–12.[105] The tool had good reliability and validity in a French study of TBI.[106] The Agitated Behavior Scale, a 14-item instrument, documents agitated behaviors.[107] It has good interrater reliability and at least face validity by including, for example, short attention span, easy distractibility, and inability to concentrate as one item and impulsivity, impatience, and low tolerance for pain or frustration as another item. Very few clinicians who care for patients with TBI use the tool, however.[108]

MEASURES OF DISABILITY

In 1999, the prevalence rate of disability in American adults found by the U.S. Bureau of the Census and the Center For Disease Con-

Table 7–12. **The Neurobehavioral Rating Scale**

COGNITION/ENERGY	
Disorientation	Fatigue
Emotional withdrawal	Motor retardation
Conceptual disorganization	Blunted affect
Memory	

METACOGNITION	
Disinhibition	Thought content
Agitation	Excitement
Self-appraisal	Poor planning

SOMATIC/ANXIETY	
Somatic concern	Hostility
Anxiety	Suspiciousness
Depression	Tension

LANGUAGE	
Expressive deficit	Comprehension deficit

trol was approximately 22%. Difficulty climbing a flight of stairs and walking three city blocks was reported by 19 million people. The great majority of these disabilities were tied to health conditions such as arthritis, back and spine pain, and heart disease. The sequelae of neurologic diseases may pose even greater disability.

Several books provide thoughtful descriptions and comparisons of instruments that measure disabilities encountered in neurologic diseases,[8,63] and many articles have reviewed the reliability, validity, and sensitivity of the most frequently employed scales.[109] A minority of functional assessment scales were specifically developed for the neurologically disabled or for a rehabilitation setting.[110] Many instruments had their reliability and validity studies determined on a pediatric or geriatric population[111] or were designed for specific nonneurological diseases, such as cancer, mental illness, and arthritis.

Much effort has been devoted to developing broadly applicable scales that emphasize ADLs and instrumental ADLs (IADLs), which include tasks commonly carried out in the community. Table 7–13 lists some of the scales that have found use in neurologic rehabilitation

Table 7–13. **Measures of Functional Disability**

GENERAL
Barthel Index
Functional Independence Measure
Program Evaluation Conference System
Level of Rehabilitation Scale
Katz Index of ADLs
Klein-Bell ADL Scale
Rivermead ADL Index
Frenchay Activities Index
OPCS Disability Scales

GLOBAL	
Rankin Disability Scale	Karnofsky Scale
Glasgow Outcome Scale	

ADL, activity of daily living; OPCS, Office Population Censuses Surveys.

studies. Most scales include 3, 4, or 7 levels for the degree of dependency for each item. When a scale exceeds the levels of "independent," "needs assistance," and "dependent," guidelines are needed to rate reliably how the patient performs during a formal screening by a trained observer. The sensitivity of existing scales to clinically meaningful change during inpatient and outpatient therapy is controversial. The *Barthel Index* (BI) has a relatively long history in North America, Great Britain, and Australia and the *Functional Independence Measure* (FIM) has gained a strong foothold in the United States. The FIM and BI were designed around the issue of dependency, which

translates into the burden of care. Less often, scales such as the *Office Population Censuses Surveys* (OPCS) reflect more about the severity and dimensions of disability.

In the future, functional assessment tools may undergo the Rasch analysis described earlier, so they can be linked together. For example, a study demonstrated the feasibility of using the admission and discharge motor skills items of the FIM and the Patient Evaluation and Conference System (PECS) and creating scale values for all of the items in the same measurement units.[112] Ratings from each scale can then be interconverted in terms of the *rehabit*, the rehabilitation functional assessment measuring unit.

Activities of Daily Living

THE BARTHEL INDEX

The BI is a weighted scale of 10 activities, with maximum independence equal to a score of 100 (Table 7–14).[113] Items considered more important for independence are weighted more heavily. Patients who score 100 on the BI are continent; they feed, bathe, and dress themselves; get up out of bed and chairs; walk at least a block; and ascend and descend stairs. This score does not imply that patients can cook, keep house, live alone, and meet the public, but they can get along without attendant care if not aphasic. Scores below 61 on hospital discharge after a stroke predict a level of dependence that makes discharge to home less likely.[114,115] The BI and the FIM have been used for patient self-reports.[116] Although a correlation exists between

Table 7–14. **The Barthel Index**

	Help	Independent
1. Feeding (if food needs to be cut up = help)	5	10
2. Moving from wheelchair to bed and return (includes sitting up in bed)	5–10	15
3. Personal toilet (wash face, comb hair, shave, clean teeth)	0	5
4. Getting on and off toilet (handling clothes, wipe, flush)`	5	10
5. Bathing self	0	5
6. Walking on level surface (or, if unable to walk, propel wheelchair)	10	15
(°Score only if unable to walk)	0°	5°
7. Ascend and descend stairs	5	10
8. Dressing (include tying shoes, fastening fasteners)	5	10
9. Controlling bowels	5	10
10. Controlling bladder	5	10

the trained observer's findings and the patient's perceptions, well-defined disability assessments are best left to a trained therapist who takes the patient through the tasks.

No other scale to date has been used as much in studies of neurologic disease and for rehabilitation. European studies have used the same 10 categories for their version of the BI, but score different items from 0 to 1 up to 0 to 3, for a total maximum score of 20.[117] The BI has high reliability and validity for inpatient rehabilitation. It has floor and ceiling effects during outpatient care.[109] The BI has been employed in epidemiologic studies such as the Framingham Study to assess patients over time after stroke and to complement impairment measures in multicenter trials of acute interventions for stroke, TBI, and SCI. The BI has its limitations and weaknesses. As with most functional assessments, a change by a given number of points does not mean an equivalent change in disability across different activities. The BI has no language or cognitive measure, so another scale must be added or a highly revised form used. The BI, however, is the scale to which new ADL measures will be compared.

The BI has also been subject to modifications to try to increase its sensitivity to changes in disability. A scoring modification with 5, rather than 3 levels of dependence, was recommended by one study.[118] The Modified BI measures the functional ability to perform 15 tasks.[119] This variation includes a limited independence score for bowel and bladder continence, divides upper and lower body dressing, and adds donning a brace and care of the perineum. The Extended BI differs almost too much from the BI to bear its name. It contains 16 dimensions scored at three or four levels of independence, includes social and cognitive dimensions, and allows a maximum time for completing each ADL.[120]

THE FUNCTIONAL INDEPENDENCE MEASURE

The Task Force to Develop a Uniform Data System for Medical Rehabilitation (UDS$_{MR}$) introduced the FIM in 1986.[121] One of the expectations in designing the FIM was that it would be more sensitive than the BI to changes in functional status in patients during their rehabilitation. The WeeFIM was developed for pediatric patients.[122] The FIM has 18 items graded on 4-level and 7-level ordinal scales (Table 7–15). The lowest score is 18; 126 is the highest level of in-

dependent function. Its popularity arises in part from the remarkable support provided for users by the UDS$_{MR}$ Data Management Service at the State University of New York at Buffalo. A manual, videotape, training workshop, newsletter that offers ongoing examples of how to rate a particular level of activity (Tables 7–16 and 7–17), and computer software accompany a subscription. Users must pass a credentialing test. Data are aggregated at the central office. An institution can compare the scores of its patients with those of all facilities for over 20 disease/impairment categories. Data such as length of inpatient stay, discharge placement, age, mean admission and discharge total scores and subscores for self-care, sphincter control, mobility, locomotion,

Table 7–15. Functional Independence Measure

ITEMS	
Self-care	
Eating	Dressing upper body
Grooming	Dressing lower body
Bathing	Toileting
Sphincter control	
Bladder management	Bowel management
Mobility/transfers	
Bed-to-chair and wheelchair-to-chair transfer	Toilet transfer Tub and shower transfer
Locomotion	
Walking or wheelchair use	Climbing stairs
Communication	
Comprehension	Expression
Social cognition	
Social interaction Problem solving	Memory

BURDEN OF CARE RATING
7 - Complete independence (timely, safely)
6 - Modified independence (device)
5 - Supervision
4 - Minimal assistance (subject = 75% +)
3 - Moderate assistance (subject = 50% +)
2 - Maximal assistance (Subject = 25% +)
1 - Total assistance (Subject = 0% +)

Table 7–16. Description of Functional Independence Measure Levels of Function

INDEPENDENT (Another person is not required for the activity [no helper]).

7. Complete independence—All of the tasks described as making up the activity are typically performed safely without modification, assistive devices, or aids and within a reasonable time frame.

6. Modified independence—The activity involves any one or more of the following: an assistive device is required, more than a reasonable amount time is needed, or there are safety (risk) considerations.

DEPENDENT (Another person is required for either supervision or physical assistance for the activity to be performed, or it is not performed [requires helper]).

Modified Dependence—The patient expends half (50%) or more of the effort. The levels of assistance required are the following:

5. Supervision or setup—The patient requires no more help than standby assistance, cueing, or coaxing, without physical contact; or the helper sets up needed items or applies orthoses.

4. Minimal contact assistance—With physical contact, the patient requires no more help than touching and expends 75% or more of the effort.

3. Moderate assistance—The patient requires no more help than touching or expends half (50%) or more (up to 75%) of the effort.

Complete Dependence—The patient expends less than 50% of the effort. Maximal or total assistance is required, or the activity is not performed. The levels of assistance required are the following:

2. Maximal assistance—The patient expends less than 50% of the effort, but at least 25%.

1. Total assistance—The patient expends less than 25% of the effort.

Table 7–17. Definitions for Ambulation for the Functional Independence Measure*

NO HELPER

7. *Independent*: Patient can be left alone to walk a minimum of 150 feet safely, within a reasonable length of time, and without assistive devices.

6. *Independent with equipment*: Patient walks a minimum of 150 feet, but uses a brace (orthosis) or prosthesis on the leg, or special adaptive shoes, cane, crutches or walker, or takes more than a reasonable amount of time.

HELPER

5. *Supervision*: Verbal cueing, demonstration, "hands-off" guarding, or standby assistance may be necessary. Patient cannot be left alone to perform the activity safely, but does not require physical assistance or contact to perform the activity. Patient walks at least 50 feet.

4. *Minimal assistance*: Patient performs 75% or more of the task. May require "hands-on" or contact guarding. Patient walks at least 50 feet.

3. *Moderate assistance*: Patient performs 25%–50% of the task. Only one person is required for physical assistance. Patient walks at least 50 feet.

2. *Maximum assistance*: Patient performs 25%–50% of the task. Only one person is required for physical assistance. Patient walks at least 50 feet.

1. *Dependent*: Patient requires total physical assistance and performs less than 25% of the task. One or more persons may be required for performance of the activity.

*Defined as the ability to walk on a level surface indoors once in a standing position (not in parallel bars) and to negotiate barriers.

communication, and social cognition provide valuable insights into important descriptors of neurorehabilitation (see Tables 9–2 and 9–11).

Interrater reliability for the 4-level and 7-level scales is good.[123] A 4-level self-reported FIM is also reliable and valid and predicts the need for inpatient care in patients with MS and with SCI.[124] The FIM, particularly its mobility and ADL subscales, also correlates with the BI.[125] A Rasch analysis of 27,000 inpatients across 13 impairment groups showed that the FIM reflects a 13-item motor and a 5-item cognitive measure of function. This study also supported the FIM's construct validity and suggests that the FIM could be scaled as an interval measure.[126] The unidimensionality of the motor score, however, is relative and controversial.[109] The raw scores are not linear, so they are not appropriate for parametric statistical analyses.

The FIM detects the severity of disability among patients with neurologic disorders, correlates with the burden of required care, and broadly demonstrates responsiveness.[127] Across neurologic diseases, the FIM score on admission to a facility is the best predictor of function at discharge.[128] For a given FIM admission score, normative standards can be calculated for average expected gains (see Table 9–12) within a FIM impairment group.[129] These findings lend support to including the FIM when one develops rehabilitation resource use models. The FIM also predicts the burden of care at home for patients with stroke[130] and multiple sclerosis.[131] A change of one point in total FIM score corresponds to approximately 3.5 minutes of help from another person each day. The FIM does not predict the hours of supervision required.[132] It is a valid and responsive tool for assessing patients with MS,[133,134] although perhaps no more so than the BI.[135]

The FIM is a sound indicator of disability, but not the ideal instrument. Although the FIM includes a cognitive scale not represented in the BI, this domain has not been especially sensitive to change in patients undergoing inpatient rehabilitation for stroke or MS. The cognitive scale is too mid-range to adequately describe patients with stroke and TBI and this scale has a substantial ceiling effect for patients with SCI.[136] The social cognition and communication subscales show a ceiling effect compared to neuropsychologic testing.[137] In an attempt to capture the disabilities of patients with TBI, the FIM has been expanded with the clinically intuitive

Table 7–18. **Dimensions of the Functional Assessment Measure**

Swallowing	Emotional status
Car transfer	Adjustment to limitations
Community mobility	Orientation
Reading	Attention
Writing	Safety judgement
Speech intelligibility	

Functional Assessment Measure (Table 7–18). The additional items are reliable and valid, but may not add substantial responsiveness.[138]

The motor scale of the FIM does not reflect fine motor function, ease of completion of a task, quality of how the task is executed, time to complete a task, and whether an affected upper extremity is used at all. For patients who are independent ambulators, walking speed is more discriminative than the FIM motor score.[139] Climbing stairs is the FIM item that best distinguishes the higher level patient. Instrumental ADLs are not included in the measure. In a clinical trial, investigators would need additional measures, when relevant to the outcome, to assess these issues. An important aim in development of the FIM was to optimize its sensitivity to changes in the functional status of disabled people. Despite including more items and item response categories than the BI, the FIM may not be any more responsive than the BI for measuring physical disability across neurologic disorders.[135,138] In addition, the FIM is most responsive during inpatient rehabilitation. Like the BI, it shows a ceiling effect during outpatient neurorehabilitation, so it may not serve as a sensitive outcomes tool for testing interventions in outpatients. None of these limitations detract from the value of the FIM as a measure of burden of care during inpatient rehabilitation.

The data reports provided by the UDS_{MR} include a calculation of the length of stay efficiency—the mean change in FIM score per day of inpatient rehabilitation.[140] That the instrument is a measure of progress related to a rehabilitation program and, thus, to program quality is not clear, although the temptation is great for programs to use their data to compare themselves to the aggregate. Most individual inpatient rehabilitation units have too variable a case mix and too few cases to be able to apply a parametric analysis to their unit's data. For example, patients with higher initial functional status for a given diagnostic category have shorter lengths of stay. Patients with lower admission function on the FIM motor score stay longer in inpatient rehabilitation in the United States and their rates of gain are slower, but they improve as much.[141]

The total FIM score or its motor and cognitive subscores, combined with a patient's disease group and age, may predict the expected length of inpatient rehabilitation stay. This FIM-Functional Related Groups (FIM-FRG) classification had been proposed as a payment scheme, like that of the Diagnostic Related Groups for acute hospital care.[142,143] Starting in 2002, the seven-level tool has been incorporated into the Inpatient Rehabilitation Facility Patient Assessment Instrument for reimbursement of care by Medicare.

OTHER SCALES

The Katz ADLs Index rates six ADLs on a three-level scale, then grades the cumulative level of independence.[144] Although once widely used across many neurologic diseases, the tool does not include a dimension for ambulation. The scale lacks evidence for reliability and validity and may be sensitive to change only at an early stage of inpatient rehabilitation and in studies of elderly patients. The BI is a better tool. The Klein-Bell scale is a weighted scale with good test–retest reliability and seems about as responsive as the BI.[145] The Patient Evaluation Conference System (PECS, Marianjoy Inc.) has 115 items[146] in a 6-step ordinal scale ranging from independence to dependence for the domains of mobility, self-care, communication, occupation and social relations, as well as a version with 44 items in 4 subscales.[147] It is designed to reveal progress in rehabilitation for specific goals. The PECS data can be transformed into interval, unidimensional measures, which improve the measurement properties of its items.[5] The items transition from ADLs to IADLs.

Instrumental Activities of Daily Living

The Frenchay Activities Index (FAI) was developed for patients with chronic stroke,[148] but it is of value for the assessment of daily activities beyond those measured by the FIM and BI for a middle-class, adult neurologic population. The Index is listed in Table 7–19 as an example of the items that may be included in IADLs. The FAI addresses a ceiling effect of the FIM in assessing disability and handicap. It takes 5–10 minutes to complete. Reliability and construct validity appear good when the test is used to discriminate between prestroke and poststroke function in domestic and outdoor activities.[149] Question 8 was a sensitive measure of outcome in a chronic stroke rehabilitation trial, although not as sensitive as the time required to walk 10 meters.[150] The Rivermead ADL Index,[151] employed primarily for patients with stroke, includes 16 self-care skills (but excludes incontinence) and 15 household and community tasks that are scored as "independent," "verbal assistance," or "dependent." It can also be scored as "independent" or "needs help." Operational definitions improve its reliability. Studies of another predominantly IADL scale, the Extended ADL Scale (EADL), have shown content and construct validity and good reliability for an outpatient stroke population.[152] The EADL's scores for important home activities correlate with measures of disability, perceived health, mood, and satisfaction. Instrumental ADL scales can be sensitive to gender, racial, cultural, and social class differences, so care must be taken when using them as outcome tools.

Mixed Functional Scales

Some scales reflect ratings of impairment and disability. The Office Population Census Survey (OPCS) Scale[63] is an even more inclusive set of disabilities that are operationally defined, weighted, and scored as "done" or "not accomplished." This scale includes dimensions related to locomotion, reaching that would be needed for dressing, dexterity with common objects, self-care, continence, vision, audition, communication, feeding, and cognitive function that, in general, have face validity for neurologic patients. Although designed for a British survey of disability, OPCS statements about functioning have a hierarchic quality that may show responsiveness to change if further studied. For example, the OPCS scales measure levels of disability in neurologically im-

Table 7–19. **The Frenchay Activities Index**

IN THE LAST 3 MONTHS

1. Preparing main meals (needs to play substantial part in organization, preparation, and cooking of main meal—not just making snacks). [1 = never, 2 = <1 time per week, 3 = 1–2 times per week, 4 = most days]
2. Washing up (must do it all after a meal, or share equally, e.g., washing or wiping and putting away—not just doing occasional item). [1 = never, 2 = <1 time per week, 3 = 1–2 times per week, 4 = most days]
3. Washing clothes (organization of washing and drying of clothes, whether in washing machine, by hand wash, or at launderette). [1 = never, 2 = 1–2 times in 3 months, 3 = 3–12 times in 3 months, 4 = ≥1 time per week]
4. Light housework (dusting; vacuum cleaning 1 room). [1 = never, 2 = 1–2 times in 3 months, 3 = 3–12 times in 3 months, 4 = ≥1 time per week]
5. Heavy housework (all housework including beds, floors, etc.). [1 = never, 2 = 1–2 times in 3 months, 3 = 3–12 times in 3 months, 4 = ≥1 time per week]
6. Local shopping (playing a substantial role in organizing and buying shopping, whether small or large amounts—not just pushing a trolley). [1 = never, 2 = 1–2 times in 3 months, 3 = 3–12 times in 3 months, 4 = ≥1 time per week]
7. Social outings (going out to clubs, church activities, cinema, theater, drinking, to dinner with friends, etc.). [1 = never, 2 = 1–2 times in 3 months, 3 = 3–12 times in 3 months, 4 = ≥1 time per week]
8. Walking outside > 15 minutes (sustained walking, approximately 1 mile, short stops for breath allowed). [1 = never, 2 = 1–2 times in 3 months, 3 = 3–12 times in 3 months, 4 = ≥1 time per week]
9. Actively pursuing hobby (must be "active" participation, e.g., knitting, painting, games, sports—not just watching sport on TV). [1 = never, 2 = 1–2 times in 3 months, 3 = 3–12 times in 3 months, 4 = ≥1 time per week]
10. Driving car/bus travel. [1 = never, 2 = 1–2 times in 3 months, 3 = 3–12 times in 3 months, 4 = ≥1 time per week]

IN THE LAST 6 MONTHS

11. Outings/car rides (coach or rail trips, or car rides, but involving some organization and decision-making by the patient). [1 = never, 2 = 1–2 times in 3 months, 3 = 3–12 times in 3 months, 4 = ≥1 time per week]
12. Gardening (light = occasional weeding, lawn mowing; moderate = regular weeding, lawn mowing; all necessary = all necessary work, including heavy digging). [1 = never, 2 = light, 3 = moderate, 4 = all necessary]
13. Household/car maintenance (light = repairing small items; moderate = some painting, decorating, routine car maintenance, and repairs; heavy = most of the necessary household or car maintenance, and repairs). [1 = never, 2 = light, 3 = moderate, 4 = all necessary]
14. Reading books (must be full-length books—not magazines, periodicals, or papers). 1 = none, 2 = 1 in 6 months, 3 = <1 in 2 weeks, 4 = >1 in 2 weeks]
15. Gainful work. [1 = none, 2 = <10 hours per week, 3 = 10–30 hours per week, 4 = >30 hours per week]

paired patients over time that are beyond the ceiling effect of the BI and were more sensitive to change in severely disabled patients.[153]

The National Highway Traffic Safety Administration proposed the adoption of its Functional Capacity Index.[154] This little-used tool employs 3–6 levels to grade eating, excretory function, sexual function, ambulation, hand and arm function, bending and lifting, vision and audition, speech, and cognition. The tool does not appear to be compromised by the floor and ceiling effects of most scales and requires patients to use the affected upper extremity. The Index deserves further study.

Several scales have been especially practical outcome measures for large clinical trials.

The Karnofsky Performance Status Scale was developed in the 1950s for oncology clinical trials and has been used occasionally in studies of patients with TBI or brain tumor. The scale ranges from normal without disease, to symptoms and signs of disease, to levels of required assistance, to death. The Rankin Scale (Table 7–20) has a special niche in stroke trials. The high interrater reliability of these 5-step scales makes them especially useful for multicenter studies. For example, the National Institutes of Health trial of tissue plasminogen activator in acute stroke revealed that use of tPA within 3 hours of onset of stroke in selected patients led to a greater percentage of patients to have a Rankin score of 0 and 1 and an almost impairment-free NIHSS. In addition, the study suggested that a score of >17 on the NIHSS at 24 hours post-stroke plus atrial fibrillation or a score >16 at 7–10 days predicts a Rankin score at 3 months of 4 or 5 or death.[155] Impairment and disability were related especially at the extremes of no impairment and great impairment. The Karnofsky and Rankin Scales mix impairment, disability, and handicap. The measures are too insensitive to detect clinically important outcomes in individuals during their course of rehabilitation. The measures may be combined with the BI, but tend to correlate with BI scores in population studies and large interventional trials for acute stroke and TBI.

DISEASE-SPECIFIC SCALES

Brain Injury

The Glasgow Outcome Scale (GOS) is a global physical, economic, and social measure, best reserved for large clinical trials (Table 7–21).[14] As a rehabilitation assessment tool, the GOS is too global to be sensitive to gradual functional progress. It does not indicate changes in specific functional, cognitive, and behavioral abilities nor neurologic impairments.

The Disability Rating Scale (DRS) is an impairment and disability measure for TBI with prognostic value for the ability to return to employability.[156] The DRS is easy to use and reliable.[156] It has concurrent and predictive validity in assessing patients with moderate to severe TBI from time of onset through 10 years of follow-up.[156] The DRS domains include the eye opening, verbalization, and motor responsiveness of the Glasgow Coma Score, the cognitive skills needed for feeding, toileting, and grooming, and the overall level of dependence and employability. The summated disability score falls within 1 of 10 categories that range from no disability (0) to death (30). The DRS is fairly sensitive to change in patients with an acute hospital admission GCS score of 4–12 who are transferred to rehabilitation. The DRS appears least sensitive to functional changes for patients with mild TBI and for patients with severe impairment in which the score exceeds 22. The DRS is more sensitive than the GOS to change.[157] During outpatient follow-up, four additional five-point scores added to the DRS assess the impact of physical and mental impairment on work and living.[156]

Table 7–20. **The Modified Rankin Scale**

Score	Outcome
0	No symptoms at all
1	No significant disability despite symptoms; able to carry out usual duties and activities
2	Slight disability: unable to carry out some previous activities, but looks after own affairs without assistance
3	Moderate disability: requires some help, but walks without assistance
4	Moderately severe disability: unable to walk without assistance and do bodily care without help
5	Severe disability: bedridden, incontinent, and requires constant nursing care and attention

Table 7–21. **Glasgow Outcome Scale**

Score	Outcome
1	Death
2	Vegetative: unresponsive and speechless
3	Severe disability: dependent on others for all or part of care/supervision because of mental or physical disability.
4	Moderate disability: disabled, but independent in ADLs and community.
5	Good recovery: resumption of normal life; may have minor neurologic or psychologic deficits

ADL, activities of daily living.

Parkinson's Disease

The United Parkinson's Disease Rating Scale (UPDRS) also mixes the concepts of impairment and disability, but it serves as one of the more standard measures of change for studies of the disease and for drug interventions. The tool is less likely to reveal changes in disability for a specific rehabilitation intervention in a clinical trial, but the UPDRS may help stratify patients for severity of disease.

Multiple Sclerosis

The Extended Disability Status Scale (EDSS) is a standard tool in MS studies that reliably and validly offers a measure of impairment and disability, loaded toward walking. The EDSS is less than optimally responsive to interventions and disease progression.[134] A change in EDSS score of 1–2 in the 20-step scale is considered significant in most large studies. A population size of approximately 45 subjects per group is required to detect, with a power of 80%, a difference of 20% in the proportion of patients changing by one point.[158] In a large cross-correlational study, the MSFC, described earlier, correlated closely to EDSS scores.[12] The Guy's Neurological Disability Scale (GNDS) was developed for interviewers to capture the more common disabilities encountered by patients with MS in the past month.[159] Initial studies suggest that the GNDS is responsive and valid and can be given over the phone or by mail.

Stroke

The Stroke Impact Scale (www2.kumc.edu/coa) is a self-report measure with 64 items that assess 8 domains, including strength, hand function, ADLs, IADLs, mobility, communication, memory, emotion, thinking, and participation.[160] Patients respond to each question on a Likert scale with five choices, for example, from "not difficult at all" to "extremely difficult." Reliability, validity, and responsiveness between 1 and 6 months poststroke are good and the tool may not have the floor and ceiling effects of the BI and the SF-36 (see below). A clinically meaningful change was estimated to be 10 to 15 points. The scale is in its third revision.

Another new offering is the American Heart Association Stroke Outcome Classification (AHA.SOC).[161] This scale rates impairments, basic self-care skills, and instrumental ADLs. The number of impairments and severity of impairments on a 3 to 0 scale are graded for motor, sensory, visual, affective, cognitive, and language deficits. Five levels, from independence to complete dependence, are graded for the combination of basic (feeding, swallowing, grooming, dressing, bathing, continence, toileting, and mobility) and instrumental (using the telephone, handling money, using transportation, maintaining a household or job, participating in leisure activities) ADLs. The scales have high interrater reliability.

Spinal Cord Injury

Although the BI and FIM can be used for studies of patients with SCI as measures of burden of care, several specific tools have been developed based on the disabilities of these patients. The Quadriplegia Index of Function (QIF) has good interobserver reliability and may be more sensitive than the BI and Kenny Self-Care Evaluation for small, but important functional gains.[162] The QIF includes 10 categories with relative weights for each component activity that add up to a normal score of 100. The Spinal Cord Independence Measure (SCIM) also includes dimensions that are relevant to patients with quadriplegia, such as the ability to use upper extremity assistive devices and to do intermittent catheterization. The tool also includes ratings for maneuvers to avoid pressure sores and mobility for indoor and outdoor distances with an electric or manual wheelchair or with assistive devices.[163]

Depression

Scales for depression and personality profiles such as the Minnesota Multiphasic Personality Inventory augment the assessment of neurologic symptoms that cause disability. These scales include vegetative symptoms, however, which may confound interpretation in disabled people who may be more sedentary and fatigable because of their physical impairments, not from a disorder of mood. The more frequently used self-rating depression scales include the 30-item Geriatric Depression Scale and the 20-item Center for Epidemiologic Studies Depression Scale. In a study of depression in geriatric stroke patients, the Zung

Scale had the highest predictive value.[164] The Beck Depression Inventory (BDI) is another reliable and valid self-administered tool to distinguish among people who are likely to be depressed.[8] A cutoff score of 13, for example, had a sensitivity of 0.71 and specificity of 0.79 for major depression in patients who have MS.[165] The BDI, like most of the self-rating scales, takes from 8 to 15 minutes to complete. Examiner rating scales with good reliablility include the Hamilton Rating Scale, the Cornell Scale, and the Comprehensive Psychopathological Rating Scale—Depression. Items from QOL scales also reflect depression and mood changes over time. All of these scales must be thought of as screening tools for depression. The scales do not make a final diagnosis for or against a mood disorder.

Pediatric Diseases

A modest number of instruments may be of value for clinical outcomes research in children.[166] The WeeFIM, mentioned earlier, includes FIM items and correlates with the degree neurologic impairments.[122] The Pediatric Evaluation of Disability Inventory (PEDI) is a longer questionnaire that includes items about caregiver assistance and environmental modifications.[167]

MEASURES OF HEALTH-RELATED QUALITY OF LIFE

Measures of QOL use the patient's perspective to assess domains that include physical, mental, social, and general health.[168] These tools evaluate the overall impact of health or of a disease and its treatment. A well-designed instrument for rehabilitation reveals what patients believe is important for them to work on and may inform clinicians about areas in need of additional support.

Scales include a variety of dimensions within each of the typical QOL domains. Some of the components are listed in Table 7–22. These measures made their first impact in oncologic and medical studies,[169,170] but should have a natural home in patient-oriented rehabilitation. The tools also provide surveillance assessments for institutional health care providers and agencies. Although the conceptualization, reliability, and validity of QOL instruments need contin-

Table 7–22. Dimensions of Health-Related Quality of Life Domains

PHYSICAL HEALTH
Mobility and self-care
Level of physical activity
Pain
Role limitations with family and work

MENTAL HEALTH
Psychological and emotional well-being and distress
Cognitive functioning and distress
Role limitations

SOCIAL WELL-BEING
Social supports
Home and social roles
Sexuality
Participation in work, hobbies
Social contacts and interactions
Role limitations

GENERAL HEALTH
Medical symptoms
Energy, fatigue
Sleep difficulty
Changes in health
Life satisfaction
Health perceptions and distresses
Overall perception of Quality of Life

ued research, measures of QOL have become one of the expected outcome measures in clinical trials of physical, pharmacologic, and surgical interventions. The tools offer interesting insights about disability as well. For example, these measures have shown that the strongest predictor of life satisfaction among disabled adults was satisfaction with leisure activities.[171] In another study, a battery of instruments revealed that following a stroke, patients had greater depression, caused more stress for their relatives, and were less socially active than a control group.[172] In a study of MS, a QOL instrument showed the impact of the disease in meaningful ways that the EDSS did not.[173]

Clinical trials, at least those that face the inspection of the U.S. Food and Drug Administration (FDA), have permitted only one primary outcome measure. That focus may work for death, stroke, or myocardial infarction as the outcome measure, but may not hold for many other medical, surgical, and rehabilitative interventions. New emphasis is being placed on what may be thought of as the *misery index* of a treatment. Even if a drug or surgical treatment lessens the risk for bad outcomes or increases the likelihood of better outcomes, is the intervention worthwhile to the individual subject? Measures of QOL may help tease apart this notion. Clinical trials reviewed by the FDA have also recently used a scale for clinicians that asks for a *global clinical impression* about the intervention and outcome, as well as a *global subject impression* scale for participants in the trial. For trials of rehabilitative interventions, reports of QOL and global impression may help researchers get a handle on outcomes that may be confounded by problems that range from the sensitivity and specificity of measurement instruments to the very different ways that individual subjects adapt to disabilities.

Disease-specific QOL tools are also being designed and tested. Greater specificity about the difficulties and expectations of patients with particular diseases that cause serious disabilities may be better reflected in the questions posed by disease-specific as opposed to generic QOL tools. Most generic instruments were developed for people with routine medical conditions or for population studies of elderly people.

For patients with chronic diseases and no serious cognitive dysfunction, physician and caregiver observations have generally not substituted for the patient's own perception of most QOL domains.[174] A patient's cognitive and communicative impairments may, however, limit the utility of QOL tools. In one study, proxy agreement was poor for the Health Status Questionnaire in people with stroke and cognitive impairment, but good between patient and caregiver for the FIM and the FAI.[175]

Instruments

The instruments in Table 7–23 offer comprehensiveness and ease of administration. They are representative of the range of ways that questions have been asked and scored.

Table 7–23. **Generic Instruments for Quality of Life**

Sickness Impact Profile
Functional Limitations Profile
Medical Outcomes Study SF-12 and SF-36
Functional Status Questionnaire
Nottingham Health Profile
Quality of Well-Being Scale

GENERAL TOOLS

The Sickness Index Profile (SIP)[176] provides 136 statements grouped into 12 categories around physical and psychosocial dimensions. The statements are weighted for scoring that reflects dependence, distress, and social isolation. The SIP primarily assesses the negative impact of disability, including the impact on work, recreation, and eating. The Functional Limitations Profile is a British version. The SIP-NH (Nursing Homes) is a 68-item scale drawn from the items in the SIP. This SIP-68 eliminates unnecesary components and has good reliability.[177] The SIP has been used in studies of stroke, TBI, SCI and other neurologic diseases. It may be more responsive to group than to individual changes.[8] A 30-item version of the SIP that retained the SIP's physical and psychosocial dimensions had similar construct, clinical, and external validities as the full version for patient with stroke.[178] Using a format similar to the SIP, the Nottingham Health Profile[8] asks about emotions more directly than does the SIP and has good reliability and validity in some populations.

The Health Status Questionnaire[179] grew out of the Medical Outcomes Study (MOS) questionnaire and another study by the RAND Corporation aimed at constructing scales sensitive to changes in functioning associated with changing health. This health-related QOL survey has taken the form of 12, 20,[180] 36, and 74 questions that cover all domains with a progressively greater number of dimensions.[181] The Short Form (SF)-12 generates the physical and mental component summary scores of the SF-36 in some groups of patients after a stroke.[182] The SF-36 version (a 39-item version includes 3 items that screen for depression) has received much support for its ability to distinguish between ill

Quality of life questions must reflect the patient's experience and personal perception. Otherwise, the questions merely rate health status, much like a disability measure.

The Functional Status Questionnaire's (FSQ) psychologic and emotional functioning questions offer six typical choices for answers, such as "Have you felt downhearted and blue (1) all of the time, (2) most of the time, (3) a good bit of the time, (4) some of the time, (5) a little bit of the time, (6) none of the time?" The physical functioning scale asks how much the subject is limited (a lot, a little, not at all) with the lowest level for mobility "walking one block." The FSQ includes questions about difficulty encountered in the past month in "moving in and out of a bed or chair" and "walking indoors" with possible responses of "(0) usually did not do for other reasons, (1) usually did not do because of health, (2) usually did with much difficulty, (3) usually did with some difficulty, (4) usually did with no difficulty."

For acute inpatient use, the physical well-being dimensions of a QOL instrument may not provide a meaningful inquiry about physical functioning. These dimensions do not strike within the ranges of function of most inpatients. The sensitivity of typical QOL questions to change with outpatient rehabilitation has not been established. Sensitivity to change may be increased with an additional patient-specific transition index.[212] Using this approach, one asks patients at baseline about their maximum physical activity, the mental activity that takes the most concentration, and their most stressful or emotionally difficult problem. At follow-up, the transition index asks whether and how these elements have changed. For example, are they much better, slightly better, the same, slightly worse, or much worse?

Visual analogue scales can also be helpful, at least as far as a single global measure can provide information. Patients mark their level of QOL from the worst to the best on a 7-step or 10-step ladder, or they may circle one of the faces on a row that gradually changes from a frown to a smile.[8] This approach serves as a helpful screen for the clinician who wants to learn how the patient perceives life with disabilities. Some investigators strongly recommend a single global rating, because it reflects the disparate values and preferences of individual patients.[213] Indeed, the notion of QOL is, at best, idiosyncratic and, at worst, merely another reflection of the questions that healthy people imagine will concern disabled people.

MEASURES OF HANDICAP

Handicap related to neurologic disease has received less attention than impairments, disabilities, and QOL. A major premise about handicap, conceptualized as the social disadvantage resulting from impairments and disabilities, is that handicap may be lessened without an attempt to diminish impairment or disability, for example, by improving access to the home. The World Health Organization Handicap Scale[214] designates 8 graded categories to describe the difference between an individual's performance or status and what that person expects of himself or herself or of people who are in a similar situation. The domains assessed include orientation and interaction with the surroundings, physical independence in ADLs, mobility, occupation, social integration, and economic self-sufficiency. Although this scale includes some guidelines for rating patients, its reliability is uncertain.

The Craig Handicap Assessment and Reporting Technique (CHART)[215] uses the same dimensions as the WHO scale and attempts to define them in measurable, behavioral terms. For example, mobility is measured by the hours per day spent out of bed and multiplied by 2, plus the days per week spent out of bed and multiplied by 5. Another 20 points are given for spending nights away from home and for independence in transportation. The answers to its 27 questions are weighted so that each of the 5 dimensions is worth 100 points when answers reflect no handicap. Reliability and validity are good when the CHART measure is applied to able-bodied persons and to patients with chronic SCI.[215] A Rasch analysis defined 11 statistically distinct handicap strata and a linearity consistent with interval data. The instrument has been employed mostly for patients with SCI.

The London Handicap Scale includes 6 self-report items about what a person may achieve in everyday life and the help required, with total scores ranging from 0 (maximum handicap) to 100 (no handicap).[216] The scale is reliable and showed responsiveness in a study of the effects of rehabilitation on patients with MS.[217,218]

The most recent World Health Organization concept of handicap is more about participation than about social disadvantage. Some instruments that assess community reintegration report on participation. The Reintegration to Normal Living Index[219] is a valid and reliable 11-item scale of participation in recreational, social, family, and community activities.[219] This tool may be a useful addendum for clinical trials in rehabilitation across diseases. The three-point scale is easier than the four-point scale for subjects to self-assess and is reliable for telephone interviews.[220] The Community Integration Questionnaire has 15 items that assess home and social reintegration and productivity primarily in patients after TBI.[221] The Community Integration Measure assesses readjustment to community life after disability with 10 items that center on belonging and participation.[222]

Many batteries and a few individual measures have been used to assess vocational rehabilitation,[223] but a more uniform measure for the ability to return to work across many types of employment is wanting.[224]

MEASURES OF COST-EFFECTIVENESS

An analysis of the ratio of the costs to the benefits of one intervention compared to another aims to establish both the value of an intervention and priorities for the allocation of resources. Measures of total direct and indirect costs, including future costs and benefits beyond the time of the intervention, may be operationally difficult and costly to obtain. For example, to fully determine the cost-effectiveness of an intervention such as outpatient day care for patients with MS or stroke, data about expenses ought to be collected for visits to physician's offices and emergency rooms, hospitalizations, pharmaceutical purchases such as antibiotics for bladder infections, and additional durable medical equipment. A bibliography of rehabilitation studies that includes a cost-effectiveness analysis is found at www.aapmr.org/memphys/cebfinala.htm. Types of cost analyses include cost effectiveness, cost benefit, cost minimization, cost utility, and length of stay.[225] The Cochrane Database of Systematic Reviews (American College of Physicians, Philadelphia, PA) also includes several rehabilitation-related analyses.

Cost-effective analyses ought to include explicit statements about the following issues: the perspective of the analysis; benefits; cost data, including program and treatment costs; costs of adverse reactions; averted costs; induced costs; the use of discounting if the timing of costs and benefits differ; a sensitivity analysis; and summary measures.[226]

The meaning of an analysis of benefit is no better than its outcome measures of disability, QOL, or complications of receiving and not receiving an intervention. The interpretation of these analyses, whether a cost is worth the benefit, depends especially upon the particular culture's socioeconomic capabilities and health agenda.

STUDY DESIGNS FOR REHABILITATION RESEARCH

Designs for research in neurologic rehabilitation began to receive much needed attention in professional journals and symposia approximately 10 years ago, particularly among physiatrists and physical therapists.[227,228] Academic and community rehabilitation programs had, in general, not fostered the activity of clinical scientists and rigorous research in rehabilitation settings and training programs. Indeed, many programs viewed rigorous research designs, such as the randomized controlled trial, as too difficult, impractical, or unethical.[229] These biases contributed to the problem that clinical research and the application of basic research have been less productive in rehabilitation medicine compared to most other fields of medicine. The National Center for Medical Rehabilitation Research at the National Institutes of Health has targeted this problem in its agenda for research and scientific training.[2] Clinical practices should be based on sound evidence for their efficacy. This burden on all rehabilitationists can also be their calling.

Clinical trials in neurorehabilitation fall into at least three general categories. These include physical, cognitive, and psychosocial training to improve function, pharmacologic and modality interventions to improve function or lessen symptoms, and neural repair strategies to enable substitutive biologic changes that enhance function. Trials of drugs and surgeries take 3 forms under the guidelines of the U.S. Food and Drug Administration and the National Institutes of Health, adding complexity at each step.

Phase I. This step involves a relatively high-risk or novel intervention for a small number of subjects. Establishing safety and examining responsiveness are the primary goals.

Phase II. This follows the Phase I trial and builds upon knowledge of risks. More subjects are involved. Safety and possible efficacy are studied. Different dosages of a medication or intensity of an intervention are determined, along with the best research methodology and outcome measures for Phase III.

Phase III. The potential efficacy of the intervention is determined by a blinded randomized trial, comparing the new intervention to another or to no intervention. The number of patients needed to show statistically significant differences may be drawn from the phase II studies.

Ethical Considerations

Clinical research often includes tensions and conflicts between the role of a clinician and the role of a scientist.[230] Several matters extend beyond the rigorous standards of creating an informed consent document and obtaining consent for participation in human research. The clinician and the volunteer who is a patient should acknowledge their conflicts of interest, and not only when the clinician or volunteer receives remuneration for participation. The clinician must balance the patient's welfare and needs for medical care with the goal of obtaining information about how to manage patients better based on the evidence gained from clinical trials. Volunteers must recognize that their participation is voluntary and their hope that participation may result in a better therapy for them is not the sole reason to engage in research. Subjects may receive a standard or placebo intervention, so they must be willing to stay on course in the trial whether or not that is their assignment.

Clinicians in a multicenter clinical trial or a trial with an outside sponsor such as a pharmaceutical company are obligated to understand for themselves the potential risks and benefits of the trial. Clinicians ought to review preliminary data and the design of the trial to convince themselves that it is well conceived, that the intervention carries at least face valid-

ity, and the trial stands a reasonable chance for successful completion. Finally, clinicians must ask themselves whether they will be able to sustain their time and energy in a trial, whether they are prepared for the tedious administrative tasks of a trial, and whether the modest opportunity for delayed gratification is adequate motivation.

DATA SAFETY MONITORING COMMITTEE

Clinical research that involves risk to subjects ought to be monitored by an external Data Safety Monitoring Committee (DSMC).[231] A DSMC participates in phase I, II, and III trials. This group usually includes a clinician familiar with the patient population and experimental and conventional interventions for the clinical problem and a statistician. The DSMC reviews the protocol, makes periodic assessments of the quality of the data, of the timeliness of data collection and entry, of patient accrual and retention rates, of the performance of each participating site, of participant risk versus benefit, of unanticipated risks, of alternate therapeutic approaches that arise during the trial, and of the methods and success of maintaining confidentiality about subjects. The committee may plan an interim analysis of the data to determine whether the study is likely to show efficacy. A DSMC may stop the trial if risks are greater than described to the subjects, if data is flawed, or if accrual rates of subjects are too slow. More often, a study is halted because an interim statistical analysis of the primary endpoints reveals that the final data are very unlikely to show benefit, sometimes called the futility of proceeding.

Types of Clinical Trials

Table 7–25 lists some of the designs used in a clinical neurologic rehabilitation setting for interventional studies. Specific designs have been explained in texts and articles.[102,232,233] When clinicians consider the results of studies for their evidence-based practices, they may classify the level of evidence based, in part, on the design of the trial.[234] Class I studies include prospective, blinded, and randomized clinical trials. Class II studies include prospective cohort studies, retrospective case-control studies,

Table 7–25. **Clinical Research Designs for Interventions**

DESCRIPTIVE

Case study

Cross-sectional survey

Cohort study

One experimental group treat and test

One experimental group treat and test versus test nonrandomized control group

One experimental group test, treat, retest

INFERENTIAL

Quasi-experimental

Multiple treated cohort groups versus multiple untreated control cohort groups

Experimental group test, treat, test versus nonrandomized control group test, no treatment, test

Experimental group test, test, treat, test, test, remove treatment or use placebo, test

Experimental group test, test, treat, test, remove treatment or use placebo, test, treat, test

Small Clinical Trials

Single-subject designs

　N-of-1 randomized, blinded trial

　　Single time series with repeated baselines

　　Time series with repeated introduction of intervention

　Sequential design

　Decision analysis-based design

Experimental

Randomized, blinded experimental versus control parallel groups

Randomized, blinded factorial design

Randomized, blinded matched pairs

Randomized, blinded withdrawal design

Randomized, blinded block design

Randomized, blinded cross-over design

and clinical series with appropriate controls. Class III studies include a clinical series without control subjects or a small series with a single-subject design. Regardless of the integrity of the trial design, an intervention does not meet the optimal standard for routine incorporation into practice until the study has been replicated by another investigator in another group of similar subjects.

In the past, too much emphasis has fallen on descriptive designs, often with retrospectively gathered data. Case studies and tests on a single group generate no more than pilot information. Such observational studies carry little strength in terms of causal inference about the intervention and its outcomes. The results of these approaches may be gutted by expected and unforseen biases. The design of an observational study must still be rigorous and ethical, by determining the appropriateness and risk of the intervention under examination for the cohort, by fixing a reasonable time to assess risks and outcomes, and by adjusting for any differences in the susceptibility to the outcomes. Quasi-experimental designs can be more inferential, but may lack scientific integrity because they do not randomize patients. Indeed, most use no control or comparison group or they rely on historical controls. Research conclusions from a quasi-experimental design may be strengthened by treatments and outcome measures performed in a blinded fashion.

RANDOMIZED TRIALS

The randomized, double-blind controlled trial is the most acceptable design to determine statistically significant differences between two interventions, one of which can be a placebo. Randomization aims to create treatment groups that are similar with respect to other potential determinants of outcome. This method allows the investigator to reach a conclusion, or an inference in the statistician's terms, about the relative merits of an intervention in the face of potential sampling bias and variations in the effects of the intervention.

A review of clinical trials outside of rehabilitation showed a significant correlation between randomized and nonrandomized studies, especially for prospective trials.[235] Discrepancies beyond chance and differences in the estimated magnitude of treatment effect were common, however, in these medical and surgical trials. Differences may be greater for rehabilitation trials, in which sampling error, the diversity of neurologic-related impairments and disabilities, and measurable outcomes pose even greater potential confounds. In a review of 124 trials in stroke rehabilitation with a meta-analysis of 36 trials, Ottenbacher and colleagues found that the type of research design affected the values for the mean effect size of the intervention.[236] In nonrandomized trials, failure to have blinded the recording of outcome measures led to smaller differences in outcomes compared to designs that included blinding. In randomized or controlled trials, the mean effect size was not affected by whether those who performed the outcome measures were blinded.

Blinding or masking the intervention lessens the risk for bias, however. Double blinding means that the subject and blinded observer who performs outcome measures do not know which treatment was assigned by the randomization procedure. The investigator also should not know the assignment when feasible. This approach works well for pharmacologic interventions, but may not be practical when the intervention involves physical therapy. Single blinding, if necessary, means that only the person who carries out the outcome measures, the blinded observer, is not aware of the intervention assignment.

Bias means a deviation of the results or inferences from the truth. Bias may arise from a conscious or unconscious selection of study procedures that produces results that depart from the truth, such as the trial's design, data acquisition, analysis, or interpretation. Deviations may also come from a unidirectional variation in measurements or flaws in measurements or analyses.

Randomized clinical trials (RCTs) with an experimental versus control group are complex affairs to develop and to carry to fruition. Table 7–26 provides a checklist of the more important features that the investigators ought to address. For reporting the results of an RCT, the *Journal of the American Medical Association* checklist provides valuable guidance.[237,238] The RCT lends itself to multicenter trials, unless the impact of the treatment is so large that its probability of detection will be high even with a relatively small representative population. Under some circumstances, a cross-over design in which the control group later receives the experimental intervention may increase the statistical power of a study.

While the RCT is nearly a gold standard, a single trial that demonstrates that one intervention is superior to another may not provide definitive evidence. Confounding issues in trials may limit their internal validity and generalizability. Several trials that demonstrate effi-

cacy by using a similar design add to the acceptability of a therapeutic intervention as being significantly better.

OTHER SMALL TRIAL DESIGNS

The Institute of Medicine has issued suggestions for the design of clinical trials that involve the small number of subjects that are often available for neurorehabilitation research.[239a] These trials will not have the statistical power, precision, and validity of larger trials. The research question must be streamlined, entry criteria strict, treatment procedures uniform, the sample group and outcomes for individuals clearly described so that a reader can relate the subjects to his or her own and so a meta-analysis can be applied one day, and alternative statistical designs may have to be explored. Most of these designs require some modeling and ongoing assessment of the probability of effectiveness of the intervention as subjects are entered.[239a] The most straightforward and naturalistic design is the n-of-1 approach.

Single-Subject Trials

Single subject or N-of-1 randomized controlled trials have been advocated to establish a definite clinical and, sometimes, a statistical answer to the question of whether or not a drug intervention alters a symptom for a particular patient.[239] For example, a patient with a SCI who has frequent, distressing flexor and extensor spasms may agree to a trial of clonidine, baclofen, or tizanidine versus a placebo. A pharmacist, with the patient's consent, can prepare the medications in unidentifiable capsules. The patient and physician are blinded to which agent the patient has been randomized for each 2-week study period. Each day, the patient grades symptoms on a 7-point scale: (1) a very great deal of trouble or distress, (2) a great deal, (3) a good deal, (4) a moderate amount, (5) some, (6) very little, and (7) no trouble or distress. The two treatments are then graphed against each other for visual inspection. The mean difference in symptom score per question between active and placebo periods can be submitted to a paired t test (Table 7–27). Other drugs or different dosages may be added in further trials. At least two pairs of treatments with similar results may be needed for each intervention to determine efficacy. Additional symptoms or interval measures can serve as outcomes.

Table 7–26. **Organizational Checklist for a Randomized Clinical Trial in Neurorehabilitation**

SPECIFIC AIMS

Importance of trial—background literature and rationale
Experimental intervention and comparison treatment
Hypotheses to be tested
Specify primary and secondary outcomes

METHODS

Define study population and criteria for inclusion and exclusion
Define potential risks and benefits
Provide training in the ethical conduct of research
Define descriptors about subjects
Rationale for specific outcome measures
   Appropriateness to intervention
   Reliability, validity, and sensitivity for the study population and intervention
Training plan to provide uniform experimental and control treatments
   Specify duration and intensity of all interventions
   Schedule of interventions
Schedule of assessment measures
Methods for blinding subjects, personnel, or those who collect outcomes
Training plan for blinded observers to uniformly collect and measure outcomes
   Plan to monitor adequacy of blinding
Plan to monitor for adverse reactions
Informed consent
   Meet Institutional Review Board requirements
   Establish common approaches across sites for presentation, advertising, maintaining privacy, and offering payments and reimbursements to subjects
   Explicitly state whether the experimental intervention is offered outside of the trial
Calculate sample size based on pilot studies
   Expected entry and dropout rates
   Demonstrate access to this sample size
Subject randomization assignment
   Check eligibility of potential subjects
   Allocation schedule and stratification criteria
   Method to generate and conceal allocation
Flow diagram for subjects by assignment, assessments, interventions, outcome measures
   Develop procedures to assure compliance by subjects and therapists with the assigned intervention
Establish data management group's responsibilities
   Develop practical data forms and transmission of forms
   Training for data entry
   Data collection assuring completeness, quality, and privacy
   Procedures for adverse reactions, dropouts, and missing data
   Interim reports
Establish an administrative oversight committee
Establish an external safety committee and set procedures
Maintain an operations manual

Continued on following page

Table 7–26.—*continued*

ANALYTIC PLAN

Rationale for statistical methods for primary, subgroup, or covariate analyses
   Intention-to-treat analysis versus efficacy analysis
   Uses of descriptor data
Plan interim analyses for safety and efficacy; specify study stop rules

RESULTS AND PUBLICATION

Describe protocol and deviations
Provide summary data including means, standard deviations, and effect size
State results in relative and absolute numbers, not just in percentages
State estimated effect on each outcome measure, including confidence intervals
Interpret findings in terms of internal validity and generalizability
Put study into the context of all available evidence

Sources: Drawn from personal experience and recommendations of CONSORT: Altman et al., 2001[260]; Moher et al., 2001.[261]

This approach is especially useful when the clinician is trying to manage a new symptom or wants to determine whether continued use of a drug is warranted. This approach also formalizes what physicians and patients already do when they experiment with a medication. A small repeated measures design takes the n-of-1 approach to its extreme. Results, of course, are not usually generalizable to other patients, as they may be in a RCT.

QUASI-EXPERIMENTAL DESIGNS

Other single-case, quasi-experimental designs that do not include randomization may come into increased use on neurologic rehabilitation

Table 7–27. **Statistical Applications**

Comparison	Nominal	Ordinal	Interval/Ratio
Group description	Frequencies Proportions Mode	Median Range	Mean (arithmetic/geometric) Variance. Coefficient of variation

Two independent samples	Fisher's Exact
	  for $n < 30$.
	  Chi-square $(1df)$ for
	  large samples and
	  expected cell
	  frequencies >5
		Mann-Whitney	Unpaired t test if
			  sample variances are
			  similar by F ratio

Two related samples	Chi-square for
	  changes with
	  continuity correction
	Fisher's for small
	  sample
		Sign test for change of
		  better/same/worse
		Wilcoxon for changes
		  ranked in order of size
			Paired t test

Multiple (k) independent samples	Chi-square (k-1df)	Kruskal-Wallis	One-way ANOVA
Multiple related samples	Cochran's Q	Friedman two-way ANOVA by ranks	Two-way ANOVA

ANOVA, analysis of variance.

services.[240,241] These designs enable the investigator to learn whether an intervention in a particular patient alters an outcome. Pretreatment baseline measures serve as the comparison for posttreatment outcomes. Multiple baseline measures must show little variability. At least 25 points in time should be measured.[242] If a treatment is expected to have an immediate effect and its withdrawal is expected to alter that effect in the opposite direction toward the baseline measure, then the design is improved by repeated introduction and withdrawal of the treatment over equal intervals of time. This circumstance requires fewer than 25 measurement points. The design is strengthened by blinding and by allowing equal intervals of time to pass between serial outcome measures.

In a multiple time series design, groups of patients, whether assigned randomly or not, are assessed before, sometimes during, and after the intervention. If the trends for each group are similar before implementation and change abruptly after a treatment begins, the change can be attributed to the intervention. Several visual analyses of data and statistical approaches can evaluate trends over time to assess whether or not the interventional program alters outcomes.[243,244]

Confounding Issues in Research Designs

The design of a clinical trial in neurologic rehabilitation must take into account many potentially confounding problems. Cognitive and physical trials are not as straightforward as a trial of a drug or surgical procedure for a well-defined medical problem that uses cure, death, or onset of a major illness as readily recognizable endpoints. Even in medical trials, recruitment of an adequately homogeneous population that has the identifiable problem, complies with the treatment, and completes the trial takes great motivation and work on the part of the subjects and the investigators.

INTERNAL VALIDITY

Issues of internal validity address the concern regarding whether a study provides a satisfactory answer to the research question. This notion involves the equality of experimental and control subjects in terms of variables that may affect the results, the integrity of the intervention, and the applicability of outcome measures.

Randomization

Random assignment to the treatment groups is more likely to achieve equalization if the size of the sample is adequate, the level of impairment or disability and the natural history of prognosis are similar, dropout is a random phenomenon, and sequential entry over a long time does not alter the prognosis as additional interventions evolve. One of potentially confounding problems of using a group-comparison approach is that facilities may not have a sufficient number of homogeneous patients who meet entry criteria and who are willing to participate. Also, sampling or selection bias may be present when subjects are recruited at a single hospital or clinic. This error may limit the generalizability of the results to other patients. Such bias is especially likely to profoundly affect a descriptive and quasi-experimental design.

In rehabilitation trials of physical and cognitive interventions, disease pathologies with a resulting range of impairments are associated with disabilities and handicaps that are equally heterogeneous. All four variables are subject to potentially unforeseen interactions. In addition, the focus of a rehabilitation trial could be at the level of pathologic process, impairment, disability, or handicap. Outcome measures may fall within any one or more of these levels. If these 4 foci of a treament intervention are the rows and the same 4 foci of outcome assessment are the columns, a total of 16 possible strategies for rehabilitation research are apparent.[245] For example, an intervention at the level of an impairment such as leg weakness in a hemiparetic patient could alter an outcome at the level of impairment (improved strength), disability (walks faster), or handicap (new ability to walk up stairs, so no further need for an elevator). If an intervention alters an impairment by improving leg strength only, but does not lessen disability (walking is still assisted or very slow), the intervention will hold little interest for rehabilitationists. On the other hand, if the outcome measure is a decrease in the number of falls related to strengthening, the outcome may be important, if that outcome measure is chosen a priori. Of course, an intervention can simultaneously be at more than one level or can affect more than one level of outcome measurement. Taking into account all of these potential relationships can produce enough wobble in a trial to flaw all but the best designs.

The control intervention, when a placebo, is often said to have an effect on up to one-third of patients in a drug, physical, or psychological trial. With any hands-on intervention, the control group should receive some defined level of attention from the therapists that is similar to the attention given to the experimental group. The notion of a large placebo-induced degree of change may lead to the mistaken concern that no experimental intervention other than a very robust one can improve outcomes in a clinical trial. The placebo effect, however, is insignificant in studies with binary outcomes and has only a small benefit in studies with continuous subjective outcomes, especially in pain studies.[246]

Integrity of an Intervention

In a rehabilitation trial, noise may arise from the style or intensity of one therapist's approach compared to the work of another therapist. Investigators must train those who carry out the experimental and control interventions so that each treatment is applied uniformly and so that the treatments do not overlap. The intensity and duration of each intervention ought to be the same to avoid showing differences between two treatments caused only by practice effects. Interventions must be defined in detail, so that they are reproducible for the study and for future use should the intervention show success. An operations manual for the trial ought to include anticipated problems and solutions, such as the way to progress a subject over time to increase the speed or accuracy of a task-oriented movement. The competing interventions are best carried out at different places or times so that subjects and therapists are not biased by what they see.

Pharmacologic interventions are often proposed for a rehabilitation trial. Should drugs be expected to stand alone as rehabilitative interventions for disabled persons? In one scenario, a drug is combined with a physical or cognitive therapy and then compared to the therapy without the drug. The combined intervention aims to affect activity-induced plasticity. A

study may fail to detect a difference that does exist if the drug's blood level is low and goes unmeasured or the peak level does not coincide with the timing of the therapy. In small trials, amphetamine plus specific therapies appears to work better than therapy alone, but the timing and frequency of dosing is uncertain.[247–249]

In another scenario, a drug is given to test its rehabilitative effect without any added therapy. For example, β_2-adrenergic agonists may exert anabolic effects on muscle. In a study of patients with facioscapulohumeral dystrophy, the agent albuterol increased lean muscle mass, but did not improve strength.[250] In retrospect, a reader may ask whether it is reasonable to expect an anabolic drug to improve muscle strength without an accompanying resistance exercise program. In the same vein, a study of an antispasticity drug to improve ADLs or walking speed may fail to do so if the drug is not augmented with therapy for the chosen endpoint and then compared to therapy alone. Subjects in a study that does not add therapy may not attempt to increase their skills when left on their own, so they do not improve functionally. The reader is left to wonder whether the drug may have had a positive effect on motor control that could have been manifested by task-oriented practice. Investigators must consider how to optimize the effects of an experimental intervention, before putting subjects into a trial. Ethical and financial considerations demand the best of possible protocols in human research.

Measurement Tools

As already noted in this chapter, outcome measures must be reliable and valid for the study population and must cover the expected consequences of the intervention. A RCT of a locomotor intervention for SCI or hemiplegic stroke may be better off using two primary outcome measures, such as the level of independence in walking based upon the criteria of the FIM for those who are less likely to recover independent walking, and walking speed for 50 feet for those who can ambulate. This approach is preferable to employing a total FIM score that includes dimensions irrelevant to walking. To assure the consistency of outcome measures, blinded observers require training and monitoring. If the outcome measure is not highly reliable, the investigators must do their own test–retest and interrater reliability studies. Data entry personnel must make sure the data fall within expected parameters and that all required data are collected.

GENERALIZABILITY

Clinical judgments, sampling procedures, and statistical inferences contribute to whether or not the results of a clinical trial may apply to other patients with the same disease, impairment, or disability. Clinical research requires screening for subjects. Clinicians establish entry and exclusion criteria in an attempt to study subjects who have the impairment, disability, or disease of interest and who seem likely to benefit from the intervention. The ideal subject has no other medical, psychologic, or psychosocial problem, takes no medication, and is highly motivated to participate. That subject does not exist in the real world. To be able to generalize the inferences from a trial, subjects ought to be as typical as possible of the population that may benefit from the intervention, should it turn out to be efficacious. In most instances, a RCT ought to be as inclusionary as possible. Of course, studying an intervention for subjects who have profound impairments or disabilities may not lead to results that apply to subjects with minimal incapacity. Including only mildly impaired subjects leads to potentially inappropriate generalization of the approach to profoundly affected patients. By being too exclusionary, investigators also create a quandry for themselves. They may not find enough cases for their trial. Indeed, the rate of finding subjects who are eligible for most RCTs often falls below the number the investigators had expected.

Sample Size and Power

For significance testing in classical fashion, the p value describes how probable or improbable the data are in their departure from expectation under the null hypothesis. It does not reflect how probable or improbable the null hypothesis is. The p value does not measure the weight of evidence against the null hypothesis relative to an alternative one, because no alternatire is included in the statistical procedure. For statisticians, a smaller p value, such as .01 compared to .001, does not mean necessarily that the evidence is stronger against the null hypothesis when no comparison hypothesis is offered.[239a] A Bayesian analysis, described later, may circumvent this concern. The *Type 1 error* probability or *alpha* describes the largest p value that will be declared statistically significant by chance alone when the null hypothesis is true.

Without a large enough sample size, tests of statistical significance can lead to a conclusion that an intervention does not work, when it really does, a phenomenon known as a *Type II error* or *beta*. This situation is in contrast to the more frequent concern of erroneous rejection of a true null hypothesis by statistical methods, which is finding that the intervention works when it really does not. This miscalculation is the *Type I error*.

Statistical power is an important concept. It is the ability of a statistical test to find a significant difference that really does exist. In statistical significance testing, power is the probability that a test will lead to the rejection of the null hypothesis when the null hypothesis should be rejected because it is false. The power of a study is 1 minus beta $(1 - \beta)$, the chance of detecting real existing differences. Low statistical power to detect small, medium, and large treatment effects has been shown to derive partly from small sample sizes in a group of clinical trials of stroke rehabilitation.[251] Larger sample sizes, more observations, and the greater treatment effects of one intervention over another reduce the risks of making a Type II error.

In planning a clinical trial, the investigators aim to detect not only a statistically significant difference if one exists, but also a clinically meaningful difference between two interventions. The *effect size* is the magnitude of the real effect to be detected. To accomplish this, the investigators need to know or must estimate the alpha, power, effect size, and sample size of the study.[252] Knowing any three allows the calculation of the fourth. The effect size is estimated as the mean result of the experimental group minus the mean of the control group divided by the standard deviation of the control group for the dependent variable. A large effect is 0.8, a moderate effect is 0.5, and a small effect is 0.2. Alpha, or the Type I error, is usually set at $p = 0.05$, although $p < 0.01$ is preferable. For a p value of 0.05, the theoretically expected minimum Type I error rate for a one-tailed comparison is actually 21%. For a two-tailed comparison, the error rate is actually 13%. The Type I error rate will be better than marginal if p is less than 0.01, especially for multiple between-group comparisons.[253] The power is most often set at 0.8. The levels of alpha and power are arbitrary, but most journals favor these choices.

Figure 7–1 assists making an estimate of the sample size needed to detect a high, intermediate, or low effect size for a two-tailed alpha of 0.05. At a power of 0.8 (beta is usually set as four times the alpha) and an effect size of 0.6, only approximately 20 subjects are needed for each arm of the trial. For rehabilitation, the detection of small differences has little meaning. For a study of stroke prevention, a small difference between two drugs may be meaningful for society, given the number of people at risk for stroke, although not necessarily meaningful for an individual.

Stratification of subjects into groups that takes into account a potentially confounding variable can help prevent a Type I error, but this method may also require a larger sample size. For ex-

ample, in a trial of a new locomotor intervention compared to a conventional one for hemiplegic stroke that starts by 2 weeks after onset, the investigators may want to stratify groups into those who had only a motor impairment and those who had sensorimotor and hemianopic impairments, especially if the primary outcome measure is the level of disability for ambulation. The concern is that most of the first group tend to become independent in gait by 12 weeks after onset and relatively few of the second group reach an unassisted level of mobility. At 12 weeks, the new treatment may not show a benefit if most of the subjects in each arm had only a motor impairment. The intervention may not improve upon the good natural history of recovery, at least by the chosen measure of functional indpendence. If each of the two impairment subgroups had been randomized in equal numbers to each of the two therapy arms, the new intervention may have revealed a benefit for the more impaired group. Another approach is to use walking speed as the primary outcome measure for subjects with only motor impairment and use the level of functional indepen-

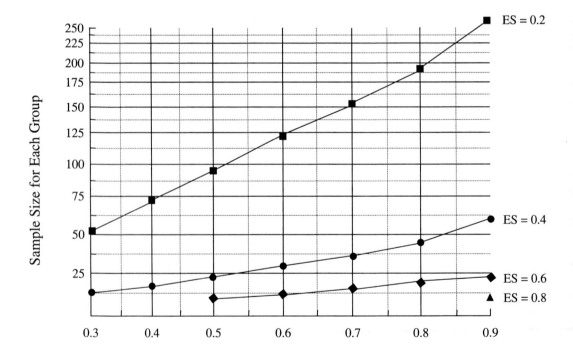

Figure 7–1. Effect size curves can be used to estimate the sample size needed for a behavioral outcome study in rehabilitation. Source: Thomas et al., 1997.[252]

dence as the primary outcome for those with far greater impairments.

Statistical Analyses

At least several schools offer approaches to statistical analyses. The frequentist mode of inference is most often employed in rehabilitation studies. This offers the triad of probabilities of interest just discussed: the p value and the Type I and Type II error probabilities. These allow the investigator to establish levels of significance, confidence intervals, and estimate bias. A Bayesian approach is rather different, because it adds a subjective criteria to find the unknown parameter q, the measure of the effect of an experimental treatment. From experience and, in some sequential designs while collecting and updating data, the investigator creates a subjective distribution of how likely it is that θ is less or equal to x, which ranges from 0–1. For small clinical trials, Bayesian and sequential analyses, hierarchical models, and other alternatives have been recommended by the Institute of Medicine.[239a] Bayesian methods are also very useful in analyzing functional neuroimaging data.

The distinctions between nominal, ordinal, interval, and ratio measures are particularly important when one considers which conventional statistical analyses can be applied to collected data. The choice of analysis must be included in the research design. For rehabilitation research, a biostatistician becomes an important team resource.

Statistical tests are conducted to determine whether the null hypothesis, which states that no difference exists between the comparison groups or conditions in a clinical trial, should be rejected. When statistical testing determines that the null hypothesis can be rejected at a chosen level of statistical significance, the clinician must keep in mind that this positive result for one intervention over another is not necessarily an indicator of the magnitude or clinical importance of the result or a sign of its reproducibility. Thus, *statistical test significance is not synonymous with clinical significance.* Rehabilitation practices are affected by repeated studies of practical interventions shown to have statistical significance and functional importance for subjects that resemble a clinician's own patients.

Table 7–27 lists some of the tests of statistical significance most commonly used in rehabilitation studies. Different mathematic approaches are needed to handle differing types of data and different assumptions are incorporated into each statistical method. For example, if an investigator wanted to compare the BI scores between two groups of patients after stroke who were randomized to different interventions, an appropriate test for ordinal data that compares two independent samples is the Mann-Whitney U test. If a researcher wants to compare 12 consecutive elderly men with stroke and left hemi-inattention to 14 females with the same impairment 2 weeks after the stroke, to study the proportion of male and female subjects who returned home, Fisher's Exact test is appropriate for these categoric data that compare two independent samples When walking speed before and after an intervention such as treadmill training is studied in patients with Parkinson's disease who are matched pairs or the same subjects, the paired t test allows a comparison of two related samples with interval data. An unpaired t test allows a comparison of treatment effects on two groups when the individuals are not paired and are different people. This method is commonly used in clinical trials that compare a treated group and a placebo group.

The t test requires that each group have a normal distribution, meaning that their measures fall within a bell-shaped curve characterized by a mean and a standard deviation. A two-tailed t test allows investigators to test the hypothesis that a treatment is significantly more or less effective than a placebo, whereas the one-tailed test allows only a test of the null hypothesis, which states that no difference exists between the treated and placebo group in one direction of change. The two-tailed test is more conservative and is employed most often. As a final example, if a therapist compared $k = 3$ different modalities in different orders to increase the range of motion at the hip in the same children with cerebral palsy, a two-way analysis of variance (ANOVA) would be a starting point for the analysis of this randomized block design with interval data. Analysis of variance allows the comparison of more than two groups at once or more than one intervention at the same time. This approach is common in rehabilitation studies.

Several other examples show the flexibility of statistical methods. The Kendall rank correlation coefficient measures the degree of association between two variables such as degree of independence in toileting and the length of inpatient stay. The Kendall partial rank correlation coefficient allows one to control for the effect of a third ordinal variable, such as attention, to see if the relation between toileting and length of stay persists. Whether parametric statistical procedures, which require a normal distribution around a mean, should be applied to nonparametric ordinal data is controversial. Calculations of the mean, standard deviation, and reliability using Pearson correlation coefficients, which are usually reserved for interval and ratio data, are sometimes reported in rehabilitation studies that use ordinal scales. In many situations, the conclusions from parametric and nonparametric analyses are similar. Thus, the application of a less appropriate method does not automatically lead to an invalid conclusion. A robust intervention with a high effect size provided to a large enough sample of patients will be revealed as significantly better by a reasonable statistical method.

SUBGROUP ANALYSIS

For subgroup analyses of the data acquired from a trial, statistical tests of interaction are more valid than inspecting the p values of subgroups.[254] Fishing in subgroup analyses and secondary outcomes often catches uninterpretable data. Despite randomization, baseline groups may not be comparable, so significance tests are inappropriate. If a baseline factor strongly influences outcome, a nonsignificant treatment imbalance may become important to any interpretation of the results of fishing. Outcomes analyses must be stated before the trial starts to prevent arbitrary post hoc data mining that ends up with samples too small and too different to provide meanigful interpretation.

META-ANALYSIS

Small sample sizes and other problems in the design of completed individual clinical trials have led to the use of a meta-analysis across neurologic rehabilitation studies. This statistical technique integrates the results of a pool of similar studies that meet certain minimal criteria, such as including randomization, to look at the efficacy of a type of intervention. The technique seems to work well, for example, when employed to study all antiplatelet trials that used the outcome variables of stroke, myocardial infarction, and vascular death in studies of patients who presented with any form of vascular disease.[255] Its utility in rehabilitation trials is uncertain, however. Composite studies may compare and aggregate patients who vary widely in their characteristics. The studies may employ different outcome parameters that vary in the reliability of their measurements. The technique may wrap together small trials of uncertain quality and is biased by the likelihood that negative trials tend not to get published.

A meta-analysis may be put into perspective if it includes a calculation of the number of negative results that would be needed to overturn a significant-seeming result. Although care in the selection of studies and complicated statistical methods are said to help prevent these and other potential biases,[236,256] the results of meta-analyses are best used to justify better designed investigations that address a hypothesis directly. In that setting, a meta-analysis may help in the estimate of the effect size of the experimental intervention.

SUMMARY

The development of clinically relevant measures of complex, integrated functional performance has been a great challenge for rehabilitationists. Issues of measurement, the choice of outcome measurement tools, the design of clinical trials, and statistical methods are conceptually and practically demanding, but manageable. If a rehabilitative intervention is truly robust in its ability to alter impairments, disabilities, or quality of life, thoughtful trial designs and outcome measures that are specific to the intent of the intervention will manifest this value.

No single, general-purpose measure is likely to meet all the needs of investigators. Available assessments of impairment, disability, and QOL that have already demonstrated clinical relevance, reliability, and validity in pilot studies of a similar population can be combined in a battery for meaningful program evaluation, for comparisons across facilities or diseases, and for research interventions. Although only one or two primary outcome measures will best serve the design of a clinical trial, insights into the factors that may account for specific and global outcomes, both successes and failures, can begin to be derived from the three-pronged approach of including instruments that capture information regarding impairment, disability, and the patient's view of change.

Methods are still under development that incorporate functional assessment and QOL measures and identify the morbidity and costs associated with particular interventions. Before health policies, payment rules, and practice guidelines based on these instruments are embraced for rehabilitation care, we will want to know that they accomplish their intended tasks. Clinicians should be wary, for example, regarding the use of FIM scores or any other disability measures as predictors of outcome when scores are used to determine eligibility for rehabilitation services. For any set of data, even data as complete as the FIM data from UDS$_{MR}$, more than one predictor equation can be used to fit the data. An extrapolation from models that are still evolving and have uncertain accuracy or are statistical inferences based on data trends could lead to unscientific conclusions, and may thereby produce health care policies derived from false premises.

One should keep in mind the possible limitations of aggregrate studies in neurorehabilitation. As in the rest of medical practice, we cannot easily transpose a clinical research finding to a particular patient. Individuals present complex medical challenges with their inherent biologic differences. Variations and biologic noise are amplified by psychosocial, personal, and societal issues. What happens to a particular patient can, of course, differ considerably from what may have been predicted from a multicenter study of 200 patients, especially if the intervention was ill defined or the study population differed considerably from the average person with that disease or disability.

On the other hand, the results of well-designed trials with an adequate sample size for interventions with a moderate effect size will serve individual patient decision-making well. Over the next 10 years, rehabilitationists will be called upon to put their best trial designs, basic therapeutic programs, and outcome instruments on the table to help test biologic interventions for neural repair. The challenge can be met with what is already available. This challenge is simply an extension of the question that neurologic rehabilitation clinicians must continue to answer: "Do we know what works best for our patients?"

REFERENCES

1. Services UDoHaH. Healthy People 2010, conference edition. Vol 1–2. Washington, D.C.: US Government Printing Office, 2000.
2. Cole T, Edgerton V. Report of the Task Force on Medical Rehabilitation Research: National Institutes of Health, 1990.
3. Clancy C, Eisenberg J. Outcomes research: Measuring the end results of health care. Science 1998; 282:245–246.
4. Johnston M, Keith R, Hinderer S. Measurement standards for interdisciplinary medical rehabilitation. Arch Phys Med Rehabil 1992; 73(suppl 12):S1–S23.
5. Silverstein B, Fisher W, Kilgore K, Harley P, Harvey R. Applying psychometric criteria to functional assessment: II. Defining interval measures. Arch Phys Med Rehabil 1992; 73:507–518.
6. Guyatt G, Bombardier C, Tugwell P. Measuring disease-specific quality of life in clinical trials. CMAJ 1986; 134:889–895.
7. Stewart A, Hays R, Ware J. The MOS short-form general health survey. Med Care 1988; 26:724–735.
8. McDowell I, Newell C. Measuring Health: A Guide to Rating Scales and Questionnaires. New York: Oxford University Press, 1996.
9. Fillyaw M, Badger G, Bradley W. Quantitative measures of neurological function in chronic neuromuscular diseases and ataxia. J Neurol Sci 1989; 92:17–36.
10. Cutter G, Baier M, Rudick R, Cookfair D, Fischer J, Petkau J, Syndulko K, Weinshenker B, Antel JP, Confavieux C, Ellison G, Lublin F, Miller A, Rao S, Reingold S, Thompson A, Willoughby E. Development of a Multiple Sclerosis Functional Composite as a clinical trial outcome measure. Brain 1999; 122:871–882.
11. Kalkers N, Bergers L, de Groot V, Lazeron R, Van Walderveen M, Vitdehaag B, Poleman C, Barkhof F. Concurrent validity of the MS Functional Composite using MRI as a biological disease marker. Neurology 2001; 56:215–219.
12. Miller D, Rudick R, Cutter G, Baier M, Fischer J. Clinical significance of the Multiple Sclerosis Functional Composite: Relationship to patient-reported quality of life. Arch Neurol 2000; 57:1319–1324.
13. Kalkers N, de Groot V, Lazeron R, Killestein J, Ader H, Barkhof F, Lankhorst G, Poleman C. MS Functional Composite: Relation to disease phenotype and disability strata. Neurology 2000; 54:1233–1239.
14. Jennett B, Bond M. Assessment of outcome after severe head injury: A practical scale. Lancet 1975; 1:480–484.
15. Nell V, Yates D, Kruger J. An extended Glasgow Coma Scale (GCS-E) with enhanced sensitivity to mild brain injury. Arch Phys Med Rehabil 2000; 81:614–617.
16. Giacino J, Kezmarsky M, DeLuca J, Cicerone K.

function of elderly outpatients. J Am Geriatr Soc 1990; 38:1105–1112.

89. Gans B, Haley S, Hallenberg S, Mann N, Inacio C, Faas R. Description and interobserver reliability of the Tufts Assessment of Motor Performance. Am J Phys Med Rehabil 1988; 67:202–210.

90. Haley S, Ludlow L, Gans B, Faas R, Inacio C. Tufts Assessment of Motor Performance: An empirical approach to identifying motor performance categories. Arch Phys Med Rehabil 1991; 72:358–366.

91. Tinetti M, Speechley M. Prevention of falls among the elderly. N Engl J Med 1989; 320:1055–1059.

92. Podsiadlo D, Richardson S. The timed "up and go": A test of basic functional mobility for frail elderly persons. J Am Geriatr Soc 1991; 39:142–149.

93. Brandstater M, deBruin H, Gowland C, Clark B. Hemiplegic gait: Analysis of temporal variables. Arch Phys Med Rehabil 1983; 64:583–587.

94. Bohannon R. Relevance of muscle strength to gait performance in patients with neurologic disability. J Neuro Rehabil 1989; 3:97–100.

95. Bohannon R, Walsh S, Joseph M. Ordinal and timed balance measurements: Reliability and validity in patients with stroke. Clin Rahabil 1993; 7:9–13.

96. Duncan P, Weiner D, Chandler J, Studenski S. Functional reach: A new clinical mesure of balance. J Gerontol 1990; 45:192–197.

97. Berg K, Maki B, Williams J, Holliday P, Wood-Dauphinee S. Clinical laboratory measures of postural balance in an elderly population. Arch Phys Med Rehabil 1992; 73:1073–1080.

98. Lehmann J, Boswell S, Price R, Burleigh A, de Lateur B, Jaffe K, Hertling D. Quantitative evaluation of sway as an indicator of functional balance in post-traumatic brain injury. Arch Phys Med Rehabil 1990; 71:955–962.

99. Winstein C, Gardner E, McNeal D. Standing balance training: Effect on balance and locomotion in hemiparetic adults. Arch Phys Med Rehabil 1989; 70:755–762.

100. Wolfson L, Whipple R, Derby C, Amerman P, Murphy T, Tobin J, Nashner L. A dynamic posturography study of balance in healthy elderly. Neurology 1992; 42:2069–2075.

101. Nashner L, Peters J. Dynamic posturography in the diagnosis and management of dizziness and balance disorders. Neurol Clin 1990; 8:331–349.

102. Ottenbacher K. Evaluating Clinical Change: Strategies for Occupational and Physical Therapists. Baltimore: Williams & Wilkins, 1986.

103. Malec J. Goal Attainment Scaling in rehabilitation. Neuropsychol Rehabil 1999; 9:253–275.

104. Cummings J, Mega M, Gray K, Rosenberg-Thompson S, Carusi D, Gornbein J. The Neuropsychiatric Inventory: Comprehensive assessment of psychopathology in dementia. Neurology 1994; 44:2308–2314.

105. Levin H, High W, Goethe K, Sisson R, Overall J, Rhoades H, Eisenberg H, Kalisky Z, Gary H. The neurobehavioral rating scale: Assessment of the behavioural sequelae of head injury by the clinician. J Neurol Neurosurg Psychiatry 1987; 50:183–193.

106. Vanier M, Mazaux J, Lambert J, Dassa C, Levin H. Assessment of neuropsychologic impairments after head injury: Interrater reliability and factorial and criterion validity of the Neurobehavioral Rating Scale-Revised. Arch Phys Med Rehabil 2000; 81:796–806.

107. Corrigan J. Development of a scale for assessment of agitation following traumatic brain injury. J Clin Exp Neuropsychol 1989; 11:261–277.

108. Fugate L, Spacek L, Kresty L, Levy C, Johnson J, Mysiw W. Measurement and treatment of agitation following traumatic brain injury: II. A survey of the Brain Injury Special Interest Group of the American Academy of Physical Medicine and Rehabilitation. Arch Phys Med Rehabil 1997; 78:924–8.

109. Cohen M, Marino R. The tools of disability outcomes research functional status measures. Arch Phys Med Rehabil 2000; 81(suppl 2):S21–S29.

110. terSteeg A, Lankhorst G. Screening instruments for disability. Crit Rev Phys Rehabil Med 1994; 6: 101–112.

111. Applegate W, Blass J, Williams T. Instruments for the functional asessment of older patients. NEJM 1990; 322:1207–1214.

112. Fisher W, Harvey R, Taylor P, Kilgore K, Kelly C. Rehabits: A common language of functional assessment. Arch Phys Med Rehabil 1995; 76:113–122.

113. Mahoney F, Barthel D. Functional evaluation: The Barthel Index. Md Med J 1965; 14:61–65.

114. Granger C, Albrecht G, Hamilton B. Outcome of comprehensive rehabilitation: Measurement by PULSES and Barthel Index. Arch Phys Med Rehabil 1979; 60:145–154.

115. Granger C, Hamilton B, Gresham G. The stroke rehabilitation outcome study—Part 1: General description. Arch Phys Med Rehabil 1988; 69:506–509.

116. Grey N, Kennedy P. The Functional Independence Measure: A comparative study of clinician and self ratings. Paraplegia 1993; 31:457–461.

117. Wade D, Collin C. The Barthel ADL index: A standard measure of physical disability? Int Disab Stud 1988; 11:64–67.

118. Shah S, Vanclay F, Cooper B. Improving the sensitivity of the Barthel Index for stroke rehabilitation. J Clin Epidemiol 1989; 42:703–709.

119. Lazar R, Yarkony G, Ortolano D, Heinemann A. Prediction of functional outcome by motor capability after spinal cord injury. Arch Phys Med Rehabil 1989; 70:819–822.

120. Jorger M, Beer S, Kesselring J. Impact of neurorehabilitation on disability in patients acutely and chronically disabling diseases of the nervous system measured by the Extended Barthel Index. Neurorehabil Neural Repair 2001; 15:15–22.

121. Granger C, Hamilton B, Sherwin F. Guide for Use of the Uniform Data Set for Medical Rehabilitation. Buffalo, N.Y.: Buffalo General Hospital, 1986.

122. Deutsch A, Braun S, Granger C. The Functional Independence Measure (FIM^{SM} Instrument) and the Functional Independence Measure for children (WeeFIM Instrument): ten years of development. Crit Rev Phys Rehabil Med 1996; 8:267–81.

123. Hamilton B, Laughlin J, Granger C, Kayton R. Interrater agreement of the seven level FIM. Arch Phys Med Rehabil 1991; 72:790(abstr).

124. Hoenig H, Hoff J, McIntyre L, Branch L. The Self-Reported Functional Measure: Predictive validity for health care utilization in multiple sclerosis and spinal cord injury. Arch Phys Med Rehabil 2001; 82:613–618.

125. Roth E, Davidoff G, Haughton J, Ardner M. Functional assessment in spinal cord injury: A comparison of the Modified Barthel Index and the 'adapted' Functional Independence Measure. Clin Rehabil 1990; 4:277–285.

126. Heinemann A, Linacre J, Wright B, Hamilton B, Granger C. Relationship between impairment and physical disability as measured by the FIM. Arch Phys Med Rehabil 1993; 74:566–573.

127. Dodds T, Martin D, Stolov W, Deyo R. A validation of the Functional Independence Measurement and its performance among rehabilitation inpatients. Arch Phys Med Rehabil 1993; 74:531–536.

128. Heinemann A, Linacre J, Hamilton B, Granger C. Prediction of rehabilitation outcomes with disability measures. Arch Phys Med Rehabil 1994; 75:133–143.

129. Long W, Sacco W, Coombes S, Copes W, Bullock A, Melville J. Determining normative standards for Functional Independence Measure transitions in rehabilitation. Arch Phys Med Rehabil 1994; 75:144–148.

130. Granger C, Cotter A, Hamilton B, Fiedler R. Functional assessment scales: A study of persons after stroke. Arch Phys Med Rehabil 1993; 74:133–138.

131. Granger C, Cotter A, Hamilton B, Fiedler R, Hens M. Functional assessment scales: A study of persons with multiple sclerosis. Arch Phys Med Rehabil 1990; 71:870–875.

132. Disler P, Roy C, Smith B. Predicting hours of care needed. Arch Phys Med Rehabil 1993; 74:139–143.

133. Brosseau L, Wolfson C. The inter-rater reliability and construct validity of the Functional Independence Measure for multiple sclerosis subjects. Clin Rehabil 1994; 8:107–115.

134. Sharrack B, Hughes R, Soudain S, Dunn G. The psychometric properties of clinical rating scales used in multiple sclerosis. Brain 1999; 122:141–159.

135. van der Putten J, Hobart J, Freeman J, Thompson A. Measuring change in disability after inpatient rehabilitation: comparison of the responsiveness of the Barthel Index and the Functional Independence Measure. J Neurol Neurosurg Psychiatry 1999; 66:480–484.

136. Hall K, Cohen M, Wright J, Call M, Werner P. Characteristics of the Functional Independence Measure in traumatic spinal cord injury. Arch Phys Med Rehabil 1999; 80:1471–1476.

137. Davidoff G, Roth E, Haughton J, Ardner M. Cognitive dysfunction in spinal cord injury patients: Sensitivity of the FIM subscales vs neuropsychologic assessment. Arch Phys Med Rehabil 1990; 71:326–329.

138. Hobart J, Lamping D, Freeman J, Langdon D, McLellan D, Greenwood R, Thompson A. Evidence-based measurement: Which disability scale for neurologic rehabilitation? Neurology 2001; 57:639–644.

139. Brock K, Goldie P, Greenwood K. Evaluating the effectiveness of stroke rehabilitation: Choosing a discriminative measure. Arch Phys Med Rehabil 2002; 83:92–99.

140. Granger C, Hamilton B. The Uniform Data System for Medical Rehabilitation report of first admissions for 1991. Am J Phys Med Rehabil 1993; 72:33–38.

141. Bode R, Heinemann A. Course of functional improvement after stroke, spinal cord injury, and traumatic brain injury. Arch Phys Med Rehabil 2002; 83:100–106.

142. Stineman M, Escarce J, Granger C, Goin J, Hamilton B, Williams S. A case mix classification system for medical rehabilitation. Med Care 1994; 32:60–67.

143. Stineman M, Hamilton B, Granger C, Goin J, Escarce J, Williams S. Four methods for characterizing disability in the formation of function related groups. Arch Phys Med Rehabil 1994; 75:1277–1283.

144. Katz R, Downs T, Cash H, Grotz R. Progress in development of the index of ADL. Gerontologist 1970; 10:20–25.

145. Klein R, Bell B. Self-care skills: Behavioral measurement with the Klein-Bell ADL Scale. Arch Phys Med Rehabil 1982; 63:335–338.

146. Harvey R, Jellinek H. Functional performance assessment: A program approach. Arch Phys Med Rehabil 1981; 62:456–461.

147. Harvey R, Silverstein B, Venzon M, Kilgore K, Fisher W, Steiner M, Harley J. Applying psychometric criteria to functional assessment in medical rehabilitation. Arch Phys Med Rehabil 1992; 73:887–892.

148. Holbrook M, Skilbeck C. An activities index for use with stroke patients. Age Ageing 1983; 12:166–170.

149. Schuling J, de Haan R, Limburg M, Groenier K. The Frenchay Activities Index. Stroke 1993; 24:1173–1177.

150. Wade D, Collen F, Robb G, Warlow C. Physiotherapy intervention late after stroke and mobility. BMJ 1992; 304:609–613.

151. Lincoln N, Edmans J. A re-validation of the Rivermead ADL scale for elderly patients with stroke. Age Ageing 1990; 19:9–24.

152. Gompertz P, Pound P, Ebrahim S. Validity of the extended activities of daily living scale. Clin Rehabil 1994; 8:275–280.

153. McPherson K, Sloan R, Hunter J, Dowell C. Validation studies of the OPCS scale—more useful than the Barthel Index? Clin Rehabil 1993; 7:105–112.

154. Bischoff D. NHTSA Functional Capacity Index. Federal Register 1992; 57:13157–13165.

155. Frankel M, Morgenstern L, Kwiatkowski T, Lu M, Tilley B, Broderick J, Libman R, Levine S, Brott T. Predicting prognosis after stroke: A placebo group analysis from the National Institute Of Neurological Disorders And Stroke rt-PA stroke trial. Neurology 2000; 55:952–959.

156. Rappaport M, Herrero-Backe C, Rappaport M, Winterfield K. Head injury outcome up to ten years later. Arch Phys Med Rehabil 1989; 70:885–892.

157. Hall K, Cope D, Rappaport M. Glasgow Outcome Scale and Disability Rating Scale: Comparative usefulness in following recovery in traumatic brain injury. Arch Phys Med Rehabil 1985; 66:35–37.

158. Solari A, Filippini G, Gasco P, Colla L. Physical rehabilitation has a positive effect on disability in multiple sclerosis. Neurology 1999; 52:57–62.

159. Sharrack B, Hughes R. The Guy's Neurological Disability Scale (GNDS): A new disability measure for multiple sclerosis. Mult Scler 1999; 5:223–233.

160. Duncan W, Wallace D, Lai M, Johnsom D, Embretson S, Laster L. The Stroke Impact Scale Version 2.0. Stroke 1999; 30:2131–2140.

161. Kelly-Hayes M, Robertson J, Broderick J, Duncan P, Hershey L, Roth E, Thies W, Trombley C. The American Heart Association Stroke Outcome Classification. Stroke 1998; 29:1274–1280.

162. Gresham G, Labi M, Dittmar S, Hicks J, Joyce S, Stehlik M. The Quadriplegia Index of Function: Sensitivity and reliability demonstrated in a study of thirty quadriplegic patients. Paraplegia 1986; 24:38–44.

163. Catz A, Itzkovich M, Agranov E, Ring H, Tamir A. SCIM-Spinal Cord Independence Measure: A new disability scale for patients with spinal cord lesions. Spinal Cord 1997; 35:850–856.

164. Agrell B, Dehlin O. Comparison of six depression rating scales in geriatric stroke patients. Stroke 1989; 20:1190–1194.

165. Sullivan M, Weinshenker B, Mikail S, Bishop S. Screening for major depression in the early stages of MS. Can J Neurol Sci 1995; 22:228–231.

166. Lollar D, Simeonsson R, Nanda U. Measures of outcomes for children and youth. Arch Phys Med Rehabil 2000; 81(Suppl 2):S46–S52.

167. Nichols D, Case-Smith J. Reliability and validity of the Pediatric Evaluation of Disability Inventory. Pediatr Phys Ther 1996; 8:15–24.

168. Staquet M, Hays R, Fayers P. Quality of Life Assessment in Clinical Trials: Methods and Practice. New York: Oxford University Press, 1998.

169. Wells K, Stewart A, Hays R, Burnam M, Rogers W, Daniels M, Berry S, Greenfield S, Ware J. The functioning and well-being of depressed patients. JAMA 1989; 282:914–919.

170. Tchekmedyian N, Cella D. Quality of life in current oncology practice and research. Oncology 1990; 4:11–233.

171. Kinney W, Boyle C. Predicting life satisfaction among adults with physical disabilities. Arch Phys Med Rehabil 1992; 73:863–869.

172. Angeleri F, Angereri V, Foschi N, Giaquinto S, Nolfe G. The influence of depression, social activity, and family stress on functional outcome after stroke. Stroke 1993; 24:1478–1483.

173. Rudick R, Miller D, Clough J, Gragg L, Farmer R. Quality of life in multiple sclerosis. Arch Neurol 1992; 49:1237–1242.

174. Sprangers M, Aaronson N. The role of health care providers and significant others in evaluating the quality of life of patients with chronic disease. J Clin Epidemiol 1992; 45:743–760.

175. Segal M, Schall R. Determining functional/health status and its relation to disability in stroke survivors. Stroke 1994; 25:2391–2397.

176. Bergner M, Bobbitt R, Carter W, Gilson B. The Sickness Impact Profile: Development and final revision of a health status measure. Med Care 1981; 19:787–805.

177. de Bruin A, Diederiks J, de Witte L, Stevens F, Philipsen H. Assessing the responsiveness of a functional status measure: The Sickness Index Profile versus the SIP68. J Clin Epidemiol 1997; 50:529–540.

178. van Straten A, de Haan R, Limburg M, Schuling J, Bossuyt P, van den Bos G. A stroke-adapted 30-item version of the Sickness Impact Profile to assess quality of life (SA-SIP30). Stroke 1997; 28:2155–2161.

179. HealthOutcomesInstitute. Health Status Questionnaire (HSQ) 2.0 User Guide. Bloomington, Minn, 1993.

180. Stewart AL, Ware JE, Greenfield S, Hays RD. Functional status and well-being of patients with chronic conditions: Results from the Medical Outcomes Study. JAMA 1989; 262:907–919.

181. Ware J, Sherbourne C. The MOS 36-item Short-Form Health Survey (SF-36): Conceptual framework and item selection. Med Care 1992; 30:473–483.

182. Pickard A, Johnson J, Penn A, Lau F, Noseworthy T. Replicability of SF-36 summary scores by the SF-12 in stroke patients. Stroke 1999; 30:1213–1217.

183. Garratt A, Rutta D, Abdulla M, Buckingham K, Russell I. The SF36 health survey questionnaire: An outcome measure suitable for routine use within the NHS? BMJ 1993; 306:1440–1444.

184. Ware J. Measuring patient's views: The optimum outcome measure. BMJ 1993; 306:1429–1430.

185. Andresen E, Meyers A. Health-related quality of life outcomes measures. Arch Phys Med Rehabil 2000; 81(Suppl 2):S30–S45.

186. Vickrey B, Hays R, Graber J, Rausch R, Sutherling W, Engel J, Brooks R. A health-related quality of life instrument for patients evaluated for epilepsy surgery. Med Care 1992; 30:299–319.

187. Vickrey B, Hays R, Genovese B, Myers L, Ellison G. Comparison of a generic to disease-targeted health-related quality-of-life measures for multiple sclerosis. J Clin Epidemiol 1997; 50:557–569.

188. Vickrey B, Hays R, Beckstrand M. Development of a health-related quality of life measure for peripheral neuropathy. Neurorehabil Neural Repair 2000; 14:93–104.

189. Jette A, Davies A, Cleary P, Rubenstein L, Brook R, Delbanco T. The Functional Status Questionnaire: Reliability and validity when used in primary care. J Gen Int Med 1986; 1:143–149.

190. Kaplan R, Bush J, Berry C. Health status: Types of validity and the Index of Well-Being. Health Serv Res 1976; 11:478–507.

191. Andressen E, Fouts B, Romeis J. Performance of health-related quality-of-life instruments in a spinal cord injured population. Arch Phys Med Rehabil 1999; 80:877–884.

192. Post P, Stiggelbout A, Wakker P. The utility of health states after stroke. Stroke 2001; 32:1425–1429.

193. Tengs T, Yu M, Luistro E. Health-related quality of life after stroke: A comprehensive review. Stroke 2001; 32:964–972.

194. Dorman P, Slattery J, Farrell B, Dennis M, Sandercock P. Qualitative comparison of the reliability of health status assessments with the EuroQol and SF-36 questionnaires after stroke. Stroke 1998; 29:63–68.

195. Vickrey B. Getting oriented to patient-oriented outcomes. Neurology 1999; 53:662–663.

196. Nortvedt M, Riise T, Myhr K-M, Nyland H. Quality of life in multiple sclerosis: Measuring the disease effects more broadly. Neurology 1999; 53:1098–1103.

197. Fischer J, LaRocca N, Miller D, Ritvo P, Andrews H, Paty D. Recent developments in the assessment of quality of life in multiple sclerosis. Mult Scler 1999; 5:251–259.

198. Nortvedt M, Riise T, Myhr K-M, Nyland H. Quality of life as a predictor for change in disability in MS. Neurology 2000; 55:51–54.

199. Vickrey B, Hays R, Harooni R, Myers L, Ellison G. A health-related quality of life measure for multiple sclerosis. Qual Life Res 1995; 4:187–206.

200. Golomb B, Vickrey B, Hays R. A review of health-related quality-of-life measures in stroke. Pharmacoeconomics 2001; 19:155–185.

201. Williams L, Weinberger M, Harris L, Clark D, Biller

J. Development of a stroke-specific quality of life scale. Stroke 1999; 30:1362–1369.

202. Hamedani A, Wells C, Brass L, Kernan W, Viscoli C, Maraire J, Awad I, Horwitz R. A quality-of-life instrument for young hemorrhagic stroke patients. Stroke 2001; 32:687–695.

203. Patrick D, Connell F, Edwards T, Topolski T, Huebner C. Age-appropriate measures of quality of life and disability among children: The youth quality of life study. Atlanta: Centers for Disease Control and Prevention, 1998.

204. Weissman M. The assesment of social adjustment: An update. Arch Gen Psychiatry 1981; 38:1250–1258.

205. McColl M, Skinner H. Concepts and measurement of social support in a rehabilitation setting. Can J Rehabil 1988; 2:93–107.

206. Spilker B. Quality of Life Assessments in Clinical Trials. New York: Raven Press, 1996.

207. Hogarty G, Katz M. Norms of adjustment and social behavior. Arch Gen Psychiatry 1971; 25:470–480.

208. Livneh H, Antonak R. Psychosocial reactions to disability: A review and critique of the literature. Crit Rev Phys Rehabil Med 1994; 6:1–100.

209. Aronson K. Quality of life among persons with multiple sclerosis and their caregivers. Neurology 1997; 48:74–80.

210. Bakas T, Champion V. Development and psychometric testing of the Bakas Caregiving Outcomes Scale. Nurs Res 1999; 48:250–259.

211. Elmstahl S, Malmberg B, Annerstedt L. Caregiver's burden of patients 3 years after stroke assessed by a novel caregiver burden scale. Arch Phys Med Rehabil 1996; 77:177–182.

211a. Denzin NK, Lincoln Y (eds.). Handbook of Qualitative Research. Sage Publ, Thousand Oaks, CA, 2000.

212. MacKenzie C, Charlson M, DiGioia D, Kelley K. A patient-specific measure of change in maximal function. Arch Intern Med 1986; 146:1325–1329.

213. Gill T, Feinstein A. A critical appraisal of the quality of quality-of-life measurements. JAMA 1994; 272:619–626.

214. World Health Organization. WHO International Classification of Impairments, Disabilities and Handicaps: A manual of classification relating to the consequences of disease. Geneva: World Health Organization, 1980.

215. Whiteneck G, Charlifue S, Gerhart K, Overholser J, Richardson G. Quantifying handicap: A new measure of long-term rehabilitation outcomes. Arch Phys Med Rehabil 1992; 73:519–526.

216. Harwood R, Jitapunkul S, Dickinson E, Ebrahim S. Measuring handicap: 1. Motives, methods, and a model. Quality in Health Care 1994; 3:54–57.

217. Freeman J, Langdon D, Hobart J, Thompson A. The impact of inpatient rehabilitation on progressive multiple sclerosis. Ann Neurol 1997; 42:236–1244.

218. Freeman J, Langdon D, Hobart J, Thompson A. Inpatient rehabilitation in multiple sclerosis: Do the benefits carry over into the community? Neurology 1999; 52:50–56.

219. Wood-Dauphinee S, Williams J. Reintegration to normal living as a proxy to quality of life. J Chron Dis 1987; 40:491–499.

220. Korner-Bitensky N, Wood-Dauphinee S, Siemiatycki J, Shapiro S, Becker R. Health-related informa-tion postdischarge: Telephone versus face-to-face interviewing. Arch Phys Med Rehabil 1994; 75:1287–1296.

221. Sander M, Fuchs K, High W, Hall K, Kreutzer J, Rosenthal M. The Community Integration Questionnaire revisited: An assessment of factor structure and validity. Arch Phys Med Rehabil 1999; 80:1303–1308.

222. McColl M, Davies D, Carlson P, Johnston J, Minnes P. The Community Integration Measure: Development and preliminary validation. Arch Phys Med Rehabil 2001; 82:429–434.

223. Crewe N, Athelstan G. Functional assessment in vocational rehabilitation: Systemic approach to diagnosis and goal setting. Arch Phys Med Rehabil 1981; 62:299–305.

224. Cornes P, Roy C. Vocational Rehabilitation Index assessment of rehabilitation medicine service patients. Int Disabil Stud 1991; 13:5–8.

225. Cardenas D, Haselkorn J, McElligott J, Gnatz S. A bibliography of cost-effectiveness practices in physical medicine and rehabilitation: AAPM&R white paper. Arch Phys Med Rehabil 2001; 82:711–719.

226. Halloway R, Benesch C, Rahillyb C, Courtright C. A systematic review of cost-effectiveness research of stroke evaluation and treatment. Stroke 1999; 30:1340–1349.

227. Braddom R. Why is physiatric research important? Am J Phys Med Rehabil 1991; 70(suppl):S2–S3.

228. DeLisa J, Jain S, McCutcheon P. Current status of chairpersons in Physical Medicine and Rehabilitation. Am J Phys Med Rehabil 1992; 71:258–262.

229. Reilly R, Findley T. Research in Physical Medicine and Rehabilitation. !V. Some practical designs in applied research. Am J Phys Med Rehabil 1989; 70(Suppl):S31–S36.

230. Miller F, Rosenstein D, DeRenzo E. Professional integrity in clinical research. JAMA 1998; 280:1449–1454.

231. Wittes J. Data Safety Monitoring Boards: A brief introduction. Biopharmaceutical Report 2000; 8:1–11.

232. Hulley S, Cummings S, Browner W. Designing Clinical Research. Baltimore: Williams & Wilkins, 2001.

233. Meinert C. Clinical Trials: Design, Conduct, and Analysis. New York: Oxford University Press, 1986.

234. Cicerone K, Dahlberg C, Kalmar K, Langenbaun D, Malec J, Berquist T, Felicetti T, Giacino J, Harley J, Harrington D, Herzog J, Kneipp S, Laatsch L, Morse P. Evidence-based cognitive rehabilitation: recommendations for clinical practice. Arch Phys Med Rehabil 2000; 81:1596–615.

235. Ioannidas J, Haidich A-B, Pappa M, Pantazis N, Kokori S, Tektonidou M, Contopoulos-Ioannidis D, Lau J. Comparison of evidence of treatment effects in randomized and nonrandomized studies. JAMA 2001; 286:821–830.

236. Ottenbacher K, Jannell S. The results of clinical trials in stroke rehabilitation research. Arch Neurol 1993; 50:37–44.

237. Editor. Instructions for authors. JAMA 1999; 281:12–16.

238. Begg C, Cho M, Eastwood S, Horton R, Moher D, Olkin I, Pitkin R, Rennie D, Schulz K, Simel D, Stroup D. Improving the quality of reporting of randomized controlled trials. The CONSORT statement. JAMA 1996; 276:637–39.

239. Guyatt G, Keller J, Jaeschke R, Rosenbloom D, Adachi J, Newhouse M. The n-of-1 randomized controlled trial: Clinical usefulness. Ann Int Med 1990; 112:293–299.

239a. Evans C, Ildstad S (eds.). Small Clinical Trials: Issues and Challenges. Washington, D.C. National Academy Press, 2001.

240. Wilson B. Single-case experimental designs in neuropsychological rehabilitation. J Clin Exp Neuropsychol 1987; 9:527–544.

241. Crabtree B, Ray S, Schmidt P, O'Connor P, Schmidt D. The individual over time: Time series applications in health care research. J Clin Epidemiol 1990; 43:241–260.

242. Kazdin A. Single-Case Research Designs. New York: Oxford University Press, 1982.

243. Sunderland A. Single-case experiments in neurological rehabilitation. Clin Rehabil 1990; 4:181–192.

244. Ottenbacher K. Analysis of data in idiographic research. Am J Phys Med Rehabil 1992; 71:202–208.

245. Whyte J. Toward a methodology for rehabilitation research. Am J Phys Med Rehabil 1994; 73:428–435.

246. Hrobjartsson A, Gotzsche P. Is the placebo powerless? New Engl J Med 2001; 344:1594–1602.

247. Walker-Batson D, Curtis S, Natarajan R, Ford J, Dronkers N, Salmeron E, Lai J, Unwin D. A double-blind placebo-controlled study of the use of amphetamine in the treatment of aphasia. Stroke 2001; 32:2093–2098.

248. Schmanke T, Avery R, Barth T. The effects of amphetamine on recovery of function after cortical damage in the rat depend on the behavioral requirements of the task. J Neurotrauma 1996; 13:293–307.

249. Crisostomo E, Duncan P, Propst M, Dawson D, Davis J. Evidence that amphetamine with physical therapy promotes recovery of motor function in stroke patients. Ann Neurol 1988; 23:94–97.

250. Kissel J, McDermott M, Mendell J, King W, Pandya S, Griggs R, Tawil R. Randomized, double-blinded, placebo-controlled trial of albuterol in facioscapulohumeral dystrophy. Neurology 2001; 57:1434–1440.

251. Matyas T, Ottenbacher K. Confounds of insensitivity and blind luck: Statistical conclusion validity in stroke rehabilitation. Arch Phys Med Rehabil 1993; 74:559–565.

252. Thomas J, Lochbaum M, Landers D, He C. Planning significant and meaningful research in exercise science: Estimating sample size. Res Q Exer Sport 1997; 68:33–43.

253. Goodin D, Frohman E, Garmany G, Halper J, Likosky W, Lublin F, Silberberg D, Stuart W, van den Noorf S. Disease modifying therapies in multiple sclerosis. Neurology 2002; 58:169–178.

254. Assmann S, Pocock S, Enos L, Kasten L. Subgroup analysis and the (mis)uses of baseline data in clinical trials. Lancet 2000; 355:1064–1069.

255. Antiplatelet Trialists Collaboration. Collaborative overview of randomised trials of antiplatelet therapy— I: Prevention of death, myocardial infarction, and stroke by prolonged antiplatelet therapy in various categories of patients. Brit Med J 1994; 308:81–106.

256. Schleenbaker R, Mainous A. Electromyographic biofeedback for the neuromuscular reeducation of the hemiplegic stroke patient: A meta-analysis. Arch Phys Med Rehabil 1993; 74:1301–1304.

257. Meythaler J, Steers W, Tuel S, Cross L, Sesco D, Haworth C. Intrathecal baclofen in hereditary spastic paraparesis. Arch Phys Med Rehabil 1992; 73: 794–797.

258. Dobkin B, Taly A, Su G. Use of the audiospinal reflex to test for completeness of spinal cord injury. J Neurol Rehabil 1994; 8:187–192.

259. Benecke R, Conrad B, Meinck H, Hohne J. Electromyographic analysis of bicycling on an ergometer for evaluation of spasticity of lower limbs in man. In: Desmedt J, ed. Motor Control Mechanisms in Health and disease. New York: Raven Press, 1983.

260. Altman D, Schulz K, Moher D, Egger M, Davidoff F, Elbourne D, Gotzsche P, Lang T. The revised CONSORT statement for reporting randomized trials: Explanation and elaboration. Ann Int Med 2001; 34:663–394.

261. Moher D, Schulz KF, Altman D. The CONSORT statement: Revised recommendations for improving the quality of reports of parallel-group randomized trials. JAMA 2001; 285:1987–1991.

Chapter 8

Acute and Chronic Medical Management

A handful of medical issues come up repeatedly during the chronic rehabilitation management of patients with neurologic diseases. This chapter reviews the mechanisms and treatment for complications within the first several months of onset of disability such as deep vein thrombosis, seizures, dysphagia, and the neurogenic bowel and bladder, and later complications from pain, spasticity, contractures, pressure sores, and sleep disorders.

DEEP VEIN THROMBOSIS

From the first day of immobility until a patient is ambulatory on the rehabilitation ward, clinicians and staff must take a forward appproach to the prevention and management of venous thromboembolism. The clinical signs and symptoms of deep vein thrombosis (DVT) and pulmonary embolism (PE) are not sensitive or specific, so they cannot be considered reliable. By impedance plethysmography and, for the calf, by radioisotope scanning with fibringoen I-125, venous thrombi have been reported in a paretic leg within 1 week of an acute stroke in over 50% of patients, although symptoms and signs are far less frequent.[1] Higher incidences have also been associated with greater severity of leg paresis, inability to ambulate,[2,3] and hypercoagulability suggested by a shortened PTT.[4] The risk of DVT appears greatest in the first 2 weeks after a SCI and reaches an incidence of 25%–50% over 12 weeks.[5] Duplex ultrasonography and venography are among the best diagnostic tests. When a PE is suspected due to unexplained dyspnea, tacycardia, or oxygen desaturation by oximetry, a ventilation-perfusion scan, CT or MRI of the pulmonary vessels with injection of

323

contrast material, or pulmonary angiography must be done.

Prevention

In controlled trials of prophylaxis after stroke, DVT has been found in 20%–75% of untreated patients within 2 weeks of stroke.[6,7] From 5% to 20% of patients suffered a PE, which was fatal in approximately 10%. Intermittent calf compression of the paretic leg, intermittent low dose heparin at 5000 units every 8 to 12 hours, and low molecular weight heparinoid were more effective than no intervention or the use of antiembolism hose. These varied interventions reduced DVT by a factor of 2–7 and PE by approximately 2 to 4. Low-dose heparin prophylaxis has been recommended by a consensus conference for all nonhemorrhagic stroke patients and external pneumatic calf compression for the rest.[8] The addition of pneumatic sequential compression devices to an anticoagulant augments the benefit of the anticoagulant.[9]

After SCI, thromboembolism was detected in 31% of patients graded Frankel A and B who were randomized to 5000 units of subcutaneous heparin twice a day within 72 hours of injury, but in only 7% of patients whose activated partial thromboplastin time was prolonged to $1-1/2$ times control values by adjusting the dose every 12 hours.[10] Over an average of 7 weeks of anticoagulation, bleeding complications were greater in the adjusted dose group, especially at sites of trauma. Mechanical and other drug interventions have also been of value for prophylaxis. Compared to intermittent heparin alone, studies suggest that low-molecular-weight heparins, a low dose of standard heparin plus electrical stimulation of the calves, and external compression stockings will each lower the incidence of positive tests for DVT.[5] Adjusted dose unfractionated heparin is still more cost-effective than enoxaparin, 30 mg twice a day.[11] Aspirin plus external leg compression may also have a benefit when heparin is contraindicated. Prophylaxis in the absence of symptoms or systemic medical complications continues for 8 to 12 weeks or until discharge from rehabilitation.[12] The incidence of DVT in persons with chronic SCI is similar or lower than the incidence in the nonambulatory surgical or medical patient, running less than 10% for acute and chronic DVT.[13]

Currently, approximately four low-molecular-weight heparins, one heparinoid, two hirudin derivatives, and one direct thrombin inhibitor are also available for use in DVT prophylaxis. Low-molecular-weight heparins are chemical or physical fractions of unfractionated heparin and have greater bioavailability, so their anticoagulant activity is more predictable. These drugs are at least as effective as fixed-dose unfractionated heparin and less likely to cause thrombocytopenia. Subcutaneous enoxaparin, 40 mg a day, given for one week after neurosurgical procedures appeared to be safe and effective in that the drug reduced the risk for venographically proven DVT by 50% without causing more bleeding complications than a placebo caused.[14] The drug is usually used as 30–40 mg every 12 hours. Fondaparinaux, which is a newer agent derived from the activated factor X-binding moiety of unfractionated heparin, was more effective than enoxaparin after hip surgery. Enoxaparin, dalteparin, and tinzaparin are effective for treating thromboembolism as well. They have a rather long half-life and require little if any laboratory monitoring.

After the diagnosis of a symptomatic DVT is made, patients with stroke or SCI are generally safe to return to rehabilitation activites after at least 3 days on a therapeutic dose of an anticoagulant.[15,16] Thus, rehabilitation efforts can usually continue without a transfer to an acute setting. Warfarin is started with heparin or a heparinoid to reach an International Normalized Ratio (INR) of 2–3 for 3–6 months for a first episode of DVT.[17,18] A vena cava filter is indicated when anticoagulation is contraindicated and in patients with a high, complete cervical SCI. A filter may not exclude the need for warfarin anticoagulation in other circumstances.

ORTHOSTATIC HYPOTENSION

Orthostatic hypotension (OH) occurs often enough in elderly patients, after stroke or SCI, after bed rest with deconditioning, from dehydration, and in relationship to drugs or diseases such as diabetes mellitus that block normal vasomotor and cardiac responses to standing that the condition may interfere with rehabilitation.

The sometimes subtle effects of standing hypotension include exercise intolerance, fatigue, dizziness, confusion, a decline in mental functioning, and of course, syncope.

After stroke, a few measures may reduce the risk for additional hypoperfusion-induced ischemic injury during initial attempts at mobilizing the patient soon after transfer for inpatient rehabilitation. The most frequent errors of commission that lead to OH include fluid restriction from initial concern about cerebral edema and, later, from inadequate fluid intake secondary to dysphagia, and medications for hypertension and heart disease, such as beta-blockers and diuretics. Deconditioning from immobility contributes to postural pressure changes. People with diabetes mellitus and a peripheral neuropathy often have baroreceptor denervation, so they cannot raise their blood pressure by increasing their heart rates. Hard stool may force patients to strain and produce Valsalva's maneuver, causing hypotension.

Postural hypotension increases with aging. An epidemiologic study of 5210 men and women 65 years and older found that 18% had asymptomatic orthostatic hypotension, defined as at least a 20 mm Hg drop in the systolic or 10 mm Hg drop in diastolic pressure.[19] This chronic postural hypotension was associated with difficulty walking, frequent falls, transient ischemic attack, isolated systolic hypertension, and the presence of a carotid stenosis. Patients with orthostatic hypotension often have undertreated supine hypertension. Their blood pressure, checked seated, is normal, but supine hypertension increases their risk for repeated stroke and for cardiovascular disease. Orthostatic hypotension is a risk factor for stroke.[20] Patients with extrapyramidal disorders such as Parkinson's disease, and with polyneuropathies, especially diabetes mellitus, are especially at risk for OH that exacerbates with bed rest. After a SCI, especially higher than the T-6 level, OH is also a common complication, not necessarily associated with autonomic dysreflexia.

Management starts with hydration with intravenous normal saline if volume depletion is suspected and oral fluids are difficult to swallow. Volume expansion can also be accomplished with fludrocortisone, 0.1 mg daily to 0.2 mg twice a day, plus at least 2 grams of salt with meals. Medications that may dehydrate, such as diuretics, are contraindicated. The dose of beta-blockers or other antihypertensive agents may have to be reduced. When the patient is in bed, placing the entire bed in reverse Trendelenberg with the head up at least 10° prevents an overnight diuresis, because the kidneys and baroreceptors appreciate an intermediate blood pressure, which is higher than when the patient is supine. Tight elastic stockings or wraps that extend above the knees and an abdominal pressure binder may improve venous return. Patients must stay out of bed, sitting and standing as much as possible, or work from a tilt-table to help build postural reflexes. Vasoconstrictors such as midodrine, 10–20 mg when out of bed every 4–6 hours, or ephedrine, 25–100 mg every 6 hours, are useful adjuncts. Midodrine, an α-agonist that acts on arteriole and venous receptors, was superior to placebo in raising systolic pressure and in reducing global symptoms when patients with neurogenic OH stood.[21]

THE NEUROGENIC BLADDER

Urine incontinence, retention, and a combination of both results from lesions at a variety of levels of the nervous system. Serious consequences include urinary tract infections, pyelonephritis, hydronephrosis, renal and bladder calculi, breakdown of skin, and social embarrassment. Incontinence and retention should be managed proactively to prevent infection and pressure sores, as well as to preserve dignity and quality of life for the patient. The incidence of neurogenic bladder is high immediately after stroke and severe TBI, then lessens over time. The incidence is very high after traumatic SCI and remains so. Patients with MS evolve a very high incidence as the disease takes on a progressive course more than 10 years after onset of the first symptoms from demyelinating plaques.

Many elderly patients have a premorbid history of bladder dysfunction. Urinary dribbling and involuntary emptying affects 30% of the healthy, noninstitutionalized population over the age of 65 years.[22] After a stroke, many of these patients decompensate further and previously asymptomatic patients with a hemiparesis become affected. In a prospective follow-up of 150 patients with all degrees of impairment after stroke, 60% were incontinent in the first week, 40% at 4 weeks, and 30% at 12 weeks.[23] Of those who had no control by 6 weeks, only 18% were continent at 1 year. Another study followed patients with a mean age of 68 years who were admitted to an inpatient rehabilitation service. By 1 month following an acute stroke, 10% with a pure motor impairment and 70% with the more severe combination of motor, proprioceptive, and visual hemianoptic deficits were incontinent of urine.[24] At 6 months, 30% of the latter group, which presumably had suffered a full middle cerebral artery territory infarction, were still incontinent. During outpatient therapy, some patients may be too embarrassed to admit that they are incontinent. The clinician must ask direct questions.

Pathophysiology

The anatomy and pharmacology of the controls for micturition provide insight for how to evaluate and manage dysfunction.[25] Conscious cortical control modulates the micturition center of the pontine reticular formation and the pudendal nerve to the striated external sphincter. The micturition center coordinates bladder and sphincter activity via inputs to the sacral spinal cord. The net effect of frontal lobe and reticulospinal control is inhibition of bladder detrusor neurons. Parasympathetic fibers from S-2 to S-4 provide motor control to the bladder detrusor muscle, as well as to the proximal urethra and the external sphincter. Parasympathetic afferents carry the sensation for bladder filling back to the sacral nuclei. Sympathetic fibers from T-11 to L-1 relax the detrusor muscle, contract the bladder neck and proximal urethra, and inhibit parasympathetic flow. Activation leads to continence and the storage of urine. The usual bladder capacity is up to 500 mL and the sensation of filling is perceived at approximately 125 mL.

Insight into the mechanism of dysfunction comes from finding a postvoid residual of more than 50 mL by catheterization. Bedside ultrasound allows nurses to quickly assess the volume of urine in the bladder. This technique eliminates urethral trauma and the risk of inducing an infection. A urodynamic study by cystometrography (CMG) shows whether the problem is primarily a failure to store or to empty urine because of bladder or urthral dysfunction. The CMG allows characterization of the bladder volume when the patient first senses the urge to void, records uninhibited detrusor contractions, measures bladder compliance, reveals external sphincter activity during filling and emptying, and measures urine flow rate. The results classify micturition as (1) normal; (2) detrusor hyperreflexia, if involuntary contractions cannot be suppressed; (3) detrusor areflexia, if contractions are poor; and (4) detrusor-sphincter dyssynergia if the urethra contracts during a detrusor contraction. In older men, the test also helps evaluate the contribution of bladder outlet obstruction from prostatic hypertrophy. In diabetic cystopathy, urodynamic studies often reveal impaired bladder sensation, decreased detrusor contractility, large bladder capacity, and impaired flow, generally in association with a peripheral neuropathy.

In a general way, clinicians may anticipate the type of bladder dysfunction from the location of a lesion. For example, a frontal lobe TBI can cause urgency and incontinence because of loss of cortical inhibitory control. Indeed, detrusor hyperreflexia, which also occurs in patients with stroke, MS, and Parkinson's disease, is the most common cause of a neurogenic bladder. Postvoid residuals are usually not high. Detrusor-sphincter dyssynergia, with either the internal or external sphincter affected, can follow a brain stem injury or MS, but most often follows SCI above the conus medullaris.

Urodynamic studies are indicated when the cause of retention or incontinence is unclear. Elevated postvoid residual volumes, over 50 mL, have been detected in 35%–50% of patients with a first stroke admitted for rehabilitation.[26] Approximately one-third of these cases of retention have bladder outlet obstruction, one-third have bladder hyporeflexia, and others have a combination of both. Cognitive dysfunction contributes in some instances. No relationship has been found between residual volume and position during voiding, whether in bed or on a commode for men or for women. Among incontinent patients admitted to one rehabilitation unit, 37% had normal CMG studies, another 37% had detrusor hyperreflexia, 21% had detrusor hyporeflexia, and 5% had detrusor sphincter dyssynergia.[27] An unstable detrusor is the most common cystometric study abnormality associated with persistent incontinence.

After SCI, rostral to the lumbosacral level, an inactive bladder evolves into bladder hyperactivity and automatic micturition.[25] Reorganization of the micturition reflex pathway involves changes in the properties of bladder afferent neurons and spinal synapses with the loss of descending inputs and a partial reversion to reflexes that were suppressed after infancy. Voiding is inefficient because of detrusor-sphincter dyssynergia. Detrusor hyperreflexia combined with dyssynergia permits large volumes of urine residuals and incontinence with high intravesical pressures, followed by the complications of bladder trabeculation, infections, and reflux up the ureters and into the kidney. Sacral spinal cord or root damage interrupts the parasympathetic excitatory input to the bladder detrusor muscle, causing an areflexic bladder and urine retention.

Management

Therapy takes many forms. The first step is to treat intercurrent urinary tract infection. Systemic antimicrobial drugs for prophylaxis, such as trimethoprim, and acidifying and alkalinizing agents do not clearly reduce the incidence of infection over the long run.[28] Of interest, 300 mL of cranberry juice did reduce the frequency of bacteriuria with pyuria in elderly women,[29] so prophylaxis might be tried after a stroke in older patients.

Behavioral techniques can be used to maintain continence in cognitively and behaviorally impaired patients, especially after a TBI. Patients with myelopathies or an areflexic bladder learn to perform intermittent catheterization of the bladder 3 to 5 times a day. Catheters can be washed, stored in plastic bags, and reused. A review of the literature of patients with MS or SCI reveals remarkably little evidence for or against differences in infection rates for sterile versus clean catheterization techniques and for differences in infections associated with indwelling versus intermittent catheterization, but it seems reasonable to encourage clean, intermittent catheterization techniques rather than indwelling catheters when feasible.[30]

MEDICATIONS

Many drugs have been tried, based on their potential effects on the alpha-adrenergic and beta-adrenergic and nicotinic and muscarinic cholinergic receptors within the micturition reflex (Table 8–1). Benign prostatic hypertrophy (BPH) may produce overflow incontinence in patients who can void and obstruction with high residual urines in patients who cannot void. Over several months, finasteride, 5 mg daily, lowers the level of 5α-dihydrotestosterone to reduce prostate size, but the effect on symptoms takes at least 6 months. Smooth muscle tone in the stroma of the prostate and in the bladder neck acompany BPH and are more quickly reduced by blockade of the α1-adrenergic receptors here. Doxazosin, for example, may improve flow within a week, but the first doses must be given with some caution to prevent symptomatic hypotension. Prostatic obstruction may have to be corrected surgically prior to inpatient discharge if catheterization and medications prove to have too many side effects.

Scheduled voids, double voiding, anticholinergics, and an external catheter in men are of value for patients who are incontinent but have less than 100 mL residuals. For urinary urge incontinence with a low storage bladder, tolterodine, which has fewer anticholinergic effects, may be better tolerated in older patients than oxybutin.[31] Dry mouth and constipation are common complaints with these drugs. Long-acting preparations are available for the anticholinergic agents, but some patients only need a short-acting preparation before sleep to prevent nocturia, which limits side effects during the day. Imipramine, when used to decrease bladder contractility and increase outlet resistance, can accentuate orthostatic hypotension. Intermittent catheterization is best for patients who cannot void. Desmopressin nasal spray taken at night has reduced overnight urine volumes enough to help relieve nocturia in people with SCI and MS.[32] Its antidiuretic effect only occasionally causes hyponatremia.

INVASIVE PROCEDURES

Neurostimulation techniques and surgical procedures, such as augmentation cystoplasty and other urinary diversions, are used mostly for people with myelopathies from SCI and MS who cannot maintain a low-pressure detrusor with intermittent catheterization. These patients run the risk of recurrent urinary infection, vesicoureteral reflux, and stone formation.

Table 8–1. **Pharmacologic Manipulation of Bladder Dysfunction**

Medication	Indication	Mechanisms of Action	Dose*
Bethanechol	Facilitate emptying	Increases detrusor contraction	25 mg bid–50 mg qid
Clonidine	Facilitate emptying; internal sphincter dyssynergia	Decreases urethral tone	0.1–0.2 mg bid
Doxazosin Prazosin Terazosin Tamulosin	Facilitate emptying due to outlet obstruction	Alpha blockade of external sphincter to decrease tone	1–8 mg qd 1–2 mg bid 1–5 mg bid 0.4–0.8 mg qd
Diazepam Baclofen Dantrolene	May facilitate emptying and decrease outlet obstruction	Decrease external sphincter tone	2–5 mg bid 10–20 mg tid 25 mg tid
Imipramine or other tricyclic	Facilitate storage; urge incontinence; enuresis	Increase internal sphincter tone; decrease detrusor contractions; anticholinergic effects	25–100 mg hs
Verapamil	Facilitate storage	Relax detrusor; decrease bladdder contractility	40–80 mg qd, intravesically
Indomethicin	Facilitate storage	Prostaglandin inhibition of detrusor	25–50 mg tid
Oxybutynin Hyoscyamine Tolterodine	Facilitate storage; urge incontinence; frequency	Relax detrusor; increase internal sphincter tone; muscurinic receptor antagonist	5 mg hs–5 mg qid 0.125 mg bid–0.25 mg qid 1–2 mg bid
Pseudoephedrine	Facilitate storage	Contracts bladder neck	30–60 mg bid to qid
Capsaicin	Facilitate storage	Blockade C-fibers	1–2 mmol/L intravesically
Desmopressin	Prevent nocturia	Antidiuretic effect	10 ug hs, intranasally 0.2–0.6 mg po

A randomized trial in patients with SCI found that urethral stents are as effective as sphincterotomy in reducing voiding pressures by almost one-half, but stents require a shorter hospitalization.[33] The bladder can be enlarged by anastomosing a piece of bowel to a resected patch of its wall. Augmentation cystoplasty has mostly replaced the sphincterotomies and other urinary diversions used more than 10 years ago. Infants and children with a meningomyelocele often require surgical diversionary methods.

Parasympathetic stimulation by electrodes placed intradurally on the anterior roots of S-2 to S-4 can reduce urine residual volumes, increase bladder capacity, and reduce fecal impaction and constipation. This approach requires a laminectomy, a posterior rhizotomy, and an implantation of a radio receiver. As described in Chapter 4, a commercial stimulator for an upper motoneuron neurogenic bladder is now available.[34] The S-3 root is most critical for bladder control. A test trial of stimulation is necessary, since some patients do not respond. Not all patients have the same underlying mechanism for detrusor hyperactivity, so stimulation of somatic afferents that then inhibit bladder reflexes in the cord may not always be effective. Stimulation is sometimes effective at other sites, including the bladder wall, pelvic floor, vaginal or anal sphincter, and over pudendal and tibial nerves, but these approaches are often not practical and results may be inconsistent.

Nonroutine management options are best discussed with a urologist who knows the patient and can evaluate surgical procedures and unusual pharmacological interventions, such as the treatment of dyssynergia with botulinum toxin injected into the bladder wall or external sphincter and intravesical instillations of capsaicin to block C-fiber afferent-induced reflexes.[35] C-fibers become mechanosensitive after SCI. Capsacin may cause pain for up to several weeks after instillation, but improves urodynamic parmeters such as bladder capacity for up to 6 months. A placebo-controlled clinical trial in patients with paraplegia showed efficacy in reducing urgency and leakage.[36] Resiniferatoxin is more potent than capsaicin in its action on the vanilloid re-ceptor of C-fiber afferents and is in clinical trials.

Long-term management of the bladder tends to be dictated by the individual's physical, vocational, and psychosocial needs. The American Paralysis Society has listed its recommendations for care.[37] Radiologic and urodynamic assessments are suggested yearly for the first 5 to 10 years after SCI and yearly cystoscopy for patients using indwelling catheters. An intravenous pyelogram or renal scan combined with renal ultrasound assess anatomy and function.

BOWEL DYSFUNCTION

Incontinence, constipation, loose stools, fecal impaction, and abdominal distention are common problems among patients with acute and chronic neurologic diseases. The prevalence of fecal incontinence in hospitalized elderly patients from all causes, with and without a normal pelvic floor, is 13%–47%.[38] Bowel incontinence develops in approximately 30% of patients after stroke, but usually resolves spontaneously by 2 weeks or is corrected by dealing with the underlying medical cause, such as diarrhea from clostridia infection.

Quality of life suffers in approximately 50% of patients with SCI from the complications of

evacuation problems and other gastrointestinal sequelae such as ileus, gastric ulcers, reflux, diverticulosis, hemorrhoids, and nausea, loss of appetite, incontinence, hours spent attempting to evacuate the bowel, and impactions. Approximately one in four patients with SCI require a hospitalization for such complications.[39]

Pathophysiology

Abnormal function at any level of the nervous system can cause incontinence. Motor innervation to the rectum and the internal and external sphincters arises from sacral roots S-2, S-3, and S-4. The internal sphincter is supplied by the hypogastric nerve and parasympathetic nerves. Continence is maintained by a closed internal anal sphincter and the acute angle of the anorectal canal. Sympathetic discharges from the upper lumber colonic nerve increase sphincter tone. Rectal dilation by stool or by digital stimulation inhibit this tone. The pudendal nerve without parasympathetic input controls the external sphincter. Colonic motility depends on chemical, neurogenic, and myogenic mechanisms. Colonic transit times are slow especially in the descending colon and anorectum after SCI. With an upper motoneuron lesion after SCI, defecation cannot be initiated by voluntary relaxation of the external anal sphincter. Reflex mechanisms, however, are intact for stool propulsion.[40]

Certain symptoms are associated with lesions at particular levels of the neuraxis. With uninhibited neurogenic bowel incontinence, patients have a sudden urge to defecate or awareness is distorted so that defecation happens without any urge. Lesions are usually cortical or subcortical. Reflex neurogenic incontinence occurs abruptly without warning or is part of a mass reflex. The lesion is within the spinal cord, above the conus medullaris. High spinal lesions cause incontinence that is more easily managed than lesions that involve the conus. A conus or cauda lesion produces an autonomous neurogenic bowel with slow stool propulsion and low external sphincter tone. Incontinence occurs with increased abdominal pressure, or it may be continuous. An autonomic or sensory neuropathy from diabetes that is superimposed upon a hemisphere stroke may produce incontinence when either lesion alone would not.

Management

Alert patients must be involved in their bowel program to achieve continence without obstipation. Constipation and impaction are common complications of inactivity, limited fluid and fiber intake, anticholinergic medication, and depression. Episodes of incontinence should be related to time of day, frequency, stool consistency, diet (fiber content, gas-forming foods like berries, constipating items like cheese and rice), fluid intake, physical activity, history of laxative abuse, and medications. Stool softeners, colonic stimulants, contact irritants, and bulk formers help in management. Optimal use of these agents takes art and patience. A blinded clinical trial in patients with SCI found a significant decrease in time for bowel care using polyethylene glycol-based bisacodyl suppositories compared to hydrogenated vegetable oil-based bisacodyl and enemas.[41] Prokinetic agents may help. Metaclopramide, for example, aids gastric emptying, but may induce extrapyramidal signs and autonomic dysreflexia.

Digital stimulation of the anal sphincter often aids the patient with SCI above the conus. Sacral root stimulation aids some patients with upper motoneuron lesions of the cord that also cause a neurogenic bladder.[34] Diarrhea not caused by an impaction or tube feedings is sometimes the residual effect of antibiotics. Live yogurt cultures can replace bowel flora and improve control. A gastrointestinal infection, particularly by clostridium or a vancomycin-resistent enterococcus, is assessed by stool culture. Persistent bowel incontinence can indicate diffuse brain injury or the inability to express the need to defecate and move to a toilet. A toileting schedule or specific communication to signal need can solve the problem. A rectal bag fastened around the anus can keep the very disabled patient clean. Education about regular routines, timing of bowel movements, and diet are critical for patient self-management.

NUTRITION AND DYSPHAGIA

Proper nutrition and caloric intake is critical for risk factor management in patients with atherosclerosis, diabetes mellitus, and chronic neuromedical disorders. During rehabilitation, optimal nutrition can offset the effects of a catabolic state. For patients whose mobility is impaired, nutritional interventions may also lessen the risk of developing skin sores, osteoporosis, and obesity. A consensus group of the American Heart Association offers reasonable dietary guidelines with rationales for recommendations that deserve review by patients.[42]

Neurogenic dysphagia means dysfunction in the mechanisms that deliver a food or liquid bolus into the esophagus. Aspiration, respiratory compromise, malnutrition, and dehydration are the serious consequences. Indeed, dysphagia is the potential cause of a pulmonary infection in any patient with stroke, TBI, motor neuron disease, cerebral palsy, MS, advanced Parkinson's disease, cervicomedullary pathologies such as a syrinx, the Guillain-Barre syndrome, myasthenia gravis, and most neuromuscular diseases.

Swallowing disorders affect 10% of acutely hospitalized, elderly patients and 30% of nursing home dwellers.[43] From 5% to 15% of cases of community-acquired pneumonia are caused by aspiration.[44] Aspiration pneumonia and inadequate caloric intake become even more likely at the time of an acute stroke. Dysphagia is diagnosed by a variety of criteria in approximately one-half of patients with acute strokes and in up to 40% of hospitalized patients in the first 2 weeks after stroke by videofluoroscopic swallow study, depending on the case mix. A prospective British study diagnosed dysphagia in 30% of 357 conscious patients within 48 hours of a unilateral hemispheric stroke.[45] Patients were rated as impaired if swallowing was delayed or they coughed on 10 ml of water. Lethargy, gaze paresis, and sensory inattention were present more often than in those who swallowed normally. By 1 week, 16% had dysphagia. At 1 month, only 2% and, at 6 months, only 0.4% of survivors were impaired. In a regional study, signs of malnutrition was found in 16% of stroke patients upon admission, with the greatest risk in women over age 74.[46] By discharge, 23% were malnourished. Elderly men and patients who had infections or received new cardiovascular drugs had the greatest risk. Persistent dysphagia correlates with greater disability and risk of death.[47] Clearly, clinicians must attend to the caloric intake of the disabled patient after stroke, as well as TBI and other illnesses that produce a catabolic state.

Dysphagia occurs in approximately one-third of patients with serious TBI, eventually in up to one-half of patients with MS, in nearly all patients with ALS, and in people with myasthenia gravis that affects oral muscles, the velopharyngeal port, and the pharynx. Aspiration is also common in people with Parkinson's disease. Fatigability may impede swallowing in any patient with a neurologic disease, but is especially apt to affect people with myasthenia. Oral secretions colonized by bacterial pathogens in dental plaque, caries, and periodontal tissue, as well as reflux of gastric fluids put patients at risk for aspiration pneumonia.

Pathophysiology

Relevant pathology can be found at multiple interacting levels of the nervous system (Table 8–2). A brain stem neural network for swallowing, related to the functionally associated network for respiration,[48] probably has the features of a pattern generator that initiates and organizes the motor sequence for automatic swallow and distributes impulses for deglutition. Stimulation of the oropharynx and laryngeal region or the superior laryngeal and glossopharyngeal nerves is the most powerful way to lower the threshold for swallowing. Higher command centers for initiation exist, of course,

in the cortex. Indeed, a prospective transcranial magnetic stimulation study found that the return of effective swallowing by 1 to 3 months after stroke correlated with an increase in the representation for the pharyngeal muscles of the unaffected hemisphere.[49]

Lesions in the pathways for swallowing interfere with the oral, oral preparatory, and reflex or pharyngeal phases of deglutition. In the first phase, chewed food particles and liquids are held in a bolus against the palate by the tongue. Bolus volume affects the timing of laryngeal and cricopharyngeal actions. During the oral phase, the tongue propels the bolus posteriorly through the pillars of the anterior fauces. A labial seal and tension in the buccal muscles prevent loss of the bolus. The reflexive swallow starts the pharyngeal phase. Velophayrngeal closure excludes the bolus from the nasophayrnx. Pharyngeal peristalsis, closure of the larynx, and the pumping action of the tongue sweeps the bolus through the cricopharyngeal sphincter. Elevation and anterior movement of the larynx under the root of the tongue, noted clinically by the superior and anterior motion of the thyroid cartilage, prevents aspiration. In addition, the epiglottis diverts a bolus into the valleculae as the aryepiglottic folds, false cords, and true vocal cords approximate to prevent aspiration. The motion of the larynx also helps open the cricopharyngeal sphincter to let the bolus pass into the esophagus. This action triggers a peristaltic wave.

Table 8–2. **Localization of Pathology Causing Neurogenic Dysphagia**

Cortex
  Inferior precentral and posterior inferior frontal gyrus
  Bilateral corticobulbar pathway interruption
Basal ganglia and cerebellum
Brain stem
  Solitary tract and adjacent reticular formation
  Lateral reticular formation near nucleus ambiguous
Cranial nerves
  V, VII, IX, X
Neuromuscular junction
Bulbar muscles

Assessment

Clinical symptoms and signs, bedside tests, and procedures identify patients with dysphagia who are at risk of malnutrition, dehydration, and aspiration. A wet-hoarse voice, drooling, and cough shortly after deglutition suggest dysphagia. Wet phonation arises from saliva or ingested material on the vocal cords or in the pyriform sinuses, but does not imply penetration of material.[50] The presence or absence of a palatal, gag, and pharyngeal reflex does not necessarily predict the safety of swallowing. Swallowing water at less than 10 mL per second[51] or coughing or a wet-hoarse quality to the voice within 1 minute of continuously swallowing 90 mL of water points to the risk of aspiration. The 90 mL water swallow test was the strongest predictor of pneumonia, recurrent airway obstruction, and death in a seven-part screening test for dysphagia during inpatient rehabilitation for stroke.[52] These complications were 7.6 times more likely in the inpatients who failed the screen than in those who passed. In the same population, the investigators also found that pneumonia was significantly more likely to develop during a 1-year follow-up of patients who aspirated a small amount, silently, or more than 10% on videofluoroscopic modified barium swallow (MBS), compared with those who did not.[53] However, from 3 to 6 times as many patients aspirated on the test and did not develop pneumonia.

The MBS reveals laryngeal penetration, as well as mechanisms of dysphagia. This evaluation usually includes attempts at swallowing 5 mL of thin and thick liquid barium, 5 mL of a barium-impregnated gel or pudding, a piece of a cookie coated with barium paste, 20 mL of thin barium liquid, and successive swallows of approximately 30 mL of thin barium liquid. Dysphagia severity has been rated as follows[54]:

1. Mild: intermittent, trace supraglottic penetration with immediate clearing
2. Moderate: repeated supraglottic penetration, stasis in the laryngeal vestibule, or 2 or less aspirations of a single viscosity
3. Moderate-severe: repeated aspiration of a single viscosity
4. Severe: repeated aspiration of more than 1 consistency.

In a study of 114 inpatients undergoing stroke rehabilitation, the MBS revealed the relative risk of developing pneumonia.[53] The risk was 7 times greater in those who aspirated compared to those who did not, approximately 5.5 times greater for silent aspirators, and 8 times greater for those who aspirated 10% or more on one or more barium swallows. Dehydration and death were not associated with the MBS findings. In alert, at-risk inpatients during stroke rehabilitation, coughing or a wet-hoarse quality of the voice within 1 minute of continuously swallowing 90 mL of water from a cup had a sensitivity of 80% and specificity of 54% for apiration demonstrated by MBS. The bedside test had a sensitivity of 88% and specificity of 44% for large amounts of aspiration that might be more clinically significant.[55] False-negative tests usually involved less than 10% aspiration of barium. Thus, this quick screen re-

veals most of those who will aspirate on the MBS and, in the study, all of those who developed a pneumonia, but will include a lot of false-positive tests. The MBS is the gold standard for screening and ought to be employed. The test offers other insights into the risks related to dysphagia. In a 1-year follow-up of 60 dysphagic patients after stroke, aspiration pneumonia occurred in patients whose videofluoroscopic studies showed a total kinematic pharyngeal transit time greater than 2 seconds, with the greatest risk if more than 5 seconds.[56] The presence or absence of vallecular or piriform pooling or penetration of the bolus through the true vocal cords did not, however, correlate with clinically apparent aspiration.

Other techniques, including auscultation during swallow, ultrasound, manometry, surface electromyography of esophageal sphincter muscles, fiberoptic endoscopy[57] or pulse oximetry during swallow,[58] and biomechanical assessments[59] have been used less often in the clinical setting. Another test may come into use at the bedside. The combination of manometry, EMG, and MBS best assess cricopharygeal dysfunction. Nebulized tartaric acid, when inhaled a few times, normally elicits a reflexive cough by stimulating receptors in the vestibule of the larynx. A weak or absent cough predicted aspiration pneumonia better than the MBS in a small group of patients admitted for rehabilitation after a stroke.[60]

Treatment

Lesions that may not ordinarily cause dysphagia may do so in patients with depressed consciousness or attention, a weak cough, loose dentures, oral candidiasis, laryngeal trauma from intubation, poor head control, reduced saliva from anticholinergic medications, a tracheostomy or nasopharyngeal feeding tube, and esophageal motility disorders or reflux esophagitis. When possible, these superimposed problems should be managed before proceeding with feeding tubes.

Aphagic patients with unilateral hemisphere lesions who will be transferred to an inpatient rehabilitation program usually should not undergo a gastrostomy for feedings. The great majority will recover spontaneously and with therapy. Patients with bihemipheric strokes and a pseudobulbar palsy, pontomedullary lesions, and unilateral lesions within the Sylvian fissure are most likely to be affected beyond the acute hospital stay. These patients become a challenge for the rehabilitation team. Figure 9–1 shows the acute diffusion-weighted MRI scan of a patient who presented with dysphasia and aphagia. She had an equivocal prior history of stroke. The imaging study revealed an old right Sylvian lesion and the new homologous cortical lesion on the left. The bilateral infarcts produced clinically unanticipated aphagia.

Most often after a hemispheric stroke or TBI, the swallowing reflex is delayed, the bolus slides over the base of the tongue and collects in the valleculae and hypopharynx, and sometimes the pharyngeal constrictor malfunctions. If oral intake is unsafe based upon a formal swallowing evaluation or provides less than 800 calories per day by 3 days after the acute admission, intravenous therapy or feeding through a small bore nasogastric tube (NGT) is indicated.

Specific treatments for neurogenic dysphagia depend in part on the impairment at each stage of swallowing.[61,62] Good motivation and cognition are necessary for successful therapy. Table 8–3 outlines some of the most frequently employed techniques. Controlled trials are few, but the efficacy of several techniques may be borne out during MBS. The need for controlled trials of any invasive or expensive therapeutic program is especially appropriate, because the natural history of dysphagia after stroke and TBI is that all but a few percent of subjects will recover. Even patients with medullary infarcts that cause unilateral paresis of the pharyngeal muscle and the adductor of the larynx, along with cricopharyngeal dysfunction, swallowing can gradually be retrained.[63]

The consistency and size of the bolus affect each stage of swallowing. For example, the patient who drools and does not move liquids in the oral preparatory and oral phases may note an improvement with liquids thickened by a gel such as *Thick-it* or added to foods such as mashed potatoes. Oral exercises, postural changes with the head turned or chin down, and thermal stimulation of the anterior faucial pillars are often used, although responses of patients differ widely. Cricopharyngeal myotomy followed by swallowing therapy can improve deglutition when the sphincter will not relax and hypopharyngeal pooling occurs, especially in patients with motor neuron disease and after a pontomedullary stroke.

Table 8–3. General Therapies for Dysphagia

COMPENSATION

Head positioning
- Head back to improve oral transit by gravity
- Chin tuck to push epiglottis and tongue posteriorly and protect airway
- Head rotation to weak pharygeal side to adduct larynx, direct bolus to strong side
- Head rotation to reduce cricopharyngeal sphincter pressure

Alter consistency of food
Thicken liquids
Alter volume of food
Alter pace of intake
Compensatory maneuvers
- Double swallow
- Supraglottic swallow
- Laryngeal elevation

SENSORIMOTOR EXERCISES

Oral sensory stimulation
- Thermal
- Vibration

Resistance and placement exercises of tongue and jaw
Chewing
Oral manipulation of bolus
Laryngeal adduction
Biofeedback

DIRECT INTERVENTIONS

Palatal prosthesis
Surgery
- Cricopharyngeal myotomy
- Epiglottopexy

A trial of three graded levels of dysphagia therapy during inpatient stroke rehabilitation randomized 115 subjects to one of three interventions:[64]

1. The therapist explained the results of MBS and gave recommendations regarding food consistency and compensatory techniques; patient and family then made their own decisions.
2. The same as above, but a therapist reassessed the diet every other week.

3. The therapist prescribed the diet and gave instructions about compensatory techniques and made recommendations daily at mealtime.

Patients who aspirated more than 50% of all food consistencies, and who continued to aspirate after attempting compensatory techniques were excluded from the trial. At discharge and at 1-year follow-up, no differences were apparent among the groups in endpoints of pneumonia, dehydration, calorie-nitrogen deficit, upper airway obstruction, and death. Fifteen percent reached an endpoint during the inpatient stay. Modified barium swallow evidence of aspiration of thick liquids and solids was associated with greater risk and earlier onset of pneumonia. No differences were found when patients were grouped by BI score, stroke impairment, or cognition. Thus, limited patient and family instruction may be as effective as daily, formal dysphagia therapy for selected inpatients.

Pharmacotherapy of dysphagia may have a role in patients with a delay in swallowing and slow pharyngeal transit times. For example, 30 mg of slow release nifedipine increased the time to initiation of pharyngeal contractions.[65] Many elderly people and patients after TBI suffer hyposmia or anosmia. Flavorings, lemon, spices, and other attempts to improve the smell or taste of foods are an important adjunct to encourage eating and nutrition.[66] Patients at risk for aspiration, especially those who are frail, immunosuppressed, diabetic, or have poor dentition require oral hygiene care supplemented by 0.12% chlorhexidine swishes, a 5000 ppm fluoride dentifrice, and when needed, oral antifungal agents such as nystatin or clotrimazole. The risk of gastric reflux is decreased by a proton pump inhibitor such as esomeprazole and by metoclopramide for gastric emptying.

TUBE FEEDINGS

Nasogastric tube feedings are not benign. They can cause gastric reflux, decrease pharyngeal sensation, get misplaced into the trachea or a bronchus, and lead to other pulmonary complications, epistaxis, and perforation of the esophagus. Nasal or pharyngeal irritation may lead to physical restraints to keep patients from pulling the tube.

A hint about the potential problems of tube feedings comes from a quality of care population study of 2824 Medicare patients who were hospitalized for first strokes in 1986.[67] In this population, 44% were unable to eat normally. Approximately 20% of patients had feeding tubes placed within the first 3 days or last 2 days of admission. The tubes were placed in 42% of comatose and 23% of noncomatose patients. The feeding tubes did not protect against the development of pulmonary infiltrates, which occurred in 10% of patients with dysphagia who did or did not receive a nasogastric feeding tube, compared to 4% who had no difficulty swallowing. Most feeding tubes remained in place at discharge and 75% of these patients were sent to nursing homes. Use of a feeding tube for comatose and alert patients was associated with higher mortality rates than found in subjects who did not have a feeding tube, even if such patients had difficulty swallowing.

During dysphagia treatment, NGT feedings supplement oral calories and fluid. The tube feedings should be given after each meal so they do not blunt the patient's appetite. Bolus feedings are preferable to continuous feedings, especially overnight feedings. Diarrhea may be managed by eliminating lactose-containing products, adding fiber, and slowing the rate of flow of the bolus. If profound dysphagia persists toward the time of discharge from inpatient rehabilitation, a gastrostomy tube is a more comfortable portal for nutrition, although the technique is probably no safer in preventing reflux aspiration than an NGT.[68]

Percutaneous endoscopic gastrostomy (PEG) has been complicated by gastric perforation, peritonitis, hematoma, fistula formation with the lung, stomal infection, cellulitis, and bleeding at the insertion site. Jejunostomy may lessen the risk for reflux. Rarely, esophagostomy or pharyngostomy are better suited for the patient with neurologic dysfunction and prior gastrointestinal disease or surgery. Clinical trials related to the efficacy of types of tube feedings and other interventions for dysphagia are monitored by the Cochrane Review (www.update-software.com/cochrane.htm).[69]

PRESSURE SORES

The incidence and prevalence of pressure ulcers is high in immobile patients with neurologic disorders and in residents of nursing homes. Patients with SCI are most apt to develop pressure sores from the combination of immobility and insensate skin. One-third of patients with acute SCI admitted to a Model Systems facility had lesions during acute care and rehabilitation and 15%–25% subsequently had pressure ulcers at annual examinations.[70] Approximately $1.3 billion and 2 million Medicare hospital days are spent on the care of decubitus ulcers yearly.[71]

Pathophysiology

Pressure sores develop primarily over bony prominences such as the occiput, heels, coccyx and sacrum, scapula, and greater trochanter. In addition to immobility, major risk factors include incontinence, poor nutrition with low serum prealbumin level, altered consciousness and poor cognition, exposure to friction and shearing forces on the skin, aged skin, anemia, diabetes, and prior skin wounds and healed ulcers. Some of these mechanisms have been studied.[72] For example, pulling a patient across a bed sheet can cause intraepidermal blisters and superficial erosions. Moisture increases the friction between two surfaces and produces maceration. Shearing forces generated when a seated person slides across a surface can stretch and angulate tissue and blood vessels, which lowers blood flow especially in elderly and paraplegic patients who tend to have compromised circulations. Both high focal pressure and lower pressures for a longer duration, as little as 60 mm Hg, compromise capillaries, produce erythema and, if not relieved, lead to irreversible cellular damage. These sequelae are the basis for surface interventions that aim to distribute and relieve pressure and for turning immobile patients every 2 hours.

The most frequently used classification of pressure sores was proposed by the National Pressure Ulcer Advisory Panel in 1989 (Table 8–4). In addition to the stage, clinicians should describe the location, size, depth, edges, exudate, necrotic tissue, eshar, surrounding skin, and signs of healing. Ulcers are photographed for serial evaluation.

Management

Clinical practice guidelines have been offered by the Agency for Health Care Policy

Table 8–4. **Pressure Ulcer Classification**

STAGE I
Nonblanchable erythema of intact skin; the heralding lesion of skin ulceration. Note: Reactive hyperemia can normally be expected to be present for one-half to three-fourths as long as the pressure occluded blood flow to the area; it should not be confused with a Stage I pressure ulcer.

STAGE II
Partial thickness skin loss involving epidermis and/or dermis. The ulcer is superficial and presents clinically as an abrasion, blister, or shallow crater.

STAGE III
Full thickness skin loss involving damage or necrosis of subcutaneous tissue that may extend down to, but not through, underlying fascia. The ulcer presents clinically as a deep crater with or without undermining of adjacent tissue.

STAGE IV
Full thickness skin loss with extensive destruction, tissue necrosis or damage to muscle, bone, or supporting structures (for example, tendon or joint capsule). Undermining and sinus tracts may be associated with Stage IV pressure ulcers.

and Research[73] and the Consortium for Spinal Cord Medicine.[72] Prevention involves dealing with the above risk factors. For example, skin should be cleansed without irritating or drying it out. Lubricants such as corn starch, protective film dressings, padding, and protective dressings such as hydrocolloids can minimize friction and shear injuries when positioning and turning techniques may compromise the patient. Pillows and wedges protect bony prominences. The heels are best lifted off the bed with pillows under the calves. Pressure-reducing devices that include foam, static air, alternating air, gel, and water mattresses, as well as similar materials for wheelchair seats, can lower the risk for sores. Costly, high-technology beds can cause dehydration, limit mobility, and they are difficult to adjust to for some patients. These beds do not eliminate the need for turning or for pressure relief.

threshold receptors whose ordinarily innocuous sensations come to be processed abnormally in a spinal somatosensory system that has evolved increased excitability, decreased inhibition, and structural reorganization.

The clinical features of neuropathic central pain after a peripheral nerve injury may include hypersensitivity at the lesion site, mechanoallodynia (low pain threshold), thermal hyperalgesia (increased response to a painful stimulus), hyperpathia (greater reaction especially to a repetitive stimulus), a regional distribution of pain as in the complex regional pain syndrome, and autonomic dysregulation.[76] The clinical examination should include having patients report on each stimulus—including touch, pin, temperature, rubbing, pressure, range of motion, and a line drawn with a blunt and a sharp object and repeatedly tapping the skin with these objects—in their own words and graded as unpleasant, painful, and as leaving an aftersensation.

MECHANISMS OF NEUROPATHIC PAIN

The ascending and descending components of the pain transmission and modulation systems are complex in their connectivity, parallel pathways, use of neurotransmitters and peptides, and functional and structural plasticity. Evidence for activity-dependent neuronal plasticity that can cause hypersensitivity to pain has been found in peripheral nociceptors, spinal dorsal horns, the thalamus, and the cortex.[77,78]

The sensation of pain is processed along with the unpleasantness of pain and the personal reflections and emotions about the long-term implications of pain and suffering. Several ascending pathways project nociception to limbic and cortical regions for such processing.[79] These projections include spinohypothalamic, spinopontoamygdaloid, and the spinothalamic pathways to medial thalamic nuclei that in turn project to the anterior cingulate and insular cortices. Spinothalamic projections to the ventral posterior nuclei of the thalamus relay nociception to the primary and secondary sensory cortices. These regions project to posterior parietal cortex, which projects to the insula and back to the amygdala and hippocampus, to converge upon the same structures as the ascending spinal pathways. The insula and especially the anterior cingulate presumably weigh attention, emotional valence, and late actions in response to nociception.

Many of these cortical and subcortical pain pathway nodes are visualized during functional neuroimaging activation studies by PET.[80,81] Indeed, event-related fMRI reveals regions of the anterior cingulate cortex that are related to stimulus perception, stimulus intensity, or to pain itself.[82] Motor-related activations are immediately posterior to the pain-related and stimulus-related cingulate activations in the supplementary motor area. Within these systems, rehabilitationists can find solid and hypothetical rationales for physical, psychologic, pharmacologic, and surgical interventions for neuropathic pain.

Pain can arise from primary afferents in peripheral nerves and dorsal and ventral roots with, for example, a diabetic neuropathy or root compression by a vertebral disk protrusion. The high thresholds of the peripheral terminals of C-fiber nociceptors are decreased by prior activation (autosensitization) or by an increase in membrane excitability by stimuli that do not activate the transducers (heterosensitization). Then, even low frequency activation of receptors by noxious stimuli allow for readily summated inputs that release neuromodulators and glutamate and build up synaptic and voltage-gated currents that create use-dependent facilitation. Clinically, this is the wind-up phenomenon in which repetitive minor stimuli induce central pain by firing dorsal horn neurons. Allodynia results from peripheral stimuli that ordinarily would not produce pain and hyperalgesia from noxious stimuli that evoke greater pain than usual.

These afferent fibers release excitatory amino acids, particularly aspartate and glutamate, and a variety of neuropeptides, endogenous opioids, and substance P. Within the layers of the dorsal horn, inhibitory amino acids including glycine and γ-aminobutyric acid (GABA), monamine neurotransmitters including histamine, serotonin, noradrenaline, and dopamine, and other peptides, especially opioids, become involved in the first spinal stage of pain transmission. Subsequent stages of the pain cascade may not involve the same neurochemicals. For example, substance P is especially important in the evocation of acute intense pain, but is not as critical in establishing nerve injury-induced mechanical and thermal allodynia within the inner part of lamina II interneurons of the dorsal horn.[83] Descending projecting fibers also contribute nociceptive inhibitory monamines that modulate pain signals in direct and indirect ways. These pathways arise from the cortex, hypothalamus, and thalamus, projecting to the periaqueductal gray (PAG) of the midbrain, and descend from the PAG and reticular formation. Within the dorsal horn, nociceptive-specific neurons encode information about the location and nature of the pain stimulus. Wide dynamic range neurons encode intensity, but are also inhibited by surrounding receptive fields for inputs that are not noxious. This differentiation contributes to a separation in the ascending circuits for discriminative pain and for the affective-motivational aspects of pain.

Potentially long-standing changes in the spinal cord are brought about by the activation of NMDA receptors, second messenger protein kinases, and oncogenes that direct protein metabolism.[78] The activation of intracellular kinases by the influx of calcium or activation of G-proteins in nociceptive dorsal horn neurons is a key step in sensitization and altered excitability that persists well beyond the time of afferent stimulation. Critical steps that may cause persistent changes in sensory processing include the expression of protein kinase C (PKC), mitogen-activated protein kinase (MAPK) system, gene activation by nerve growth factor (NGF), which induces gene expression for substance P, brain-derived neurotrophic factor (BDNF) and other growth factors, and phosphorylation of cAMP response element binding protein (CREB). All of these cascades play a role in regulating neuronal plasticity. Indeed, several of these cascades unfold during normal learning and the induction of long-term potentiation (Chapter 1). These fluxes produce anatomical changes in the peripheral nerve, dorsal root ganglia, and dorsal horn over the course of prolonged states of pain. Touch fibers invade the dorsal horn layers once innervated by C-fibers. Sympathetic nerves sprout and form baskets around touch neurons that switch to pain neurons in the dorsal root ganglia. Interneurons may even die in the outer dorsal horn laminae. A major therapeutic thrust will be to interfere with one or more of the cascades associated with chronic neuropathic pain.

Pain inputs at one dermatome can spread to other dorsal spinal segments, which can produce widespread painful sensations. This plasticity leads to changes in the spinothalamic and spinoreticular inputs and representational maps for pain within the somatotopically organized thalamus. For example, repeated pain signals sensitize spinal neurons to future signals, in part via effects on the NMDA receptor. The pain response gets turned up. Pain signals then may fail to trigger the GABA-producing neurons in the thalamus that ordinarily mute incoming pain sensation. Changes in responsiveness of pronociceptive projecting neurons that go to the thalamus can subsequently cause pain independent of afferent input or of inputs that had previously not been associated with pain.[84] Thalamic disinhibition appears to help explain burning pain and allodynia to cold in people with central pain.[77]

Thalamic Pain

Central pain follows a brain stem, thalamic, or thalamocortical stroke in approximately 2% of patients and tends to cause greater symptoms in the arm than the leg. This pain must be distinguished from an unpleasant coldness of the hemiparetic hand or arm associated with reduced blood flow.[85] Dysesthetic thalamic pain arises from damage to the pain and temperature representations in the ventral part of the ventral medial nucleus of the thalamus.[86] Cell loss here appears to disinhibit specific spinothalamic signals that reach the anterior cingulate via a neighboring thalamic nucleus. The anterior cingulate gyrus is involved in the motivational-affectve aspects of pain, but not in feeling a burning dysesthesia. Thus, within the spinal cord, thalamus, and thalamocortical projections to the somatosensory and anterior cingulate cortex,[87] pronociceptive and antinociceptive plasticity is found. These changes presumably account for peripheral neurogenic pain and the not uncommon syndrome of central pain that develops with a variety of neurologic diseases (Table 8–7). After SCI, at-level and below-level of injury central pain affects one-third of patients. Mechanisms of onset are likely similar to the dorsal root ganglia, dorsal horn, and loss of ascending and descending fiber actions discussed. This debilitating condition and its occasional surgical management is reviewed in Chapter 10, but the medical management is similar to that for neuropathic pain.

Table 8–7. **Prevalence of Central Pain**

Disorder	Percentage (%)
Stroke	5
Parkinson's disease	10
Multiple Sclerosis	20
Spinal Cord Injury	30

Reflex Sympathetic Dystrophy

Sympathetically maintained pain, usually of the hand or foot, has been associated with stroke, MS, SCI, radiculopathies, and peripheral neuropathies. Trauma to bone, soft tissue, a major nerve or a plexus, and immobilization are other predisposing causes. Approximately 1 of every 2000 traumatic injuries leads to chronic *reflex sympathetic dystrophy* (RSD), also called *complex regional pain syndrome* type 1 (CRPS).[88] Following stroke, the incidence is less than 2% for patients who are closely monitored during their rehabilitations.[89] Symptoms include poorly localized burning, boring pain, hyperesthesia, mechanical or thermal allodynia, patchy bone demineralization, and autonomic dysfunction with hyperhydrosis, abnormal skin color, intermittent warm and cold sensations, increased nail and hair growth, and edema. Atrophy is a late feature. Weakness, tremor, muscle spasms, and dystonia may precede the pain or occur on the side contralateral to the pain. After a peripheral nerve injury, the syndrome is often called causalgia of CRPS type 2. Table 8–8 describes the clinical stages through which many patients pass. Diagnostic tests include skin plethysmography, skin conductance, thermography, and X-ray studies. The 3-phase technetium bone scan has a sensitivity of 45%–95% and specificity of 85%–92% for RSD.[90] The test may also have predictive value about subsequent symptoms in asymptomatic patients with upper extremity sensorimotor loss after stroke.[91]

Successful treatment by intravenous regional sympathetic blockade with drugs such as reserpine and guanethidine, or with stellate ganglion blocks and surgical sympathectomy, reflect the sense that the pain of RSD is maintained by the sympathetic system. Central autonomic dysfunction includes abnormal respiratory and thermoregulatory sympathetic neurogenic reflexes.[92] One possible mechanism is that a peripheral nerve injury results in sprouting of normal postganglionic sympathetic fibers around large axotomized dorsal root ganglion neurons, which are the myelinated, low-threshold mechanoreceptors.[93] Innocuous inputs become noxious. Injury also releases NGF, which enables the growth of these sympathetic connections in animal models. Nerve growth factor-neutralizing compounds are being studied to try to reduce the proliferation and, in turn, diminish pain. Diminished presynaptic inhibition of nociceptive afferents by GABAergic inhibitory neurons may be responsible for the dystonic posturing and myoclonic jerks in some patients. This notion was partially confirmed by the finding that some patients with RSD and dystonia affecting the hands improved with intrathecal baclofen.[94]

OVERVIEW OF MANAGEMENT

Pain can be managed with medications, physical therapies and modalities, behavioral interventions and counseling, and more invasive intrathecal, electric stimulation, and surgical approaches. The aims are to eliminate pain or at least make discomfort tolerable and to restore physical and social functioning. People with chronic debilitating pain are sometimes best managed as inpatients, especially if they need to be withdrawn from high doses of narcotic analgesics and have poor exercise toler-

Table 8–8. **Stages of Reflex Sympathetic Dystrophy**

Stage 1	Develops in first month; lasts 3–6 months	Edema, burning, warm and dry or cold and sweaty skin
Stage 2	Follows stage 1; lasts 3–6 months	Atrophic skin, osteoporosis, spreading pain, joint fibrosis, muscle wasting
Stage 3	Duration varies	Resolving pain, contractures, cool skin, atrophy

ance. Outpatient chronic pain management programs include a team that can carry out behavioral modification, relaxation, and cognitive, physical, and occupational therapies to increase activity and reduce pain behavior. In addition, the team may adjust medications, deal with mood disorders, and provide education. Claims about the efficacy of pain treatments that have not been subjected to a clinical trial must be considered in relation to the nonspecific placebo effects provided by the team's interest, attention, and overall approach to the patient. Hands-on therapies such as soft tissue manipulations and ultrasound are less likely to affect neuropathic compared with musculoskeletal sources of pain. However, nociceptive pain from muscles and joints commonly accompanies neurologic diseases, causes disability, and degrades quality of life, and can exacerbate neuropathic sources of pain.

The dimensions of pain that are unique to individuals include quality, intensity, duration, course, personal meaning, and impact on function and roles. Their measure poses challenges. Subjective personal assessments of pain are used most often. These measures are supported by scales of motor performance, ADLs, work history, mood, and quality of life. Clinicians most often record the frequency of pain-related behaviors and employ visual analog scales for pain, verbal pain rating scales, the McGill Pain Questionnaire,[95] the Minnesota Multiphasic Personality Inventory, and the Sickness Index Profile (see Chapter 7).

Remarkably few placebo-controlled, randomized clinical trials with more than 20 subjects who had a similar etiology or type of chronic central pain have been reported. Table 8–9 includes a few of the better studies. Most drug trials that show a benefit reveal this for some pain sensations more than others, such as diminishing cold-induced allodynia or hyperalgesia, or the drug helps at-level pain more than below-level pain after a SCI. For peripheral neuropathies such as diabetes mellitus that cause pain, the tricyclics, anticonvulsant sodium channel blockers, and NMDA antagonist dextromethorphan, followed by gabapentin, tramadol, SSRIs, and capsaicin seem most efficacious.[96] Although some animal studies do not point to an increase in GABA with the use of gabapentin, magnetic resonance spectroscopy in healthy persons reveals that GABA levels rise approximately 50%

by 6 hours after a dose and levels rise by over 25% after 4 weeks of the anticonvulsants topiramate, lamotrignine, or gabapentin.[97]

For postherpetic neuralgia, clinical trials show that lidocaine patches, gabapentin, and tricyclics work best. For HIV-associated distal sensory neuropathy, tricyclics and lamotrigine were shown in controlled trials not to be useful. Unfortunately, the efficacy of the drugs used to treat neuropathic pain is low. The clinician will have to treat from 3 to 6 patients with any one drug to see a partial benefit in 1 patient.[96]

MEDICATIONS

Details about the use of medications for pain are readily available. I emphasize the nonnarcotic analgesic drugs that act within the inhibitory neurotransmitter mechanisms for pain control just discussed (Table 8–9). Opiates, however, may be especially valuable when combined with modest doses of a GABAergic agent or tricyclic, or when used only at night to enable sleep. The nonnarcotic medications often cause CNS and systemic side effects that may increase if combinations of drugs become necessary. These drugs should be initiated at low doses and gradually increased, usually no faster than at weekly intervals.

Antidepressants

Norepinephrine has a marked tonic inhibitory effect on nociceptive neurons in the dorsal horn. Indeed, because all of the monamines released by descending pain pathways inhibit pain, the tricyclic antidepressants that affect norepinephrine and serotonin uptake have been valuable for the treatment of chronic neuropathic pain. These drugs also have local anesthetic effects and potentiate opioid-induced analgesia. Doses are usually much less than needed for antidepressant therapy. All these agents are worth trying for peripheral and central causes of neuropathic pain. Amitriptyline has been studied the most. When taken about an hour before bedtime, this tricyclic's sedating action becomes useful for patients who sleep poorly. Trazadone can also aid sedation using from 50 to 200 mg taken an hour before bedtime. Desipramine tends to have the fewest anticholinergic side effects, so it is better for those with prostatic hypertrophy that causes out-

Table 8–9. Classes of Medication for Neuropathic Pain

Class	Possible Mechanisms	Range of Dosage	Randomized Clinical Trials
ANTICONVULSANTS			
Carbamazepine	Blocks voltage-dependent Na$^+$ channel	100–400 mg tid	
Phenytoin	Blocks voltage-dependent Na$^+$ channel	100–400 mg qd	
Valproate	Enhances GABA;Blocks voltage-dependent Na$^+$ channel	250–500 mg tid	
Gabapentin	Indirect GABA enhancer; L-type calcium channels.	300–800 mg qid	
Topiramate	Enhances GABA	25–400 mg bid	
Lamotrigine	Inhibits presynaptic Na$^+$ channels and glutamate release	50–200 mg bid	Central poststroke pain decreased[271]
ANTIDEPRESSANTS			
Amitriptyline	Blocks uptake of norepinephrine, serotonin; anticholinergic sedation	10–200 mg hs	Poststroke central pain decreased[272]
Desipramine	Blocks uptake of norepinephrine, serotonin	25–200 mg	
Trazadone		25–200 mg hs	
Fluoxetine Other SSRIs	Blocks uptake of serotonin	10 ≯ 60 mg	
Venlafaxine	Blocks uptake of norepinephrine, serotonin	50–150 mg	
ADRENERGICS			
Clonidine	Alpha-2 receptor agonist	0.05–0.2 mg tid IT titration	Intrathecal morphine plus clonidine post SCI decreased at/below level pain[273]
ANESTHETICS			
Mexilitene	Na$^+$ channel blockade	75–200 mg tid	
Lidocaine		IV	Brief decrease of pain poststroke and SCI[274]
BENZODIAZEPINES			
Clonazepam	GABA receptor binding	0.5–4 mg tid	
CALCIUM CHANNEL BLOCKERS			
Nifedipine	Calcium flux	30–120 mg sustained release	

Continued on following page

Table 8–9.—*continued*

Class	Possible Mechanisms	Range of Dosage	Randomized Clinical Trials
GABAERGICS			
Baclofen	GABA-B receptor agonist	10–40 mg qid;IT	
NMDA ANTAGONISTS			
Dextromethorphan	Inhibit receptor	40–80 mg qid	
NONSTEROIDAL ANTIINFLAMMATORIES			
	Prostaglandin inhibition; potentiate opioids		
OPIATES			
Fentanyl transdermal	Binds opioid receptors	25–100 mcgm	
Morphine		IT	
Methadone	μ-agonist	5–40 mg bid	
Tramadol	Blocks opioid receptors and monamine uptake	50–100 mg qid	

GABA, γ-aminobutyric acid; SSRI, selective serotonin reuptake inhibitor; SCI, spinal cord injury; NMDA, N-methyl-D-aspartate; IT, intrathecally.

let obstruction and for patients bothered by dry mouth. The more selective serotonergic nontricyclic antidepressants tend to have a similar profile for pain relief, are generally less sedating, and can be included among first-line drugs. Placebo-controlled trials have shown the efficacy of these agents in the treatment of tension and migraine headache, diabetic neuropathy,[98] postherpetic neuralgia,[99] and myofascial pain.

Anticonvulsants

Phenytoin and carbamazepine probably act on pain mechanisms by suppressing paroxysmal discharges, by blocking ion channels, by preventing the spread of ectopic discharges, and by other commonly invoked anticonvulsant effects. These drugs seem especially good at reducing the lancinating and dysesthetic pain of trigeminal and glossophayrngeal neuralgia, postherpetic neuralgia, traumatic neuropathies, MS, and SCI. Some patients respond to clonazepam or valproate. Several of the newer anticonvulsants that tend to increase GABA availability, such as gabapentin and vigabatrin, have come into increasing use, with gabapentin often the first drug of choice. Topiramate has generally been less effective across all types of central pain.[100] Side effects from each of the anticonvulsants can be limited by building up doses slowly and keeping blood levels at or below the therapeutic range used for treating seizure disorders.

Anesthetics

Intravenous administration of local anesthetics and antiarrhythmics can limit chronic peripheral neuropathic pain. These agents are less likely to affect pain caused by a central injury.[101] The analgesic mechanism includes suppression of ectopic impulse generators in the damaged peripheral nerve. In postherpetic neuralgia, both injection and topical application of lidocaine into the sensitive, painful skin has reduced the pain in some patients, which suggests that the cutaneous terminals play a role.[102] Mexiletene, given orally at up to 750 mg/day, has also shown a benefit in, for example, diabetic neuropathy.[103]

person's cognitive evaluation of the emotions evoked by pain.

The clinician can get some insight into cognitive barriers by listening to the way patients think about their pain. Patients may discount positive experiences, see their pain management as worthless if less than a full cure, consider every setback as part of a never-ending pattern of failure, express guilt, feel worthless, and state that if this most recent approach does not work, and it almost certainly will not, then the pain will never go away. Such patients need more than pain medication. Although the approach has served the management of patients with chronic headache and back pain well, the strategies have not been reported in clinical trials for patients with chronic neuropathic and central pain who have neurologic diseases.

Weakness-Associated Shoulder Pain

Pain in the upper extremity often limits therapy and function and interferes with sleep, so it requires immediate attention. Indiscriminate traction on a paretic arm and shoulder during bed mobilization and transfers can start the pain. In the shoulder, some level of pain has been noted in up to 75% of patients by approximately 2 months after a hemispheric stroke. Subluxation of 1 or more cm, found in 50%–85% of hemiplegic patients, may contribute, though studies have not always shown this relationship. Glenohumeral subluxation is lessened by a variety of slings, but these do not necessarily prevent shoulder pain.[121] Sources of pain include biceps tendonitis, capsulitis, rotator cuff impingement or tear, myofascial pain, brachial plexopathy, suprascapular neuropathy, heterotopic osssification, osteoporosis and fractures, contractures, flaccidity or spasticity, overuse, degenerative joint disease, and RSD. Most patients have inflammation of the rotator cuff tendons and subacromial bursa. Magnetic resonance imaging of the shoulder and brachial plexus region can help diagnosis the cause of unrelenting pain.

At 3 months after a stroke, debilitating shoulder pain was found in 5% of all survivors.[122] During a controlled trial of upper extremity therapies, 26% of patients with severe impairments who received conventional therapy developed pain, whereas 47% receiving more intensive therapy had pain.[123] The dif-

ferences, however, were not statistically significant in this small sample population. Induction of pain during constraint-induced movement therapy is a potential drawback, so the therapist must monitor for discomfort. Repeated shoulder abduction or use of an overhead pulley that allows soft tissue impingement between the acromium and greater tuberosity is likely to induce pain, regardless of the presence of subluxation.

Pain can usually be managed with some combination of nonsteroidal anti-inflammatory medications, TENS, range of motion (ROM), physical modalities, a humeral sling, and tender point injections with a local anesthetic and steroids. A clinical trial showed that treatment with NSAIDs and range of motion decreased pain more than exercise alone.[124] A small randomized trial that compared ROM exercises alone to ROM and ultrasound or to ROM and placebo ultrasound showed no added benefit of ultrasound on lessening shoulder pain.[125] Ultrasound may be of greater benefit for calcific tendonitis.[126] In another trial, patients received physical therapy plus high intensity TENS 3 times a week for 4 weeks at 100 Hz and at 3 times the sensory threshold, enough to produce a muscle twitch. The procedure improved pain-free range of motion significantly more than TENS done at the sensory threshold or physical therapy alone.[127] Two randomized trials show that from 2 to 6 hours of functional electrical stimulation of the posterior deltoid and supraspinatus muscles for 5–6 weeks significantly reduces the amount of shoulder subluxation and pain compared to physical therapy alone.[128,129] Injections into tender and trigger points can be both diagnostic and lead to relief. For example, a subscapularis muscle motor point or nerve block can produce an immediate increase in pain-free abduction, flexion, and external rotation in a spastic hemiplegic shoulder. Surprisingly, a trial that compared injected triamcinolone to placebo did not reveal efficacy.[130]

Neck, Back, and Myofascial Pain

Fibromyalgia and myofascial pain is characterized by chronic, palpably painful areas within muscle and perhaps tendon insertions, and in ligaments. Commonly affected sites in patients during neurorehabilitation include the suboccipital musculoligamentous tissues; upper trapezius, levator scapula, supraspinatus, and medial scapular rhomboid muscles; the upper outer buttocks; tissues around the sacroiliac joints; and the transverse and interspinous ligaments from C-3 to T-1 and L-1 to S-1. The original, if scientifically unexamined notion from Travell and Simons, was that taut bands or nodules developed local twitch responses and that pain could radiate from pressing on trigger points. The reproducibility of such findings by different examiners has usually failed.[131] Rheumatologists have tried to formalize criteria for a diagnosis by consensus, but the exercise led to rather circular reasoning. A committee decided that a diagnosis of fibromyalgia requires widespread pain involving 3 or more body segments and at least 11 of 18 designated tender points.[132] Proponents of myofascial trigger spots suggest that spinal mechanism causes the problem and the release of acetylcholine causes a local twitch on abnormal muscle end plates.[133] Just how muscle fiber sources of pain persist and how palpably tender areas come to be associated with headaches and cervical and lumber pain is far from clear. Often, however, approaches that focus on and manipulate tender areas will reduce pain.

Physical treatments include injection into tender areas, tissue stretching and range of motion, postural education, exercise conditioning, and strengthening. Local injection of short-acting anesthetics such as procaine, with or without a steroid, often helps painful trigger points, tender areas, and taut bands asociated with myofascial pain. A review of needling with and without injecting the muscle could not support or refute any efficacy; the design of nearly all trials is poor.[134] Injection of as little as 1 mL of 1% procaine does eliminate a palpably tender area in some patients. The local anesthetic presumably alters C-fiber activity. Physical therapy should follow. A randomized trial showed that for cervical myofascial pain, neck stretches combined with either ultrasound or tender point injections into the trapezius muscle are both better than no treatment.[135]

Neck and back pain that persist for more than 3 months and interfere with attendance affect at least 10% of working people across Western countries.[136] Interventions have proliferated. A variety of educational and physical therapies have been studied for managing chronic neck and back pain without radiculopathy. Thera-peutic exercise appears to be most useful.[137,138] A randomized trial of strengthening, stretching, relaxation, and education about back care for 6 weeks was superior to usual primary care physician management with pain still comparatively reduced at 1 year.[139]

Recent randomized trials with good designs add to the potential armamentarium of interventions, although all of these results require confirmation by additional trials. For low back pain, osteopathic manual care and standard medical care produce equivalent results;[140] bipolar magnets were no better than sham magnets;[141] low energy laser treatment 3 times per week for 4 weeks is modestly better than sham treatment;[142] 40 units of botulinum toxin injected into 5 paralumbar sites is better than placebo for up to 8 weeks of less pain;[143] neuromuscular electrical stimulation and TENS for 5 hours per day at 2-day intervals is better than placebo stimulation;[144] percutaneous electrical nerve stimulation with acupuncture-like needles in the paraspinal muscles reduces the need for opioid analgesics more than sham treatment, TENS, or exercise;[145] and facet injections with methylprednisolone are no better than placebo in patients who reported less pain after the facet was injected with local anesthetic.[146] Back schools and cognitive and behavioral interventions are useful, although the specific elements of value are uncertain.[147] Evidence about the efficacy of acupuncture is equivocal. Of interest, physical therapy, chiropractic manipulation, and provision of an educational booklet produced similarly good outcomes in patients with acute low back pain.[148]

Similar approaches for chronic, nonradicular neck pain generally reveal no advantages to any modality other than stretches and exercise. Traction has no apparent value based on multiple studies. The loads and EMG levels induced in cervical and shoulder girdle muscles increase markedly with head-forward postures.[149] These tense postures are common in stressed people. Thus, these muscles and their related structures may fatigue from overuse and become a source of pain. Simple exercises that reduce an exaggerated cervical lordosis and increase cervical flexion and rotation, postural education about positions that increase cervical dysfunction, and passive joint mobilization techniques are often used with success. Improved head and neck positioning was associated with reduced neck pain in one con-

loading joints as soon as possible after onset of an UMN lesion may limit certain negative changes in muscle and connective tissue that add to the manifestations of spasticity. An overall approach to hypertonicity includes reversing any noxious stimulus that contributes, using simple physical interventions before experimenting with medications or muscle endplate injections, and reserving more invasive techniques such as intrathecal drugs, nerve blocks, and orthopedic or neurosurgical procedures to recalcitrant situations.

The approach to treatment also depends on whether the hypertonicity affects a single group of muscles such as the wrist flexors, affects a region such as the lower extremities, or diffusely affects the body as in patients with quadriplegia from TBI with bulbar dysfunction as well. Adverse reactions and trade-offs for benefits versus side effects, risks, and costs must be weighed by clinicians and patients.

PHYSICAL MODALITIES

Patients are educated about how slow movements and daily passive range of motion stretches reduce motion sensitive symptoms of spasticity. Noxious stimuli exacerbate hypertonicity and may trigger flexor and extensor spasms. Even ordinarily innocuous stimuli, such as tight clothing or a sunburn, can abruptly increase tone, much as they can cause autonomic dysreflexia in patients with cervicothoracic SCI. Treatable noxious sources include bowel and bladder distention, irritation from an indwelling catheter, urinary tract infection, rectal fissure or abcess, gastrointestinal gas, epididymitis, joint inflammation or pain especially on range of motion, or unrecognized vertebral fractures, pressure sores, ingrown toenails, and deep vein thrombosis.

Static stretching during the day or over night with splints and by serial casting can reduce stretch reflex activity and contractures. For example, tonic toe flexion, which is a plantar grasp reflex, is reduced with a toe spreader. This correction can significantly increase gait velocity and cadence by reducing pain with stepping and by altering tone.[159] Repetitive, externally imposed flexion-extension movements of the elbow held for 10 seconds every minute for 30 stretches produced a 50% decrease in the initial torque elicited.[160] This adaptation varied considerably across hemi-

paretic subjects. Thus, stretching has at least a transient quantifiable effect on reducing resistance, as most patients and clinicians appreciate. Mechanisms of action of passive stretch include changes in the mechanical properties of the joint, muscles, and tendons; a reduction in spindle afferent discharges; and central habituation that reduces excitability.

Muscle cooling with an ice pack for 20 minutes will decrease spasticity for approximately an hour,[161] so cryotherapy is commonly used to prepare for other modalities such as stretching, range of motion, and gait. Tendon vibration, reflex-inhibiting postures when seated and especially in bed, and EMG biofeedback can complement a stretching program, but formal studies of their use are too limited to judge any added benefit. Patients with spastic paraplegia from MS and SCI often report that standing in a support frame for as little as a $\frac{1}{2}$ hour a day reduces spasms. The effect may be related to modulation by afferent inputs from prolonged stretching and from loading the joints. Formal studies of standing in nonambulatory patients, however, have not clearly demonstrated efficacy on clinical measures of hypertonicity or on limiting contractures and osteoporosis.[162]

PHARMACOTHERAPY

Drug approaches to spasticity generally aim to alter spinal or muscular mechanisms associated with hypertonicity and spasms (see Table 2–3). Across randomized controlled trials of various drugs, the target symptoms of patients vary or go unstated, assessments are limited to a change in tone across one or more joints and are not related to any change in functional use of a hand, ADLs, or mobility; only a particular neurologic disease is studied, and many patients do not tolerate the side effects of a drug, so they drop out before an individualized approach to dosing is undertaken. Dose-response studies for individuals within a trial would allow a more practical assessment of potential benefits, but this approach was rarely taken prior to the mid-1980s. The outcomes of nearly all trials generally do not, when explored, reveal functional gains related to locomotion and upper limb use. The impact of a purported benefit should be weighed. For example, if an intervention diminishes extensor spasms by 50% over a placebo, but spasms still thrust a

Table 8–10. **Initial and Maximum Dosages of Medications for Spasticity**

FIRST LINE
Dantrolene—25 mg bid–50 mg qid
Baclofen—5 mg bid–40 mg qid
Clonidine—0.05 mg qd–0.2 mg tid
Tizanidine—2 mg bid–8 mg qid
Clonazepam—0.5–2 mg bid–tid

USEFUL ADDITIONS
Gabapentin—300 mg tid–600 mg qid
Tiagabine—4 mg bid–8 mg qid
Cyproheptadine—4 mg bid–8 mg qid
Levodopa/carbodopa—25/100 mg bid–25/250 mg tid
Phenytoin—serum concentration 10%–20% mg
Chlorpromazine—10 mg qd–25 mg bid
Cannabinoids—5 mg THC qd–10 mg tid

INJECTABLES
Intramuscular botulinum toxin A or B
Intramuscular phenol
Intrathecal baclofen—50–75 ug trial dose, then titration
Intrathecal clonidine or morphine titration

patient out of his wheelchair 3 times a day and make every transfer dangerous, the reduction does not achieve a critical goal.

The average range of dosages for drugs that may lessen spasticity is shown in Table 8–10. Incremental increases in dose can usually be made at 4–7-day intervals, but patients may need a longer baseline for each dose change to be able to assess positive and negative effects. The combination of low dosages of two agents may lessen side effects of a high dose of one agent. Whenever a drug appears to be useful for an individual, it is worth tapering the dose every 4 months, so that the patient can judge continued benefits. Many claims are implied by the companies that vigorously market drugs, injectables, and intrathecal pumps. Clinicians and patients must appreciate the rather limited role of agents.

Dantrolene (Dantrium)

Muscle relaxants such as methocarbamol and cyclobenzaprine are occasionally tried for hy-

pertonicity. Dantrolene is the only antispastic agent that operates on muscle. The agent competitively blocks the release of calcium from the sarcoplasmic reticulum to active myosin fibers in a dose-response fashion. This action decreases the force produced by electrical excitation–contraction coupling by approximately 5% in normal muscle. The drug acts on both intrafusal and extrafusal fibers with a half-life of 9–15 hours. Adverse reactions include lethargy, nausea, diarrhea, lightheadedness, and paresthesias. In early trials, a reversible hepatotoxicity developed in 1.8% of users with fatalities in 0.3%. A surveillance study of reports uncovered by the manufacturer estimated 9 asymptomatic and symptomatic cases per 100,000 perscriptions with 0.8 fatal hepatic reactions.[163] Liver biochemical tests should be monitored monthly for the first few months and at 3-month intervals, especially if more than 200 mg per day is used.

Small clinical trials of patients with chronic myelopathies,[164,165] stroke,[166] multiple sclerosis,[167] and cerebral palsy (CP)[168] show that dantrolene can decrease passive resistance, clonus, and spasms, but may cause weakness that impairs mobility. Studies have not been designed to reveal beneficial effects on ADLs and ambulation. A 14-week, placebo-controlled crossover study of 31 patients with hemiparesis and no initial spasticity entered at onset of stroke rehabilitation revealed no change in functional assessment and no reduction in tone by clinical or mechanical measures after patients reached 200 mg per day, but the trial did determine a reduction in the maximal torque developed by the unaffected arm and leg.[169] Thus, the drug can weaken paretic and normal muscle.

Dantrolene is most commonly used for spasticity from a cerebral injury, especially for the hemiplegic patient's dystonic flexed arm or stiffly extended leg. The induction of paresis may assist hygiene and nursing care in immobile patients with severe arm or leg adduction.

Baclofen (Lioresal)

This GABA-B-receptor agonist restricts the influx of calcium into presynaptic terminals in dorsal horn laminae. The agent depresses monosynaptic and polysynaptic reflexes and gamma efferents by the presynaptic inhibition of the release of excitatory neurotransmitters, including those released from nociceptive peripheral afferents that cause flexor and extensor spasms. The drug may also have a glycine-mediated postsynaptic action for reciprocal inhibition.[170] A physiologic study of its effects on soleus motoneurons in patients with spasticity from MS show that the drug, by oral or intrathecal administration, depresses the H(max)/M(max) ratio (see Chapter 7), suggesting direct depression of motoneuron excitability, more so than an effect on presynaptic inhibition.[171] Baclofen's half-life is 4 hours. Side-effects of oral or intrathecal administration include fatigue, weakness, drowsiness, nausea, dizziness, paresthesia, confusion, concentration, and memory. Abrupt withdrawal can cause hallucinations, confusion, and generalized seizures. Seizures are avoided by tapering half the total dose every 3 days. Physostigmine may partially antagonize an intrathecal overdose.

The drug is perhaps most effective in reducing involuntary flexor and extensor spasms, clonus, and the resistance to passive movements associated with myelopathies from SCI and MS.[172] It did not quantitatively reduce the viscous and elastic stiffness produced by the reflexive response to sinusoidal motion of the ankle joint in moderately spastic patients with a SCI.[173] When combined with a modest stretching program, baclofen improved scores on the Ashworth Scale and on a quantitative measure of quadriceps hypertonicity, but did not improve ADLs.[174]

Baclofen has been used intrathecally (IT) in patients with SCI,[175] MS,[176] TBI,[177] stroke,[178] hereditary spastic paraparesis,[179] and CP[180] when oral therapies failed to lessen spasms or dystonic postures. For example, intrathecal baclofen significantly decreased the Ashworth score and frequency of spasms in a randomized double-blind crossover study of 20 subjects with severe spasticity from SCI or MS.[175] Their spasticity had interfered with ADLs when taking from 60 to 200 mg of oral baclofen. On doses ranging from 60 to 750 ug per day infused by a programmable implanted lumbar pump, the lower Ashworth scores persisted in the patients for 19 months of follow-up. The modest decrease in resistance to passive movement has no clear clinical impact. In many of these patients, transfers and self-care improved, however. In another randomized, double-blind trial of baclofen infusion versus placebo for 3 months in 22 patients disabled by MS or SCI, the baclofen group substantially improved in Ashworth scores and pain, as well as on quality of life subscales for physical and mental health, mobility, and sleep using the Sickness Impact Profile.[181] All patients were then treated with IT baclofen and had significant gains 1 year later.

Baclofen presumably penetrates the substantia gelatinosa of the dorsal horn. Continuous infusion by a programmable pump with a catheter in the lumbar subarachnoid space avoids fluxes in CSF concentration and tends to reduce the side effects of high oral doses. Patients may use larger doses when needed, such as during sleep when spasms may awaken them. The peak effect of a bolus occurs approximately 4 hours after injection and maximum activity during continuous infusion is found at 24 to 48 hours.

Tolerance develops to intrathecal baclofen, probably caused by either downregulation of the number of receptors or by a change from high to low affinity receptors brought on by the high local concentrations of drug. Interference with flow from the catheter tip could also decrease effectiveness. Higher infusion rates, often a doubling in the first year, do maintain the effect on suppressing spasms. In a follow-up of 100 patients with MS and SCI treated for up to 6 years, spontaneous spasms and muscle tone continued to be decreased in 95 patients and 23 of 41 bedridden patients became able to use a wheelchair.[182] In terms of morbidity, 20 required a catheter revision, 3 had a wound infection, and 3 suffered an overdose of baclofen.

Benzodiazepines

This family of agents augments the postsynaptic actions of GABA by increasing the affinity of GABA to GABA-A receptors. Activation of the receptor site initiates the opening of the chloride channel for presynaptic inhibition of the release of excitatory neurotransmitters from spinal afferents, as well as inhibition of polysynaptic descending brain stem facilitatory inputs.[170]

Although adverse effects vary within the family of drugs, all can produce sedation, depression, weakness, fatigue, psychomotor slowing, antegrade amnesia, lightheadedness, and imbalance. A short-acting benzodiazepine may work for nighttime relief of spasms, although an untapered withdrawal of drug after chronic use can cause self-limited symptoms of anxiety and insomnia. Diazepam and clonazepam, which have long and moderate effects, respectively, are used most often.

Small, less than optimal clinical studies suggest that diazepam can modestly decrease spasms and the resistance to passive movement in patients with SCI, MS, stroke, and CP, but, when specifically evaluated, the drug does not improve upper limb function or ambulation. GABA-A receptors are downregulated by benzodiazepines and modulated by barbiturates. The former open the chloride channel more often and the latter helps keep it open longer. The combination may be useful in immobile patients with uncontrolled spasms. One of the concerns with using an antispasticty agent that acts on the GABA receptor such as a benzodiazepine is that the drug may affect molecular mechanisms such as long-term potentiation and may inhibit new learning.[183,184]

Clonidine (Catapres)

Clonidine is a presynaptic and postsynaptic alpha-2 adrenergic receptor agonist that is active in the locus coeruleus and within the substantia gelatinosa of the dorsal horns at nociceptive sites. It restores noradrenergic input to the cord, perhaps best in patients with myelopathies. The agent decreases motoneuron excitability, especially by enhancing alpha-2–mediated presynaptic inhibition of sensory afferents.[185] Thus, clonidine, like baclofen, may have a clinically important ability to modulate peripheral pain inputs and noxious sensory inputs that cause spasms.

When used as an adjunct to baclofen, oral clonidine led to subjective improvement in hypertonicity in approximately half of a group of 55 SCI subjects.[186] Peak plasma levels occur in approximately 4 hours and the half-life is 5–18 hours. The transdermal clonidine patch also seems effective, starting with a dose of 0.1 mg released for a week. Intrathecal clonidine is an infrequently used alternative to baclofen and has improved characteristics of walking in patients with incomplete paraplegia, probably by presynaptic inhibiton of group II afferents.[187] The drug suppresses EMG activity from the leg muscles in patients with severe to complete SCI during locomotion with BWSTT.

Tizanidine (Zanaflex)

This alpha-2 receptor agonist is similar to clonidine in its structure and mechanisms of action. The agent has greater muscle relaxant properties, acting upon spinal polysynaptic reflexes.[188] The serum concentration peaks in 2 hours and has a half-life of 4 hours. In some studies, tizanidine is comparable or better than baclofen in clinical and functional measures for patients with SCI and MS[189] and better than diazepam in spastic hemiplegia.[190] Other small studies suggest that tizanidine is comparable to baclofen and diazepam in efficacy, but these drugs have different profiles for side effects.[191] Hypotension, lightheadedness, fatigue, dry mouth, sedation, haalucinations, and elevated transaminases (up to 5% of patients) but not weakness, are occasional adverse reactions. Tizanidine significantly decreased the number of spasms in placebo-controlled trials of patients with MS[192] and SCI.[193] An open-label study of patients with chronic hemiplegic stroke showed improvement in the Ashworth score and on global pain and quality of life measures in subjects who could tolerate the drug.[194] Somnolence affected 63% of these patients.

Secondary Agents

A variety of other medications have been tried to manage spasticity. Monaminergic agents ought to have a modulatory effect on dorsal horn neurotransmission as the sensorimotor pools reorganize their activity when descending influences that carry 5-hydroxytryptomine (5-HT) and noradrenaline are diminished or lost. As discussed in Chapter 1, these neuromodulators play an important role in spinal reflex and locomotor functions.[195] Cyproheptadine, a serotonin antagonist, decreased clonus and spasms and enhanced aspects of gait in a small group of well-studied patients with MS and SCI.[196] Its action on 5-HT receptors could give it an adjunctive role with the alpha-2 agonists on the spinal motor pools. Dopamine may depress transmission by group II afferents to reduce spasticity.[197] Both agents have been valuable adjuncts with few side effects in my management of dystonic postures and spasms.

The anticonvulsants phenytoin and carbamazepine have multiple effects, including presynaptic inhibition of afferent fibers that may lessen the excitability of spinal cord motor pools. Gabapentin, the anticonvulsant that finds use for management of pain as well as for seizures, reduced painful spasms and improved global assessments of spasticity-related symptoms and signs in a small placebo-controlled crossover trial of patients with MS.[198] For 10 of 14 severely impaired children with epilepsy and spasticity, tiagabine at approximately 0.45 mg/kg/day improved the Ashworth Score and range of motion.[199] This agent decreases neuronal and glial uptake of GABA, which increases GABA availability at spinal synapses.

Presumably by inhibiting spinal polysynaptic pathways, oral cannaboids have reduced spasms in patients with MS.[200] Marijuana has altered spasticity in some paraplegics after SCI. Epidural and intrathecal opioids have also reduced the frequency of spasms, presumably by acting on lumbar multisynaptic reflexes mediated by A-delta and C-fibers.[201] The phenothiazines may inhibit the discharge of fusimotor fibers to reduce spasticity or, more likely, to act at dopaminergic sites and in the brain stem reticular formation.[170]

Glycine crosses the blood-brain barrier and acts on receptors on motoneurons and interneurons of the brain stem and spinal cord. The inhibitory neurotransmitter acts on strychnine-sensitive receptors to hyperpolarize membranes, decrease cell firing, and dampen reflex excitability. This action occurs when released by spinal inhibitory interneurons and Renshaw cells. Oral doses of up to 1 gm qid have been used in anecdotal reports with favorable clinical results, but without good measures of outcome.[202] Threonine has been used to try to increase levels of glycine. In a crossover trial of 24 patients with MS who could ambulate and had flexor spasms or spasticity that was felt to interfere with ADLs, the amino acid had no effect on the Ashworth score, electrophysiologic measures of spasticity, gait, or symptoms, but reduced clinical signs of spasticity.[203]

To limit drug-induced lethargy, confusion, weakness, hypotension, and other side effects, dosages of all of these medications must be titrated up from very low starting points and increased, in general, no more often than 1–2 times a week. A diary of the number of episodes of spasms, clonus, or unwanted involuntary movements during daily activities is most helpful in making decisions about whether a drug at a particular dose is efficacious. A global pain assessement may be of value if completed 1 week after each change in medication. Measuring the benefits of other possible goals for antispasticity therapy, such as improved ambulation or upper extremity function, requires an objective assessment. An improvement in walking speed over a distance of 50 feet or in the distance walked in 3 minutes may work for ambulatory patients. A change in range of motion, reach, or speed of a functional arm movement helps in making drug adjustments. Clinicians need to be creative at times and try combinations of drugs, such as baclofen and dantrium that act at different sites, or baclofen with clonidine or cyproheptadine to affect related spinal mechanisms, or tizanidine with levodopa/carbidopa to amplify action at a similar site. When disabling spasms still do not respond, intrathecal drug therapy with baclofen is indicated.

CHEMICAL BLOCKS

Chemical agents can be injected into a nerve, motor point, or muscle to reduce localized clonus, inappropriate muscle activity, velocity-dependent tone, and, sometimes, dystonic postures.[204] Motor point and nerve blocks are usually of less value in diminishing nonvelocity-dependent tone, rigidity, and flexor or extensor spasms. Since motor point blocks can partially spare voluntary movement and reduce reciprocal inhibition when given to an antagonist muscle, this approach may in theory improve some aspects of motor control. The short-term effects of chemical agents can also allow physical therapies and oral medications to have a greater ancillary effect.

Botulinum Toxin

The success of treating focal dystonias such as torticollis led to the use of botulinum toxin (BX) for focal symptoms and signs of spasticity. Botulinum toxin type A (*Botox*) and type B (*MyoBloc*) are among seven serotypes of the toxin. The agents have quickly become a new wrinkle in the fashion of managing the local effects of spasticity.

The toxin exerts its paralytic action within a few hours by binding to presynaptic cholinergic nerve terminals and then entering them by endocytosis. The cleaved BX chains are cleaved and in turn cleave one or more of the many proteins involved in acetylcholine exocytosis.[205] When the neurotransmitter fails to be released, the muscle fiber becomes paralyzed. The muscle becomes functionally denervated and atrophies, but axon terminals sprout to make new synaptic connections to neighboring muscle fibers and to repair paralyzed end plates by approximately 3 months after the injury.[206] Retrograde transport probably puts some of the drug into spinal segments, where it can block recurrent inhibition mediated by Renshaw cells. The onset of the botulinum effect takes up to 72 hours. Side effects include weakening of the affected and, if diffusion occurs, of neighboring muscles, malaise, and local discomfort.

Botulinum toxin type A is supplied in the United States in vials in which 100 Mouse Units equal 400 ng of type A toxin. The toxin is diluted to 10 U per 0.1 ml or less. The lethal parenteral dose in primates is 39 U/kg.[207] In adults, up to 400 U has been given safely in one or more muscles at one visit. The optimal dose is uncertain. As in its use for movement disorders, the quantity, usually in increments of 40 U, depends upon the mass of the target muscle. Botulinum toxin type B uses approximately 10–15 times the number of arbitrary units as the commercial BX A form. Needle EMG studies that identify the region of the muscle's motor end plate will localize injections to where they have the greatest efficacy.

Clinical trials of BX for spasticity suggest some practical uses. Injected into the leg adductors in a divided dose of 200 U, BX improved manual abduction and perineal hygiene for up to 3 months.[208] Across 25 patients with stroke and TBI, injections into single muscles of the arm or leg reduced hypertonicity in 80% and gave functional improvements to 68%, with gains in range of motion, brace tolerance, and pain relief.[209] An injection of 400 U by EMG guidance into the soleus, tibialis anterior, and both heads of the gastrocnemius reduced plantar flexor spasticity in hemiplegic patients for at least 8 weeks.[210] Gait improved in velocity, stride length, loading on the foot, and in push-off in many of these patients. In several small controlled trials of children with CP, injection into a variety of spastic paretic leg muscles improved aspects of their gaits for 6 weeks to 4 months.[207,211] Although subsequent trials tend to show gains in stride length and speed by approximately 8%–10% (a common outcome of nearly every drug and inva-

sive treatment for spastic diplegic children), kinematic and kinetic measures and functional outcomes are not affected.

Of the 10 reported double-blind, placebo-controlled randomized clinical trials of BX for spasticity, all show a decrease in the Ashworth score and only one shows any effect on disability.[212] The outcome measures in most trials would not be expected to reveal functional improvements, however. In addition, most trials do not include any physical therapy to try to take advantage of greater range of motion or passive motion. The decision not to offer rehabilitation seems to rest with the pharmaceutical companies that sponsor most trials. A trial that had a very good design to get at the issue of functionally meaningful outcomes used a goal-attainment scale related to the injection site's hoped for effect. Objective measures of function were not found for the arm and modest gains were reported for distal leg muscle injections, but goal attainment was no different for the experimental and placebo groups.[213] If BX is going to be injected several times a year at great expense and with induction of antibodies to the drug, functional gains, not just more range of motion, ought to be a required aim.

Phenol

No well-designed clinical trials of phenol blocks to muscle or nerve have been reported[214] and no functional gains are evident. Blocks with phenol as a 2%–10% solution and ethyl alcohol have been used for over 30 years.[215] The nerve or motor point is most often located by percutaneous electrical stimulation via a hypodermic needle cathode, but an intraneural injection by an open procedure is also advocated.[216] An initial injection of a long-acting local anesthetic such as bupivacaine helps predict the efficacy of a subsequent phenol block. The most commonly injected nerves include the posterior tibial nerve to decrease equinovarus positioning of the feet and to decrease clonus, the obturator nerve to reduce adductor scissoring with gait but mostly to improve skin care management for immobile patients, and the sciatic nerve to allow better positioning of a patient with very spastic paraplegia. In the upper extremity, blocks of the musculocutaneous, median, or ulnar nerves may improve resting position of the arm and hand. Painful dysesthesias can follow a nerve trunk injection. The effect of a nerve block persists for 12 months or more and can be repeated. Intrathecal and epidural phenol are rarely used today. Motor point blocks by intramuscular infiltrative injections of 50% ethanol have reduced spasticity for up to 6 weeks in the tibialis posterior, triceps surae, hamstrings, and subscapularis muscles, and in the flexors of the wrist and fingers.

ELECTRICAL STIMULATION

Electrical stimulation of motor and sensory nerves, muscles, and dermatomes by a variety of paradigms has, in general, reduced spasticity at the ankle and knee.[217] A single stimulation session decreases resistance and clonus for a few hours. Studies of chronic use show a range of responses that, in part, result from variations in patient characteristics, outcome measures, location of the stimulation, and parameters of the electrical stimuli. For example, after twice daily 20-minute stimulations of the quadriceps muscle for 4 weeks, an increase in spasticity was found, based on the leg relaxation time after a pendulum drop test, especially in patients with incomplete paraplegia and quadriplegia who had been more spastic prior to the stimulation program.[218] Stimulation over the surface of the tibialis anterior muscle for 20 minutes decreased the viscoelastic stiffness in patients with TBI and SCI for up to 24 hours, although a functional benefit was found only for the SCI patients who had ankle clonus.[219]

A study of spastic hemiparetic subjects with chronic stroke showed that 15 daily low intensity, high frequency, TENS applications for 1 hour over the proximal common peroneal nerve decreased a clinical measure of spasticity, increased vibratory inhibition of the H-reflex of the soleus muscle, improved voluntary dorsiflexion force, and reduced the magnitude of the stretch reflex in the affected ankle.[220] Enhanced presynaptic inhibition was considered a contributing mechanism. Stimulation of flexor reflex afferents (FRAs) via peroneal and sural nerve stimulation may account for similar positive results in subjects with myelopathies.[221,222] Electrostimulation for 5–10 minutes by a rectal probe to elicit ejaculation had the added effect of reducing spasms and tone in 10 of 14 subjects for approximately 9 hours.[223]

Changes in tone have not been systematically reported during functional electrical stimulation (FES) studies of muscle where the primary aim is to increase muscle mass, improve conditioning, or assist ambulation, but some patients with SCI report less spasticity.[224] The rather subjective measures of spasticity, variations in stimulation techniques, and the lack of a control therapy during trials make the clinical usefulness of neuromuscular stimulation equivocal until more research is completed. Electrical stimulation of the forearm muscles can at least transiently reduce flexor tone in the hand. Also, a chain-link glove that conducts electrical impulses has decreased finger flexor postures in the hemiplegic upper extremity in some patients.[225]

Dorsal column stimulation of the spinal cord, using techniques similar to those tried for pain control, has been of value in some anecdotal reports. Epidural stimulation over the upper lumbar cord, primarily affecting the dorsal roots, with quadripolar electordes in the range of 50–100 Hz can reduce physiologic measures of lower extremity spasticity in patients with chronic severe hypertonia.[226] These approaches are extraordinary measures even for the management of disabling flexor and extensor spasms that are refractory to oral medications. Intrathecal antispasticity medications are generally a better option.

SURGICAL INTERVENTIONS

Ablative neurosurgical procedures and orthopedic surgeries that correct deformities and improve function by a tendon lengthening, tenotomy, or tendon transfer can improve range of motion and decrease hypertonicity or some of its consequences. Altering the action of a tendon or muscle may also decrease sensory inputs that increase reflexive spasms. Surgeries seem to work best when followed by physical therapy. Patients with CP, stroke, SCI, or TBI are occasionally candidates. A gait analysis with EMG helps determine which procedure may aid mobility.

A variety of interventions have been used based on the patient's age, amount of strength and sensation, and disabilities. Both an obturator neurectomy and an adductor tenotomy will relieve severe spasms in the hip adductors. Tendon transfers and lengthenings preserve some function, whereas ablative procedures tend to eliminate any residual motor control.

For example, a hamstrings tendon release, transfer or lengthening will improve a spastic knee flexion deformity or contracture. An Achilles lengthening can decrease an equinus deformity. A tibialis posterior tendon transfer can reduce a varus deformity of the foot.

Spinal Cord Approaches

Microsurgical lesions at the dorsal root entry zone were reported to reduce spasticity in 75% of subjects with paraplegia and pain in 90% of the 47 patients.[227] Joint range of motion and positioning especially improved in the most handicapped patients, allowing them to sit and sleep in comfort. Minor and more serious complications, however, affected half of the patients and five died. A longitudinal myelotomy that divides the cord into anterior and posterior halves from T12 to S1 will preserve some function, unlike a cordotomy. The invasive procedure will usually, but not always, eliminate spasticity over the long run.[228]

Posterior Rhizotomy

Dorsal rhizotomy for reduction of spasticity was first introduced in 1913 and has been modified to improve its safety and efficacy. The procedures has been mostly confined to children with cerebral palsy. Selective division of posterior nerve rootlets of the second lumbar to first or second sacral level is based on intraoperative electromyographic responses of lower extremity muscles to posterior nerve rootlet stimulation.[229] Those rootlets associated with hyperactive responses deemed to be abnormal are divided, whereas those associated with more normal responses are spared. Abnormal neural responses have been characterized by incremental, multiphasic, or clonic activity to a steady 1-second train of stimuli. Additional abnormalities include spread of the response to muscle groups not innervated by the root being tested, as well as sustained responses that continue beyond the 1-second stimulus interval. Some of these responses may be valid criteria of an abnormality,[230] but the criteria are controversial. Depending on the severity of the spasticity, approximately 25%–50% of the posterior nerve rootlets are cut. By dividing only selected posterior nerve rootlets, the influence of excitatory (primarily Ia) afferents on the alpha motoneuron pools

can be diminished while preserving sensory function.

Practitioners state that appropriate patient selection is vital to the success of the selective posterior rhizotomy procedure. Patients with the most dramatic functional improvements have been bright and motivated ambulatory youngsters with spastic diplegia who had minimal fixed contractures and good strength.[231] Children with selective control of movement and freedom from synergistic movement patterns are more likely to improve their movement patterns following rhizotomy.

The claims for a positive effect have been supported by H-reflex studies, EMG assessment, and measures of resistance to passive motion using a force transducer. In addition, gait analyses reveal greater range of motion at the hip, knee, and ankle with accompanying increases in stride length and speed of walking, as well as more normal relationships between movement of limb segments during gait.[231,232] A randomized trial in children with CP, however, did not find rhizotomy to be better than the same intensity of physical therapy given to the surgically and nonsurgically treated groups (see Chapter 12).

CONTRACTURES

It is far easier to prevent contractures than to treat them. Success depends upon manual stretching of joints twice a day when active ranging and strengthening exercises cannot be done, proper bed and wheelchair positioning, early weight bearing, and aggressive treatment of limb pain. Lower limb orthoses can decrease muscle tone in response to cutaneous and postural reflexes. Static splints for the hand and wrist are most commonly used when tone increases. Splints aim to prevent contractures and pain by stretching elastic tissues and maintaining the normal adaptation of muscle to elongation. Orthotics may also inhibit flexor reflexes via cutaneous stimulation. Many small clinical trials across diseases suggest subjective value for the use of almost every variation of hand orthotic (Table 8–11). Dynamic splints for the hands and continuous passive motion devices for the arm or leg are more expensive. Schedules of wearing time for a device vary from 2 to 24 hours a day. The optimum time has not been established. Any approach that

Table 8–11. Hand Splints to Reduce Hypertonicity and Contractures

Volar or dorsal wrist and forearm splint
Foam finger spreader
Inflatable pressure splint (Johnson)
Firm cone in palm

lengthens the affected tissues is worth a try. Unfortunately, no particular approach has been put to a good clinical trial.

Impaired range of motion of a joint associated with an UMN disorder develops along with spasticity and with pathologic changes in the joint and surrounding connective tissue and muscle. Immobilization produces degenerative changes within a joint. Eventually, the cartilage thins, hyaluronate and other components decrease, vessels proliferate, and fibrous adhesions form.[233] Collagen fibers around the joint shorten when not passively loaded or stretched. The fibers stiffen by increasing their crosslinks. Collagen within muscle also changes, along with a reduction in the number and length of sarcomeres in muscle across the shortened position of a joint.[234] Thus, passive resistance at a joint from a contracture is closely related to the spastic resistance from muscle and connective tissue that contributes to hypertonicity.[235]

In one study,[236] 15% of patients with SCI admitted for rehabilitation and, in another study, 84% of patients with TBI[237] had lost more than 15% of the normal range of motion of at least one joint. Hemiparetic patients with stroke fall between these extremes. Contractures are found especially in the lower extremities in neuromuscular diseases, affecting at least 70% of outpatients with Duchenne's muscular dystrophy.[238] Contractures limit functional use of a limb and impair hygiene, mobility, and self-care. Serious contractures can cause pressure sores, pain, and, especially in youngsters, emotional distress when odd postures distort their bodies.

A number of strategies have been tried to manage contractures (Table 8–12). A local anesthetic block of the motor point may help separate the effects of spasticity from a contracture fixed by bone and soft tissue pathology. If the joint's range of motion greatly improves with a block, any of the therapies for spasticity can be applied. All such interventions must include manual stretching performed for at least a $1/2$-hour a day and appropriate joint positioning. Ultrasound applied to the joint capsule and musculotendinous junction can make stretching more effective. Serial splinting or casting when the contracture is fixed may gradually stretch tissue under a low load, but the tension must be monitored to prevent pressure sores, compression neuropathies, and connective tisssue injury. Casts are usually reapplied every 2 to 5 days for plantarflexion and knee and elbow flexion contractures.

A variety of surgeries and chemical blocks have been described to reduce contractures at most joints (Table 8–12). Electromyographic studies of a partially functioning hand and, in an ambulatory patient, during a formal gait analysis, are mandatory before attempting an invasive intervention. Otherwise, selection of the optimal procedure for the right muscle is guesswork and can lead to iatrogenic complications. For example, if the hip adductors are used for stepping, an obturator neurectomy for an adductor contracture could prevent the subject from ambulating. Surgeries in the leg must also take into account that muscles such as the hamstrings and rectus femoris cross both the hip and knee and the gastrocnemius crosses the knee and ankle. For instance, if the long head of the biceps femoris were lengthened too much for a knee contracture, the hip may lose stability. Overcorrection of an equinovarus foot by heel cord lengthening can cause a calcaneovalgus foot deformity and require heel stabilization. Surgeries and blocks are followed by vigorous physical therapy for ranging, strengthening, and to improve functional activities.

The optimal physical methods to maintain the range of motion of a joint in normal and spastic or paretic subjects has yet to be clarified.[239]

MOOD DISORDERS

Posttraumatic Stress Disorder

Motor vehicle accidents, assaults, falls, drive-by shootings, and injury during a natural disaster may produce posttraumatic stress disorder (PTSD) in addition to a TBI, SCI, or other neurologic impairment. Although little is yet known about the risk in a rehabilitation population, the rate of PTSD among urban young adults is 24% and the lifetime prevalence is 9%.[240] A 2-month follow-up of patients hospitalized after serious

Table 8–12. **Therapies for Joint Contractures Usually Associated with Spasticity**

Joint	Range of Motion Exercise	Splints/Orthotics	Chemical Blocks	Surgeries
Shoulder	Abduction and external rotation; manipulation under anesthesia		Pectoralis major; teres major	Tendon transection
Elbow	Continuous passive ROM	Low load dynamic splint; turnbuckle orthotic; serial casting	Musculocutaneous nerve; brachioradialis motor point	Brachioradialis muscle release; biceps tendon lengthening; aponeurotic section of brachialis; anterior capsulotomy
Forearm	Supination/ pronation		Pronator teres	Pronator teres release or tendon transfer for supination
Wrist and hand	Extension, rotation, sliding fingers; elastic gloves, massage, elevation for edema	Air splint for entire upper extremity	Differential temporary median, radial, ulnar nerve blocks; percutaneous phenol nerve blocks	Release of individual muscles or elevate all forearm muscles from bone and interosseus membranes; tendon transfers or lengthening for thumb function
Hip	Assess for subluxation; hip extension and abduction		Temporary or phenol blocks of obturator nerve, L-2–3 roots, sciatic nerve or branches, quadriceps motor points	Iliopsoas, tensor fasciae latae, rectus femoris release; adductor longus and gracilis tenotomy or transfer to ishial tuberosity; adductor myotomy; neurectomy of obturator nerve branches
Knee	Hamstring stretch	Serial casting; plastic AFO	Phenol block of femoral nerve	Hamstrings lengthening; femoral or tibial osteotomies; rectus femoris transfer
Ankle and foot	Ambulation; gastrocnemius stretch	AFO—double upright versus molded with lateral flare for varus tilt; metatarsal arch support; serial casting for severe equinovarus posture	Temporary or phenol blocks of tibial nerve or motor points of gastrocnemius, soleus tibialis posterior, flexor digitorum longus, flexor hallucis longus	Achilles tendon lengthening; split anterior tibial tendon transfer; release/transfer long toe flexors; arthrodese

ROM, range of motion; AFO, ankle-foot orthoses.

trauma found that 24% met full criteria for PTSD and an aditional 22% had two of the three symptom clusters.[241] Early symptoms of heightened arousal and coping with disengagement were early predictors of PTSD. Posttraumatic stress disorder does interfere with functional gains after SCI in affected youth.[242]

Symptom crteria include (1) emotional numbing with loss of interest and avoidance of any activity related to the trauma, (2) the phenomenon of reexperiencing aspects of the traumatic event by intrusive thoughts, flashbacks and, nightmares, and (3) hyperarousal with startle reactions, irritability, insomnia, or hypervigilance, and (4) symptoms lasting more than a month that impair daily functioning. It may take considerable detective work to identify environmental events that symbolize or resemble the traumatic event and produce the equivalent of a startle response. Posttraumatic amnesia and other memory, cognitive, and behavioral disorders can mask or delay onset of PTSD in patients. The syndrome is also associated with impairment in attention and working memory. A PET study using the n-back test (see Chapter 7) as an activation procedure and suggested differences in patients with PTSD compared to healthy control subjects in regions that interact with the working memory system.[243]

The National Center for PTSD Clinician-Administered PTSD Scale helps evaluate the frequency and intensity of symptoms and their

EXPERIMENTAL CASE STUDIES 8–1:
Posttraumatic Stress Disorder

Several examples reveal how difficult it can be to make the diagnosis of PTSD unless the physician looks for the problem. A young man suffered a cervical SCI when he injured his neck in a surf board accident. Six months later, he walked well and had only mild weakness in his hands and lower extremities, along with variably unpleasant tingling sensations in the legs. He had not returned to work, however. Exercise caused him to feel weak. He admitted to outbursts of anger and difficulty with concentration. Oddly, he would spend several days in bed every week, saying that his body felt tired after he tried to exert himself by taking a walk. He had stopped swimming, which had been a favored activity before the accident. On questioning, he recalled terrible nightmares in the first 2 months after his injury, a time when he was regaining control of his leg and arm movements. He described his accident with a very flat affect. He was driven off his surfboard by a wave and suddenly could not move. He floated in water for several minutes unable to call out. A friend realized he needed help and pulled him onto the beach. Shadows of people around him, sun glaring in his eyes, muffled voices, a sensation of floating on sand, derealization, and salt water in his mouth all later became recurrent thoughts, parts of nightmares, and cues for panic attacks. Moreover, he said that he was sure that if he had struggled in the ocean, he would have drowned. The sense of fatigue in his body rerepresented his powerlessness and loss of control in the water, so he retreated to his bed. Counseling and psychiatric care that included sertraline and education about how the myelopathy and the psychic terror of his accident were related to his mental and physical problems, along with a graded exercise program, helped relieve his symptoms over the next 3 months. He returned to work.

While driving on a freeway, an elderly couple was suddenly confronted by an 18 wheeler truck that plowed into the road divider and toppled onto the roof of their car. The wife dropped below the level of the window, but the husband felt the roof of the car collapsing on his head. The roof partially held, but they could not get out of the car. All was quiet for moments, then the roof and truck groaned and compressed the roof to the level of the bottom of the window before stopping again. He heard the voices of several men trying to figure out how to get to the car under the long cargo container that completely obscured it. One voice said, "Nobody can be alive in there." The couple was pulled out several hours later by a crew of fireman and rescue workers. He had neck pain and arm weakness that led to the removal of a centrally herniated cervical disk. During the acute hospital stay, he seemed very anxious and detached from his wife, who had no injuries. He recalled little about the accident. He startled at noises in the evening and could not sleep. He became preoccupied with residual arm numbness and a sense of imbalance during walking that was related to modest residual of the myelopathy. He repeatedly asked to have another MRI scan of his neck to be sure he was at no risk for paralysis. Along with his outpatient rehabilitation, psychiatric care, sertraline, and a benzodiazapine led to a remission of his symptoms over several months.

impact.[244] Experimental Case Studies 8–1 describe several patients who suffered with PTSD during inpatient and outpatient rehabilitation.

Counseling with an eye on environmental stimuli that evoke panic may be important for recovery. The symptoms appear easier to limit if treatment starts early after onset of symptoms. The mean duration of illness is 3–5 years, which is associated with poor psychosocial functioninng.[245] A randomized controlled trial of sertraline compared to placebo in patients with long-duration PTSD found a significant reduction in symptoms using from 50 to 200 mg daily for 12 weeks, although the drug did not prevent intrusive thoughts related to reexperiencing details of the traumatic event.[245]

Depression

Epidemiologic studies show that many of the affective, cognitive, and somatic symptoms of depression show up in 15% of community dwellers over age 65 years. The prevalence of major depression is approximately 2% in community studies, rises to 3% in late life and to a rate of 13% per year in nursing homes.[246] The severity and duration of community-wide untreated depression vary widely. The additive effects of psychosocial and medical problems, physiologic changes with aging, functional disabilities, and other factors that may contribute to depression remain uncertain. Differences among studies of depression after stroke, SCI, TBI, and other neurologic disease arise from factors that include the age of subjects, socioeconomic factors, and how the mood disorder is identified.[247–249] The location of a new lesion such as an infarct also increases the risk for depression (see Chapter 9).

Studies of the incidence of depression also vary in the timing of the assessment for depression following a neurologic disability and in the assessment instrument or interview technique used to make a diagnosis. Although many self-rating and examiner-rated scales are sensitive to the presence of depression, particularly in geriatric stroke patients, a formal interview seems best. The diagnosis of a major depressive episode can be made with some confidence if patients meet at least five of the nine criteria in the Diagnostic and Statistical Manual of Mental Disorders (Table 8–13) for daily symptoms that last at least 2 weeks and

Table 8–13. DSM-IV Criteria for Major Depressive Episode

Depressed mood most of the day, nearly every day, by subjective report or the observation of others

Loss of interest or pleasure in most activities almost daily

Large change in weight, appetite, or both

Insomnia or hypersomnia nearly daily

Fatigue or loss of energy

Psychomotor retardation or agitation observed by others

Feelings of worthlessness or excessive or inappropriate guilt

Impaired concentration, thinking, or decisiveness

Recurrent thoughts of death or suicide

Source: Diagnostic and Statistical Manual of Mental Disorders, Fourth Edition (DSM-IV, American Psychiatric Association).

represent a change from previous functioning. These symptoms must include a depressed mood or loss of interest or pleasure. Clinicians may classify patients who are depressed after a stroke as meeting the criteria for DSM-IV 293.83, which is a Mood Disorder Due to a General Medical Condition.

A confounding problem arises in distinguishing depression from the neurobehavioral sequelae of stroke, TBI, and MS. With a right cerebral lesion, some patients minimize impairments and distress and appear indifferent. This affect can mask depression. Minor and major depression take some leg work to detect in patients with anosognosia.[250] Aprosodia and nonverbal vegetative behavior can be mistaken for depressive signs in patients who are not depressed. Many of the somatic and cognitive complaints that suggest depression can reflect treatable problems particularly during inpatient hospitalization. For example, a noisy neighbor or shoulder pain may lead to sleep deprivation, fatigue, and poor concentration. Adverse reactions to any centrally acting medication may produce loss of energy, poor appetite, and systemic somatic complaints. Somatic complaints after stroke or any serious illness are common. In isolation, they do not imply a mood disorder.

Rehabilitationists need to be alert to premorbid affective disorders, alcohol abuse, inadequate psychosocial supports, and poor socioeconomic status as contributing causes to depression. Elderly patients require special attention. Patients who present with a new onset of depression should be checked for hypothyroidism, a low B_{12} or high methylmalonic acid level, hearing loss, substance dependence, death of a spouse or family member in the past few months, comorbid chronic illness, and prior history of depression or anxiety disorder.

Minor depression, dysthymia, and subsyndromal symptomatic depression (SSD) may also be premorbid risk factors for depression following new disability. The 1-month prevalence of SSD in the general population is approximately 4%, compared to minor depression in 1.5% and major depression in 2.3% of people.[251] Subsyndromal symptomatic depression defines patients who suffer from a cluster of depressive symptoms, but the number of symptoms, duration, or quality is insufficient to meet DSM IV criteria for major depression.[252] Insomnia, fatigue, thoughts of death, impaired concentration, slowed thinking, and hypersomnia are the most frequent symptoms. Subsyndromal symptomatic depression predisposes to major depression and to psychosocial impairments, but often responds to psychotherapeutic and psychopharmacologic treatments.

Anxiety is also common with cortical lesions in studies of stroke-related affective disorders. Mania has been associated with right cerebral lesions, particularly if limbic projections are involved.[253]

Positron emission tomography studies have also begun to show a relationship between depression and metabolic activity in a left limbic-thalamo-prefrontal cortical circuit that includes the amygdala.[254] The medial ventral frontal regions tend to respond to antidepressant treatment, as well as to placebo in patients whose symptoms lessen. Cortical and subcortical lesions may also contribute to hypometabolism of this region and perhaps to depression.

A biochemical marker for depression or for who may best respond to medication has been sought especially in patients after stroke.[255] The dexamethasone suppression test is considered positive if a nighttime dose of 1 mg fails to suppress the next day's 4 PM cortisol level below 5 ug/dL. Among reports that used a variety of measures of poststroke depression, the sensitivity of the test ranged from 15% to 75%. Its specificity varied from 15% to 90%.[256] For an individual patient, then, the suppression test may have little meaning.

TREATMENT

All of the SSRI agents are about equivalent in reducing the symptoms of depression.[257] A Cochrane Library Review of controlled trials shows that antidepressants significantly lessen the symptoms of depression compared to no treatment or placebo in patients with a range of physical illnesses, including stroke, MS, TBI, and SCI.[258] The efficacy is such that the clinician will have to treat approximately 4 patients to produce one recovery. A controlled trial in older adults with minor depression or dysthymia (many would qualify as having SSD) with comorbid medical conditions found that paroxetine, 10–40 mg, had a moderate benefit on depressive symptoms and mental health, whereas problem-solving therapy had a smaller impact over placebo. These participants are, perhaps, not unlike the patients who may suffer a stroke and find themselves in rehabilitation, leading to greater symptoms and signs of depression.

In nonrandomized comparisons, the trend is for tricyclics to be more effective than the SSRIs, but more patients stop these drugs due to side effects compared to SSRIs.[258] For patients undergoing rehabilitation, drugs that have fewer potential cardiovascular and cognitive side effects, such as the SSRIs, are best for first-line use. Of interest, the SSRIs normalize indices of platelet activation and aggregation in patients with ischemic heart disease.[259] Mirtazepine, 5–45 mg, is an inhibitor of both serotonin and noradrenaline reuptake and may improve appetite, especially in elderly patients.

Another drug that has significantly decreased the symptoms of depression in men who have longstanding erectile dysfunction is sildenafil. A randomized trial of 152 men showed that 73% who received the drug compared to 14% who received a placebo had a large improvement in depression scores in close association with improved erectile function.[260]

The treatment of depression is also potentially important for secondary prevention of stroke and coronary heart disease.[260] Mortality rates during 10-year follow-up are significantly higher in depressed patients after a stroke or myocardial infarction and the rates of stroke and heart attack are 2–3 times higher in depressed adults.

Close clinical monitoring for adverse reactions to the antidepressants is important during inpatient and outpatient rehabilitation. Sedation, insomnia, anticholinergic effects on bowel, bladder, and salivation, orthostatic hypotension, cardiac arrhythmias, anxiety, and extrapyramidal symptoms can be especially deleterious to the elderly stroke patient.[261] The serotonin syndrome can develop within a day after initiating or increasing the dose of any of the tricyclics except desipramine, all of the SSRIs, and when these are combined with medications such as bromocriptine, tryptophan, meperidine, amphetamine, and dextromethorphan.[262] Excess synaptic serotonin and modulation of serotonin's regulation of dopamine in the striatum and hippocampus probably cause the syndrome. Clonus, confusion, and agitation may result. Extrapyramidal features include rigidity, restlessness, movement disorders, and tremors. Autonomic symptoms include shivering, low-grade fever, autonomic instability, nausea, diarrhea, flushing, and sweating. Rhabdomyolysis, coma, and death have been reported as well. Clinically, this syndrome looks similar to the neuroleptic malignant syndrome that rarely develops approximately 1 week after starting or increasing a dopamine receptor blocker.

SLEEP DISORDERS

Insomnia often accompanies anxiety and depression. From 12% to 25% of healthy people over age 65 years report chronic insomnia with the greatest disturbance in maintaining sleep. Hospitalization with its new noises and discomforts and impaired bed mobility from neurologic disease may add to this difficulty. Over the short run, both behavioral and pharmacologic approaches, using temazepam for example, are significantly better than placebo management.[263]

Sleep apnea is reported in 4% of middle-aged men. Obesity and alcohol and cigarette use are risk factors. During rehabilitation, one-third of patients with TBI of less than 3 months duration who scored higher than level 3 on the Rancho Los Amigos Scale (see Table 11–7) had

central and obstructive sleep apnea.[264] After SCI, sleep apnea is more prevalent in people with quadriplegia than paraplegia and in patients with motor-incomplete injuries, affecting from 15% to 45% of patients with chronic SCI.[265] Impaired sensory feedback from respiratory muscles, sleeping in a supine position, and antispasticity agents may contribute. Central and obstructive sleep apnea or a mix of both can develop from brain stem and cortical lesions, especially with bulbar dysfunction, or in relation to a superimposed toxic-metabolic encephalopathy. These disorders may have preceded the stroke, given that they have been associated with a higher risk for stroke.[266] Pharyngeal muscle weakness and impaired neural control during sleep of nasophayrngeal and pharyngolaryngeal muscles caused by a stroke contributes to the risk for obstructive apnea. From one-third to two-thirds of inpatients with stroke may have a sleep disorder when formally tested by polysomnography.[267]

Sleep apnea may cause severe oxygen desaturation, pulmonary hypertension, and is associated with causing hypertension, stroke, and myocardial infarction. Patients often complain of poor concentration, memory impairment, malaise, and disinterest. A polysomnagram is indicated when the rehabilitation team observes a hypersomnolent, confused, and snoring or apneic patient. More than 5 apnea episodes per hour or 30 per night is abnormal. One study found an average of 52 sleep-disordered breathing events per hour in selected subjects within 1 year of stroke.[268] The number of oxygen desaturation events and the oximetry measures during sleep disordered breathing have correlated with BI scores at 1 and 12 months after stroke.[269]

Tilting the head of the bed up 45° can lessen obstructive apnea. Approximately 70% of affected people will tolerate the use of continuous positive airway pressure therapy. Continuous positive airway pressure (CPAP) devices improve both central and obstructive apneic conditions. A randomized trial during inpatient stroke rehabilitation found that nasal CPAP lessened depression, but compliance was poor in patients with delirium and marked cognitive impairment.[270] Drugs such as protriptyline may increase upper airway muscle activity. Surgical interventions that include uvulopalato-pharyngoplasty can lessen oropharyngeal obstruction, although this procedure may be contraindicated in patients with bulbar muscle weakness.

SUMMARY

Acute and long-term prevention and management of neuromedical complications falls within the bailiwick of physicians and other members of the neurorehabilitation team. Approaches to the care of some of the more frequent management issues are described. Continued improvements in methods for surveillance of risk factors for these complications and for physical and pharmacologic interventions are needed. The measurement and treatment of spasticity to achieve functionally important goals remains a particularly vexing problem. The rehabilitation team must try to assure compliance in preventative care by patients, families, and family physicians, so that serious complications can be avoided. If successful, the quality of life of patients is less likely to be unnecessarily compromised by bed sores, contractures, incontinence, malnutrition, infections, pain, and social isolation.

REFERENCES

1. Sioson E. Deep vein thrombosis in stroke patients: An overview. J Stroke Cerebrovasc Dis 1992; 2:74–78.
2. Oczkowski W, Ginsberg J, Shin A, Pauju A. Venous thromboembolism in patients undergoing rehabilitation for stroke. Arch Phys Med Rehabil 1992; 73: 712–716.
3. Bromfield E, Reding M. Relative risk of deep vein thrombosis or pulmonary embolism post stroke based on ambulatory status. J Neurol Rehab 1988; 2:51–57.
4. Landi G, D'Angelo A, Boccardi E, Candelise L, Mannucci PM, Morabito A, Orazio EN. Venous embolism in acute stroke: Prognostic importance of hypercoagulability. Arch Neurol 1992; 49:279–283.
5. Merli G, Crabbe S, Paluzzi R, Fritz D. Etiology, incidence, and prevention of deep vein thrombosis in acute spinal cord injury. Arch Phys Med Rehabil 1993; 74:1199–1205.
6. Turpie A, Hirsh J, Jay R, Powers PJ, Andrew M, Magnani HN, Hull RD, Gent M. Double-blind randomised trial of ORG 10172 low-molecular-weight heparinoid in prevention of deep-vein thrombosis in thrombotic stroke. Lancet 1987; 1:523–526.
7. Turpie A, Gent M, Cote R, Levine MN, Ginsberg JS, Powers PJ, Leclerc J, Geerts W, Jay R, Neemeh J. A low-molecular-weight heparinoid compared with unfractionated heparin in the prevention of deep vein thrombosis in patients with acute ischemic stroke. Ann Int Med 1992; 117:353–357.
8. Office of Medical Applications Research N. Consensus conference: Prevention of venous thrombosis and pulmonary embolism. JAMA 1986; 256:744–749.
9. Kamran S, Downey D, Ruff R. Pneumatic sequential compression reduces the risk of deep vein thrombosis in stroke patients. Neurology 1998; 50:1683–1687.
10. Green D, Lee M, Ito V, Cohn T, Press J, Filbrandt PR, Vandenberg WC, Yarkony GM, Meyer PR. Fixed vs adjusted dose heparin in the prophylaxis of thromboembolism in SCI. JAMA 1988; 260:1255–1258.
11. Wade W, Chisholm M. Venous thrombosis after acute spinal cord injury. Am J Phys Med Rehabil 2000; 79:504–508.
12. Consortium for Spinal Cord Injury. Clinical Practice Guidelines: Prevention of Thromboembolism in Spinal Cord Injury. Washington, D.C.: Paralyzed Veterans of America, 1997.
13. Kim S, Charallel J, Park K, Bauerle LC, Shang CC, Gordon SK, Bauman WA. Prevalence of deep venous thrombosis in patients with chronic spinal cord injury. Arch Phys Med Rehabil 1994; 75:965–968.
14. Agnelli G, Piovella F, Buoncristiani P, Severi P, Pini M, D'Angelo A, Beltrametti C, Damiani M, Androli GC, Pugliese R, Iorio A, Brambilla G. Enoxaparin plus compression stockings compared with compression stockings alone in the prevention of venous thromboembolism after elective neurosurgery. N Engl J Med 1998; 339:80–85.
15. Kiser T, Stefans V. Pulmonary embolism in rehabilitation patients: Relation to time before return to physical therapy after diagnosis of deep vein thrombosis. Arch Phys Med Rehabil 1997; 78:942–945.
16. Hull R, Raskob G, Rosenbloom D, Panju AA, Brill-Edwards P, Ginsberg JS, Hirsh J, Martin GJ, Green D. Heparin for 5 days as compared with 10 days in the initial treatment of proximal venous thrombosis. N Engl J Med 1990; 322:1260–1264.
17. Weinmann E, Salzman E. Deep-vein thrombosis. N Eng J Med 1994; 331:1630–1641.
18. Schulman S, Rhedin A-S, Lindmarker P, Carlsson A, Larfars G, Nicol P. A comparison of six weeks with six months of oral anticoagulant therapy after a first episode of venous thromboembolism. N Engl J Med 1995; 332:1661–1665.
19. Rutan G, Hermanson B. Orthostatic hypotension in older patients-the Cardiovascular Health Study. Hypertension 1992; 19:508–519.
20. Eigenbrodt M, Rose K, Couper D, Arnett D, Smith R, Jones D. Orthostatic hypotension as a risk factor for stroke. Stroke 2000; 31:2307–2313.
21. Low P, Gilden J, Freeman R, Sheng K-N, McElligott M. Efficacy of midodrine vs placebo in neurogenic orthostatic hypotension. JAMA 1997; 277:1046–1051.
22. Teasdale T, Taffet G, Luchi R, Adam E. Urinary incontinence in a community-residing elderly population. J Am Geriatr Soc 1988; 36:600–606.
23. Borrie M, Campbell A, Caradoc-Davies T, Spears G. Urinary incontinence after stroke: A prospective study. Age and Ageing 1986; 15:177–181.
24. Reding M, Winter S, Thompson M. Urinary incontinence after unilateral hemispheric stroke. J Neurol Rehabil 1987; 1:25–30.
25. de Groat W, Kruse M, Vizzard M, Cheng C, Araki I, Yoshimura N. Modification of urinary bladder function after spinal cord injury. In: Seil FJ, ed. Advances

in Neurology. Vol. 72. Philadelphia: Lippincott-Raven, 1997:347–364.

26. Gelber D, Jozefczyk P, Good D. Urinary retention following acute stroke. J Neurol Rehabil 1994; 8: 69–74.

27. Gelber D, Good D, Laven L, Verhulst S. Causes of urinary incontinence after acute hemispheric stroke. Stroke 1993; 24:378–382.

28. Morton S, Shekelle P, Dobkin B, Adams J, Montgomerie J, Vickrey B. Antimicrobial prophylaxis for urinary tract infection in persons with spinal cord dysfunction. Arch Phys Med Rehabil 2002; 83:129–138.

29. Avorn J, Monane M, Gurwitz J, Glynn RJ, Choodnovskiy I, Lipsitz LA. Reduction of bacteriuria and pyuria after ingestion of cranberry juice. JAMA 1994; 271:751–754.

30. Vickrey B, Shekelle P, Morton S, Dobkin B. Prevention and management of urinary tract infections in paralyzed persons. Evidence Report/Technology Assessment No. 6. Rockville, MD: Agency for Health Care Policy and Research Publication No. 99-E008, 1999.

31. Abrams P, Freeman R, Anderstrom C, Mattiasson A. Tolterodine, a new muscarinic agent: As effective but better tolerated than oxybutin in patients with an overactive bladder. Brit J Urol 1998; 81:801–810.

32. Chancellor M, Rivas D, Staas W. DDAVP in the urological management of the difficult neurogenic bladder in spinal cord injury. J Am Paraplegia Soc 1994; 17:165–167.

33. Chancellor M, Bennett C, Simoneau A, Finocchiaro MV, Kline C, Bennett JK, Foote JE, Green BG, Martin SH, Killoran RW, Crewalk JA, Rivas DA. Sphincteric stent versus external sphincterotomy in spinal cord injured men: Prospective randomized multicenter trial. J Urol 1999; 161:1893–1898.

34. Creasey G, Grill J, Korsten J, H, Betz R, Anderson R, Walter J, UHS. An implantable neuroprosthesis for restoring bladder and bowel control to patients with spinal cord injuries: A multicenter trial. Arch Phys Med Rehabil 2001; 82:1512–1519.

35. Ozawa H, Jung S, Fraser M. Intravesical capsaicin therapy: A review. J Spinal Cord Med 1999; 22: 114–118.

36. Wiart L, Joseph P, Petit H, Dosque JP, de Seze M, Brochet B, Deminiere C, Ferriere JM, Mazaux JM, N'Guyen P, Barat M. The effects of capsaicin on the neurogenic hyperreflexic detrusor. A double blind placebo controlled study in patients with spinal cord disease. Spinal Cord 1998; 36:95–99.

37. Linsenmeyer T, Culkin D. APS recommendations for the urological evaluation of patients with spinal cord injury. J Spinal Cord Med 1999; 22:139–142.

38. Madoff R, Williams J, Caushaj P. Fecal incontinence. N Eng J Med 1992; 326:1002–1007.

39. Consortium for Spinal Cord Medicine. Clinical Practice Guidelines: Neurogenic bowel management in adults with spinal cord injury. Washington, D.C.: Paralyzed Veterans of America, 1998.

40. Stiens S, Bergman S, Goetz L. Neurogenic bowel dysfunction after spinal cord injury: Clinical evaluation and rehabilitative management. Arch Phys Med Rehabil 1997; 78:S86–S102.

41. House J, Stiens S. Pharmacologically initiated defecation of persons with spinal cord injury: Effectiveness of three agents. Arch Phys Med Rehabil 1997; 78:1062–1065.

42. Krauss R, Eckel R, Howard B, Appel LJ, Daniels SR, Deckelbaum RJ, Erdman JW Jr, Kris-Etherton P, Goldberg I, Kotchen TA, Lichtenstein AH, Mitch WE, Mullis R, Robinson K, Wylie-Rosett J, St Jeor S, Suttie J, Tribble DL, Bazzarre TL. AHA dietary guidelines. Stroke 2000; 31:2751–2766.

43. Elliot J. Swallowing disorders in the elderly. Geriatrics 1988; 43:95–113.

44. Marik P. Aspiration pneumonitis and aspiration pneumonia. N Engl J Med 2001; 344:665–661.

45. Barer D. The natural history and functional consequences of dysphagia after hemispheric stroke. J Neurol Neurosurg Psychiatry 1989; 52:236–241.

46. Axelsson K. Nutritional status in patients with acute stroke. Acta Med Scand 1988; 224:217–224.

47. Smithard D, O'Neill P, Park C, Morris J, Wyatt R, England R, Martin DF. Complications and outcome after acute stroke: Does dysphagia matter? Stroke 1996; 27:1200–1204.

48. Smith J, Greer J, Liu G, Feldman J. Neural mechanisms generating respiratory pattern in mammalian brainstem-spinal cord in vitro. J Neurophysiol 1990; 64:1149–1169.

49. Hamdy S, Aziz Q, Rothwell J, Power M, Singh K, Nicholson DA, Tallis RC, Thompson DG. Recovery of swallowing after dysphagic stroke relates to functional reorganization in the intact motor cortex. Gastroenterol 1999; 115:1104–1112.

50. Warms T, Richards J. "Wet voice" as a predictor of penetration and aspiration in oropharyngeal dysphagia. Dysphagia 2000; 15:84–88.

51. Nathadwarawala K, Nicklin J, Wiles C. A timed test of swallowing capacity for neurological patients. J Neurol Neurosurg Psychiatry 1993; 55:822–825.

52. DePippo K, Holas M, Reding M. The Burke Dysphagia Screening Test: Validation of its use in patients with stroke. Arch Phys Med Rehabil 1994; 75:1284–1286.

53. Holas M, DePippo K, Reding M. Aspiration and relative risk of medical complications following stroke. Arch Neurol 1994; 51:1051–1053.

54. Daniels S, Ballo L, Mahoney M, Foundas A. Clinical predictors of dysphagia and aspiration risk: Outcome measures in acute stroke patients. Arch Phys Med Rehabil 2000; 81:1030–1033.

55. DePippo K, Holas M, Reding M. Validation of the 3-oz water swallow test for aspiration following stroke. Arch Neurol 1992; 49:1259–1261.

56. Johnson E, McKenzie S, Sievers A. Aspiration pneumonia in stroke. Arch Phys Med Rehabil 1993; 74:973–976.

57. Leder S. Serial fiberoptic endoscopic swallowing evaluations in the management of patients with dysphagia. Arch Phys Med Rehabil 1998; 79:1264–1269.

58. Collins M, Bakheit A. Does pulse oximetry reliably detect aspiration in dysphagic stroke patients? Stroke 1997; 28:1773–75.

59. Reddy N, Thomas R, Canilang E, Casterline J. Toward classification of dysphagic patients using biomechanical measurements. J Rehabil Res Dev 1994; 31:335–344.

60. Addington R, Stephens R, Gilliland K, Rodriguez M. Assessing the laryngeal cough reflex and the risk of developing pneumonia after stroke. Arch Phys Med Rehabil 1999; 80:150–154.

61. Logemann J. Approaches to the management of dis-

ordered swallowing. Clin Gastroenterol 1991; 5:269–280.

62. Park C, O'Neill P. Management of neurological dysphagia. Clin Rehabil 1994; 8:166–174.

63. Logemann J, Kahrilas P. Relearning to swallow after stroke-application of maneuvers and indirect biofeedback. Neurology 1990; 40:1136–1138.

64. DePippo K, Holas M, Reding M, Mandel FS, Lesser ML. Dysphagia therapy following stroke: A controlled trial. Neurology 1994; 44:1655–1660.

65. Perez I, Smithard D, Davies H, Kalra L. Pharmacological treatment of dysphagia in stroke. Dysphagia 1998; 13:12–16.

66. Schiffman S. Taste and smell losses in normal aging and disease. JAMA 1997; 278:1357–62.

67. Kahn K, Rubenstein L, Draper D, Kosecoff J, Rogers WH, Keeler EB, Brook RH. The effects of the DRG-based prospective payment system on quality of care for hospitalized Medicare patients. JAMA 1990; 264:1953–1955.

68. Finucane T, Christmas C, Travis K. Tube feeding in patients with advanced dementia. JAMA 1999; 282:1365–1370.

69. Bath P, Bath F, Smithard D. Interventions for dysphagia in acute stroke. In: Review C, ed. The Cochrane Library: Oxford: Update Software, 2001.

70. Yarkony G. Pressure sores: A review. Arch Phys Med Rehabil 1994; 75:908–917.

71. Staas W, Cioschi H. Pressure sores: A multifaceted approach to prevention and treatment. West J Med 1991; 154:539–544.

72. Consortium for Spinal Cord Injury. Clinical Practice Guidelines: Pressure Ulcer Prevention and Treatment Following Spinal Cord Injury. Washington, D.C.: Paralyzed Veterans of America, 2000.

73. AHCPR. Agency for Health Care Policy and Research. Pressure ulcers in adults: Prediction and prevention. Washington, D.C.: U.S. Department of Health and Human Services, 1992.

74. Sumpio B. Foot ulcers. N Engl J Med 2000; 343:787–793.

75. Malmberg A, Yaksh T. Hyperalgesia mediated by spinal glutamate or substance P receptor bloked by spinal cyclooxygenase inhibition. Science 1992; 257:1276–1278.

76. Schwartzman R, Grothusen J, Kiefer T, Rohr P. Neuropathic central pain. Arch Neurol 2001; 58:1547–1550.

77. Lenz F, Gracely R, Baker F, Richardson R, Dougherty P. Reorganization of sensory modalities evoked by stimulation in the region of the principal sensory nucleus (ventral caudal—Vc) in patients with pain secondary to neural injury. J Comp Neurol 1998; 399:125–138.

78. Woolf C, Salter M. Neuronal plasticity: Increasing the gain in pain. Science 2000; 288:1765–1772.

79. Price D. Psychological and neural mechanisms of the affective dimension of pain. Science 2000; 288:1769–1772.

80. Tolle T, Kaufmann T, Siessmeier T. Region-specific encoding of sensory and affective components of pain in the human brain: A positron emission tomography correlation analysis. Ann Neurol 1999; 45:40–47.

81. Derbyshire S. Exploring the pain "neuromatrix." Curr Rev Pain 2000; 4:467–77.

82. Buchel C, Bornhovd K, Quante M, Glauche V, Bromm B, Weiller C. Dissociable neural responses related to pain intensity, stimulus intensity, and stimulus awareness within the anterior cingulate cortex. J Neurosci 2002; 22:970–976.

83. Basbaum A. Spinal mechanisms of acute and persistent pain. Reg Anesth Pain Med 1999; 24:59–67.

84. McMahan S, Koltzenburg M. Novel classes of nociceptors: Beyond Sherrington. Trends Neurosci 1990; 13:199–201.

85. Wanklyn P, Ilsley D, Greenstein, Hampton IF, Roper TA, Kester RC, Mulley GP. The cold hemiplegic arm. Stroke 1994; 25:1765–1770.

86. Craig A, Bushnell M, Zhang E-T, Blomqvist A. A thalamic nucleus specific for pain and temperature sensation. Nature 1994; 372:770–773.

87. Roland P. Cortical representation of pain. Trends Neurosci 1992; 15:3–5.

88. Ribbers G, Geurts A, Mulder T. The reflex sympathetic dystrophy syndrome: A review. Int J Rehabil Res 1995; 18:277–295.

89. Petchkrua W, Weiss D, Patel R. Reassessment of the incidence of complex regional pain syndrome type 1 following stoke. Neurorehabil Neural Repair 2000; 14:59–63.

90. Davidoff G, Werner R, Cremer S, Jackson MD, Ventocilla C, Wolf L. Predictive value of the three-phase technetium bone scan in diagnosis of reflex sympathetic dystrophy syndrome. Arch Phys Med Rehabil 1989; 70:135–137.

91. Weiss L, Alfano A, Bardfeld P, Weiss J, Friedmann LW. Prognostic value of triple phase bone scanning for reflex sympathetic dystrophy in hemiplegia. Arch Phys Med Rehabil 1993; 74:716–719.

92. Schwartzman R. New treatments for reflex sympathetic dystrophy. N Engl J Med 2000; 343:652–653.

93. McLachlan E, Janig W, Devor M, Michaelis M. Peripheral nerve injury triggers noradrenergic sprouting within dorsal root ganglia. Nature 1993; 363:543–545.

94. van Hilten B, van de Beek W-J, Hoff J, Voormolen J, Delhaas E. Intrathecal baclofen for the treatment of dystonia in patients with reflex sympathetic dystrophy. N Engl J Med 2000; 343:625–630.

95. Melzack R. The McGill pain questionnaire: Major properties and scoring methods. Pain 1975; 1:275–299.

96. Sindrup S, Jensen T. Pharmacologic treatment of pain in polyneuropathy. Neurology 2000; 55:915–920.

97. Kuzniecky R, Ho S, Pan J, Martin R, Gilliam F, Faught E, Hetherington H. Modulation of cerebral GABA by topiramate, lamotrigine, and gabapentin in healthy adults. Neurology 2002; 58:368–372.

98. Max M, Lynch S, Muir J, Shoaf SE, Smoller B, Dubner R. Effects of desipramine, amitriptyline, and fluoxetine on pain in diabetic neuropathy. N Eng J Med 1992; 326:1250–1256.

99. Watson C, chipman M, Reed K, Evans RJ, Birkett N. Amitriptyline versus maprotiline in postherpetic neuralgia. Pain 1992; 48:29–36.

100. Canavero S, Bonicalzi V, Paolotti R. Lack of effect of topiramate for central pain. Neurology 2002; 58:831–832.

101. Galer B, Miller K, Rowbotham M. Response to intravenous lidocaine infusion differs based on clinical diagnosis and site of nervous system injury. Neurology 1993; 43:1233–1235.

102. Rowbotham M. Managing post-herpetic neuralgia with opioids and local anesthetics. Ann Neurol 1994; 35(suppl):S46–S49.

103. Chabal C, Jacobson L, Mariano A, Chaney E, Britell CW. The use of oral mexiletine for the treatment of pain after peripheral nerve injury. Anesthesiol 1992; 76:513–517.

104. Verdugo R, Ochoa J. 'Sympathetically maintained pain'. Neurology 1994; 44:1003–1014.

105. Drummond P, Finch P, Smythe G. Reflex sympathetic dystrophy: The significance of differing plasma catecholamine concentrations in affected and unaffected limbs. Brain 1991; 114:2025–2036.

106. Kemler M, Barendse G, Van Kleef M, de Vet HC, Rijks CP, Furnee CA, van den Wildenberg FA. Spinal cord stimulation in patients with chronic reflex sympathetic dystrophy. N Engl J Med 2000; 343:618–624.

107. Taira T, Tanikawa T, Kawamura H, Iseki H, Takakura K. Spinal intrathecal baclofen suppresses central pain after a stroke. J Neurol Neurosurg Psychiatry 1994; 57:381–382.

108. Allan L, Hays H, Jensen N, Donald R, Kalso E. Randomised crossover trial of transdermal fentanyl and sustained release oral morphine for treating chronic non-cancer pain. BMJ 2001; 322:1154–1158.

109. Boucher T, Okuse K, Bennett D, Munson J, Wood J, McMahon S. Potent analgesic effects of GDNF in neuropathic pain states. Science 2000; 290:124–127.

110. Ji R, Woolf C. Neuronal plasticity and signal transduction in nociceptive neurons: implications for the initiation and maintenance of pathological pain. Neurobiol Dis 2000:1–10.

111. Waxman S, Cummins T, Dib-Hajj S, Black J. Voltage-gated sodium channels and the molecular pathogenesis of pain: A review. J Rehabil Res Dev 2000; 37:517–528.

112. Guieu R. Analgesic effects of vibration and TENS applied separately and simultaneously to patients with chronic pain. Can J Neurol Sci 1991; 18:113–119.

113. Biella G, Sotgiu ML, Pellegata G, Paulesu E, Castiglioni I, Fazio F. Acupuncture produces central activations in pain regions. NeuroImage 2001; 14:60–66.

114. Van Buyten J-P, Van Zundert J, Vueghs P, Vanduffel L. Efficacy of spinal cord stimulation. Eur J Pain 2001; 5:299–307.

115. Katayama Y, Fukaya C, Yamamoto T. Poststroke pain control by chronic motor cortex stimulation: Neurological characteristics predicting a favorable response. J Neurosurg 1998; 89:585–591.

116. Peyron R, Garcia-Larrea L, Deiber M, Cinotti L, Convers P, Sindou M, Mauguiere F, Laurent B. Electrical stimulation of precentral cortical area in the treatment of central pain: electrophysiological and PET study. Pain 1995; 62:275–286.

117. Mertens P, Sindou M. Surgery in the dorsal root entry zone for treatment of chronic pain. Neurochirurgie 2000; 46:429–446.

118. Morley S, Eccleston C, Williams A. Systematic review and meta-analysis of randomized controlled trials of cognitive behavioral therapy for chronic pain in adults, excluding headache. Pain 1999; 80:1–13.

119. Sullivan M, Stanish W, Waite H, Sullivan M, Tripp D. Catastrophizing, pain, and disabiolity in patients with soft-tissue injuries. Pain 1998; 77:253–260.

120. Engel J, Schwartz L, Jensen M, Johnson D. Pain in cerebral palsy: The relation of coping strategies to adjustment. Pain 2000; 88:225–230.

121. Zorowitz R, Idank D, Ikai T, Hughes MB, Johnston MV. Shoulder subluxation after stroke: A comparison of four supports. Arch Phys Med Rehabil 1995; 76:763–771.

122. Parker V, Wade D, Langton-Hewer R. Loss of arm function after stroke: Measurement, frequency and recovery. Int Rehabil Med 1986; 8:69–74.

123. Sunderland A, Tinson D, Bradley E, Fletcher D, Langton Hewer R, Wade DT. Enhanced physical therapy improves recovery of function after stroke. A randomised controlled trial. J Neurol Neurosurg Psychiatry 1992; 55:530–535.

124. Poduri K. Shoulder pain in stroke patients and its effects on rehabilitation. J Stroke Cerebrovasc Dis 1993; 3:261–266.

125. Inuba M, Piorkowski M. Ultrasound in treatment of painful shoulders in patients with hemiplegia. Phys Ther 1972; 52:737–741.

126. Philadelphia Panel. Evidence-based clinical practice guidelines on selected rehabilitation interventions for shoulder pain. Phys Ther 2001; 10:1719–1730.

127. Leandri M, Parodi C, Rigardo S. Comparison of TENS treatments in hemiplegic shoulder pain. Scand J Rehabil Med 1990; 22:69–72.

128. Faghri P, Rodgers M, Glaser R, Bors JG, Ho C, Akuthota P. The effects of functional electrical stimulation on shoulder subluxation, arm function recovery, and shoulder pain in hemiplegic stroke patients. Arch Phys Med Rehabil 1994; 75:73–79.

129. Chantraine A, Baribeault A, Uebelhart D, Gremion G. Shoulder pain and dysfunction in hemiplegia: Effects of functional electrical stimulation. Arch Phys Med Rehabil 1999; 80:328–331.

130. Snels I, Beckerman H, Twisk J, Dekker J, de Koning P, Koppe PA, Lankhorst GJ, Bouter LM. Effect of triamcinolone acetonide injections on hemiplegic shoulder pain: A randomized clinical trial. Stroke 2000; 31:2396–2401.

131. Bohr T. Problems with myofascial pain syndrome and fibromyalgia syndrome. Neurology 1996; 46:593–597.

132. Wolfe F, Ross K, Anderson J, Russell I, Hebert L. The prevalence and characteristics of fibromyalgia in the general population. Arth Rheum 1995; 38:19–28.

133. Hong C-Z, Simons D. Pathophysiologic and electrophysiologic mechanisms of myofascial trigger points. Arch Phys Med Rehabil 1998; 79:863–872.

134. Cummings T, White A. Needling therapies in the management of myofascial trigger point pain: A systematic review. Arch Phys Med Rehabil 2001; 82:986–992.

135. Esenyel M, Caglar N, Aldemir T. Treatment of myofascial pain. Am J Phys Med Rehabil 2000; 79:48–52.

136. Andersson G. Epidemiological features of chronic low-back pain. Lancet 1999; 354:581–585.

137. Philadelphia Panel. Evidence-based clinical practice guidelines on selected rehabilitation interventions for low back pain. Phys Ther 2001; 81:1641–1674.

138. Philadelphia Panel. Evidence-based clinical practice guidelines on selected rehabilitation interventions for neck pain. Phys Ther 2001; 81:1701–1717.

139. Moffett J, Torgerson D, Bell-Syer S, Jackson D, Llewlyn-Phillips H, Farrin A, Barber J. Randomised controlled trial of exercise for low back pain. BMJ 1999; 319:279–283.

140. Andersson G, Lucente T, Davis A. A comparison of osteopathic spinal manipulation with standard care for patients with low back pain. N Engl J Med 1999; 341:1426–1431.
141. Collacott E, Zimmerman J, White D, Rindone J. Bipolar permanent magnets for the treatment of chronic low back pain. JAMA 2000; 283:1322–1325.
142. Basford J, Sheffield C, Harmsen W. Laser therapy: A randomized, controlled trial of the effects of low-intensity Nd:YAG laser irradiation on musculoskeletal back pain. Arch Phys Med Rehabil 1999; 80: 647–652.
143. Foster L, L C, Erickson M, Jabbari B. Botulinum toxin A and chronic low back pain: A randomized, double-blind study. Neurology 2001; 56:1290–1293.
144. Moore S, Shurman J. Combined neuromuscular electrical stimulation and transcutaneous electrical nerve stimulation for treatment of chronic back pain: A double-blind, repeated measures comparison: Arch Phys Med Rehabil 1997; 78:55–60.
145. Ghoname E, Craig W, White P, Ahmed H, Hamza M. Percutaneous electrical nerve stimulation for low back pain. JAMA 1999; 281:818–823.
146. Carette S, Marcoux S, Truchon R, Grondin C, Gagnon J, Allard Y, Latulippe M. A controlled trial of corticosteroid injections into facet joints for chronic low back pain. N Engl J Med 1991; 325:1002–1007.
147. Haigh R, Clarke A. Effectiveness of rehabilitation for spinal pain. Clin Rehabil 1999; 13 (suppl 1):63–81.
148. Cherkin D, Deyo R, Battie M, Street J, Barlow W. A comparison of physical therapy, chiropractic manipulation, and provision of an educational booklet for the treatment of patients with low back pain. N Engl J Med 1998; 339:1021–1029.
149. Schuldt K. On neck muscle activity and load reduction in sitting postures. Scand J Rehabil Med 1988; Suppl 19:1–49.
150. Revel M, Minguet M, Gergoy P. Changes in cervicocephalic kinesthesia after a proprioceptive rehabilitation program in patients with neck pain. Arch Phys Med Rehabil 1994; 75:895–899.
151. Holroyd KA, O'Donnell FJ, Stensland M, Lipchik GL, Cordingley GE, Carlson BW. Management of chronic tension-type headache with tricyclic antidepressant medication, stress management therapy, and their combination. JAMA 2001; 285:2208–2215.
152. Banovac K, Gonzalez F, Renfree K. Treatment of heterotopic ossification after spinal cord injury. J Spinal Cord Med 1997; 20:60–65.
153. Buschbacher R. Heterotopic ossification: A review. Crit Rev Phys Rehabil Med 1992; 4:199–213.
154. Altkorn D, Vokes T. Treatment of postmenopausal osteoporosis. JAMA 2001; 285:1415–1418.
155. Bohannon R. Relationship between active range of motion deficits and muscle strength and tone at the elbow in patients with hemiparesis. Clin Rehabil 1991; 5:219–224.
156. Fellows S, Kaus C, Thilmann A. Voluntary movement at the elbow in spastic hemiparesis. Ann Neurol 1994; 36:397–407.
157. Dietz V. Human neuronal control of automatic functional movements: Interaction between central programs and afferent input. Physiol Rev 1992; 72:33–69.
158. Lamontagne A, Malouin F, Richards C. Locomotor-specific measure of spasticity of plantarflexor muscles after stroke. Arch Phys Med Rehabil 2001; 82: 1696–1704.
159. Rogers de Saca L, Catlin P, Segal R. Immediate effects of the toe spreader on the tonic toe flexion reflex. Phys Ther 1994; 74:561–570.
160. Schmit B, Dewald J, Rymer Z. Stretch reflex adaptation in elbow flexors during repeated passive movements in unilateral brain-injured patients. Arch Phys Med Rehabil 2000; 81:269–278.
161. Price R, Lehmann J, Boswell-Bessette S, deLateur B. Influence of cryotherapy on spasticity at the human ankle. Arch Phys Med Rehabil 1993; 74:300–304.
162. Kunkel C, Scremin E, Eisenberg B, Garcia JF, Roberts S, Martinez S. Effect of "standing" on spasticity, contracture, and osteoporosis in paralyzed males. Arch Phys Med Rehabil 1993; 74:73–78.
163. Chan C. Dantrolene sodium and hepatic injury. Neurology 1990; 40:1427–1432.
164. Basmajian J, Super G. Dantrolene sodium in the treatment of spasticity. Arch Phys Med Rehabil 1973; 54:60–64.
165. Luisto M, Moller K, Nuutila A. Dantrolene sodium in chronic spasticity of varying etiology. Acta Neurol Scand 1982; 65:355–362.
166. Ketel W, Kolb M. Long term treatment with dantrolene sodium of stroke patients with spasticity limiting the return of function. Curr Med Res Opin 1984; 9:161–169.
167. Tolosa E, Soll R, Loewenson R. Treatment of spasticity in multiple sclerosis with dantrolene. JAMA 1975; 233:1046–7.
168. Haslam R, Walcher J, Lietman P. Dantrolene sodium in children with spasticity. Arch Phys Med Rehabil 1974; 55:384–388.
169. Katrak P, Cole A, Poulos C, McCauley J. Objective assessment of spasticity, strength, and function with early exhibition of dantrolene sodium after cerebrovascular accident: A randomized double-blind study. Arch Phys Med Rehabil 1992; 73:4–9.
170. Davidoff R. Antispasticity drugs: Mechanisms of action. Ann Neurol 1985; 17:107–116.
171. Orsnes G, Crone C, Krarup C, Petersen N, Nielsen J. The effect of baclofen on the transmissin in spinal pathways in spastic multiple sclerosis patients. Clin Neurophysiol 2000; 111:1372–1379.
172. Feldman R, Kelly-Hayes M, Conomy J, Foley J. Baclofen for spasticity in multiple sclerosis: Double blind crossover and three-year study. Neurology 1978; 28:1094–1098.
173. Hinderer S, Lehmann J, Price R, White O, DeLateur B, Deitz J. Spasticity in spinal cord injured persons: Quantitative effects of baclofen and placebo treatments. Am J Phys Med Rehabil 1990; 69:311–317.
174. Brar S, Smith M, Nelson L, Franklin G, Cobble N. Evaluation of treatment protocols on minimal to moderate spasticity in multiple sclerosis. Arch Phys Med Rehabil 1991; 72:186–189.
175. Penn R, Savoy S, Corcos D, Latash M, Gottlieb G, Parke B, Kroin JS. Intrathecal baclofen for severe spinal spasticity. N Eng J Med 1989; 320:1517–21.
176. Azouvi P, Mane M, Thiebaut J-B, Denys P, Remy-Neris O, Bussel B. Intrathecal baclofen administration for control of severe spinal spasticity: functional

improvement and long-term follow-up. Arch Phys Med Rehabil 1996; 77:35–39.

177. Meythaler J, Renfroe S, Grabb P, Hadley M. Long-term continuously infused intrathecal baclofen for spastic-dystonic hypertonia in traumatic brain injury: 1-year experience. Arch Phys Med Rehabil 1999; 80:13–19.

178. Meythaler J, Guin-Renfroe S, Hadley M. Continuously infused intrathecal baclofen for spastic/dystonic hemiplegia. Am J Phys Med Rehabil 1999; 78:247–254.

179. Meythaler J, Steers W, Tuel S, Cross LL, Sesco DC, Haworth CS. Intrathecal baclofen in hereditary spastic paraparesis. Arch Phys Med Rehabil 1992; 73: 794–797.

180. Albright A, barron W, Fasick M, Polinko P, Janosky J. Continuous intrathecal infusion for spasticity of cerebral origin. JAMA 1993; 270:2475–2477.

181. Middel B, Kuipers-Upmeijer H, Bouma J, Staal M. Effect of intrathecal baclofen delivered by an implanted programmable pump on health related quality of life in patients with severe spasticity. J Neurol Neurosurg Psychiatry 1997; 63:204–209.

182. Ochs G, Delhaas E. Aspects of long-term treatment with intrathecal baclofen for severe spasticity (abstr). Neurology 1992; 42 (Suppl 3):466.

183. Boroojerdi B, Ziemann U, Chen R, Butefisch C, Cohen L. Mechanisms underlying human motor system plasticity. Muscle Nerve 2001; 24:602–613.

184. Donchin O, Sawaki L, Madupu G, Cohen L, Shadmehr R. Influence of agents affecting synaptic plasticity on learning of reaching movements. Soc For Neurosci Abstr 2001; 27:302.2.

185. Bedard P, Tremblay L, Barbeau H, Filion M, Maheux R, Richards CL, DiPaolo T. Action of 5-hydroxytryptamine, substance P, thyrotropin-releasing hormone and clonidine on motoneurone excitability. Can J Neurol Sci 1987; 14:506–509.

186. Donovan W, Carter R, Rossi C, Wilkerson M. Clonidine effect on spasticity: A clinical trial. Arch Phys Med Rehabil 1988; 69:193–194.

187. Rémy-Néris O, Barbeau H, Daniel O, Boiteau F, Bussel B. Effects of intrathecal clonidine injection on spinal reflexes and human locomotion in incomplete paraplegic subjects. Exp Brain Res 1999; 129:433–440.

188. Coward, D. Tizanidine: Neuropharmacology and mechanism of action. Neurology 1994; 44(Suppl 9): S6–S11.

189. Hoogstraten M, van der Ploeg R, Van der Berg W, Vreeling A, van Marle S, Minderhoud JM. Tizanidine versus baclofen in the treatment of multiple sclerosis patients. Acta Neurol Scand 1988; 77:224–230.

190. Bes A, Eysette M, Pierrot-Deseilligny E. A multicentre, double-blind trial of tizanidine in spasticity associated with hemiplegia. Curr Med Res Opin 1988; 10:709–718.

191. Lataste X, Emre M, Davis C, Groves L. Comparative profile of tizanidine in the management of spasticity. Neurology 1994; 44(suppl 9):S53–S59.

192. Smith C, Birnbaum G, Carter J, Greenstein J, Lublin FD. Tizanidine treatment of spasticity caused by multiple sclerosis. Neurology 1994; 44(Suppl 9):S34–S43.

193. Nance P, Bugaresti J, Shellenberger K, Sheremata W, Martinez-Arizala A. Efficacy and safety of tizanidine in the treatment of spasticity in patients with spinal cord injury. Neurology 1994; 44(Suppl 9): S44–S52.

194. Gelber D, Good D, Dromerick A, Sergay S, Richardson M. Open-label dose-titration safety and efficacy study of tizanidine hydrochloride in the treatment of spasticity associated with chronic stroke. Stroke 2001; 32:1841–1846.

195. Schmidt B, Jordan L. The role of serotonin in reflex modulation and locomotor rhythm production in the mammalian spinal cord. Brain Res Bull 2001; 53:689–710.

196. Wainberg M, Barbeau H, Gauthier S. Quantitative assessment of the effect of cyproheptadine on spastic paretic gait: A preliminary study. J Neurol 1986; 233:311–314.

197. Eriksson J, Olausson B, Jankowska E. Antispastic effects of L-dopa. Exp Brain Res 1996; 111:296–304.

198. Cutter N, Scott D, Johnson J, Whiteneck G. Gabapentin effect on spasticity in multiple sclerosis: A placebo-controlled randomized trial. Arch Phys Med Rehabil 2000; 81:164–169.

199. Holden K, Titus M. The effect of tiagabine on spasticity in children with intractable epilepsy: A pilot study. Pediatr Neurol 1999; 21:728–730.

200. Petro D, Ellenberger C. Treatment of human spasticity with delta-9-tetrahydrocannabinol. J Clin Pharmacol 1981; 21:413S–416S.

201. Erickson D, Blacklock J, Michaelson M, Sperling K, Lo J. Control of spasticity by implantable continuous flow morphine pump. Neurosurgery 1985; 16:215–217.

202. Stern P, Bokonjic R. Glycine therapy in 7 cases of spasticity. Pharmacology 1974; 12:117–119.

203. Hauser S, Doolittle T, Lopez-Bresnahan M, Shahani B, Schoenfeld D, Shih VE, Growdon J, Lehrich JR. An antispasticity effect of threonine in multiple sclerosis. Arch Neurol 1992; 49:923–926.

204. Skeil D, Barnes M. The local treatment of spasticity. Clin Rehabil 1994; 8:240–246.

205. Hallett M. One man's poison—clinical applications of botulinum toxin. N Engl J Med 1999; 341:118–120.

206. De Paiva A, Meunier F, Molgo J, Aoki K, Dolly J. Functional repair of motor endplates after botulinum neurotoxin type A poisoning. Proc Natl Acad Sci USA 1999; 96:3200–3205.

207. Chutorian A, Root L. Management of spasticity in children with botulinum-A toxin. Int Pediatr 1994; 9: 35–43.

208. Snow B, Tsui J, Bhatt M, Varelas M, Hashimoto SA, Calne DB. Treatment of spasticity with botulinum toxin: A double-blind study. Ann Neurol 1990; 28: 512–515.

209. Pierson S, Katz D, Tarsy D. Botulinum toxin A in the treatment of spasticity. Neurology 1994; 44(suppl2): A184.

210. Hesse S, Lucke D, Malezic M, Bertelt C, Friedrich H, Gregoric M, Mauritz KH. Botulinum toxin treatment for lower limb extensor spasticity in chronic hemiparetic patients. J Neurol Neurosurg Psychiatry 1994; 57:1321–1324.

211. Koman L, Mooney J, Smith B, Goodman A, Mulvaney T. Management of spasticity in cerebral palsy with botulinum-A toxin. J Pediatr Orthop 1994; 14: 299–303.

212. Brashear A, Gordon M, Elovic E, Kassicieh D. In-

tramuscular injection of botulinum toxin for the treatment of wrist and finger spasticity after a stroke. N Engl J Med 2002; 347:395–400.

213. Richardson D, Sheean G, Werring D, Desai M, Edwards S, Greenwood R, Thompson A. Evaluating the role of botulinum toxin in the management of focal hypertonia in adults. J Neurol Neurosurg Psychiatry 2000; 69:499–506.

214. Beckerman H, Lankhorst G, Verbeek A, J B. The effects of phenol nerve and muscle blocks in treating spasticity: Review of the literature. Crit Rev Phys Rehabil Med 1996; 8:111–124.

215. Halpern D, Meelhuysen F. Phenol motor point block in the management of muscular hypertonia. Arch Phys Med Rehabil 1966; 47:659–664.

216. Garland D, Lucie R, Walters R. Current uses of open phenol nerve block for adult acquired spasticity. Clin Orthop 1982; 165:217–222.

217. Stefanovska A, Rebersek S, Bajd T, Vodovnik L. Effects of electrical stimulation on spasticity. Crit Rev in Phys Rehabil Med 1991; 3:59–99.

218. Robinson C, Kett N, Bolam J. Spasticity in spinal cord injured patients: 2. Initial measures and long-term effects of surface electrical stimulation. Arch Phys Med Rehabil 1988; 69:862–868.

219. Seib T, Price R, Reyes M, Lehmann J. The quantitative measurement of spasticity: effect of cutaneous electrical stimulation. Arch Phys Med Rehabil 1994; 75:746–750.

220. Levin M, Hui-Chan C. Relief of hemiparetic spasticity by TENS is associated with improvement in reflex and voluntary motor functions. EEG Clin Neurophys 1992; 85:131–142.

221. Petajan J. Sural nerve stimulation and motor control of tibialis anterior muscle in spstic paresis. Neurology 1987; 37:47–52.

222. Petersen T, Klemar B. Electrical stimulation as a treatment of lower limb spasticity. J Neuro Rehabil 1988; 2:103–108.

223. Halstead L, Seager S. The effects of rectal probe electrostimulation on SCI spasticity. Paraplegia 1991; 29:43–47.

224. Granat M, Ferguson A, Andrews B, Delargy M. Role of functional electrical stimulation in the rehabilitation of patients with incomplete spinal cord injury: Observed benefits during gait studies. Paraplegia 1993; 31:207–215.

225. Dimitrijevic M, Stokic D, Wawro A, Wun C-C. Modification of motor control of wrist extension by meshglove electrical afferent stimulation in stroke patients. Arch Phys Med Rehabil 1996; 77:252–258.

226. Pinter M, Gerstenbrand F, Dimitrijevic M. Epidural electrical stimulation of posterior structures of the human lumbosacral cord: 3. Control of spasticity. Spinal Cord 2000; 38:524–531.

227. Sindou M, Jeanmonod D. Microsurgical DREZ-otomy for the treatment of spasticity and pain in the lower limbs. Neurosurgery 1989; 24:655–670.

228. Putty T, Shapiro S. Efficacy of dorsal longitudinal myelotomy in treating spinal spasticity: A review of 20 cases. J Neurosurg 1991; 75:397–401.

229. Vaughan C, Berman B, Peacock W. Cerebral palsy and rhizotomy: A 3 year follow-up with gait analysis. J Neurosurg 1991; 74:178–184.

230. Steinbok P, Keyes R, Langill L, Cochrane D. The validity of electrophysiological criteria used in selective functional dorsal rhizotomy for treatment of spastic cerebral palsy. J Neurosurg 1994; 81:354–361.

231. Peacock W, Staudt L. Functional outcomes following selective posterior rhizotomy in children with cerebral palsy. J Neurosurg 1991; 74:380–385.

232. Cahan L, Asams J, Perry J, Beeler L. Instrumented gait analysis after selective dorsal rhizotomy. Develop Med Child Neurol 1990; 32:1037–1043.

233. Akeson W, Amiel D, Abel M, Garfin SR, Woo SL. Effects of immobilization on joints. Clin Orthop 1985; 219:28–39.

234. Bell K, Halar E. Contractures: Prevention and management. Crit Rev Phys Rehabil Med 1990; 1:231–246.

235. Dietz V. Spastic movement disorder. Spinal Cord 2000; 38:389–393.

236. Yarkony G, Bass L, Keenan V, Meyer P. Contractures complicating spinal cord injury. Paraplegia 1985; 23:265–269.

237. Yarkony G, Sahgal V. Contractures: a major complication of craniocerebral trauma. Clin Orthop 1987; 219:93–98.

238. Johnson E, Fowler W, Lieberman J. Contractures in neuromuscular disease. Arch Phys Med Rehabil 1992; 73:807–810.

239. Liebesman J, Cafarelli E. Physiology of range of motion in human joints: A critical review. Crit Rev Phys Rehabil Med 1994; 6:131–160.

240. Breslau N. Traumatic events and posttraumatic stress disorder in an urban population of young adults. Arch Gen Psychiatry 1991; 48:216–222.

241. Mellman T, David D, Bustamante V, Fins A, Esposito K. Predictors of post-traumatic stress disorder following severe injury. Depress Anxiety 2001; 14:226–231.

242. Boyer B, Knolls M, Kafkalas C, Tollen L. Prevalence of posttraumatic stress disorder in patients with pediatric spinal cord injury: relationship to functional independence. Top Spinal Cord Inj Rehabil 2000; 6(suppl):125–133.

243. Shaw M, Strother S, McFarlane C, Morris P, Anderson J, Clark CR, Egan GF. Abnormal functional connectivity in posttraumatic stress disorder. NeuroImage 2002; 15:661–674.

244. Yehuda R. Post-traumatic stress disorder. N Engl J Med 2002; 346:108–114.

245. Brady K, Pearlstein T, Asnis G, Baker D, Rothbaum B, Sikes CR, Farfel GM. Efficacy and safety of sertraline treatment of posttraumatic stress disorder. JAMA 2000; 283:1837–1844.

246. NIH Consensus Development Panel. Diagnosis and treatment of depression in late life. JAMA 1992; 268:1018–1024.

247. Wiart L, Petit H, Joseph P, Mazaux J, Barat M. Fluoxetine in early poststroke depression; a double-blind placebo-controlled study. Stroke 2000; 31:1829–1832.

248. Robinson R. Depression and anxiety in the context of physical illness. Depress Anxiety 1998; 7:147–165.

249. Krause J, Kemp B, Coker J. Depression after spinal cord injury: Relation to gender, ethnicity, aging, and socioeconomic indicators. Arch Phys Med Rehabil 2000; 81:1099–1109.

250. Starkstein S, Fedoroff J, Price T, Leiguarda R, Robinson RG. Anosognosia in patients with cerebrovascular lesions. Stroke 1992; 23:1446–1453.

251. Judd L, Akiskal H, Maser J, Zeller P, Endicott J, Coryell W, Paulus MP, Kunovac JL, Leon AC, Mueller TI, Rice JA, Keller MB. A prospective 12-year study of subsyndromal and syndromal depressive symptoms in unipolar major depressive disorders. Arch Gen Psychiatry 1998; 55:694–700.

252. Sadek N, Bona J. Subsyndromal symptomatic depression: A new concept. Depress Anxiety 2000; 12: 30–39.

253. Starkstein S, Robinson R. Affective disorders and cerebral vascular disease. Brit J Psychiatry 1989; 154: 170–182.

254. Drevets W, Videen T, Price J, Preskorn SH, Carmichael ST, Raichle ME. A functional anatomical study of unipolar depression. J Neurosci 1992; 12:3628–3641.

255. Reding M, Orto L, Winter S, McDowell F. Antidepressant therapy after stroke. Arch Neurol 1986; 43:763–765.

256. Grober S, Gordon W, Sliwinski M, Hibbard MR, Aletta EG, Paddison PL. Utility of the dexamethasone supression test in the diagnosis of poststroke depression. Arch phys Med Rehabil 1991; 72:1076–1079.

257. Kroenke K, West S, Swindle R, Gilsenan A, Eckhert GJ, Dolor R, Stang P, Zhou XH, Hays R. Similar effectiveness of paroxetine, fluoxetine, and sertraline in primary care. JAMA 2001; 286:2947–2955.

258. Gill D, Hatcher S. Antidepressants for depression in people with physical illness. In: Review C, ed. The Cochrane Library. Oxford: Update Software, 2000.

259. Laghrissi-Thode F, Wagner W, Pollock B, Johnson P, Finkel M. Elevated platelet factor 4 and beta-thromboglobulin plasma levels in depressed patients with ischemic heart disease. Biol Psychiatry 1997; 42:290–295.

260. Roose S, Glassman A, Seidman S. Relationship between depression and other medical illnesses. JAMA 2001; 286:1687–1690.

261. Potter W, Rudorfer M, Manji H. The pharmacologic treatment of depression. New Eng J Med 1991; 325: 633–642.

262. Bodner R, Lynch T, Lewis L, Kahn D. Serotonin syndrome. Neurology 1995; 45:219–223.

263. Morin C, Colecchi C, Stone J, Sood R, Brink D. Behavioral and pharmacological therapies for late-life insomnia. JAMA 1999; 281:991–999.

264. Webster J, Bell K, Hussey J, Natale T, Lakshminarayanan S. Sleep apnea in adults with traumatic brain injury: A preliminary investigation. Arch Phys Med Rehabil 2001; 82:316–321.

265. Burns S, Little J, Hussey J, Lyman P, Lakshminarayanan S. Sleep apnea syndrome in chronic spinal cord injury: Associated factors and treatment. Arch Phys Med Rehabil 2000; 81:1334–1339.

266. Partinen M, Palomaki H. Snoring and cerebral infarction. Lancet 1985; 1:1325–1326.

267. Bassetti C, Aldrich M, Quint D. Sleep-disordered breathing in patients with acute supra- and infratentorial strokes. A prospective study of 39 patients. Stroke 1997; 28:1765–1772.

268. Mohsenin V, Valor R. Sleep apnea in patients with hemispheric stroke. Arch Phys Med Rehabil 1995; 76:71–76.

269. Good D, Henkle J, Gelber D, Welsh J, Verhulst S. Sleep-disordered breathing and poor functional outcome after stroke. Stroke 1996; 27:252–259.

270. Sandberg O, Franklin K, Bucht G, Eriksson S, Gustafson Y. Nasal continuous positive airway pressure in stroke patients with sleep apnoea: A randomized treatment study. Eur Respir J 2001; 18:630–634.

271. Vestergaard K, Andersen G, Gottrup H, Kristensen B, Jensen T. Lamotrigine for central poststroke pain. Neurology 2001; 56:184–190.

272. Leijon G, Boivie J. Central poststroke pain—a controlled trial of amitriptyline and carbamazepine. Pain 1989; 36:27–36.

273. Swiddall P, Molloy A, Walker S, Rutkowski S. The efficacy of intrathecal morphine and clonidine in the treatment of pain after spinal cord injury. Anesth Analg 2000; 91:1–6.

274. Attal N, Brasseur G, Dupuy M, Guirimand F, Parker F, Bouhassira D. Intravenous lidocaine in central pain. Neurology 2000; 54:564–574.

PART III

REHABILITATION OF SPECIFIC NEUROLOGIC DISORDERS

Chapter 9

Stroke

Apoplexy convolutes the lives of young and old, rising with each decade of untreated risk factors. Across national boundaries, the disease kills 15%–35% of its victims and causes serious disability in more adults who survive than any other medical disease. The sudden burdens of disability, the prospect of a life diminished by a "dead" hand, by a gimpy leg, or by grimacingly difficult speech swell most victims with the confusion and fear of helplessness for the first time in their lives. For a retired person beached in bed with hemiplegia, the shade of stroke encloses dark worries about losing all dignity and cherished independence. The rehabilitation team offers immediate hope. Its assessment and management of impairment and disability is the most responsible therapeutic environment for enhancing outcomes for patients who need inpatient care. Stroke rehabilitation calls for creative problem-solving by rehabilitationists, patients, families, and increasingly, by neuroscientists and bioengineers.

EPIDEMIOLOGY

The prevalence of stroke is from 500 to 800 cases per 100,000 adults. From 550,000 to 700,000 Americans suffer strokes each year with an incidence of approximately 120 per 100,000 adults. Rates are highest in white men and black women. Age-standardized rates are

38 per 1000 men and 28 per 1000 women over 55 years of age. By age 85, rates are approximately 10% per year. Approximately 20% of these strokes are repeated ones and most often by the same mechanism as the initial stroke. A population study in Auckland found that 460 per 100,000 report incomplete recovery at any given time, but the prevalence of survivors who need physical help in at least one ADL is approximately 175 per 100,000.[1] Approximately 27% of women and 16% of men need assistance. On average, across age groups, patients survive approximately 6 years after a stroke, with a mean survival of 3 years for men and 1.5 years for women over 75 years of age.

Mortality at 30 days after a stroke runs approximately 20% in Western countries. A prospective study of a multiethnic population in New York City found a 5% rate at 1 month, although the subjects were younger than most studies and many had small vessel disease.[2] Cumulative mortality was 16% at 1 year, 29% at 3 years, and 41% at 5 years, but vascular causes of death accounted for only approximately 43% of deaths beyond the first month. Of interest, mortality was twice as great in Carribean Hispanics as in black or white patients. One-year survivors in Perth died at the rate of 10% per year over the next 4 years, about twice the expected rate for a matched nonstroke population, mostly because of a recurrent stroke or cardiovascular disease.[3] In the Oxfordshire Community Stroke Study,[4] the relative risk of death after infarction for those of all ages, compared to controls, was 4.8 in the first year and 2.1 for the next 5 years. The cumulative risk of death in a region of Copenhagen County was 28% at 28 days, 41% at 1 year, which was double the risk for the general population, and 60% at 5 years.[5] At age 65, the risk for dying was about the same regardless of type of stroke. The probability of survival for patients age 65 who were admitted between 1987 and 1991 was 75% at 1 year, 70% at 2 years, and 55% at 5 years poststroke. In the Framingham Study,[6,7] those who survived the first year and did not have hypertension or cardiac disease had no subsequent excess mortality. Vigorous attempts at secondary prevention of vascular disease over the long run must be part of any rehabilitation effort. This management may reduce mortality from vascular causes and total mortality at 5 years by 50%.

In China and India, stroke accounts for approximately 40% of all deaths in adults. Whereas Western countries have experienced a decline in the incidence of stroke into the early 1990s despite aging populations, central and eastern Europe are seeing a rise. Higher rates seem related to inadequate management of treatable risk factors. Stroke causes almost 10% of the 50 million deaths around the world. Based on the reported 5% absolute decrease in mortality for patients managed in a stroke unit,[8] organized management of 80% of the world's cases of stroke could prevent approximately 200,000 deaths a year.

Overall, then, approximately one-third of people who suffer a stroke die within a year, one-third make at least fair gains, and one-third remain disabled.

Fiscal Impact

In the United Kingdom, 5% of all health services pay for the care of people with stroke, although only 55% of people with a stroke are admitted to an acute care hospital.[9] Estimates of the total costs of stroke in the United States depend on simplifying assumptions. The approximate distribution of costs is shown in Table 9–1.[10–12] Estimates on the cost for federally sponsored patients, developed by the Patient Outcomes Research Team Study (PORT) for the Agency for Health Care Policy and Research, suggested that the direct cost of stroke in 1993 was $13 billion and the indirect cost,

Table 9–1. **Estimated Distribution of Costs for Stroke Patient Care**

DIRECT COSTS	(%)
Acute hospital care	19
Nursing homes	10
Medical and social services	9
Inpatient rehabilitation	5
Physician services	<2
Chronic hospital care	2
Assistive devices	0.4
INDIRECT (LOST INCOME)	
Disability	6
Premature death	48

taking into account caregiver burden, was another $17 billion.[10] Medicare actually paid an average of $15,000 per patient or over $6 billion for the first 90 days of care. Of this amount, initial hospital care accounted for 43%, rehospitalizations for 14%, and rehabilitation for 16%. Approximately 78% of patients with strokes are covered by Medicare. The lifetime cost of stroke in the United States based on the year 1990 was $228,00 for subarachnoid hemorrhage, $124,000 for intracerebral hemorrhage, and $104,000 for ischemic stroke, which adds up to an aggregate total of $81 billion.[11] Care for the first 2 years accounted for 45% of costs, ambulatory care for 35%, and nursing home care for 17%. In countries where cost containment measures are less imposing, social factors such as placement problems, more than the need for additional diagnostic and medical care, can account for longer lengths of hospital stay and greater costs.

Briefer inpatient acute hospital and rehabilitation stays are a product of Medicare reimbursement schemes and capitated care. The mean cost across regions of the United States for inpatient rehabilitation is approximately twice the cost of an acute hospital stay, but only a minority of stroke survivors receive this level of care. In different regions, from 10% to 17% of Medicare patients receive inpatient stroke rehabilitation.[13] Starting in 2002, the average reimbursement for each patient who receives inpatient stroke rehabilitation under Medicare will be from $12,000 to $16,000.

Stroke Syndromes

The incidence of stroke syndromes in westernized white populations does not differ much between countries. In the World Heath Organization's MONICA project, cities in 10 countries reported that 75%–85% of strokes are thrombotic, 10% are caused by parenchymatous hemorrhage, 2%–5% are because of subarachnoid hemorrhage, and 5%–15% are from uncertain causes. Investigators in the Stroke Data Bank, which prospectively collected data from four American university hospitals, used its own rules to classify the cause of stroke in 1800 patients admitted between 1983 and 1986.[14] Infarcts accounted for 70%, which included large artery stenosis or occlusion in 6%, tandem occlusive lesions in 4%, and lacunes in

19%. A cardioembolus was diagnosed in 14% and an infarct of undetermined cause in 28%. Intracerebral hemorrhages were found in 13% and subarachnoid hemorrhages in another 13%. The category of undetermined cause arises in at least 20% of cases across studies, usually because diagnostic tests are incomplete or offer ambiguous results. The diagnosis of an artery-to-artery embolus or cardioembolus may require more invasive testing than some physicians are willing to order, such as a cerebral angiogram within the first 6 hours after onset or a transesophageal echocardiogram.

Five-year recurrence rates for stroke ran 40% for men and 25% for women in the Framingham study, in which no special effort was made to manage risk factors.[7] In the 675 patients registered with a first stroke in the Oxfordshire Community Stroke Project, the actuarial risk of suffering a recurrence was 30% by 5 years, 9 times the risk in the general community.[15] The risk was 13% in the first year, then 4% per year, without a clear relationship to age or stroke type. These recurrent strokes caused significant functional disability in 60% of cases. The second stroke is most often the same type as the first stroke, so knowledge gained about the initial cause may determine subsequent risk factor management. Silent stroke may be another risk factor for clinical stroke, for a decline in cognition, and for other unexpected neurologic impairments at the time of a definite stroke, such as dysphagia or pseudobulbar palsy (Fig. 9–1).[16] Magnetic resonance imaging reveals subclinical deep gray and white matter lesions from 3 to 15 mm in diameter that are presumably associated with a vasculopathy or emboli to small artery branches.

MEDICAL INTERVENTIONS

With shorter acute care hospital stays encouraged by the Diagnostic Related Groups (DRG)-based Prospective Payment System for Medicare reimbursement and by managed care organizations, physicians in the United States and, increasingly around the world, may have less time to monitor and adjust their initial therapies. Fine tuning of medications, elimination of some, and the need to begin others, has become a daily routine on inpatient services. In 1994, the length of stay covered for

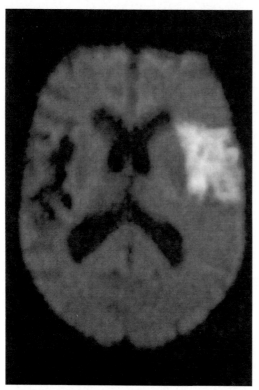

Figure 9–1. Diffusion-weighted magnetic resonance imaging (DWI) study of a 70-year-old woman who presented with a moderate nonfluent aphasia and unexpectedly profound aphagia from a cardioembolic stroke. The scan revealed causation. She had an old, clinically silent right cerebral infarct that had not altered swallowing. The second infarct, which affected a similar perisylvian region, eliminated any compensatory oromotor control. DWI and T-2–weighted studies may reveal old and new lesions to explain impairments that usually do not arise from just the newly visible infarct.

Table 9–2. **First Admission for Stroke Rehabilitation: Typical Functional Independence Measure Results Reported by Uniform Data System for Medical Rehabilitation**

Average Scores	Admission	Discharge
Self-care	3.5	5.2
Sphincter	3.7	5.4
Mobility	3.0	5.0
Locomotion	2.1	4.3
Communication	4.2	5.2
Social Cognition	3.5	4.6
Total FIM	62	86
Age (years)	70	
Onset (days)	12	
Stay (days)		20
DISCHARGE STATUS (%)		
Community	76	76
Long-term care	15	14
Acute care	7	6

FIM, Functional Independence Measure.

Frequency of Complications

In a study of patients transferred to a rehabilitation center within a mean of 10 days after a stroke, the incidence of serious medical complications found upon admission rose from 22% before to 48% the year after institution of DRGs.[18] Many of these complications derived from altering or starting medications during the acute hospitalization, especially antihypertensives, antiarrhythmics, platelet antiaggregants, anticoagulants, steroids, hypoglycemics, antibiotics, anticonvulsants, analgesics, and sedatives. Azotemia, hypoglycemia, hyponatremia, orthostatic hypotension, and a drug-induced encephalopathy were among the most common problems encountered. These problems delayed rehabilitative therapies and contributed to additional medical morbidity.

Neuromedical complications are commonly encountered during inpatient rehabilitation (Table 9–3). From the onset of a stroke, medical complications that gradually accumulate over 30 days include falls, pressure sores, urinary tract and pulmonary infections, deep vein thrombosis and pulmonary embolism, and de-

stroke without serious complications (DRG 14) was approximately 7.5 days. Average stay is now fewer than 7 days. Prior to 1983, American stroke rehabilitation programs that published the functional outcomes of their patients reported the average time from onset of stroke to transfer to their unit as ranging from 14 to 48 days.[17] For 1992, the Uniform Data Service for Medical Rehabilitation (UDS$_{MR}$) reported a mean stroke onset to transfer of 20 days. This data include non-Medicare patients, patients who developed lengthy medical complications, and, of course, those who were so disabled by the stroke that they needed inpatient rehabilitation. By 2001, the onset of stroke to transfer reported by the UDS$_{MR}$ had declined to 12 days (Table 9–2).

pression.[19] A randomized trial in the United Kingdom compared stroke management on general wards with that on a stroke unit starting 2 weeks poststroke. The investigators detected medical complications in 60% of 245 patients, which included one-third with aspiration, another third with musculoskeletal pain, and nearly a third with urinary tract infections and with depression.[20]

In one free-standing American rehabilitation facility in 1990, patients with an average stroke onset to transfer delay of 37 days and an average 52-day stay had a mean of 3.6 medical and

Table 9–3. **Percentage of Rehabilitation Inpatients with New and Exacerbated Medical Complications**

Complication	Percent (%)
Urinary tract infection	30–40
Musculoskeletal pain	15–30
Depression	20–40
Urine retention	20–30
Medication adjustments for stroke risk factor	20–30
Falls	15–25
Dehydration, azotemia	10–20
Electrolyte abnormality	10–15
Hyperglycemia/hypoglycemia	10–20
Fungal rash	10–20
Adverse drug reaction	10–20
Anemia	10
Hypotension	10
Toxic-metabolic encephalopathy	10
Pneumonia	5–10
Arrhythmia	5–10
Pressure sore	5–10
Malnutrition	5
Congestive heart failure	5
Angina	5
Thrombophlebitis	5
Pulmonary embolus	<5
Myocardial infarction	
Recurrent stroke	
Seizure	
Gastrointestinal bleeding	

Source: Data comprised of studies from Dobkin, 1987[18]; Dromerick and Reding, 1994[21]; Langhorne et al., 2000[22]; Roth et al., 2001.[23]

0.6 neurological complications.[21] These complications were more frequent in patients with sensorimotor and hemianopic visual loss than in those with only motor or sensorimotor impairments. Complications were also higher in patients with the lowest admission BI scores and in those with the longest rehabilitation hospital stays. Nearly all patients required physician interventions for conditions that could limit rehabilitative therapies. Greater disability is associated with a higher incidence of infections, pressure sores, and anxiety.[22] In another American study of 1029 admissions for inpatient rehabilitation, medical complications arose most often in patients who had greater neurologic impairments, rising from an incidence of 60% with mild impairment on the NIHSS to 93% with severe impairment.[23] Hypoalbuminemia, which suggests chronic or a severe acute illness and a history of hypertension, also predicted complications. Of the 2027 medical complications in this group, infections, deep vein thrombosis, symptomatic heart disease and new strokes accounted for most of the 263 transfers to an acute hospital ward. Across rehabilitation centers, from 5% to 15% of patients require transfer back to an acute hospital setting. The UDS$_{MR}$ reports an incidence of approximately 7% across many types of rehabilitation sites.

Some potential medical problems must be sought proactively. When specifically monitored during physical therapy, up to one-half of patients experience cardiac arrhythmias and wide variations in blood pressure, especially during stair climbing, walking, stationary bicycling, and tall kneeling.[24,25] Although many patients with stroke have some heart disease, the symptoms of fatigue and exercise intolerance from congestive heart failure, chronic obstructive lung disease, anemia, deconditioning, exertional angina, sleep apnea, and orthostatic hypotension limit therapy the most. The combination of congestive heart failure and a systolic blood pressure below 130 also predicts cognitive impairment that may interfere with learning during rehabilitation.[26]

SEIZURES

Prospective studies of patients drawn from a single community and across multiple university centers find an incidence of seizures no greater than 5% within 2 weeks of a stroke and

Table 9–4. **Secondary Prevention of Ischemic Stroke**

Category	Goal
Define type of first stroke *Evaluate cause of subclinical infarcts*[383]	Manage specific risk factors for stroke type, e.g., symptomatic carotid stenosis for endarterectomy, atrial fibrillation for anticoagulation, hypertensive arteriopathy for blood pressure intervention
Define cardiovascular disease	Manage coronary artery disease, arrythmias, congestive heart failure, valve disease, septal defects
Physical activity	Brisk walk 30–60 minutes (>6 METs), 4 times weekly[488,489]
Hypertension	Blood pressure 120–140/70–80[55,491,492]
Angiotensin-converting enzyme inhibitor	Protect endothelium, especially in diabetics
β-blocker (metoprolol 25 mg bid)	Cardiac protection
Diuretics[490]	
Exercise and weight reduction	
Self-monitor blood pressure at home	
Platelet aggregation	Antiplatelet effect[66]
Aspirin 80 mg–325 mg	
Ticlopidine 250 mg bid	
Clopidogrel 75 mg	
ASA/dipyridamole sustained release 25 mg/200 mg bid	
Anticoagulation	Prevent thrombus
Warfarin	Atrial fibrillation: INR 2.5–3
	Myocardial infarct; patent foramen ovale >5 mm, or with atrial septal aneurysm;[493] arterial dissection: INR 2–2.5
	Anticardiolipin antibody: INR 3–3.5
	Noncardioembolic stroke INR 1.4–2.8[67]
	Factor V von Leiden defect
Cholesterol	Optimize lipid levels, especially with coronary artery disease to a total cholesterol <200 mg/dl; HDL-C >50 mg; LDL-C <100 mg
Diet, fiber and exercise	
Niacin	
Cholestyramine	Trigycerides <100 mg
	Lipoprotein-a <30 mg
	Apolipoprotein b/Apo a-1 <1
Statins[41]	Plaque stabilization; improve endothelial function; lower LDL-C; anti-inflammatory
Gemfibrozil	
Glucose	Normoglycemia;[494,495] monitor hemoglobin A1C
Diet with 24 g fiber and exercise	
Hypoglycemic agent	
Homocysteine	Homocysteine <8 μmol/l[43,496]
Folate 1–2 mg	Reduce endothelial injury
B$_{12}$ 400 μg	
Pyridoxine 10 mg	
Cigarettes	No smoke exposure
Nicotine substitute, bupropion[497]	
Behavioral modification	
Alcohol	Lipid lowering and antiplatelet effects
1–2 oz.[498]	Greater risk of hemorrhage if >4 oz/day
Orthostatic Hypotension[499]	Monitor supine and standing blood pressure; manage >20 mm fall
Sleep Apnea[500]	CPAP or BiPAP to lessen hypertension, hypoxia
C-Reactive Protein	Exercise, weight loss
High serum fibrinogen	Exercise

Continued on following page

Table 9–4.—*continued*

Category	Goal
Hematocrit over 55%	Manage chronic hypoxia, polycythemia
High leptin level	Manage diabetes and hypertension
Chronic infections	Atherosclerotic plaque associated with periodontal disease and chlamydia pneumoniae
Postmenapausal estrogen/progestin	Contraceptives reduce lipoprotein-a,[501] but no effect on stroke recurrence[502]
Antioxidants[503] E 400 u C 250 mg Selenium, beta-carotene	Possibly lessen risk for atherosclerosis

INR, International Normalized Ratio; HDL-C, high density lipoprotein-cholesterol; LDL-C, low density lipoprotein-cholesterol; CPAP, continuous positive airway pressure; BiPAP, bilevel positive pressure ventilation.

Sources: Hess et al., 2000[41]; Homocysteine Lowering Trialists' Collaboration, 1998[44]; Perry et al., 2000[55]; Albers et al., 1998[66]; Mohr et al., 2001[67]; Bernick et al., 2001[383]; Hu et al., 2000[488]; Kiely et al., 1994[489]; Klungel et al., 2001[490]; Perindopril Group, 2001[491]; Rogers et al., 1997[492]; Mas et al., 2001[493]; Boushey et al., 1995[496]; Jorenby, 1999[497]; Sacco et al., 1999[498]; Eigenbrodt et al., 2000[499]; Mohsenin, 2001[500]; Shilpak et al., 2000[501]; Viscoli et al., 2001[502]; Willett and Stampfer, 2001.[503]

folate, pyridoxine, cyanocobalamin, and probably with betaine, another methyl donor. The Vitamin Intervention in Stroke Prevention clinical trial is testing the effect of folate, B12 and pyridoxine supplementation on the prevention of repeated stroke.

Unusual risk factors should be sought when the cause of an ischemic stroke is not readily explained. A circulating antiphospholipid antibody can cause a procoagulant state. Although antiplatelet agents might suffice for risk reduction in asymptomatic people and after a TIA, warfarin anticoagulation may be more protective after an ischemic stroke.[45] Clinical trials are in progress. Other therapies may be needed for migraine-induced stroke,[46] a coagulopathy,[47] collagen-vascular disease and vasculitis, the small risk of oral contraceptives as a cause of stroke,[48] drug abuse-induced stroke, a vascular dissection, atrial and ventricular septal defects, and genetic predispositions to atherosclerosis and vascular disease.

Prevention of recurrence of an intracerebral hemorrhage requires defining and managing an aneurysm, vascular anomaly, venous thrombosis, or neoplasm. When not present, the most important approach is strict management of hypertension. More than 60 grams/day of alcohol and a total serum cholesterol of less than 160 mg/dl may increase risk. Phenylpropanolamine in appetite suppressants (now removed from over-the-counter cold remedies) and abuse of other sympathomimetics such as ephedra and cocaine must be stopped. Elderly patients with lobar hemorrhages from amyloid angiography should not use antiplatelet and anticoagulant medications if possible. The association of hemorrhage and the apolipoprotein-ϵ allele in these patients may some day lead to a therapeutic intervention.

Teaching during rehabilitation should include information about how to modify the risk factors associated with stroke and cardiac disease. Physicians and nurses start to manage these factors with full explanations about benefits and potential adverse reactions of each intervention.

MANAGEMENT

One estimate suggested that optimal treatment of hypertension in the United States could prevent up to 246,000 strokes. Imagine the profound benefit a diuretic such as hydrochlorothiazide for the treatment of hypertension would accomplish in a third world country to inexpensively and effectively help prevent stroke and myocardial infarction. The elimination of cigarettes would cut another 62,000 strokes a year in the United States, which would save $20 billion in the nation's health care costs.[49] The excessive risk for stroke among female former smokers largely disappears by 4 years after cessation[50] and the rate

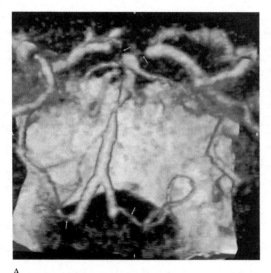
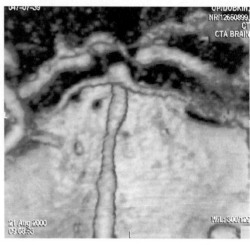

A   B

Figure 9–3. (A) Spiral computed tomography angiogram shows a mid to distal basilar artery high grade stenosis in a patient who presented with a stroke in the distribution of the posterior inferior cerebellar artery (PICA). The patient has bilateral PICA stenoses (small arrows at bottom). (B) One year later, the basilar artery stenosis has regressed. The patient's medical management included a statin agent, 80 mg of aspirin, coumadin with an INR kept approximately 2–2.5, and an angiotensin-converting enzyme inhibitor.

of progression of carotid atherosclerosis slows in people who quit, compared to those who continue.[51] Risk reduction is best viewed as the absolute reduction provided by an intervention when compared to a placebo or another intervention. For warfarin and carotid endarterectomy after a stroke, the reduction is approximately 7%–9% per year. For antiplatelet agents, absolute risk is decreased by 3% over a placebo. Statin agents reduce risk approximately 0.8%. Does optimal management really work for secondary prevention of stroke? Figure 9–3 shows the reversal of an atherostenosis of the basilar artery within 1 year in a patient with a brain stem stroke who was vigorously managed for his risk factors.

Hypertension

Vigorous therapy of hypertension reduces the risk of first stroke, recurrent stroke, and coronary artery disease. For repeated stroke, risk reduction is at least 30% by lowering the blood pressure by 5–10 mm Hg.[52] Recurrence rates for stroke decreased in one epidemiologic study as diastolic blood pressure control increased in patients with hypertension at the time of the initial stroke.[53] Remarkably, this population-based study found that 44% of pa-

tients who had no history of hypertension had an elevated blood pressure 4 months after the first stroke and 65% with a history of hypertension still had uncontrolled hypertension.[54]

Diuretics are still very effective antihypertensives for stroke prevention.[55] The angiotensin-converting-enzyme inhibitors (ACE-Is) appear valuable in patients with coronary artery disease for managing hypertension, but also for their effects on the process of atherosclerosis. A randomized trial of 6000 subjects compared the ACE-I perindopril (4 mg daily) to placebo in both hypertensive and nonhypertensive patients with a prior stroke or transient ischemic attack (TIA).[56] The hypertensive patients also took medications for hypertension that were not ACE-Is. The ACE-I reduced the blood pressure by $5/3$ mm Hg, but did not reduce the risk of stroke. Perindopril plus the diuretic indapamide (2.5 mg) reduced the pressure by $12/5$ mm Hg and the risk for all subtypes of stroke by 43%, as well as a significant reduction in risk for myocardial infarction and vascular death. *This risk reduction was apparent for both hypertensive and nonhypertensive subjects.* Five years of treatment with the combination of medications would avoid 1 fatal or major nonfatal vascular event for every 11 patients treated.

Hypertensive patients after a stroke ought to be instructed in how to check their own blood pressure with a digital cuff, so they can bring a daily series of pressure measurements to the attention of their physicians. Patients and physicians must check both supine and standing blood pressure to rule out supine hypertension and upright hypotension. Hypotension, either orthostatic or diurnal, may be a risk factor for recurrent stroke, especially in the presence of occlusive vascular disease.[57–59] Borderline hypertension at 140/85 probably ought to be treated especially after a stroke, even in elderly persons.[60,61]

Antithrombotics

Antiplatelet and anticoagulant treatments are perhaps the most frequent interventions for patients following a stroke to prevent recurrence. The level of risk reduction for an individual patient is quite modest, however. After a TIA or minor stroke, aspirin reduces the absolute rate of death and dependency by no more than 2% yearly. One needs to treat 83 patients to prevent one of these outcomes, or, in a population of 1 million people who have 2000 strokes in a year, aspirin eliminates 19 deaths or cases of dependency. Some of the nonsteroidal anti-inflammatory agents such as ibuprofen may block the effect of aspirin on serum thromboxane B_2 levels, which is an index of the inhibition of cyclooxygenase-1 activity in platelets.[62]

Ticlopidine has a modest advantage over aspirin or placebo in reducing stroke rates after TIA and first stroke by approximately 30% over several years. The absolute reduction is approximately 3%–4%.[63] Diarrhea, a reversible neutropenia, and rare thrombocytopenia have limited its use as other medications in addition to aspirin have become available.

Clopidogrel reduces the absolute rate of recurrent stroke, myocardial infarction and death by 0.5% per year compared to aspirin in patients who presented with stroke, myocardial infarction, or severe peripheral vascular disease.[64] The physician would have to treat 200 patients with the drug for 1 year to prevent one of these outcomes. The combination of aspirin and clopidogrel for stroke prevention is in a clinical trial, based on the 1% absolute benefit of the combination, compared to aspirin alone, in a study of coronary ischemia.[65]

Long-acting *dipyridimole* with aspirin has a somewhat greater benefit than aspirin alone.[66] Over 2 years, one would have to treat 33 poststroke patients with *Aggrenox* instead of aspirin alone to prevent one stroke.

Warfarin may be about equal to aspirin for secondary thrombotic stroke prevention.[67] The anticoagulant reduces the risk of repeated cardioembolism in patients with atrial fibrillation by over 65%.

In summary, the patient who has a stroke associated with systemic atherosclerosis or hypertension may be most effectively managed to prevent another stroke with the prescription of a statin, an ACE-inhibitor, an antiplatelet agent, vitamin B complex, and a beta-blocker if coronary heart disease is present; compulsively monitored therapies for hypertension, diabetes, and cardiac disease; and lifestyle changes that include exercise, a balanced diet with fiber, measures to reach optimal body weight, and cessation of the use of tobacco. Since cardiac mortality is even higher than the 30%–50% death rate over 5 years from a second stroke, clinicians should consider evaluating selected patients who had a good recovery after stroke for a noninvasive heart study, such as an exercise stress test.

INPATIENT REHABILITATION

Eligibility for Rehabilitation

Criteria recommended by an American consensus group's review of the literature for rehabilitation placement following a stroke (Table 9–5)[68] were found to have fair to good interrater reliability when operationalized for 60 patients with moderate to severe strokes and good cognition.[69] Figure 9–4 is a flow chart derived from these recommendations of the Agency for Health Care Policy and Research, now known as the Agency for Healthcare Research and Quality. A study of compliance with these guidelines in a veterans population suggests that greater levels of adherence to the guidelines in Table 9–5 leads to significantly better outcomes measured by the Functional Independence Measure (FIM) and the Stroke Impact Scale.[70] For this mostly male population, compliance in the setting of a nursing home was significantly worse than for an inpatient rehabilitation service.

Table 9–5. **Dimensions of Stroke Care Developed by the U.S. Agency for Healthcare Research and Quality**

ACUTE CARE

1. Multidimensional team coordination
2. Baseline assessment
3. Early initiation of rehabilitation
4. Management of general health functions
5. Prevention of complications
6. Prevention of recurrent stroke
7. Use of standardized scales appropriate for stroke
8. Screening for rehabilitation placement

POSTACUTE CARE

1. Multidisciplinary team coordination
2. Baseline assessment
3. Goal setting
4. Treatment plan
5. Monitoring progress
6. Management of impairments and disabilities
7. Prevention of complications
8. Prevention of recurrent stroke
9. Family involvement
10. Patient and family education
11. Discharge planning

Many issues affect decisions about the most appropriate placement, assuming that these options are available in a community. Table 9–6 includes types of placements for more seriously diabled patients. For inpatient rehabilitation, the evaluator must estimate the ability of the patient to tolerate at least 3 hours of therapy and glean from the family whether they have the resources to provide home support for someone who may require a minimal to moderate level of assistance for ADLs by the time of discharge.

Eligible patients require more than minimal assistance for ambulation and self-care and have adequate motivation for the work of therapy and adequate cognition and language function to be able to learn. Patients in the United States who already function too independently to qualify for inpatient rehabilitation are eligible for home therapies, if they are physically unable to leave the house. Others attend outpatient physical, occupational, and speech therapy until their functional progress plateaus,

based upon the observations of physician and therapist, but subject to retroactive review by Medicare and most payors. Geriatric patients who are at too low a level to participate on an inpatient unit or to return home may still be eligible for less intensive therapies at a skilled nursing facility. These patients may later qualify for transfer to an inpatient unit.

Strategies that take into account functional levels have been suggested for determining admission to an inpatient service.[71–75] For example, in patients with FIM scores over 80, a well-designed outpatient rehabilitation program may be more appropriate than inpatient care, except when the partially disabled patient has inadequate supervision at home. A clinical trial of patients with a high admission FIM score who are randomized to the same intensity of therapy as inpatients versus outpatients would be of great interest. Patients over the age of 75 years who have rehabilitation admission FIM scores of less than 60 are at highest risk for eventual placement in a nursing facility, especially if they have suffered a stroke in the full distribution of the right middle cerebral artery. Except for people who have the resources to obtain costly care in the home upon rehabilitation discharge or who have a reversible medical problem that has made their FIM score much lower than it will be after a medical intervention, clinicians may consider nursing facility placement with less intensive attempts at therapy. This group should be reassessed for eligibility for inpatient care every few weeks for up to several months.

Patients who are eligible for admission and have FIM scores of 40–80 are most likely to improve and return home. These patients should, in general, be admitted for inpatient therapy. This group may be most appropriate for clinical trials of a particular therapeutic approach to one or more disabilities. Patients with this level of function can also serve to compare organized hospital-based rehabilitation to treatment in a less expensive, skilled nursing facility.

In practice, a minority of stroke survivors are referred for inpatient rehabilitation. Table 9–7 reflects data from American and British studies and recent Medicare data for the DRG stroke. For example, when American medical centers reported the discharge sites of their patients who survived a stroke between 1971 and 1982 54%–63% went home, 29%–36% were sent to a long-term care facility, and 3%–17%

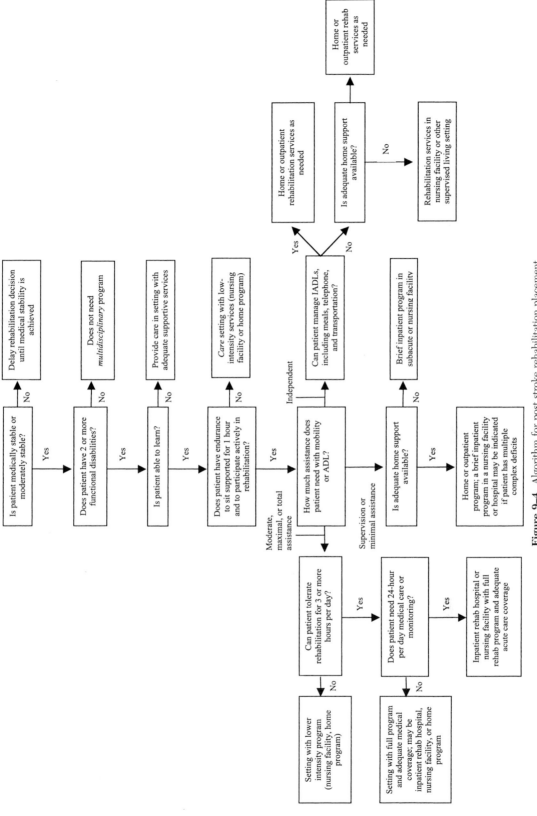

Figure 9–4. Algorithm for post stroke rehabilitation placement.

Table 9–6. Possible Rehabilitation Placements for Patients with Moderate to Severe Disability from an Acute Stroke

SINGLE OR NOT MULTIDISCIPLINARY SERVICES
Home
Nursing facility
Outpatient

MULTIDISCIPLINARY PROGRAM
High intensity inpatient
Low intensity subacute or nursing facility
Low intensity home
Low intensity outpatient

went to a rehabilitation inpatient program.[76] At a Rochester, Minnesota center that followed 251 1-week survivors of a first stroke between 1975 and 1979, approximately 50% received evaluations by rehabilitation physicians and physical therapists; 26% of these patients were referred to inpatient rehabilitation programs, 40% were seen by occupational therapists, and 13% by speech therapists.[77] Thus, 14% of the entire group received inpatient rehabilitation after a median acute hospitalization of 17 days. Of 1094 acute stroke admissions to a British district hospital around the same time, 33% died in the hospital, 20% had fully recovered by discharge, 30% were too frail or ill to be offered participation in an outpatient rehabilitation trial of 4 whole days a week, leaving 11% able to participate.[78]

Trials of Locus of Treatment

A number of studies have tried to establish the best locus and time for acute and subacute re-

Table 9–7. Placement after Hospitalization for Acute Stroke

Location	Percentage
Nursing home care	15–30
Rehabilitation unit	10–20
Home	45–65

habilitation care. A prospective study showed that patients with stroke admitted to a rehabilitation hospital were significantly more likely to return to the community and recover ADLs than patients sent to subacute or traditional nursing facilities for therapy and management.[79] Such comparisons may also depend heavily on additional factors. For example, in the United States, some studies find that investor-owned nursing homes provide significantly less care and worse care than not-for-profit nursing facilities or public homes.[80] Chain ownership deficiencies were even greater. Not-for-profit facilities accounted for less than 30% of ownership in 2000.

The use of thrombolysis and angioplasty for the management of early cerebral ischemia has increased the call to create community stroke centers to provide emergency care and manage peristroke complications.[81] A related approach has already improved important outcomes. At least 20 trials have compared patients managed on specialized stroke units to management on general medical wards.[82]

The mean age for patients in these trials was 65–75 years. Subjects were randomized within a few days to 2 weeks after the stroke. Outcome measures were almost never blinded to the treatment allocation. These trials show that a dedicated stroke unit that provides rehabilitation or a dedicated rehabilitation unit improves at least several important outcomes. The organized milieu decreases dependency, institutionalization, and mortality at 1 year poststroke. Studies of stroke units show an absolute reduction of 6.6% (66.4% in controls vs. 59.8% in patients on the unit) in death or dependency.[9] Thus, approximately 15 patients would have to be treated on a stroke unit to prevent one of these negative outcomes. Five-year mortality is still significantly higher in patients treated on a general medical or neurology ward, running 71% after ward care versus 64% after stroke unit care in a study by Jorgensen and colleagues in Copenhagen[83] and 71% versus 59% in the study by Indredavik in Norway.[84]

Although some of the benefit of a specialty service relates to acute care interventions,[8] which may include better hydration, control of blood pressure, and management of fever,[85] most of the benefit derives from the focus on prevention of medical complications related to immobility, on earlier onset of skills training for mobility,[85] on training functional activities,[86] on family training, on the intensity of retraining,[87,88] on early recognition of mood disorders, and perhaps on outpatient follow-up.[89] Of interest, the trial by Indredavik and colleagues[85] provided stroke unit patients with much more education and a motor relearning approach, whereas the general medical ward patients received a Bobath approach to therapy, although total therapy time was similar. Even with the same type and intensity of physical and occupational therapy services provided by people with the same level of experience, functional recovery on BI tasks was greater and more rapid on the dedicated unit that directed therapy toward adapting the patients' residual abilities to their future needs in their homes.[90,91] Indeed, in the British trial by Kalra and colleagues, patients who reached the median BI score associated with discharge had significantly shorter lengths of stay after having reached that level of function when managed on the stroke unit compared to those who were just as functional on a medical unit.[91] This finding suggests a better organization of assessment and goal-oriented services on a dedicated unit. Two years after admission to a stroke unit, patients are more independent in ADLs, if they had been independent prior to the stroke, than patients managed initially on a general medical ward.[92] Case management may not add any benefit to a multidisciplinary approach.[93]

The literature suggests that the earlier the onset of an inpatient rehabilitation program, the better the outcomes.[94–96] Most studies are potentially tainted by the levels of disability or severity of stroke that come to be counted among the early versus late recipients. A case-control design by Italian investigators assigned 145 subjects to an inpatient program within 20 days, 20–40 days, or 41–60 days after onset of stroke by matching each triad of subjects for age and subscores on the BI.[96] The average length of stay was approximately 67 days across groups. Treatment begun within 20 days (average 15 days) had a 6 times greater likelihood of a high response on the BI, even though 60% of the delayed subjects received exercise instruction at home several times a week while on the waiting list.

Discharge

Discharge should occur when the patient becomes independent enough to be managed at home. When feasible, this goal includes controlled bowel and bladder function and minimally assisted, or better, transfers and ambulation. Long inpatient rehabilitation stays have been associated with lower admission ADL scores, along with private funding for hospitalization and admission from places other than the home.[97] Patients under age 55 who have low admission FIM scores, usually under 50, may have the longest stays.[71]

One argument for the use of focused rehabilitation programs, as opposed to care on a medical ward, is that patients are more likely to be discharged from the less organized setting without adequate warning and family preparation, without durable medical equipment, and without immediate follow-up medical care or disability-oriented community care. The discharge plan should include these important features.

OUTPATIENT REHABILITATION

Functional performance improves significantly during inpatient rehabilitation, but patients generally continue to improve for at least another 3 to 6 months, especially in mobility and compensatory techniques for ADLs. Follow-up studies of patients discharged to outpatient care or to no formal therapy vary greatly. For example, trials differ in the time from onset of stroke to discharge, in the residual impairments and disabilities of the patients, in the level of available psychosocial support, and perhaps most important, in the style, intensity, and duration of therapies.

In the 3 months after discharge, UDS_{MR} data show approximately 10% gains in FIM scores. At 6 months to years later, most patients discharged to home report maintained or modestly improved gains.[98,99] When self-care skills decline after discharge, the cause, in the absence of new neuromedical problems, is often the caregiver's ability to provide more efficient and convenient assistance for ADL than the patient can accomplish independently.

Locus of Treatment

One of the first studies to assess the organization for outpatient care randomized 133 patients upon discharge from acute hospitalization to 4 days of outpatient rehabilitation therapies per week, versus 3 half-days, versus regular home visits that encouraged patients to carry out what had been taught in the hospital.[78] By 6 months after the stroke, the greatest improvement in ADL occurred in the group that received the most intensive therapy, intermediate gains were made by the conventionally treated group, and the untreated patients deteriorated . The maximum benefit was achieved by 3 months.

A Nottingham study randomly allocated three groups of inpatients who had been discharged from acute and rehabilitation hospitals to either a domiciliary team or to hospital-based outpatient care.[100] No differences in ADL and scores on a quality of life profile were apparent at 6 months with these modestly different levels of organization for therapy and support. In addition, no differences were found in 6-month outcomes for 140 elderly patients requiring outpatient stroke rehabilitation who were randomly assigned to domiciliary care or day-hospital care after the acute hospital stay.[101] Social activity was low for both groups. The amount of therapy was a bit greater for the domiciliary group, but time in therapy was modest for all participants.

Most trials have compared home therapy to hospital clinic or day programs for outpatient rehabilitation. The Bradford Community Stroke Trial randomized 124 new stroke patients to rehabilitation therapy in a day hospital twice a week or to home therapy for up to 20 hours over 8 weeks.[102] This British study also stratified patients using two levels of functional severity. Subjects were over age 60 and had new, residual disability at the time of hospital discharge. The interval between stroke and acute hospital discharge was fewer than 4 weeks for 16%, 4–7 weeks for 31%, 8–11 weeks for 23%, and more than 12 weeks for 30%. Thus, over half these patients were more than 2 months poststroke at entry. At 8 weeks, both groups showed small, significant gains. The home-treated group, which received less therapy, did better on stairs. Presumably, they practiced more at this task. Over one-third of both groups were depressed. A general health questionnaire showed that one in four caregivers felt stressed. At 6 months, both groups had improved compared to function at discharge, but gains on the BI and Motor Club assessment were greater for the home-treated

group. Depression and emotional stress remained the same. For the modest resources expended, home physiotherapy was somewhat more beneficial, but neither approach addressed psychosocial functions very well.

Most studies that compare one locus of care to another either immediately or late after an inpatient stay reveal modest or no differences in clinical outcomes. The designs have flaws, such as no control group, uncertain randomization scheme, small sample size, unclear primary outcome measure, unblinded observers of outcomes, rather low intensities of therapy, and limited generalizability because of the level of disability of the sample.[103] One large randomized trial compared rehabilitation at home after an average 12-day inpatient stay to another week of inpatient care followed by hospital-based outpatient treatment.[104] All subjects were independent in transfers when they left the hospital if they lived alone or were assisted by a caregiver. Similar outcomes at 12 months poststroke were achieved at lower costs because of less use of hospital beds by the early discharge group. An intention-to-treat randomized trial with 250 subjects showed that rehabilitation on an inpatient unit following a brief stay in an acute stroke unit or general medical ward produced better outcomes in moderate to severely disabled patients (BI score <50) compared to rehabilitation treatment in the community.[105] No differences in QOL were found and instrumental ADLs were not measured. Smaller trials confirmed similar outcomes at 3 to 6 months for home versus various forms of outpatient care with the home group having fewer in-hospital days,[106] greater gains in instrumental ADLs,[107] and greater caregiver stress.

Indredavik and colleagues initially treated their patients on a stroke unit, then randomly assigned 320 patients to an ordinary or extended stroke service.[89] The extended service included closer interaction with the primary health care system. A mobile team with a nurse, therapists, and a physician began its activities to coordinate home care while patients were still hospitalized. After 26 weeks, 60% who received extended care compared to 49% who did not were independent in ADLs. The average length of stay in the hospital was significantly less for the extended care group, 19 days versus 31 days. Of potential importance, this trial included patients who were quite disabled compared to most other trials of early discharge to home.

As a clinical generalization, formal therapy provided at least three times a week, accompanied by home practice for specific disabilities, seems more likely to get patients to their highest plateau of function in the least time than informal instruction and services that put limits on the specificity and intensity of training.

Pulse Therapy

Community mobility, cooking and cleaning skills, leisure activities, social isolation, and support for caregivers often continue to be problematic for 2-year stroke survivors.[108] The clinician ought to ask about instrumental ADLs or use an assessment that asks patients to rate the difficulty they perceive in carrying out these tasks,[109] so an appropriate rehabilitation prescription may be ordered. A pulse of therapy carried out beyond 6 months poststroke, especially if focused on training specific skills such as walking speed or using the affected arm, often improves the practiced ADLs.[110,111] The physician should recommend conditioning exercises and task-oriented practice. Muscle strengthening and aerobic training counteract many of the potentially debilitating physiologic changes associated with aging and with a sedentary lifestyle. At every follow-up visit, patients should be encouraged to walk more at home over ground or on a treadmill,[112] set up a circuit training course,[113] or pedal on a stationary bicycle for at least 20 minutes a day. Along with their routine stretches and home therapy program, patients can improve balance and leg muscle strength simply by repeatedly standing up from a chair and walking on uneven surfaces. In addition, therapy that restarts a year or more after a stroke with a specific goal may benefit motivated patients.

CLINICAL TRIALS

In a randomized, crossover trial with repeated measures of walking speed and functional activities related to ambulation, patients who were 2–7 years poststroke and who still walked slowly (>10 seconds to go 10 meters if under age 60, >12.5 seconds if 60–69 years old, >16.5 seconds if over 70 years old) spent from 1 to 6 sessions with a physiotherapist.[114] The interventions, mostly problem-solving, included reeducation for gait deviations, practice on uneven surfaces and going from sit to stand, adjustments and provision of aids, and exercise to increase fitness. This very modest approach led to a significant increase in speed after 3 months for the treated group while the other half of the cohort declined. When the second group was treated, these patients improved over the subsequent 3 months, whereas the first group declined. Speed increased 9% and declined about 12%. Functional measures related to mobility did not change.

A small trial for community ambulators with chronic stroke provided a 30-session program for muscle strengthening by resistance training and physical conditioning by aerobic exercise and walking.[115] Significant gains were found for walking speed, general activity and, quality of life. A trial of constraint-induced movement therapy for a paretic upper extremity improved the functional use of the arm.[116]

In a quasi-experimental design in which subjects, on average 3 years after a stroke, were their own controls, significant improvements were demonstrated in weight shifting, balance, and ADL scores after 8 hours of physical and occupational therapy a week for 1 month.[117] The treatment emphasized skills required by the outcome measures in these motivated, ambulatory patients. Far more intensive therapy was given to 51 selected patients who could not walk and had BI scores below 60 at 3 months after a stroke.[118] Subjects received 20–30 hours a week of physical and occupational therapy for 1-month to 3-month intervals, repeated for up to 2 years. At 6 months after their strokes, 25% achieved BI scores over 70 and 18% reached independent ambulation. At 1 year, 68% and 64% did so, and at 2 years, 79% and 74% achieved these remarkable levels of function, respectively. Changes for the group were statistically significant at 1 year, but not at 2 years. A briefer regimen of treadmill walking may also benefit conditioning, leg strength, and walking speed.[119,120]

Thus, patients maintain functional gains and can make some additional improvements in ambulation and ADLs with a directed refresher program. Brief, "pulse" rehabilitation therapy aimed at a specific functional need should be considered even years after a stroke. The goal and the intervention must be well-defined and success should aim to improve the quality of life of the patient.

410 patients from the Stroke Data Bank, 23% of patients with a pure motor stroke had improved by 10 days, whereas 5% with other stroke syndromes had deteriorated compared to the examination on admission.[133] The mean relative improvement in those in each group with improved strength at the shoulder, wrist, hip, and ankle was also greater in the pure motor stroke subjects, by 52% versus 40%. Most of them had lacunar infarcts. In a trial of acute heparinization versus placebo to prevent progressing stroke, in which most subjects appeared to have suffered lacunar infarcts, approximately one in four patients also improved in the first week in neurologic scores that emphasized strength.[134]

In a longitudinal study of 41 patients starting within 1 week of a right cerebral infarction, behavioral and motor abnormalities were followed at 2-week to 4-week intervals by repeated measures with specific tests, until the patients recovered or plateaued.[135] Most patients received an unspecified amount of physical and occupational therapy. Using a life-table analysis method, recovery curves showed that arm and leg weakness recovered in approximately 40% by week 16; sensory extinction recovered in 80% by week 46; hemianopsia in 65% by week 33; unilateral spatial neglect on drawing in 70% by week 13; anosognosia and neglect in nearly all by week 20 with half of those affected recovering by week 10; motor impersistence in all by week 55 with 45% recovering by week 8; and prosopagnosia and constructional apraxia on the Block Design and Rey figure in 80% by week 20. Patients with smaller lesions (less than 6% of right hemispheric volume), hemorrhages, and younger patients tended to recover faster for some of these impairments. The amount of recovery for many of these behaviors, compared to motor function, is consistent with the notion that recovery is better for impairments that have the most diffuse neural substrate for reorganization (see Chapter 1).

The Unaffected Limbs

Loss of the use of an arm and hand, especially of the dominant upper extremity, impedes everyday activities. For some stroke survivors, what they call the "dead arm" acts as an im-

mutable reminder of disability and of vulnerability to stroke. They constantly fidget with the paretic hand, pulling on the wrist and straightening the fingers with their "good hand." Even patients who regain selective movements over mass flexion of the fingers with slow, if any, finger extension, often do not recover their ability to finely coordinate and efficiently manipulate objects. Compensation through use of the unaffected hand and by using assistive devices is a mainstay of rehabilitative interventions.

The nonparetic arm of the patient with hemiplegia, which often serves as a contol in clinical studies, also appears to be affected in subtle ways after an ipsilateral stroke. Studies[136] of the "normal" arm have shown slower EMG recruitment patterns, reduced speed and strength of hand actions, paretic proximal and distal muscles, and impaired sensory discrimination in the hand. Tests that require continuous sensory feedback, such as reaction times and tracking, seem especially impaired, even 12 months after a stroke.[137] Possible mechanisms, discussed in Chapter 1 in the context of the hierarchical and distributed organization of the brain, include loss of commissural fiber inputs from the involved to the uninvolved hemisphere, contributions of uncrossed pathways to bilateral upper limb functions, and alterations in the modulation of subcortical, brain stem, and spinal sensorimotor regions that receive bilateral inputs. These findings help explain why upper and lower extremity functions that were initially impaired by a contralateral stroke sometimes worsen after a subsequent ipsilateral stroke, with or without an accompanying pseudobulbar palsy. Rehabilitationists must identify any ipsilateral impairments that interfere with compensatory training of the "unaffected" arm.

Impairment-Related Functional Outcomes

The degree and type of impairment strongly influence functional outcomes. The Copenhagen Stroke Study revealed a close parallel between impairment measured by the SSS and disability on the BI.[138] The severity of motor impairment is perhaps the strongest predictor of outcome for ADLs, but sensory and visual field loss also contribute when one controls for the severity of motor loss.[139]

IMPAIRMENT GROUPINGS

Reding and Potes[140] related impairment groups to their functional outcomes in a prospective study of 95 consecutive inpatients admitted to a rehabilitation center after a hemispheric stroke. The study did not control for severity of motor impairment. The patients were divided into 3 categories of impairment and examined at 2-week intervals until they reached a plateau in recovery. The investigators constructed Kaplan-Meier life-table analyses of the probability of recovering mobility and overall BI ADLs. Over 90% of patients with a pure motor (M) deficit became independent in walking 150 feet by week 14. Only 35% with motor and proprioceptive (SM) loss were independent by week 24 and 3% with motor, sensory and hemianopic deficits (SMH) were independent by week 30. The probability of walking over 150 feet with assistance increased to 100% with M impairment by week 14 (80% by week 8), and to over 90% in those with SM loss by week 26 and with SMH deficits by 28 weeks after the stroke. Approximately 65% achieved a BI score over 95 by 15 weeks if they had only M deficits and by 26 weeks with SM loss. Only 10% scored that high with SMH deficits after 18–30 weeks. However, 100% achieved a score of >60 by 14 weeks with M loss only, 75% by 23 weeks with SM deficits, and 60% by 29 weeks with SMH loss. Both the life-table analyses and this clinical grouping of patients make good sense for some experimental designs of stroke rehabilitation interventions.

Duncan and colleagues also showed the value of relating impairment groups to functional and quality of life outcomes.[139] The investigators examined the cumulative probabilities of achieving a BI score over 60 or over 90 within 14 days of stroke and 1, 3, and 6 months after stroke for four impairment groups: motor (M) only, motor and sensory (SM), motor and hemianopia (MH), and sensorimotor and hemianopia (SMH). The 360 patients who survived the stroke represented all eligible stroke patients from 12 hospitals in greater Kansas City. The patients were alert and had been living at home at the time of the first evaluation. The investigators employed the lower extremity portion of the Fugl-Meyer index as their measure of motor impairment, using a cutoff score of 28 points out of a possible 34 points to identify patients with less than normal hip flexor power (see Chapter 7). The level of disability correlates especially with motor function of the leg.[141] Sensory and visual field function was defined as present or absent based on the NIH Stroke Scale (NIHSS). Between 1 and 3 months after the stroke, the probability of achieving a BI score of 60 or greater (often adequate for a discharge to the home) rose from 80% to 90% for M, from 70% to 85% for SM, from 35% to 70% for MH, and from 12% to 53% for SMH.

Table 9–9 compares the cumulative probabilities of reaching a BI score of 60 and of 90 or better at 6 months for the patients in the

Table 9–9. Cumulative Probability of Reaching Barthel Index Scores of Greater Than 60 and 90 at 6 Months After Stroke Based on Impairment Group

	SCORE ≥ 60		SCORE ≥ 90	
	All Stroke Cases (%)	Stroke Cases in Rehabilitation (%)	All Stroke Cases (%)	Stroke Cases in Rehabilitation (%)
Motor	95	100	70	65
Sensorimotor	85	75	62	65
Motor, hemianopia	72	—	45	
Sensorimotor, hemianopia	52	60	35	10

Source: Data from Kaplan-Meier graphs in Patel et al., 2000[139] and Reding and Potes, 1988.[140]

Table 9–10. **Recovery of Walking by Impairment Group after Stroke**

Impairment Group	Onset (%)	1 Month (%)	3 Months (%)	6 Months (%)
Motor	18	50	75	85
Sensorimotor	10	48	72	72
Motor, hemianopsia	7	28	68	75
Sensorimotor, hemianopsia	3	16	33	38

Source: Data from Kaplan-Meier graphs in Patel et al., 2000.[139]

Reding and the Duncan studies. For independent walking (a 6 or 7 on the FIM), the probabilities based on the study of Kansas City stroke cases are shown in Table 9–10. In comparison to the data for patients admitted for rehabilitation, the data for all stroke patients reveal a similar likelihood for independent walking for the M group, but a higher likelihood for the other impairment groups. This difference may be related to referral patterns and greater case severity, especially for motor impairment and absent proprioception, for admissions to the rehabilitation unit.

The strong correlation between the NIHSS and FIM measures for patients with stroke holds for both admission and discharge scores.[142] In their study of 400 patients admitted for inpatient rehabilitation, Roth and colleagues found that 85% of their patients experienced little or no change in their NIHSS score. The 15% who did improve included a significantly greater proportion of patients with intracerebral hemorrhage. The subgroup that had less impairment by discharge had a similar decline in level of disability as the subgroup whose NIHSS changed minimally. Thus, the NIHSS may not be sensitive enough to reflect changes in impairment that are important for reducing disability on the FIM, or, more likely, rehabilitation efforts aimed at reducing disability are successful without an accompanying decline in impairments.

IMPAIRMENT MODELS

Although survivors of acute stroke do improve, for any individual patient, studies of early impairments do not provide clear-cut information for the selection of patients for inpatient and outpatient rehabilitation efforts. Even carefully constructed equations that seek to help predict outcome at 6 months have not been powerful enough to anticipate the outcome for a particular patient.[143] Rehabilitationists may, however, consider prognosticators of poor recovery when designing a clinical interventional trial, as well as an individual patient's program. For example, one multivariate model compared impairments found within 48 hours of stroke and functional outcomes at 6 months in 205 patients with acute stroke.[144] Leg and arm power and function, mental status, level of consciousness, score on a line-cancellation test for hemineglect, and electrocardiographic abnormalities predicted functional outcome with 67% accuracy and death with 83% accuracy.

A review of 33 studies found certain impairments to be potentially unfavorable for recovery, if present at the time of transfer to a rehabilitation unit.[17] In addition to advanced age, the prognosticators include profound paresis, loss of proprioception, visuospatial hemineglect, and bowel and bladder incontinence. In patients over the age of 75, the Orpington Prognostic Score of impairments, measured 2 weeks post stroke, had a strong correlation with functional outcome.[145] Patients who scored <3.2 were discharged within 3 weeks, whereas those with scores >5.2 required long-term care (see scoring system Table 7–9). Persistently poor attention span, judgment, memory, and carryover skills negatively influence outcome as well. Motor impersistence and impaired $1/2$-hour recall have predictive value for poorer functional outcome.[146] For inpatients during rehabilitation, impairments in comprehension, judgment, short-term memory, and abstract thinking, determined by the Neurobehavioral Cognitive Status Examination, led to longer stays, lower scores for ADLs, and more outpatient therapy and home services, compared to a control group of orthopedic rehabilitation patients.[144] A study of 440 patients admitted for rehabilitation divided the subjects into subgroups of severe, medium, and moderate impairment based on the Canadian Neurological Scale score.[147] With severe impairment and global aphasia, the risk of no improvement in ADLs was 4–6 times greater than in the other 2 groups. Age over 65 years, hemineglect, and depression also had negative consequences in a multiple regression analysis of 32 variables.

Even with any combination of these potential prognosticators, many individuals still improve enough to reach a functional level that allows them to live at home. Up to several variables such as sensory, motor, and visual field impairment groupings, severity of motor impairment, hemineglect, global aphasia, incontinence, and perhaps severe depression and poor sitting balance may be useful to stratify patients who participate in clinical trials.

ASSESSMENTS BY TECHNOLOGIES

Sensory and motor gains may be predicted by studies using evoked potentials, transcranial magnetic stimulation, and anatomic and functional neuroimaging. The sensitivity and specificity of these tests are rather limited, but of some interest especially for understanding mechanisms of recovery. Chapter 3 reviews these approaches. Several of the techniques may help anticipate gains or lack of gains.

Anatomic Imaging

A few distinctions that may not be intuitively appreciated by the clinician relate differences in outcome to the location of the lesion, despite the same initial impairments. For example, sparing of 60% or more of the cerebral peduncle predicts recovery of finer hand functions.[148] The presence or absence of Wallerian degeneration (see Figure 2–3) visualized by MRI of the brain stem following a subcortical stroke does not lead to different impairment or disability outcomes.[149] Infarction of the basal ganglia and internal capsule may predict less motor recovery and lower scores on the FIM, especially related to poorer leg function and walking, than patients with a cortical infarction or a combined cortical and subcortical infarction.[150] Lesions confined to the basal ganglia often cause a flaccid hemiplegia, along with memory, visuospatial, and other cognitive impairments that may interfere with learning and motivation during rehabilita-

tion.[151] Patients with infarctions within the distribution of the middle cerebral artery that spare the premotor cortex in BA 6 may have better proximal leg control and be more likely to walk than patients with damage to this region.[152] Sparing of BA 6 probably allows some corticospinal and corticoreticulospinal input to proximal muscles and permits better motor planning (see Chapter 1).

Evoked Potentials

Somatosensory evoked potentials (SEP) and motor evoked potentials (MEP) have been used to try to predict the recovery of upper extremity function. The median nerve stimulated SEP can recover or increase its amplitude or conduction time to become more symmetric with the SEP of the unaffected hemisphere over the first 6 to 8 weeks after a stroke.[153] The presence of an SEP was shown to correlate with a higher BI score at discharge,[154] with recovery of hand function, and, in 70% of cases, with independent gait.[155] These studies do not, however, reveal a clear prognostic advantage of the SEP over the clinical examination that assesses for impaired sensation and strength.[156] The combination of a motor impairment score and presence of the SEP had good prognostic value for short-term gains, but the motor score and MEP were a better predictor for long-term outcome when performed 2 months after the stroke.[157] A poor prognosis for motor recovery of the hand 4 weeks after a stroke is more robustly predicted by persistent absence of movement than by an absent SEP. As an assessment tool, the SEP can be helpful in its quantitative approach to somatic sensation and when, for example, an aphasic or obtunded patient cannot report on sensory appreciation.

The MEP has been elicited by transcranial electric and transcranial magnetic stimulation (TMS) (see Chapter 3). Stimulation provides the equivalent of a central motor nerve conduction study. A subcortical infarct along the corticospinal tract can delay, prolong, or abolish the MEP.[158] Poor movement and no functional recovery of the upper extremity tends to be predicted by an absent response in the patient who presents with a plegic hand,[159] whereas a normal or a delayed, but present MEP identifies the patient who is most likely to improve.[160] A study of 118 patients with stroke found that a normal or delayed central motor conduction time in the first 12 to 72 hours identified the group with a high probability of survival and functional recovery at 1 year by the BI and Rankin Scale.[161] Absence of a cortical response or a very high threshold for stimulation was associated with poor function and greater probability of a stroke-related death. A smaller study related an improvement in central motor conduction time between day 1 and day 14 after a stroke to improved impairment and ADLs scores, whereas a decline in conduction was associated with greater impairment and disability.[162]

Overall, TMS studies suggest that the presence or absence of an MEP has greater meaning than conduction time, absence of a response carries a poorer prognosis for motor gains, better MEP responses and impairment outcomes may depend upon the subject's ability to produce slight target muscle contraction, and motor thresholds may increase over the first few weeks after ischemia. Elicitation of an MEP in the affected biceps muscle or hand by TMS over the contralesional motor cortex may point to a poor recovery, corresponding to activation of corticoreticulospinal or propriospinal pathways or to dorsal premotor cortical activation.[163] Transcranial magnetic stimulation also reveals cortical representational plasticity and reorganization after a cortical or subcortical stroke (see Chapter 3).

Less clinically applicable techniques that have looked at prognostic features include magnetoencephalography, electroencephalography–electromyography coherence between cortical motor and muscle signals, and TMS studies that examine the silent period that follows stimulation, as well as TMS stimulation that inhibits activation.

Functional Imaging

Both resting metabolic and activation paradigms may help predict changes in impairments. Neurologic outcome at 2 months, based on the Mathew Scale of impairments, has been correlated with cerebral blood flow and oxygen consumption by PET performed at 5 to 18 hours after onset of a middle cerebral artery distribution infarction.[164] The pattern of a large cortical–subcortical area of greatly reduced perfusion and oxygen consumption carried a poor prognosis. A pattern of increased perfusion, equivalent to hyperemia, with only a small area of focally reduced oxygen consumption anticipated a good recovery. PET[165] and diffusion–perfusion magnetic resonance imaging[166] may reveal spared tissue that later contributes to sensorimotor reorganization and gains. A negative predictor for motor recovery is the depression of regional cerebral glucose metabolism[167] or blood flow by single-photon spectroscopy[168] in the thalamus ipsilateral to the infarct. Single-voxel proton magnetic resonance spectroscopy revealed a positive correlation between the decrease in N-acetylacetate signal (reflecting neuronal death) within a week of stroke and the SSS score at 6 months.[169]

Activation studies offer perhaps greater prospects for prognostication, because these paradigms may reveal spared nodes in a network and representational plasticity that underlie the potential for restitution or substitution of function. For example, transcranial doppler insonation of the middle cerebral arteries was shown to reveal bilateral increases in flow velocity during a mental object recognition task in patients who improved their scores on the Canadian Stroke Scale.[170] No increase in flow in the affected hemisphere correlated with poor recovery. Positron emission tomography and fMRI studies rather consistently show that activation within sensorimotor regions of the affected hemisphere[171] or of primary language regions[172] correlates best with a decrease in impairment. Chollet and colleagues found that higher intensity of activation in primary sensorimotor cortex, SMA and inferior BA 40 contralateral to the affected moving finger correlates with good recovery, whereas activation of ipsilateral homologous regions suggests poorer gains.[173] The activation of the unaffected hemisphere may disappear months after the stroke, at the time of better gains in hand function.

Metabolic activation studies may find use as physiologic markers of whether therapy has achieved as much as possible in, for example, improving motor control or improving ambulation. As described in detail in Chapter 3, an fMRI activation study used ankle dorsiflexion to monitor and relate the combination of burst characteristics of the EMG activity of the tibialis anterior muscle, the representational plasticity of the foot region of the ipsilateral and contralateral primary motor and supplementary motor cortices, and the behavior of walking speed.[174] Repeated epoques of BWSTT continued to resculpt the cortical activation, the EMG, and improve walking speed, until the activation approached the level in control subjects.

OUTCOMES OF DISABILITIES

Overview of Outcomes

Geriatric victims of acute stroke often present with premorbid impairments and disabilities that may confound assessment, treatment, and expected outcomes. People over the age of 65 have twice the disability and four times the limitation in their activities as those who are 45 to 64 years old. Chronic impairments and diseases cause the need for assistance in walking, bathing, and dressing to rise from 5% between ages 65 and 74 to 11% between 75 and 84, then to 35% over the age of 85. For these three age groups, assistance in shopping, chores, preparing meals, and handling money rises from 6% to 14% to 40%.[175]

A yearly report of first admissions for stroke rehabilitation from hospital programs that subscribe to the UDS_{MR} shows some interesting trends about functional gains after stroke. For 1992, approximately 27,000 patients were reported.[176] For 1998, UDS reported data about admission and discharge FIM scores for 67,000 patients admitted in 1 year.[177] In 1992, the mean time from onset of stroke to admission for rehabilitation was 20 days; in 1998, the mean fell to 12 days. In 1992, the mean length of stay was 28 days; in 1998, this fell to 20 days. In 1992, the mean total FIM score was 62 on admission and 86 on discharge; in 1998, the scores were unchanged at 63 and 87, respectively. About the same percentage of patients have returned home over this time. Thus, the level of functional dependence has not increased, based on the FIM, despite the significant decline of 16 days in the total time from onset of stroke to discharge from rehabilitation. The national trend continues to fall, approaching acute stays of 7 days for patients who are referred for rehabilitation, followed by rehabilitation stays of 18 days.

Table 9–2 shows the FIM subscores reported by UDS_{MR} in recent years. These scores provide good insight into the average gains made by patients during inpatient therapies. A FIM motor score above 62 and cognitive scores

Table 9–11. **Percentage of Stroke Patients Discharged to the Community in Relation to Discharge Functional Independence Measure Score**

Score	Percentage (%)
18–29	25
30–39	30
40–49	37
50–59	45
60–64	55
65–69	58
70–74	59
75–79	67
80–84	77
85–89	80
90–99	87
100–109	92
110–119	97
>120	98

Source: Uniform Data Service Newsletter, 1993.

of 30 by discharge from inpatient rehabilitation correlates with independence in most tasks.[178] Table 9–11 shows that higher FIM scores at discharge increase the likelihood of a return to the community. The admission FIM motor score is proportional to the daily rate of gains, the total FIM discharge score, and the likelihood of a home discharge when large numbers of patients fall into these categories (Table 9–12). This UDS_{MR} data also reveals that patients with higher motor FIM scores have briefer lengths of stay. For groups who have high FIM motor scores, the cognition score plays a greater role in determining the length of stay and gains during inpatient care. This data can be interpreted as consistent with other studies that correlate the need for inpatient stroke rehabilitation with motor impairments and dependence in toilet or tub transfers and in ambulation.

COMMUNITY STUDIES

Community-based populations of acute stroke survivors also provide insight into functional recovery. The prospective Framingham Study examined the 148 people in their cohort who

Table 9–12. **Classification and Regression Tree Analysis of Outcomes by the FIM On Admission to Inpatient Rehabilitation for Stroke Based on National UDS$_{MR}$ Data**

FIM Motor Group	Motor 13–26	Motor 27–41	Motor 42–52; Onset >7 days	Motor 42–52; Onset <7 days	Motor 53–91; Cognitive 5–29	Motor 53–91; Cognitive 30–35
FIM Daily Point Gain	1.0	1.4	1.7	2.0	2.2	2.6
Length of Stay (days)	29	23	18	16	12	10
Total FIM at Discharge	60	84	96	98	103	113
Percent Community Discharge	51	74	86	88	92	97

FIM, Functional Independence Measure; UDS$_{MR}$, Uniform Data System for Medical Rehabilitation.
Source: C. Granger and K. Ottenbacher in ADVANCE For Directors in Rehabilitation, January, 2002.

survived for 6 months after an acute nonhemorrhagic stroke.[179] The Framingham investigators compared functional disabilities in survivors of stroke with a control group matched for age and sex. As mentioned earlier, 52% of stroke survivors had no motor impairment. Some persisting disability was related to comorbid problems and not directly to the stroke. Gresham and Granger analyzed the study's stroke-related disability with and without these comorbid conditions. For those limited in household tasks, the number disabled by the stroke alone fell from 56% to 28% upon "removal" of comorbidities; in patients who were dependent in self-care, those disabled only from their new impairments decreased from 32% to 14%; in those dependent in mobility, from 22% to 9%; in those socializing less, from 59% to 32%; and in those living in an institution, from 15% to 4%.

A subgroup of 46 long-term Framingham Study survivors whose mean age was 77 years had further evaluations. The subjects were given a neurologic examination, Mini-Mental State Examination, and the BI at onset of stroke and 3, 6, and 12 months later.[180] Statistically significant recovery occurred in the first 3 months in the total BI score and in self-care, mobility, and language. Lesser gains were made in continence and toileting, cognition, and strength. Only language continued to improve beyond 6 months. The 12 patients in this group of 46 people who received rehabilitation were more disabled at onset (BI scores were 36 vs. 68) and improved an average of 30 points in the BI in the first 3 months compared to an increase of 16 for those not sent to inpatient rehabilitation. The best predictor of institutionalization after stroke for men was single status; for women, it was age and severity of disability. This cultural phenomenon has shown up in other studies, including the NINDS Pilot Stroke Data Bank.

The prospective Frenchay Health District study found that 47% of survivors were functionally independent and 21% showed moderate to severe dependence at 6 months after their stroke. The ADLs recovered in a consistent order at 3 weeks and 6 months. The evolution of gains went from walking to dressing, stair climbing, and then bathing.[181]

In a retrospective study that drew upon the record linkage system of the Mayo Clinic, Rankin scores (see Table 7–18) were determined for the 251 patients who survived more than 1 week after a first stroke.[77] Their mean age was 70 years. The mean Rankin Score increased from 1.7 before the stroke to 2.8 (moderate disability) in survivors at discharge from the acute hospital stay. Before their strokes, 20% were rated at 3 to 5 (moderate to severe disbility). This percentage increased to 75% at onset, then decreased to 57% at discharge from the acute hospital. This level of disability fell to 40% at 6 months and to approximately 35% at 1–3 years, although half the cohort had been lost to follow-up by then. Age over 75 years was highly associated with a Rankin Score at 1 year after stroke of 3 or more, even in the elderly with no comorbid conditions.

The Copenhagen Stroke Study, described earlier, offers insights into outcomes for unselected, acute stroke cases when a multidisciplinary team provides a Bobath approach and keeps patients in the hospital until further rehabilitation progress appears to be unlikely.[130] At the time of discharge from inpatient care, 20% of patients had severe disability, 8% had moderate disability, 26% had mild disability, and 46% had no disability, based on the BI. Functional recovery was completed by 12.5 weeks after onset in 95%. Best ADLs were reached in 95% of patients by 11.5 weeks with initially very severe impairments, by 17 weeks with severe impairments, by 13 weeks with moderate impairments, and by 8.5 weeks with mild impairments. The BI, however, does not measure walking distance beyond 150 feet or use of the paretic limb when performing ADLs.

Upper Extremity Use

In studies of selected stroke survivors, approximately 10% recover normal function of the upper extremity, approximately 33% recover useful function, approximately 25% have no recovery, and 33% have some movement and limited function.[182,183] Follow-up studies vary in the timing of examinations and in the tests used to measure strength and function.

In one series, 20% of patients with an upper extremity that remained flaccid 2 weeks after a stroke regained functional use of the hand. No one regained use if isolated motion of the fingers and some grip strength had not returned by 1 month.[184] Increases in grip

age, dysphasia, and weakness of any limb had varying effects over time. With this model, the predicted BI score at a given time was within 3 points of the observed score on the 20-point variation of the index approximately 70% of the time.

The admission score on the FIM may be used to anticipate the burden of care on the provider and the discharge placement. A classification and regression tree analysis revealed a mean rate of increase of 1.7 points per day across all patients regardless of admission FIM score. Thus, the efficiency or rate of improvement of inpatient gains in ADLs is independent of initial disability.[97] The FIM motor score, however, does correlate with the daily FIM point gain (Table 9–12).

A retrospective American study of 464 nonhemorrhagic stroke patients admitted in 1991 to 1 inpatient rehabilitation unit after a mean acute hospitalization of 18 days examined many variables.[71] Patients spent an average of 34 days at the facility. Admission FIM scores and age were analyzed in relationship to discharge FIM and placement. Admission FIM positively correlated with discharge FIM and admission FIM negatively correlated with length of stay. Lesser gains on the FIM followed a right, compared to a left, cerebral infarct in patients with the lowest admission FIM scores, less than 40. The greatest FIM change over time occurred in patients with admission FIM scores of 4 to 80. Patients with admission scores over 80 and age less than 55 years returned home. A score of less than 40 and age over 65 produced a nursing home discharge for 62%. For the rest of the FIM-age subgroups, only 13% went to nursing facilities.

A few predictors for functional outcome were found in the Copenhagen Stroke Study for patients with the most severe impairments who survive for at least 3 months.[83] Decreasing age, having a spouse, and greater gains in neurologic impairments at 1 week predicted a higher BI score.

QUALITY OF LIFE

A study assessed quality of life (QOL) in 442 patients with a mean age of 73 years using the Sickness Index Profile 6 months after a stroke.[200] The investigators found that 60% reported mildly diminished QOL, 33% reported more dysfunction on the physical and psychosocial dimensions, and 7% had marked psychosocial dysfunction. Comorbidities, severity of stroke, and supratentorial location produced the most impaired pattern of QOL. No differences were found for patients with intracerebral hemorrhage and supratentorial infarct. Patients with lacunar infarcts had significantly less dysfunction, with the exception of emotional discomfort, than patients with other subcortical lesions.

FUNCTIONAL IMAGING

Metabolic and functional activation studies may reveal information relevant to functional recovery (see Chapter 3). For example, a higher global and contralateral cerebral metabolic rate for glucose within 1 to 2 weeks of an acute stroke correlated with a better functional outcome in survivors at a mean of 3 and 50 months.[201] Low glucose consumption within the unaffected hemisphere in hypertensive patients was associated with poorer ADLs, perhaps because of a subclinical hypertensive arteriopathy producing tissue damage that limited compensation. Perilesion metabolic activation and activations associated with greater motor recovery tend to correlate with functional gains, but too few serial studies have been completed to establish meaningful predictors. Activations that change over the course of training, especially for a motor task or a working memory task, may come to serve as physiologic markers of the capacity for improvement in ADLs and the effectiveness of rehabilitative training.

CLINICAL TRIALS OF FUNCTIONAL INTERVENTIONS

Aside from trials aimed at the locus for rehabilitation interventions, clinical trials of stroke rehabilitation had most often been designed to learn whether overall stroke rehabilitation is efficacious. For the better,[202] rehabilitationists have been improving the designs of trials that examine whether a particular therapeutic approach is more effective than another. Increasingly, the literature reflects theory-based interventions (see Chapter 5) and more scientific study designs with outcome measures that reflect the likely consequences of the intervention (see Chapter 7). Many good ideas about therapy for impairments and disabilities have yet to be tested in enough subjects.

After reviewing 124 investigations drawn from a literature search of studies done from 1960 to 1990, Ottenbacher and Jannell carried out a meta-analysis of 36 trials.[203] These studies met the criteria of including hemiparetic patients with stroke who were given a rehabilitation service in a design that compared at least two groups or conditions for change in a quantifiable functional measure. Outcomes included gait, hand function, ADLs, response times, and visuoperception. From 173 statistical evaluations recorded on the 3717 acute and chronic patients in the 36 trials, the analysis showed that the average patient who received a program of focused stroke rehabilitation or a particular procedure performed better than approximately 65% of the patients in the comparison group. Larger treatment effect sizes were associated with an earlier intervention and younger patients.

No association was found in the meta-analysis between the duration of a program and its outcomes. Most of these interventions were, however, rather brief. The authors point out that this synthesis of data is imperfect. The review could not assess the intensity of the interventions or how well they were carried out to be able to judge the integrity of each research study. The authors would not be in a position to detect systematic biases or account for missing data while evaluating the individual studies. In addition, the real impact of the changes in the wide variety of outcome mea-sures used to assess an even wider variety of stroke-related functional problems is unknown. Statistical significance in this meta-analysis does not imply that a change has clinical or functional importance and does not reveal how long a benefit lasted. None of the investigations led to an accepted intervention among therapists. Could the same outcome have been facilitated by any physical or behavioral art? If improvement depends on specific training methods, do gains in one neurologic impairment, say visuoperceptual skills, generalize to decrease disability, for example, in dressing and ambulation? Future clinical trials can draw upon the limitations of prior designs.

Trials of Schools of Therapy

Early studies compared one school of physiotherapy (see Chapter 5) to another to determine whether a particular technique improves functional performance. Small randomized trials during inpatient or outpatient therapy revealed no significant differences between conventional therapy and proprioceptive neuromuscular facilitation (PNF),[204] conventional exercise and Bobath's technique,[205] conventional exercise versus Bobath and Rood,[206] conventional versus PNF versus Bobath,[207] electromyographic biofeedback (EMG BFB) versus Bobath technique,[208] sensorimotor integration versus functional treatment in occupational therapy,[209] and, in an alternating treatment design, Bobath compared to the Brunnstrom method.[210] One of Johnstone's neurophysiologic techniques applies an air splint to the extended upper extremity and aims for the subject to push back with the affected proximal arm as a rocking chair leans the subject forward. A half-hour treatment for 30 days was compared to passive rocking in a well-designed trial with 100 subjects who had an acute stroke.[211] The Fugl-Meyer score for the proximal arm was significantly higher at 6 and 12 months postintervention, but upper extremity function did not differ between the groups.

Another trial gave all 75 patients functional training and stretching, then randomized the patients into 3 groups. One group continued this training, another performed additional active exercises, and the third performed additional resistive exercises.[212] The latter group was more independent at 1 month, but no difference was apparent by 2 months. Strength increased in the resistive-exercise group. Although selective muscle strengthening has not been a focus of most schools of therapy, this trial alone warrants further exploration of potential links between the rate of early recovery and methods for selective muscle strengthening. An increasing variety of studies point to the feasibility and functional benefit of using general exercise and resistance training to increase strength in hemiparetic subjects.[120,213,214]

A well-designed trial compared traditional Bobath, Johnstone, and related techniques to a series of more intensive treatments. These included behavioral methods to increase family and patient participation in therapy and to prevent learned nonuse of the arm. The therapists also facilitated the learning of new motor skills with tasks of graded difficulty, provided feedback on performance, used EMG BFB, and trained patients with microcomputer games.[215] It took 3 years to enroll subjects and 5 years to complete the trial. Patients were evaluated by a variety of tests at a median of 10 days after the stroke and retested at 1, 3, and 6 months. Subgroups of 64 severe and 57 mildly affected patients were also compared. The primary effect of the enhanced intervention, that included about twice the amount of therapy time, was improved arm function at 1 month. At 6 months, the mildly affected, but not the severely impaired subgroup that received enhanced therapy, had significantly improved in the 9-Hole Peg Test and a motor score. Thus, a moderate addition to usual interventions had some benefit in patients with selective upper extremity movement at entry. Perhaps a better defined and more intensively applied set of enhanced interventions and measures with less serious floor and ceiling effects would generate greater efficacy.

The individual trials comparing schools of therapy include many methodologic flaws.[216,217] For example, the studies entered too few subjects, given the spectrum of impairments and disabilities of stroke patients, to detect real differences if such differences exist. Thus, they are at risk for a type II statistical error. The trials did not clearly address principles for training skills. The therapists concentrated on movement, rather than upon the ADLs that served as the measure of efficacy. The trials did not include outcomes related to how the therapists' efforts affected behavioral compensation for the hemiplegia, compared with changes in the performance of the affected limbs. Indeed, indices of independence in ADLs, the primary outcome measure in these trials, may reflect poorly the primary intention of the schools of physiotherapy, which traditionally has been to improve patterns of movement.[202]

Task-Oriented Approaches

The school of physiotherapy may not matter as much as the provision of a thoughtful across-the-board approach that aims to enhance mobility and self-care skills, while it provides individual and family psychosocial support. The amount and type of practice in relearning a skill may be most critical.[88] The optimal style, daily intensity, and overall duration of training, and

the best outcome measures in terms of sensitivity to change and relevance to useful movements, are a work in progress for all interventions for hemiparetic patients. Task-oriented approaches take these issues to heart. A task-oriented approach toward retraining ADLs has recently become a growing portion of what therapists do, supplemented by Bobath and other techniques.

How much opportunity for practice do patients actually receive? On an inpatient service, it is remarkable how little formal therapy time may be spent with each patient in the course of a day. Although the definition of active therapy time for stroke rehabilitation is debatable, reports range from 13% to 30% of the working day.[218,219] A lot of time is spent beginning to get started, talking about therapy, and resting. Almost any type of clinical trial for a rehabilitation approach could include a dose-response comparison of differing intensities of a specific therapy.

ARM FUNCTION

The evidence favoring task-specific practice is increasing, especially for patients with modest impairments. One trial randomized 185 patients within 1 month of a stroke to either up to 5 months of home-based therapy with an occupational therapist or to no therapy.[220] The number of visits ranged from 1 to 15 with a mean of only 6 visits per patient. None of the subjects had been admitted to a hospital for the stroke. Their median BI scores were 18 (approximately 90 on the American version of the test), so they were minimally disabled. Blinded outcomes revealed significant gains made by the group that received therapy. Instrumental ADLs were clearly better and handicap decreased. The investigators also found a significant if modest gain in ADLs, along with a decrease in reported caregiver strain. The quality of life measure did not differ between groups.

A well-defined approach for patients with mild residual hemiparesis, called Arm Ability Training (AAT), employs practice in aiming, tapping, writing, turning over coins, tracking through a maze, picking up bolts, and placing small and large objects. Sixty subjects who offered at least mild resistance in most hemiparetic muscles, were randomly assigned to no treatment, a $1/2$-hour of daily AAT for 15 sessions, or to the AAT provided with knowledge of results feedback.[221] The AAT groups were significantly faster in performing a series of functional outcomes tasks for the upper extremity and the benefit persisted a year later. The outcome measure, the TEMPA (see Chapter 7), includes tasks that are similar to the tasks of AAT. Thus, a brief task-oriented program of modest intensity led to gains on related tasks in patients with good motor control. The skills training did not further improve with knowledge of results feedback, perhaps because the number of possible strategies for carrying out the movements were limited.

AMBULATION

Two well-designed trials demonstrate the impact of the specificity of practice for locomotor outcomes. Dean and colleagues randomly assigned 12 chronic stroke subjects to either 1 hour of locomotor circuit training or upper extremity exercise.[113] The subjects started with a large range of walking speeds from approximately 15 cm/second to 110 cm/second. The 10 workstations of the circuit stressed sit-to-stand, reaching while standing, ankle and knee flexor and extensor strengthening, treadmill walking, and walking on uneven ground and stairs. All of the tasks had individually been shown in prior studies to improve an aspect of leg function. The circuit-trained group significantly improved in walking speed (mean of 10 cm/second) and leg strength by 4 weeks and retained its gains 2 months later.

Kwakkel and colleagues randomized 100 patients by 14 days after a stroke who initially could not walk alone to one of 3 interventions for 30 minutes a day for 20 weeks: upper extremity training in reaching and gripping items and strengthening: leg exercise with strengthening, weight-bearing, walking, and treadmill walking when feasible; or to the control condition in which the affected arm and leg were immobilized with inflatable splints.[88] All subjects also received 15 minutes of arm and 15 minutes of leg therapies daily and 1.5 hours of training in ADLs weekly. At 20 weeks, no differences were found between the arm and leg training groups. The leg training group performed significantly better than the controls in ADLs by the BI, in walking speed, and in hand dexterity by the Action Research Arm Test. Walking speed at weeks 6 and 20 was 17 meters/second and 37 meters/second for the control group, 21 meters/second and 55 meters/second for the arm training group, and 40 meters/second and 65 meters/second for the leg training group. The arm trained group performed better than the control group on dexterity tests only.

The effect of additional therapy was studied in already mobile patients from the community.[222] At entry, 148 recent stroke patients walked at least 20 meters independently without an assistive device. Their minimum BI was 75 and cognition and language were unimpaired. After 5 hours of Bobath-based physiotherapy a week for 4 weeks, plus occupational therapy, the group showed statistically significant gains in stance duration and in the symmetry of swing and push-off of both legs. The symmetry of ground reaction forces did not change. Speed over a 10-meter distance and maximum distance walked changed slightly. Thus, functional mobility did not improve with a modest intervention that emphasized balance and symmetry of movement, but not practice to increase walking speed in rather high functioning patients.

If walking speed and walking distance are important outcomes, then perhaps therapy ought to emphasize practice at varying speeds and aim to build endurance. These are important, if underplayed outcomes. Mean ranges for walking speed in several studies of recovery from hemiplegic stroke were 25–50 cm per second,[223] which is about one-third the normal walking speed of geriatric persons. In a large group that received conventional inpatient rehabilitation for stroke, the mean walking speed increased from 18 cm per second at 30 days poststroke to 38 cm per second at 140 days.[224] Although household ambulation may be achieved by patients who walk at 25 ± 10 cm per second, unrestricted community ambulation is achieved by those who walk at speeds of 80 ± 15 cm per second, by 3 months after hemiparetic stroke.[194] Thus, gait speed and endurance for walking longer distances than required by the BI and FIM test of 150 feet should become a focus for mobility interventions.

Concentrated Practice

Massing or concentrating task-oriented practice for upper extremity functions and for walking has increasingly revealed its value in stroke rehabilitation. Learning a new skill may take many hours of practice (see Chapter 5). The most popularized approach for the affected arm is Constraint-Induced Movement Therapy (CIMT). For walking, body weight–supported treadmill training (BWSTT) offers intensive bouts of practice aimed at optimizing the kinematics and timing of phases of the gait cycle.

Massed practice may include *mental practice* and *imagery* (see Chapter 1). Before attempting to enhance motor gains with physical and mental practice, the clinician may ascertain if this approach is viable in the patient with stroke. Lesions of the dorsolateral prefrontal cortex, superior parietal lobules, striatum, and other regions of the observation and imagery networks may have been damaged by the stroke. After a parietal stroke, patients may imagine a movement, but the affected arm moves slower than the unaffected one.[225] To test for imaginability, a patient is asked to perform the requested mental movement, such as reaching for a cup and bringing it to the mouth, a few times. If each trial takes the same time to complete, the patient probably is imaging the task.[226] Mental practice may help maintain a cerebral representation for movements at a time of limb paralysis and later help prime the movement. Physical practice is more powerful than imagery, however. Imagery may augment practice, but the proprioceptive feedback of physical actions drives sensorimotor integration and learning.

ARM FUNCTION

Constraint-Induced Movement Therapy

Failed early attempts to use the affected upper extremity may lead to behavioral suppression of its incorporation into daily activities. Forced use of the affected hand and gradual shaping of a variety of functional movements to overcome what is theorized as learned nonuse may increase the incorporation of the affected arm into daily manual tasks.[227] No data reveal the frequency of nonuse. Experience suggests it is uncommon in patients with at least 3/5 strength of shoulder and hand.

A study of 25 chronic hemiplegic stroke and head injured patients who could overcome a flexor synergy used a multiple baselines design to look for an effect of enclosing the normal hand in a sling for 2 weeks.[228] For a series of simple functional tasks, repeated measures showed significant increases in speed and greater applied force, including grip. The quality of the shoulder, elbow, and hand movements did not appear to improve based on observer ratings. At 1-year follow-up, these gains persisted or increased.

A trial with nine highly selected chronic stroke patients who could extend the fingers at least 10° and the wrist 20° randomized four to CIMT and five to encouragement to make use of the affected hand at home.[229] The experimental group practiced a variety of guided upper extremity movements across many tasks for 7 hours a day at a rehabilitation site for 2 weeks. The CIMT subjects wore a sling or glove that prevented use of the unaffected upper extremity for the rest of the day. Much of the improvement in daily use of the affected arm in the study was evident within a day or 2 of restraint of the unaffected arm plus therapy, which suggests that a latent capability had succumbed to learned nonuse.[229] The restrained subjects showed a significant 30% decrease in the timed performance of a series of upper extremity functional tasks and a significant increase in the amount of use of the affected hand during daily activities.

Two uncontrolled trials of CIMT also reported a large effect on subsequent use of the paretic arm in patients with chronic stroke.[230,231] Uncontrolled trials do, however, tend to overestimate the effects of a treatment (see Chapter 7). A larger, well-designed randomized trial of 66 subjects with chronic stroke compared CIMT to bimanual hand training based on the neurodevelopmental program of Patricia Davies.[116] After 2 weeks of training, the CIMT group scored minimally better on functional use and amount of daily use of the affected arm, as well as dexterity of the hand. The difference in amount of use did not persist 1 year later. The study assessed primarily the possible benefit of constraining the affected hand, rather than attempting to provide a large difference in the intensity of therapy for each group. Subjects with sensory loss and hemiinattention appeared to do better with CIMT, which bears further study. Patients with higher levels of residual arm function improved more than those with less function.[232]

A pilot study of 20 acute patients with stroke compared 2 hours of daily CIMT for 2 weeks to standard occupational therapy that did not emphasize use of the affected arm.[233] The CIMT patients scored better on the Action Research Arm Test and its pinch scale. This small trial points to the feasibility of a large randomized clinical trial of this intervention in subjects with minimal upper extremity movement. The study also emphasizes what the actual benefit of CIMT may be. The intervention stresses mass practice of task-oriented activities. Nonuse is not the critical feature for employing CIMT. Good motor control and practice are critical for success. Thus, many other forms of mass practice, styles of therapy that do not glove the unaffected hand, for instance, or that require only 2 hours of treatment a day, may be equally as valuable.

A large randomized trial of CIMT is in progress in the United States for subjects who are 3–9 months poststroke and can extend several fingers and the wrist at least 10°. The small trials to date do not provide information about upper extremity functions that had improved and then were lost between the onset of stroke and entry into a forced-use protocol. The trials do confirm that strong motivation, good cognition, and some selective hand movement is needed if gains are to be made. Training interventions need to be further developed to determine whether more specific learning paradigms and activities can unmask latent function, train compensatory motor actions, and take advantage of the potential for neuronal representational plasticity.

Constraint-induced movement therapy is a form of intensive, task-oriented practice for patients who have at least modest motor control of the upper extremity. The intervention does not prescribe a particular approach to motor learning. For example, what is the best schedule of reinforcement and best form of feedback during training? A shaping procedure has been suggested,[111] but no study has shown the reproducibility or efficacy of that operant conditioning approach. Should an effort be made to retrain reaching, grasping, and pincer movements so that the CNS perceives the most normal visual and proprioceptive input from the arm that is feasible? In any controlled trial, CIMT must be compared to an equally active program of upper extremity management. Taub and colleagues have suggested an intensive 2-week, 60–80 hour program with one patient managed by one therapist for patients with chronic upper extremity paresis and nonuse. Other investigators have begun to test the effects of fewer hours of massed practice, practice monitored intermittently by a therapist, small group practice, and less time spent at home with arm restraint, in order to reduce the cost of the intervention.[234]

Constraint-induced movement therapy received a lot of fanfare when studies showed that the intervention was associated with primary motor cortex reorganization in a small study that included transcranial magnetic stimulation (TMS) and fMRI studies, suggesting the induction of activity-dependent plasticity.[235,236] Rapid, transient changes in representational plasticity may be observed with TMS soon after practice, so the meaning of a change related to CIMT is debatable. Other functional imaging studies have been less convincing about representational plasticity when the comparison is made to control subjects. Indeed, task-oriented training without CIMT compared to passive training in patients with recent stroke also led to neuroimaging improvements in synaptic efficacy in primary sensorimotor cortex.[237] The intensity of training necessary to reap maximum benefit from repetitive practice for upper and lower extremity activities needs much experimental study.

Focused Retraining

When brief, intensive therapy of various types has been provided to subjects with recent or chronic stroke, upper extremity function related to the practiced task has usually improved.[88,211,215,238–240] When the amount of practice is modest, gains may not be found. For example, one trial randomized 280 subjects with recent stroke to three groups—a Bobath approach commonly used in Great Britain for up to 45 minutes a day for 5 weeks, this treatment plus 2 hours a week of additional facilitation treatment by a senior physiotherapist, or the additional 2 hours of treatment provided by an assistant physiotherapist.[241] No differences were found up to 6 months after completion of the interventions in outcomes across a variety of scales of upper extremity impairment and disability. Only about half of the subjects in the more intensive therapy groups received the extra 10 hours of therapy, however. Compared to most trials of an intervention, the subjects in this well-designed trial were more impaired than most. Many would not have fit into the required wrist and finger extensor movement set by studies of CIMT. Also, 35% either could not tolerate the additional therapy or died during the period of the intervention, so both the intention-to-treat and efficacy analyses may have been compromised. This trial offers a note of caution for future trials. Greater intensity of practice, perhaps more like 10 hours a week for several weeks, rather than 10 hours spread over 5 weeks, may be a better goal for a study that aims to show a difference between two approaches.

Bimanual retraining also has a solid theoretical basis.[242,243] Aspects of movement, such as timing, may transfer from one arm to another. A pilot study of 14 patients with chronic hemiparesis had subjects practice pushing and pulling movements in an apparatus gripped by each hand.[244] A metronome cued the phase of movement. After training 3 times a week for 6 weeks, wrist and elbow strength and function significantly improved and gains persisted 2 months later. These effects were specific to the muscle and joints that were trained. Although the task seems trivial, several reasonable motor learning parameters were met. The trainers set goals for subjects within the task and the rhythmic auditory cues may have helped entrain the motor skill. Another controlled trial of 36 patients with marked hemiplegia of less than 3 months or from 1 to 11 years after stroke did not find improvements after mass practice of bilateral contractions of the deltoid and extensor carpi radialis longus muscles.[245] Fatigue may have interfered with the ability of subjects to participate fully, however.

Practice also improves aspects of motor function in the ipsilesional upper extremity,[246] which is often a bit weak or slow in its movements compared to those of control subjects, owing to the partial bihemispheric control of proximal movement (see Chapter 1).[136] Indeed, bimanual practice that is as intensive as CIMT may be as effective as CIMT for many patients.

Apraxia

Apraxia means a deficiency in the ability to understand an action or to perform an action by imitation or in response to a verbal direction in the absence of sensorimotor impairments that would prevent either understanding or performance. At least a dozen forms of apraxia have been defined.[247] Ideational and ideomotor limb apraxia affect approximately 20% of patients after a stroke. Ideational apraxia is an impairment in the sequential use of multiple items such as lighting a candle. The term often refers to impairment in the concept of an action, but the term conceptual apraxia serves this form better. Ideomotor apraxia implies impaired performance of skilled movements on verbal command or by imitating another person. Patients make spatial and temporal errors when they try to execute a movement. The former is usually tested with a battery that aims to demonstrate the use of objects as told and the latter by having subjects reproduce symbolic and meaningless gestures or show how to use an imaginary item. Limb apraxia refers to an ideomotor apraxia of primarily hand and finger movements.[248] Orofacial or buccofacial apraxia implies impaired performance of tongue, mouth, or facial actions to command or by imitation. The examiner looks for errors in sequencing, perseveration, or omission as well as spatiotemporal errors in tests for any of the apraxias. The underlying complexity of neural networks related to the apraxias is brought out by dissociations in the ability to perform meaningful versus meaningless actions, to respond to verbal versus visual commands, and to conceptualize versus carry out an act.

A form of dyspraxia may be found in up to one-half of patients with a left hemisphere stroke and approximately 10% of patients with right hemisphere lesions, especially when the parietal region is affected (see Chapter 1). Careful studies, however, suggest that injury to either hemisphere leads to errors when patients try to pantomime what an examiner does.[249] The left hemisphere is important for representing actions in terms of knowledge about bodily structure. The right hemisphere is involved in the visuospatial analysis of gestures. The gestural errors related to planning an action and using items with conceptual appropriateness typical of an ideational apraxia tend to resolve by 1 month after stroke. The difficulty in executing a gestural motor program related to spatial and timing errors typical of ideomotor apraxia may still persist at least mildly 1 year later.[250]

Imitative learning and the ability to draw upon the concept of movement and past use of items is important for practice in ADLs. Limb apraxia seriously interferes with self-care. Rehabilitation interventions for apraxia may improve daily gesturing, aid gestural communication by aphasic patients, and improve the ability of patients to relearn motor skills. One approach is to verbalize steps or try compensatory strategies.[251] Specific aspects of apraxic impairments have responded to 10–35 hours of practice in those gestures and actions.[252,253] Related interventions ought to aim to activate the action-observation and imitation system discussed in Chapter 1.

Sensory Retraining

Sensory stimulation is commonly used by therapists. For example, a proprioceptive neuromuscular facilitation technique applies resistance to the affected arm in the path of movement or increases the load on the knee during stance. The inability to discriminate temperature, texture, or shape and to use proprioception for sensorimotor integration often impedes functional use of the hand after a stroke. Visual input allows some compensation. Often, even when subjects cannot tell the direction of a joint movement, they are able to recognize joint and muscle stretch signals that provide information about the presence of motion. Training may benefit some patients, especially those who retain some awareness of pressure or motion in the fingertips.

Sensory input such as transcutaneous nerve stimulation has been applied to chronic stroke patients for 1 hour a day to accomplish afferent stimulation. A controlled trial found that this intervention improved the Fugl-Meyer motor score in subjects who had less impairment, starting at baseline scores above 30, than with greater impairment.[254] The electrical stimulation was used daily in the experimental group for 3 months, but not necessarily provided during 2 therapy sessions received by all subjects weekly. Electrical stimulation of the median nerve of the affected hand in 1 Hz trains each with 5 single pulses lasting 1 ms delivered at 10 Hz for 2 hours led to a brief increase in key pinch strength and subjective transient gains in functional use of the hand for up to 1 day.[255] The trial did not include practice, but raises the possibility that peripheral sensory stimulation plus task-oriented practice

with the stimulated hand may enhance contingent sensorimotor associations and augment representational plasticity. Protocols of functional electrical stimulation for grasp and release could also explore these relationships (see Chapter 4).

An exploratory study design showed gains in the ability of a chronic stroke patient to use utensils after a series of interventions over the course of a year.[256] A 100-Hz current was applied to finger surfaces at intensities that evoked appreciation of the stimulus and aimed to allow the patient to identify which finger was stimulated. Velcro strips attached to a variety of objects and utensils and in geometric patterns on cardboard were used to stimulate moving touch-pressure inputs. The patients were highly motivated to accomplish their defined functional goals.

A series of four single-case study designs with multiple baselines showed significant improvements in wrist proprioception and tactile discrimination of the fingers.[257] For discrimination, the investigators used finely graded ridges and grooves that were explored by one finger with graded progression of stimuli and no visual input. The trainers used a learning paradigm with quantitative feedback on performance and summary feedback on judgements and on the method of exploration. The training effects were specific to the individual tasks.

In another protocol, investigators trained chronic stroke patients to relearn sensory information and compared this group to an untreated, matched control group. Subjects correlated tactile input with what they saw in their affected hand and attempted to make purposeful exploratory movements with the hypesthetic fingers.[258] By training subjects 3 times a week for 6 weeks on a variety of problem-solving tasks, the patients improved their ability to identify the location of a touch to the fingers, the position of the elbow, and to discern 2-point discrimination and stereognosis.

Although these trials have flaws in their designs, they do suggest that rehabilitationists should explore further the use of multisensory inputs with learning paradigms and functional tasks. The location of the lesion will affect that strategy. For example, an injury to somatosensory cortex may impair learning new motor skills from loss of sensorimotor integration, but not alter the execution of existing ones.[259]

AMBULATION

In addition to the compensatory and reeducation approaches described in Chapters 5 and 6 for mobility and gait training, therapists have tried a variety of methods of concentrated exercise for hemiparetic subjects, such as bicycling,[260-262] muscle strengthening,[263] and balance training after stroke. The amount of practice in transferring weight onto the paretic leg during stance to improve extensor strength may improve ambulation, but balance training on a forceplate to improve the symmetry of weight bearing on each leg does not generalize to improve gait.[264] Electrical stimulation of leg muscles is sometimes used, mostly to aid ankle dorsiflexion. Rhythmic practice entrained by the temporal elements of music [265] may also improve walking speed and the symmetry of the stance and swing phases of gait.

Treadmill Training

Treadmill training for ambulatory patients with a hemiparesis may improve walking speed,[223] reduce the energy cost of walking,[119] improve strength in the hemiparetic leg,[120] and improve physiologic measures of fitness.[266] A 5-week, randomized trial with acute hemispheric stroke patients compared two traditional approaches and intensities of treatment to a more intensive and focused set of interventions that included treadmill gait training.[223] At 6 weeks after stroke, the latter group had a 40% greater gait speed than the conventional groups. At 3 months, the investigators found no differences, though all three groups had continued to improve. One conclusion was that a trial for gait training should proceed for 3 months following a stroke.

Safety improves by placing patients in a harness connected overhead. The therapist may better be able to provide verbal cues and physical assistance for kinematic, kinetic, and temporal features of the gait cycle, along with using higher treadmill speeds in patients who cannot safely step on a treadmill, by providing partial body weight support.

Body Weight-Supported Treadmill Training

Treadmill walking is a task-oriented approach for ambulation. In patients with stroke, small studies and a larger clinical trial[267] suggest that BWSTT increases the likelihood of achieving more independent ambulation and at greater speeds than by conventional locomotor therapy.[110] Body weight-supported treadmill training, if carried out optimally by therapists, allows the spinal cord and supraspinal locomotor regions to experience sensory inputs akin to ordinary stepping rather than the atypical inputs created by compensatory gait deviations and difficulty with loading the paretic leg. The therapist employs different levels of weight support and treadmill speeds, and, most importantly, assists the step pattern with physical and verbal cues to optimize the temporal, kinematic, and kinetic parameters of the step cycle. The more normal input may improve the timing and increase the activation of residual descending locomotor outputs on spinal motor pools. As discussed in Chapters 1 and 6, sensory inputs related to the level of loading and to treadmill speed have been shown to modulate the EMG output during BWSTT, even when the legs are fully assisted during the step cycle.[268,269] Most importantly, BWSTT allows massed practice with many repetitions guided by the cues of the therapist. This approach ought to enhance motor relearning.

Pilot studies have been limited to patients who are 2 to 12 months or more poststroke who walk overground poorly or not at all. Hesse and colleagues added 25 sessions of BWSTT to ongoing physiotherapy in 8 stroke patients who could not ambulate independently 2–14 months after onset.[270,271] Initial treadmill training speeds were often 7–11 cm/second (0.2 mph) and usually reached a maximum of 12–23 cm/second (0.5 mph) by day 8. Patients often were felt not to require weight support on average at day 6 (range of 4 to 20 days). Swing and stance times of each leg became more symmetric, and gait became more independent. Mean overground velocities increased significantly from 12 (SD 8) cm/s to 42 (SD 23) cm/second, which is a mean of less than 1 mph.

A large randomized clinical trial by Visintin and colleagues compared treadmill training to BWSTT. Fifty subjects were randomized to each 6-week intervention, but 21 subjects did not complete the trial and were not included in the data analysis. Entry criteria included the ability to flex the hip and take a step with assistance if needed. The average time from onset of stroke to entry into the trial was 50 days.

Even after that long delay, patients had an average inpatient stay of 70 days, mostly because no outpatient therapy was available to them. The average time spent stepping on the treadmill for each group was approximately 15 minutes daily, so the intensity of practice was modest, but equal. By week 3, almost 50% of the BWSTT group were trained with little or no weight support. By week 6, 79% practiced without weight support. Thus, the difference in the interventions disappeared rather quickly. Treadmill speeds were slower for the no-BWS group initially and at completion. At week 6, speeds were 0.95 ± 0.49 mph for the BWSTT group and 0.76 ± 0.42 mph for the no-BWS group. The BWSTT group had significantly better scores for balance (Berg Balance Scale), motor recovery, overground walking speed (10-meter walk), and walking endurance over ground (no time limit). Overground walking speed for the BWS compared to no-BWS group reached 34 ± 4 cm/second versus 25 ± 4 cm/second. Three months after completing the intervention, 52 subjects were available for follow-up. Significant differences for the BWSTT group persisted in walking speed (52 ± 6 cm/second vs. 35 ± 4 cm/second) and motor recovery, but not balance or walking endurance. Thus, the final walking speeds were modest and not good enough for community ambulation. Of interest, patients who initially walk slower than 30 cm/second increased their walking speeds significantly more with BWSTT than patients who practiced without BWS. Both groups improved significantly in their walking speed over time when initial speed was over 60 cm/second,[272] suggesting a general practice effect of treadmill training for patients who can step on a moving treadmill belt at greater than 1.5 mph.

Kosak and Reding randomized 56 patients during inpatient rehabilitation at approximately 40 days after onset of stroke to either BWSTT or aggressive bracing with knee-ankle-foot or ankle-foot orthoses and training overground and at a hemibar.[273] Subjects received 45 minutes of gait training under each condition 5 days a week in addition to their routine physical therapy. Treadmill speeds ranged from 0.6 to 1.8 mph. The duration of therapy was the time until inpatient discharge or until the subject walked overground with no physical assistance. The investigators did not report the number of treatment sessions. Both groups

tripled their walking endurance and doubled their overground walking speed, increasing from 9 cm/second to 18 cm/second, which is quite slow (see Table 6–3; 45 cm/second equals 1 mph). A subgroup analysis of subjects who had large hemisphere strokes with sensorimotor and visual field deficits and who received more than 12 sessions of BWSTT showed significantly better walking speed compared to the braced group (20 cm/second vs. 14 cm/second) and endurance. The limited gains in speed in all subjects suggest that training intensity and duration were too little to judge the comparative benefits of the interventions.

Another randomized trial entered 73 subjects admitted for inpatient rehabilitation at a median of 20 days after a stroke to either BWSTT or to the Motor Relearning Programme of Carr and Shepherd (see Chapter 5). The median age was 54 years. The length of stay was a median of 68 days with a range of 21–137 days. Patients were treated for one-half hour a day, 5 days a week until discharge. Treadmill speeds started at a mean of 0.45 mph and reached a mean of 0.9 mph. At discharge and 10 months after onset of stroke, no differences were found for the groups (total of 60 subjects) in walking speed, balance, and Fugl-Meyer Assessment. At 10 months, 90% of patients were independent walkers. Walking speeds for the groups improved a mean of 40 cm/second from admission to 10 months, which included the change in patients who could not walk at all on admission. The mean walking velocity of each group reached 60 ± 35 cm/second. The great range in time of onset of stroke to entry, very slow treadmill training speed for the BWSTT group, variations in the duration of therapy across patients, and lack of an intention-to-treat analysis make the conclusion that the two approaches are equivalent rather debatable.

Figure 9–5 shows several relationships between treadmill speed and speed attained for overground ambulation over the course of BWSTT for stroke patients who were 1 year post-onset.[274] At slow speeds, usually below 0.8 mph, many patients describe a highly cognitive approach to their stepping in which they have to pay attention to more details during each step than when pushed to walk at higher speeds. One mechanism that affects automaticity of stepping during BWSTT is related to the angular velocity and degree of hip extension induced by the treadmill and the tim-

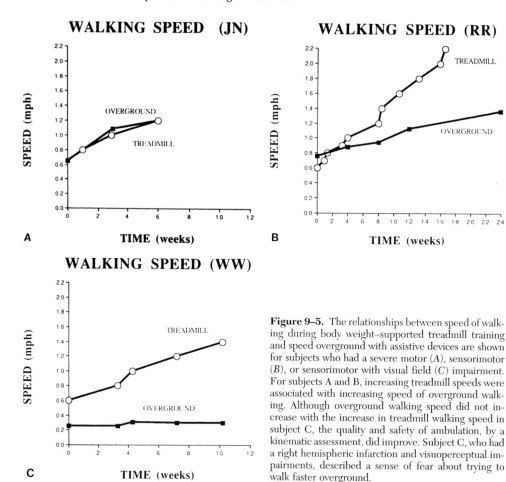

Figure 9–5. The relationships between speed of walking during body weight–supported treadmill training and speed overground with assistive devices are shown for subjects who had a severe motor (*A*), sensorimotor (*B*), or sensorimotor with visual field (*C*) impairment. For subjects A and B, increasing treadmill speeds were associated with increasing speed of overground walking. Although overground walking speed did not increase with the increase in treadmill walking speed in subject C, the quality and safety of ambulation, by a kinematic assessment, did improve. Subject C, who had a right hemispheric infarction and visuoperceptual impairments, described a sense of fear about trying to walk faster overground.

ing of loading and unloading the stance leg. This finding is consistent with the load and hip extension studies described for spinal transected cats and patients with SCI (see Chapter 1). To test the effects of optimizing these kinematic and kinetic details of gait, we trained 24 patients with chronic hemiparetic stroke who walked slowly. The subjects were randomized to training at one of 3 treadmill speeds: slow (their overground walking speed), fast (approximately 2 mph) and varied (0.5–2 mph) speeds for 30–60 minutes per session as tolerated for 3 sessions of BWSTT weekly for 4 weeks. All improved their overground speed, but the patients assigned to fast treadmill training at 2 mph increased overground walking speed by 30%–50%.[275] This approach also led to reorganization of activity in the supplementary motor cortex and primary sensorimotor cortex, as overground walking speed and selective control of ankle dorsiflexion improved (see Color Fig. 3–8 in separate color insert).[174,276]

Another study supports the positive impact of training at faster treadmill speeds. Pohl and colleagues randomized 60 ambulatory patients who were a mean of 16 weeks postonset of stroke to conventional gait training, treadmill training with incremental increases in speed of 10% within sessions and rising to as much as the subject could manage, or to treadmill walking with a maximum 5% per week increase in speed.[277] Subjects in the fast training group increased treadmill walking speeds by an average of 3.7 ± 1.9 times their initial speed. After 12 treatment sessions, this group achieved faster overground walking speeds (163 ± 80 cm/s) compared to the other 2 groups. The steady 5% increment group walked significantly faster (122 ± 74 cm/s) than the conventionally trained group (97 ± 64 cm/s). Stride length, cadence, and functional level for walking also significantly improved over conventional treatment. The maximum average belt speed for the last training session was 4.7 mph! Thus, training at walking speeds typical of at least the casual walking speed of healthy subjects, over 2 mph, may be essential, if faster overground walking is a goal of therapy.

Other treadmill studies of hemiparetic patients after stroke show that patients can safely exercise at a level of effort that provides a conditioning response[266] and that the energy cost of walking may decrease by approximately 50% as walking speeds increase from 0.4 to 1.5 meters/second.[278] This decline in energy cost especially holds for treadmill speeds ≥ 2 mph. As with any task-oriented approach, the intensity and specificity of practice drive functional gains for the practiced motor skill.[279] Body weight-supported treadmill training is also being combined with functional neuromuscular stimulation with surface[280] or implanted electrodes for patients with chronic stroke.[281] The results to date show modest improvements in walking speed and kinematics within subjects, but the design of clinical trials with the combined approach seems premature, given that the optimal use of BWSTT has not yet been demonstrated.

Additional trials that compare BWSTT to conventional methods are needed before the approach can be generally recommended. Attention must be given to the use of continued weight support to allow training at higher treadmill speeds (progressing patients up to at least 2 mph) and to the details of how the therapists cue their patients. A study of patients entered within the typical time frame of 10–15 days poststroke, inclusion of subjects who cannot yet step, a combination of inpatient and outpatient training for 8–12 weeks, and an intention-to-treat analysis may produce more generalizable results.[110]

Assistive Trainers

Robotic and other assistive training devices have also improved performance for reaching, usually in the plane of practice or across the joints most used (see Chapter 4).[244,282,283] Robotic trainers for walking (Fig. 4–2) are also being tested.[284] Trials that do not succeed in augmenting the amount of practice time generally produce negative results.[241] Functional electrical stimulation (FES) devices for hand grasp and opening (see Chapter 4) could also augment retraining, or simply allow greater functional use of a profoundly weakened hand.[285] Five weeks of FES may also reduce shoulder pain related to subluxation arising from paresis. The FES may improve shoulder function,[286] perhaps by allowing pain-free practice. Virtual reality systems that augment feedback about the position of the hand in space offer a potentially powerful form of practice for hemiparetic subjects. This computerized approach can be programmed to provide feedback information regarding knowledge of performance and knowledge of results using parameters such as velocity, trajectory, and accuracy of the reaching movement.

Unilateral and bimanual practice with the upper extremities may be enhanced with robotic and mechanical assistive devices. Devices aim to allow subjects to practice movements to increase motor control and functional use of the arm with only intermittent therapist oversight. The MIT-MANUS manipulates a patient's paretic elbow and shoulder much as a therapist might provide hand-over-hand therapy for reaching in a plane over a table.[283] The interactive device measures a subject's forearm motion and, when necessary, augments and completes a stereotyped movement that enables the subject to control an object on a computer monitor that provides visual feedback. In a randomized trial that began approximately 3 weeks after onset of stroke in 56 subjects undergoing inpatient rehabilitation, robot-trained subjects received approximately 25 hourly sessions and 1500 repetitions of assisted movement, whereas the control group used the device for the unaffected arm or with the affected arm without a robotic assist.[287] The robotic-trained group, which had significantly less motor and cognitive impairment by the FIM at the start, had a modest, but significantly greater increase in FIM motor score over the control group. The FIM tasks were not necessarily carried out by the affected arm, however. In addition, motor power and control improved at the shoulder and elbow with robotic training, consistent with the greater intensity of practice using those muscle groups. A device that could allow movement in multiple planes and incorporate the hand may be of yet greater value for training. Although a no-practice control may be

parent by 3 weeks and may last up to 3 months. Drawbacks of most trials include the failure to provide physical therapy to increase range of motion or strength after the injection, no benefit on functional use of the hand, and a change in the Ashworth score that has statistical, but not necessarily clinical significance. Gait speed may increase if pain is lessened or a foot flat phase in stance is achieved.

FUTURE STUDIES

These and other unpublished small trials raise the possibility that certain neuromodulators may be of value when given at some ideal interval after stroke, in a dose and frequency yet to be configured. The peak effect of a drug ought to coincide with a period of task-oriented therapy and intensive practice, if a mechanism related to enhancing learning underlies the efficacy of adjuvant treatment. Pharmacologic trials aimed at rehabilitation-related outcomes, however, are challenging to design and accomplish.

Entry criteria for trials to date have been too selective. Inclusion criteria should be broad and exclusion criteria minimal. Stratification by impairment levels may improve the power to detect differences among patients. Functional imaging may some day help screen subjects for whether a particular medication affects cerebral activity. After properly conducted imaging studies, this information may allow investigators to allocate only patients who have a particular pattern of postneuromodulator activation into a trial.

Most trials to date have focused upon a motor outcome. Future trials must also reveal gains in the functional activities related to what is practiced when the medication is on board.

Functional Electrical Stimulation

Electrical stimulation of the peroneal nerve to increase ankle dorsiflexion during the swing phase has been used for decades in some institutions, but has not come into wide use. An AFO usually substitutes quite well for walking, but may not encourage motor control timed to the gait cycle.

Many case studies of EMG-triggered neuromuscular stimulation have revealed modest gains in wrist extensor strength, but the change may not generalize to functional use of the affected hand. One theory behind the intervention is that when the subject initiates a slight contraction, followed by electrically induced contraction, sensorimotor integration may improve. Two randomized trials provided from 15 to 24 sessions of neuromuscular stimulation of the wrist and finger extensors during inpatient rehabilitation for stroke.[310,311] Functional wrist extension improved compared to routine therapy, but the positive effects did not persist by 24 weeks after stimulation stopped. Also, approximately 25% of subjects who received stimulation dropped out, mostly from pain induced by the electrical impulse. A randomized study of 11 subjects with chronic hemiparesis showed significantly better extensor strength when managed with movement-triggered electrical stimulation and, in a rare demonstration, this improved the ability to pick up small objects.[312] Orthotic devices (see Chapter 4) placed across the wrist have been designed to stimulate a grasp or pinch.[313,314] Better trials need to be designed.

Biofeedback

Biofeedback, particularly EMG BFB, has been used during inpatient therapy to increase or decrease selective muscle activity, but has found its greatest use during outpatient care (see Chapter 5). Feedback plays an important role in learning motor skills. It improves error detection and correction, helps guide the patient towards the desired movement, and motivates the patient. Biofeedback should work best for motor learning in a task-specific paradigm. The clinical value of the approach, however, is moot.

A meta-analysis of EMG BFB for neuromuscular reeducation of the arm or leg included 8 randomized or matched control group studies with 190 patients. It found a significant range of gains in a variety of outcome measures.[315] Range of motion on the affected side appeared to benefit from EMG BFB in another meta-analysis of the literature.[316] However, this type of analysis, the quality of the studies included, and the clinical significance of the outcome measures leave the efficacy of BFB still in doubt. Blinded outcome measures, dropouts, and lack of control subjects also limit any interpretation. A more strict meta-analysis of 79 studies of EMG BFB for the lower extremity found 8 that met reasonable citeria for design. The only outcome superior to conventional therapy was strength of ankle dorsiflexion in ambulating subjects.[317] The analysis suggested that larger numbers of patients with stroke in well-designed trials may be able to show efficacy for the pattern and speed of walking. Activation of the tibialis anterior for foot clearance and of the gastrocnemius-soleus muscles for push off are prime targets for improving the gait pattern.

Many of the studies of its use for the upper extremity suggest that BFB may improve performance during training, but not necessarily when visual or auditory guidance stop. An intermittent, rather than continuous feedback schedule may increase the likelihood of transfer of the training to the non-EMG BFB condition. Other results raise the issue of whether EMG feedback is likely to be more or less useful than, say, kinematic or kinetic feedback. Although approaches have been as creative as electromyography-triggered electrical stimulation of the wrist and finger extensor muscles,[311,312,318] no single paradigm has been proven to be efficacious for a particular population and for improving functional reaching, gripping or pinching. Some techniques may impede gains. For example, in a single training session of pursuit tracking movements in 16 hemiparetic subjects, continuous EMG BFB from the spastic elbow flexors did not improve tracking any more than the control group's performance. Indeed it negatively affected the transfer of gains in speed and accuracy when the BFB was discontinued.[319] Electromyographic BFB that aimed to reduce activity in a cocontracting muscle and recruit activity in the agonist was compared to having the paretic arm copy the output during movements of the same muscles of the unaffected arm.[320] The investigators found no clear differences in the integrated EMG from each proximal and distal muscle, in joint range of motion, or in the time taken to complete specific functional tasks.

A 6-week randomized trial for gait dysfunction compared a control group with groups receiving one of 3 interventions: EMG BFB, FES, and FES plus BFB.[321] With only 8 subjects in each group, the investigators found a significantly better outcome on 2 measures in the FES-plus-BFB group compared to the control group, but no differences between the control and other groups. Even this one positive finding may have been related to chance alone, given the multiple outcome measures. On the other hand, the sample size may not have been large enough to detect differences, if they ex-

isted. Another approach converted the EMG signal for a normal person's muscle activation pattern during gait to a changing sound pitch. The investigators asked the hemiparetic subjects to match the timing of the sounds throughout their own gait cycle.[322] This BFB led to a reduction of the flexor synergy through relaxation of the tibialis anterior at onset of the swing phase, but changes are difficult to interpret without a control group. Audio monitoring of the EMG signal did decrease foot-drop during the swing phase after 15 training sessions in a small experimental group compared to a group of chronic stroke patients treated with the Bobath method alone, although step length and velocity did not change.[323]

Feedback from changes in the joint angles of the leg has also shown promise in improving hemiplegic gait. In a randomized study of 26 patients with recent stroke who ambulated with standby help, electrogoniometric BFB was used during training for stance and gait to correct genu recurvatum.[324] An auditory signal activated at the moment of hyperextension increased in pitch proportional to the degree of recurvatum. The BFB led to a statistically significant reduction in knee hyperextension over the subsequent 4 weeks of physical therapy, compared to the group that had physical therapy without BFB for 8 weeks. Gait velocity and level of independence in this small group did not improve.

Thus, BFB for specific hemiplegic motor problems can complement the training of discrete motor control for gait. Larger controlled clinical trials with well-defined paradigms and outcome measures that establish whether gains carry over to real-world settings when BFB is discontinued will determine whether the approach plays a more important role in stroke rehabilitation.

Acupuncture

Acupuncture has been used in China for managing acute stroke and for rehabilitation for centuries, but modern reports from Asia are, at best, descriptive of poorly measured changes in uncontrolled trials.[325] Possible mechanisms for a positive effect include the special attention given to the acupuncture patients, effects of the release of systemic or CNS peptides and neurotransmitters on neuronal networks, and the greater sensory stimulation that may, for example, modulate the size of neuronal representational sensorimotor maps. Acupuncture appeared to improve motor impairments or functional outcomes in several quasi-experimental and randomized clinical trials.[326–330]

Two well-designed randomized trials that used a sham procedure did not find any benefit on ADLs.[331,332] One of the research groups had previously reported significant improvements in ADLs and motor function based on a similar approach, but that study had not included a sham or alternative intervention.[333] Treatments have been given from 2 to 4 times a week for up to several months and all studies claim to employ traditional oriental acupuncture points. A randomized trial of acupuncture with 106 Chinese patients in Hong Kong stratified subjects based on severity of impairment from 3 to 15 days after a stroke.[334] All patients received inpatient rehabilitation. The experimental group received 5 sessions a week during inpatient care and 3 sessions a week during outpatient care for a mean of 35 sessions in 10 weeks. Ten acupoints were needled, but not the scalp. The blinded observers found no differences in outcomes at 10 weeks on the Fugl-Meyer Assessment or the FIM. A review of 9 Western controlled trials with 538 patients, carried out by investigators from a department of complementary medicine in Britain, concluded that no compelling evidence shows acupuncture to be effective for the rehabilitation of stroke.[335] Despite 12 positive randomized trials reported in the Chinese literature,[334] the results of very well-designed clinical trials do not support the use of this intervention.

Whereas sensory stimulation may alter cortical reorganization, acupuncture, electroacupuncture, and transcutaneous stimulation may not drive activity-dependent plasticity unless combined with skills learning. If extrinsic cortical stimulation can drive activity-dependent plasticity, perhaps this can only be demonstrated by direct electrical stimulation of the primary sensorimotor cortex or of a peripheral nerve during training.

TRIALS OF INTERVENTIONS FOR APHASIA

Across a range of studies, 20%–40% of acute stroke patients have impaired language at onset and 10%–20% of long-term survivors remain aphasic. Poor communication skills have a negative impact on mood, new learning, socialization, quality of life, and caregiver burden. Chapter 5 reviews the traditional aphasic syndromes (see Table 5–5) and therapeutic approaches.

Although speech therapy may offer a psychotherapeutic benefit, the randomized trial of language therapy from Lincoln and colleagues revealed no differences in measures of the mood of treated and untreated patients and their families.[336] Only 10% of patients were rated as depressed, but nearly half the spouses had depressive symptoms 22 weeks after the stroke. The investigators found no relationship between the Porch Index of Communicative Abilities (PICA) score and mood. A case control study, however, found minor or severe depression in 70% of aphasic and 46% of nonaphasic patients 3 months after a stroke and a significantly greater incidence of depression in aphasic patients at 12 months.[337] Depressed aphasic patients had significantly greater handicap and disability than aphasic patients who were not depressed. Thus, trials for aphasia may need to include the management of depression and monitor for success.

Rate of Gains

A British health district of 250,000 people detected 202 cases of aphasia per year. By 1 month poststroke, the 165 who had survived, but had not recovered, were candidates for speech therapy.[338] Wade and colleagues screened over 900 consecutive acute stroke patients in a British health district using a simple battery to test comprehension, expression, reading, and writing.[339] The investigators found that at least 24% of testable patients were aphasic in the first week, 20% at 3 weeks, and only 12% of survivors remained aphasic at 6 months. Thus, approximately 40% who tested as being aphasic at 3 weeks after onset recovered by 6 months. Of relevance to other studies, 44% of patients and 57% of caregivers thought that speech was still abnormal.

The community-based Copenhagen Stroke Study reported that 38% of 881 patients were aphasic on admission and 20% of the admissions were rated as severe, based on the SSS.[340] Nearly one-half of the severe aphasics died early after onset and one-half of the mild aphasics recovered by 1 week. Only 18% of community survivors were still aphasic at the time of their acute and rehabilitation hospital discharge. Up to 28% received early speech therapy as needed. Patients were retested for 6 months. The best predictor of recovery was a less severe aphasia close to the time of the stroke. Ninety-five percent with a mild aphasia reached their best level of recovery by 2 weeks, with a moderate aphasia by 6 weeks, and with severe aphasia by 10 weeks. Only 8% of the severe aphasic patients fully recovered on the scoring system by 6 months. Mild language deficits and changes below the limited sensitivity of the SSS were not ascertained. Functional communication was not assessed. The reported peak time to maximum gains should not imply that aphasic patients cannot improve in aspects of comprehension and expression for months or years after onset.

Over the range of aphasia severities found by testing with the PICA, patients in a typical series improve in total scores throughout the 1st year after a stroke and then level off during the 2nd year.[341] Most gains in overall function are made in the first 3 months, except for global aphasics, who tend to improve in more subtle ways over a longer time.[342,343] In the first 3 months, aphasic patients from a stroke tend to improve by a fixed amount, rather than in proportion to the initial severity of aphasia.[344]

Prognosticators

The best outcomes, as expected, come to patients with the least severe aphasia near the time of the stroke. Age, gender, and handedness matter less than the extent and location of the injury, the severity of language impairments at onset, and the degree of recovery by 1 month after onset.[345] A few individual features of aphasia, such as agnosia for environmental sounds, serve as a poor prognostic sign for gains in comprehension.

A few studies offer insights into gains over time. Helm-Estabrooks and colleagues tested 17 patients with severe global aphasia and 5 patients with severe Wernicke's aphasia starting 1 to 2 months after onset.[341] The investigators monitored the patients with the Boston Assessment of Severe Aphasia (BASA) at 6-month intervals for 2 years. Higher subscores for praxis (the ability to carry out bucco-facial and limb commands) and for oral and gestural expression at 6 months best predicted overall BASA performance at 24 months. Praxis improved significantly in the first 6 months, whereas reading and auditory comprehension scores increased between 6 and 12 months. Language gains, then, may continue over several years. Some global aphasics evolve into less severe forms of a nonfluent aphasia, but most remain within the same classification.[346] Most long-term studies of aphasia recovery suggest that auditory comprehension tends to improve more than speech output across all aphasics.[347]

LOCATION OF LESIONS

Anatomic neuroimaging sometimes provides insights about recovery. Single-word and sentence level comprehension appear especially likely to improve by 1–2 years in the global aphasic whose frontoparietal infarct extends only to the isthmus of the subcortical temporal lobe, compared to having a lesion that includes at least half of Wernicke's area (BA 22).[348] On an axial CT scan, this sparing corresponds to the temporal lobe seen from the level of the maximum width of the third ventricle to its roof, often visualized with the pineal gland. Wernicke's aphasics also tend to have better recovery of auditory comprehension by 6 to 12 months if less than half of Wernicke's cortical area is infarcted.[349] These patients may develop a milder fluent aphasia, such as a conduction or anomic aphasia.

Patients with aphasia involving Broca's area also recover in ways that are partly predicted by analyzing the location of the injury and its language sequelae. For example, many of the variations in the nonfluent aphasic person's speech and language arise from differential lesions of the frontal operculum, the lower motor cortex, and subjacent subcortical and periventricular white matter.[350] Damage to the frontal operculum affects its function as an integrator for the limbic activational aspects of speech, the posterior temporal and inferior parietal semantic inputs for language, and the frontal motor areas for planning. The resultant impairment may not be permanent, however. The finding of sparse and effortful speech, along with dysnomia and semantic paraphasias, involves more extensive damage to adjacent cortex and white matter projecting from limbic and posterior language-associated regions.

Lesion localization may help predict the response to a specific intervention for aphasia. In patients who have a chronic, profound aphasia with no meaningful spontaneous speech, certain lesion patterns correspond to the ability to train and respond to nonverbal, icon-based computer assisted visual communication programs (see Chapter 5).[351] For example, patients with the best response spare either large regions within Wernicke's area and its temporal isthmus or portions of the anterior language regions such as the supplementary motor cortex and cingulate gyrus in area 24, which are motor and limbic-related regions.

Acute stroke structural assessments by magnetic resonance imaging are complemented by diffusion-weighted and perfusion-weighted (PWI) imaging. The volume of relative hypoperfusion on PWI or the diffusion-perfusion mismatch in patients with acute stroke affecting Wernicke's area predicted errors in spoken word comprehension.[352] The relative delay in regional blood flow may parallel the magnitude of impairment of the cognitive and language function attributed to the region.

METABOLIC IMAGING

Resting and especially activation studies using PET and fMRI reveal changes over time in both hemispheres that parallel improvements or the failure to improve in language tasks after a stroke (see Chapter 3). These approaches may reveal functional reorganization as a subject practices a specific language task.[353] As an overall summary, preilesional activation in the affected language cortex is most important for gains of speech and language that follows a focal injury. Homologous cortical regions of the unaffected, usually right hemisphere may play a role in long-term reorganization and gains, though activations most often arise in patients with limited gains.[354,355] For example, in patients with aphasia of all types who could speak spontaneously, a higher left hemisphere regional metabolic rate for glucose by PET during speech activation at 2 weeks postonset strongly predicted a better recovery at 4 months.[356] In patients with moderate to severe impairments within 3 weeks of a stroke, receptive language dysfunction that persisted for 2 years on the Token Test correlated with low metabolic rates for glucose in the superior temporal cortex.[357] Poor word fluency correlated

with low rates in the left prefrontal cortex. These findings are consistent with the contribution of these regions to the neurocognitive networks for comprehension and speech production (see Chapter 1).

Transcranial doppler insonation of the middle cerebral artery during a word-fluency task may also help predict gains. An increase in the mean flow velocity between rest and the task in the left hemisphere was associated with gains in language with rehabilitation 2 months later.

Results of Interventions

Studies of the efficacy of aphasia therapy after a stroke have usually set out to learn whether nonspecific approaches improve language functions. Most studies suffer from the methodological shortcomings found in clinical trials of stroke rehabilitation interventions for mobility and self-care. Design problems include the lack of randomized controls, failure to stratify subjects by particular aphasia syndromes, inadequate assessment of the extent of the cortical and subcortical lesion or of the presence of a contralateral lesion that might affect compensation, and assessment and outcome tools of uncertain precision and reliability. In addition, studies include wide variations among patients in the time since onset of stroke, in age and education, and in comorbidities that affect cognition and learning. The investigators may not specify the type, intensity, or duration of language therapy. Also, aphasia assessment tests often do not reflect changes in functional communication with family and friends. By reporting an overall outcome score, investigators may not detect clinically important gains in language and nonlanguage subskills.

Table 9–13 summarizes some of the better designed, large clinical trials of aphasia therapy for stroke. Treatments averaged 45 to 60 minutes, provided up to 3 times a week in most instances. Dropouts were due to illness, death, disenchantment with the program, or satisfaction with the level of recovery. Overall, subjects showed average gains of 20% in scores on the Functional Communication Profile (FCP) and a 10–20 percentile change on the PICA. Aphasics improved on test scores spontaneously and with nonspecific, traditional interventions. Gen-

Table 9–13. Clinical Trials of General Aphasia Therapy After Stroke

Trial	Comparison (No. Subjects)	Intervention	Duration of Therapy	Outcomes	Comments
Basso et al.[507]	Traditional therapy, emphasis on verbal responses (162) versus no therapy (119)	<2 months: 137 / 2–6 months: 86 / >6 months: 58	≥3 therapies/week × 6 months	On standard tests: gains in expression and comprehension in therapy groups	Not randomized; 85% had a stroke
David et al.[508]	Traditional therapy (71) versus untrained volunteer support (84)	Median: 4 weeks; range: >50 weeks	2 therapies/week × 15–20 weeks	On FCP: no difference in gains	Randomized; 30% dropout; poorly defined cases
Shewan and Kertesz[347]	Linguistic (25) versus facilitation by therapist (25); versus stimulation by trained nurse (25) versus no treatment (25)	2–4 weeks	Therapy to maximum gain or 1 year (mean = 68 therapies)	On WAB: therapy groups gains are greater than no therapy group	Subgroups too small to see therapy group differences; auditory comprehension changed the least
Lincoln et al.[509]	Traditional therapy (104) versus no therapy (87)	10 weeks	2 therapies/week × 24 weeks	On PICA and FCP: no difference	15% dropout; many received less than planned therapies; in 47 matched pairs who completed >50% of therapy: no difference
Wertz et al.[510]	Traditional therapy (29) versus therapy with a trained family (36) versus deferred 12 weeks then traditional therapy (29)	7 ± 6 weeks	8–10 hours/week × 12 weeks	On PICA: traditional therapy was better than no therapy at 12 weeks; no difference in gains between groups at 24 weeks	23% dropout; no harm apparent for delayed therapy
Hartman and Laudau[511]	Traditional therapy (30) versus supportive conversation (30)	1 month	2 therapies/week × 6 months	On PICA: no difference in gains at 7 and 10 months	Equal gains in fluent and nonfluent cases

FCP, Functional Communication Profile; WAB, Western Aphasia Battery; PICA, Porch Index of Communicative Abilities.

eral gains continued for 6 months. These studies did not examine whether different patterns of improvement arose from each therapeutic approach.

A meta-analysis performed on 55 interventional trials of speech/language therapy in aphasic patients after stroke offers insights into the effectiveness of language therapies.[358] Significant gains were found for treated over untreated patients at all stages of recovery. The benefit appeared most evident in patients who started speech therapy soon after their stroke. Treatments in excess of 2 hours per week gave greater gains than lesser amounts of therapy. Severe aphasics improved when treated by a speech-language pathologist, rather then by family or assistants. Only one defined intervention, multimodal stimulation, was tested in enough cases to show its greater average effect. Any differential effects of treatment for differing types of aphasia could not be assessed since too few studies have been published. Indeed, after reviewing 60 studies done through 2000 and examining the best 12, the Cochrane Library's sytematic review of group trials in stroke (http://update-software.com/cochrane.htm) concludes that speech and language therapy for aphasic people after stroke has not been shown to be clearly effective or ineffective within a randomized clinical trial.[359]

INTENSITY AND SPECIFICITY OF INTERVENTIONS

The modest, sometimes equivocal effects of conventional therapy suggest the need to find techniques to assess and treat better defined types of communication disorders. Single-case and small group studies have shown that interventions developed for specific impairments can improve outcomes beyond the time of spontaneous improvements. The intensity and specificity of practice may be most important in testing the efficacy of a particular language intervention. For example, a well-designed study employed a picture card game in which a group of aphasic subjects were prompted to request and provide a card of depicted objects in their hands. The results suggest that, compared to less intensive and formalized therapy, behaviorally relevant mass practice for at least 3 hours a day for 10 days that constrains the use of nonverbal communication and rein-

forces appropriate responses within a group setting can improve comprehension and naming skills.[360]

A multiple baselines study of moderate aphasic patients from 6 to 12 months after a stroke tested a specific lexical and a nonlexical therapy to improve written naming and writing words from dictation.[361] Significant gains in writing tasks were made after 20 to 24 treatment sessions lasting 1 hour over 5 to 6 weeks of each intervention, including improved functional communication by reading and writing, but not for oral language. Computer software offers the opportunity for intensive practice. An uncontrolled case series of chronic aphasic patients showed that repetitive practice with a therapist and at home with a microcomputer-based symbolic language device improved performance on several language tests.[362] A visual iconic computer-based interface also improved the ability of chronic aphasic subjects to relearn the use of past tense verbs and to comprehend passive-voiced sentences, pointing to an approach to lessen agrammatism and syntactic deficits.[363] Generalization to other language tasks should not be anticipated, given that a focused intervention will be constrained by the overall pattern of impairments for each aphasic patient.

More work is needed to test such specific approaches and determine whether they allow practical gains in social communication (see Chapter 5). In addition, the cortical responses to an intervention may be monitored during activation studies using functional neuroimaging (see Chapter 3).[353,364,365] This potential means of physiologic monitoring may help guide the applicability of a particular intervention.

Pharmacotherapy

Clinical trials in modest numbers of patients with amphetamine,[366] piracetam,[364,367] and cholinergic[368] and dopaminergic[369,370] agents have shown suggestive efficacy for particular aphasic syndromes and language impairments. The neurotransmitter systems stimulated by such drugs affect a variety of pathways for attention, memory, reward, and learning (see Chapter 1).[371–373] The decrease in hesitations and better word finding reported in some trials may arise from drug-induced increases in activity in dopaminergic and noradrenergic pathways for arousal, attention, and intention, after interruption of projections from the ventral tegmental tract and from diffuse frontal projections. These drugs may also alter mood.

DOPAMINERGIC AGENTS

Several open label, uncontrolled small group studies suggested that bromocriptine, in an average dose of 30 mg, or with carbidopa/levodopa, may improve the fluency of chronic, moderately affected patients with Broca's and transcortical motor aphasia.[374,375] Bromocriptine, 15 mg, improved word retrieval deficits in 4 patients with chronic nonfluent aphasia in a 10-week, ABBA design (see Chapter 7).[370] Subjects did not receive therapy. A placebo-controlled trial using 15 mg of bromocriptine in 20 chronic nonfluent aphasics, however, reported no change in speech, language, and cognitive skills.[369] Hemidystonia on the paretic side, sometimes with painful spasms, developed in 5 of 7 chronic nonfluent aphasic subjects given from 30 mg to 60 mg of bromocriptine daily.[376]

NORADRENERGIC AGENTS

A randomized trial stratified 21 moderate and severe aphasic patients within 2–6 weeks after a stroke to 10 treatments of 10 mg of dextroamphetamine or to placebo for 5 weeks.[366] Subjects received 1 hour of stimulation/facilitation speech therapy approximately a $\frac{1}{2}$ hour after receiving a pill and a total of approximately 30 hours of speech therapy during the trial. The investigators screened 859 subjects for inclusion over 4 years. One week after conclusion of the interventions, the dextroamphetamine group scored significantly better on the PICA. Gains persisted 6 months later. The optimal dose and timing of the noradrenergic agent and its efficacy is a work in progress. The noradrenergic agent may improve cortical signal-to-noise ratio and working memory.[373]

CHOLINERGIC AGENTS

Piracetam, a derivative of γ-aminobutyric acid, but with no GABA activity, may facilitate cholinergic and aminergic neurotransmission. This nootropic agent has been available in Eu-

rope for several decades. The drug did not alter outcomes when employed within 12 hours of acute stroke, although the subgroup of patients with aphasia performed better.[377] A randomized, placebo-controlled trial included 50 moderately aphasic patients who had a stroke more than 1 month (mean of 10 months) before starting the 6-week intervention of 10 hours of speech therapy weekly.[367] The drug-treated group had a significantly better total score on the Aachen Aphasia Test, though the clinical impact is not clear. In a randomized trial of 24 patients, piracetam was also associated with some language subtest gains, as well as higher left language area cerebral blood flow during a word repetition task.[364] Other cholinergic agents improved naming in moderately severe Wernicke's aphasic patients, especially by reducing perseveration.

These studies suggest that intensive therapy combined with a drug that enhances vigilance or learning may benefit patients who have adequate language comprehension.

TRIALS FOR COGNITIVE AND AFFECTIVE DISORDERS

From anosognosia to dementia, from not shaving one side of the face to mistaking a wife for a hat, cerebrovascular disease produces as many neuropsychologic sequelae as clinicians can differentiate. Subtle and profound cognitive disorders increase disability and limit gains in mobility, ADLs, and social reintegration. After discharge from inpatient rehabilitation, patients and their families often become aware of modest cognitive limitations, but they cannot always articulate what is wrong. The paucity of brief, uniform, standardized tests with alternate forms that can be given serially to a predominantly elderly population makes the formal investigation of cognitive dysfunction difficult.

Cognitive disorders are common after ischemic stroke and can be formidable after subarachnoid hemorrhage. A prospective study of 227 patients in New York City with ischemic stroke revealed cognitive impairments 3 months after onset in 35% of patients and 4% of controls.[378] Memory, orientation, language, and attention were most often affected, especially following large dominant and nondominant hemisphere infarcts. As in other studies, greater intellectual impairment correlated with dependent living after hospitalization, even after adjusting for age and physical impairment. Impairment in performing sequential tasks such as the Trailmaking Test B correlated with lesser quality of life on the Sickness Impact Profile 9 months after stroke in patients living at home with a mean age of 56 years.[379] A South African study of 955 alert, mostly impoverished patients found cognitive impairments in 64% at admission for stroke using a standard set of bedside tests.[380] The impairments included aphasia in 25%, apraxia in 15%, memory impairments in 12%, and executive dysfunction in 9%. Twenty-two percent of affected patients had no sensorimotor or visual field deficit.

The Canadian Study of Health and Aging found vascular cognitive impairment without dementia to be the most prevalent type of vascular cognitive impairment in people age 65–85 years, affecting 26 per 1000 persons.[381] Vascular dementia affects 15 per 1000 people, Alzheimer's disease with a vascular component affects approximately 9, and Alzheimer's disease alone affects 51. The burden of the vascular impairments is high, carrying a significant risk for death and institutionalization compared to people the same age who have normal cognition.

Prior to a clinically evident stroke, some patients will have had silent infarcts, appreciated by imaging studies (Fig. 9–1). Premorbid lesions that partially disconnect neurocognitive networks can lessen the patient's ability to compensate for the new stroke or produce greater dysfunction than expected from the location of the new injury. A community study of subjects who were approximately 70 years old and free of stroke showed that risk factors for cerebrovascular disease independently correlated with impaired abstract reasoning, memory, and visuospatial function.[382] Silent strokes presumably led to these impairments and to greater risk for a stroke.[383]

Memory Disorders

Patients are called upon to encode and retrieve new information during rehabilitation. Memory disturbances may have a proportionately negative influence on the compensatory learning that underlies much of the rehabilitation process.

INCIDENCE AND PREVALENCE

The incidence and risk factors for memory loss and for dementia caused by one or more strokes have become increasingly appreciated.[378,381,384–386] Up to 30% of all stroke survivors have a disturbance in memory. In a population study, dementia was 9 times greater in the 1st year after a stroke compared to the expected incidence in an age-controlled group and twice the risk for the stroke population each subsequent year.[387] In other community-based studies, the incidence ranged from 15% to 30% within 3 months to 1 year after a stroke and 33% within 5 years.[386,388,389] In a prospective follow-up of 169 patients who had a stroke, but no dementia by testing, 29% were diagnosed with a dementia by the 3rd yearly evaluation.[390] Most cases were apparent by 6 months after the stroke. Vascular dementia accounted for two-thirds of cases. Independent predictors of dementia included greater age, diabetes mellitus, silent infarcts (leuokoaraiosis) on imaging, some cognitive disturbance at entry, and the severity of the impairments from the stroke. The frequency of dementia across studies varies with the definition used to designate a dementia.

Wade and colleagues followed a community cohort of 138 3-month survivors of stroke who were not too confused or aphasic to participate. This restriction eliminated 50 of their initial cases.[391] Using the Wechsler Memory Scale subtests, these investigators found no difference in immediate digit span recall when patients were compared to age-matched healthy persons. Abnormally low scores were found, however, in 29% on the immediate recall of a story on the Logical Memory test, as well as in 39% on drawing four shapes recently presented, a visual memory test. Delayed recall at 30 minutes correlated with immediate recall impairments. Significant improvements were made in these two tests by 6 months after the stroke. Poor visual recall or a related cognitive ability not directly assessed, such as visuoperception, was associated with poor performance of ADLs. The Oxfordshire Stroke Project found that 14% of 328 long-term stroke survivors were severely impaired on the Rivermead Behavioral Memory Test at a mean of 4 years after their stroke.[4] None of the control group scored as poorly.

LESION-RELATED IMPAIRMENTS

Specific disorders in memory have been related to the location of the infarction. For example, left cerebral lesions tend to affect verbal recall while right-sided lesions can diminish visual memory. Even a mild aphasia may affect verbal memory and interfere with verbal learning during rehabilitation.[392] The number and location of subcortical ischemic lesions found on CT scan has been associated with poorer scores on neuropsychologic tests.[393] Impairments of visuospatial function and concentration were significantly related to the number of small lesions (an average of three). Periventricular lucencies and ventricular enlargement corresponded most to impaired performance on tests that depended upon memory and language. Lesions in the caudate nucleus and basal ganglia often cause memory impairment.[151] Bilateral posterior cerebral artery infarctions that damage the hippocampi or their immediate connections may cause antegrade and retrograde memory impairment. Indeed, cognitive impairment on neuropsychologic testing across all domains may better correlate with a decrease in hippocampal and cortical gray matter volume in patients with vascular dementia and Alzheimer's disease than the presence of subcortical lacunes.[394] The volume of white matter lesions in 157 subjects who had no dementia, some impairment, or dementia was a better indicator of cognitive impairment than the presence of subcortical lacunes.

Confabulation

Antegrade and sometimes lesser retrograde amnesia with confabulation may follow the rupture of an anterior communicating artery aneurysm, along with a wide range of other cognitive impairments.[395] Figure 3–4 shows an orbitofrontal medial infarction accompanied by spontaneous confabulation in a patient with almost no retention of new information. The profound deficit persisted more than a year following the rupture and clipping of an anterior communicating aneurysm. The patient failed tests of new learning, acted on the basis of past memories and habits, could not attend to current information, composed details in a fluid,

if chaotic fashion drawn from elements of events that preceded the stroke, and could not suppress evoked, often inaccurate memories that were not relevant to present conversation.[396,397] The PET scan (Color Fig. 3–4 in separate color insert) reveals the functional anatomy of this impairment; the left frontal lobe and its subcortical connections with the basal ganglia and thalamus are profoundly hypometabolic. Irle and colleagues[398] found severe mnemonic impairments when inferior and medial frontal lesions included more than 1 cm of the head of the caudate nucleus, extended into the anterior limb of the internal capsule, and damaged the cholinergic cells of the diagonal band of Broca, the substantia innominata, and the ventral striatum. Bromo-criptine, but not noradrenergic or cholinergic medications, improved learning in a patient with a mediobasal forebrain injury by enhancing the ability to make verbal associations after a confined mediobasal forebrain injury.[399] Other impairments from limited lesions that selectively interfere with a particular neurotransmitter projection might partially respond to drug interventions.

INTERVENTIONS

The optimal rehabilitation strategy to enhance learning after a stroke depends upon the type and severity of memory, attention, or other cognitive processes affected. In general, patients after stroke have good motor learning abilities,[240,400] but more frequent feedback or errorless learning may improve retention in patients who have difficulty retaining new information during their rehabilitation. Cognitive remediation for memory disorders involves the training of compensatory strategies such as rehearsal, visual imagery, semantic elaboration, and memory aids including notebooks, calendars, and electronic devices. Procedural learning often proceeds better than declarative learning. In normal subjects who are learning a new skill, constant feedback enhances immediate performance, but an intermittent schedule of reinforcement that allows errors and gradual processing of how to perform may improve long-term retention. Amnestic subjects and at least some subjects with impaired episodic memory do worse with trial-and-error training. More frequent feedback and errorless learning may improve retention.[401] The spontaneous confabulator cannot respond to these compensatory approaches until able to suppress chaotic, self-certain evoked memories.

Anticholinesterase inhibitors have been less effectve on improving memory in patients with vascular-related cognitive dysfunction compared to their benefits in patients with Alzheimer's disease, but clinical trials that include the use of donezepil are ongoing. Most of the drugs that have been tried for treating Alzheimer's disease, such as hydergine, piracetam, and ginkgo biloba, have been tried in patients with vascular dementia with about as little success.[402] Pharmacologic memory molecules will also come to clinical trials (see Chapter 2).

Visuospatial and Attentional Disorders

Patients with left hemineglect may nonchalantly push their wheelchairs into a wall or run over a person on the unattended side, smack into doorway frames, look off to the right to find a voice that comes from their left, ignore food on the left side of a plate, and finish shaving with cream still matted to the left side of the face. The families of these patients smile at the quirky errors, and despair.

Clinical findings include hemispatial neglect, hemibody neglect, hemiakinesia, extinction of simultaneous stimuli, and anosognosia, the denial of impairment. Hemispatial neglect in patients with right cerebral lesions may be accompanied by impairments in facial recognition and in producing or appreciating emotionally toned speech. The presence of aphasia can limit testing for any of these disturbances. Severe left visual neglect in peripersonal space can coexist with minimal inattention to items in extrapersonal space.[403] Hemisensory and visual field impairments often accompany neglect and anosognosia, but are not essential.[404] Some patients with neglect sit with their trunks leaning toward their affected side, although their strength is no worse than patients who sit in the midline and do not have a neglect syndrome.[405]

LESION-RELATED IMPAIRMENTS

Directed attention arise from within distributed parallel neural networks of the parietal, frontal, and cingulate cortices, along with subcortical structures that include the striatum, superior colliculus, reticular formation, and anterior thalamus (see Chapter 1). Destruction or disconnection of components produces both overlapping and clinically distinct symptoms and signs. Unilateral neglect arises from injuries of the posterior parietal cortex, the prefrontal cortex that encompasses the frontal eye fields, and the cingulate gyrus. These regions include representations for sensory integration, for motor activities such as visual scanning and limb exploration, and for motivational relevance, respectively. Contralesional attentional neglect is most associated with parietal lesions. Patients are unaware of stimuli or the stimuli are less salient. Contralesional intentional neglect tends to occur with frontal lesions. Patients have a directional or hemispatial hypokinesia or even akinesia.

Lesions of the right inferior parietal lobule (BA 39 and 40) are particularly associated with neglect. This region appears necessary for awareness of external stimuli and serves as a critical node in the modular cortical-limbic-reticular network that directs attention.[406,407] Incoming and outgoing neural activity in this posterior region helps integrate the localization and identification of a stimulus, as well its importance to the person. Subcortical areas such as the thalamus, the striatum, and the superior colliculus interact with these networked cortical regions, perhaps coordinating the distribution of attention, so lesions in these areas may also cause impairment.

Atrophy of frontal white matter and the diencephalon contributes to persistent anosognosia.[408] The anterior and posterior extent of a lesion may augment impairments in attentional and intentional processes that contribute to neglect.[409]

INCIDENCE

A community-based study of 281 3-week survivors of a first stroke who had only unilateral signs detected visual neglect in approximately 10%.[410] Subjects were tested for their ability to copy a Greek Cross and to use visual reasoning to complete the Raven's Colored Progressive Matrices. Only about one-half had a hemianopsia or visual extinction. The neglect was modestly associated with poorer ADL scores and slower recovery. Severe neglect was rare beyond 6 months. The NINDS Stroke Data Bank also looked at the effect of hemineglect on the ADL scores at 7 to 10 days and

1 year after onset of a first stroke.[411] Patients who had anosognosia, visual neglect, tactile extinction, motor impersistence or auditory neglect had the lowest BI scores at 1 year, as low as aphasic and hemiplegic patients, even after adjusting the data for initial ADL scores and for poststroke rehabilitation. Another large study found visual neglect in 38% of 150 consecutive patients with moderate disability after a new stroke, but severe neglect rarely persisted beyond 6 months.[412]

In a serial follow-up study of patients with right hemispheric stroke, recovery occurred in unilateral spatial neglect tested by drawing in 70% by week 13 and in anosognosia and neglect in nearly all by week 20. The mean time to recovery of hemineglect was 11 weeks.[135] Visual neglect, documented on a battery of 7 tests by 3 days after a stroke, was greater in right than left hemisphere lesions.[413] In this report and others, right-sided inattention on testing has been detected in 15%–40% of non-aphasic patients with acute left cerebral infarcts, although the attentional deficit is clinically most prominent after a right brain injury. Recovery was most rapid within 10 days, regardless of side of stroke, and plateaued at 3 months, when most patients had little visual neglect. Severe visual neglect and anosognosia at 3 days was a predictor for persistent impairment at 6 months. Only 14 out of 84 patients with initial neglect showed moderate or severe dependence in ADLs on the BI in follow-up.[414] Interventional studies ought to consider matching subjects by scores on this test battery and by the time from onset of stroke to the time of testing.

Unilateral neglect, then, has multiple components. When the most clinically obvious components resolve, the patient may seem cured. However, many patients have lingering impairments. The detection and grading of a hemi-inattention syndrome depend on features of the test. For example, early after a right hemisphere stroke, a group of patients with stroke showed a strong and consistent rightward attentional bias in addition to an inability to reorient their attention leftward.[415] Twelve months later, the attentional bias continued, but the patients could fully reorient to left hemispace when performing line bisection and cancellation tasks. Unilateral spatial neglect is associated with sensorimotor and cognitive impairments and disabilities in ADLs and instrumental ADLs that are not found in patients with right hemisphere lesions who can attend to the left.[416] Patients with ongoing spatial neglect always require a caregiver.

INTERVENTIONS

Table 9–14 includes a range of interventions, most of them used in only a handful of subjects in any one study. For most of these clever treatment approaches, however, benefit is modest or may not last much longer than the active intervention. The choice of interventions is based upon the theory of unilateral spatial neglect that best applies to the patient.[417,418] Treatments may aim to engage attention to the left, disengage attention to the right, shift spatial coordinates to the left, and increase arousal.

Table 9–14. **Interventions Employed to Reduce Hemi-inattention**

Multisensory visual and sensory cues, then fading cues[422]

Verbal elaboration of visual analysis[400]

Left limb movement in left hemispace[412,430]

Head and trunk midline rotation[405,429,432,433,512]

Visual imagery[513]

Environmental adaptations—bed position,[434] red ribbon at left margin of printed page

Video feedback[514]

Monocular and binocular patches[437,441,442,515]

Prisms[437,438]

Left frontal transcranial magnetic stimulation[450]

Vestibular caloric stimulation[447–449]

Left optokinetic stimulation[516]

Contralesional cervical transcutaneous nerve stimulation[517]

Reduce hemianopic defects[444]

Computer-assisted training[439,518]

Pharmacotherapy[451,457]

Sources: Hanlon, 1996[400]; Taylor et al., 1994[405]; Kalra et al., 1997[412]; Ben-Yishay and Diller, 1993[422]; Wiart et al., 1997[429]; Robertson and North, 1992[430]; Karnath et al., 1997[432]; Mennemeier et al., 1994[433]; Loverro and Reding, 1988[434]; Rossi et al., 1990[437]; Rossetti et al., 1998[438]; Robertson et al., 1990[439]; Butter and Kirsch, 1992[411]; Beis, et al., 1999[442]; Kerkhoff et al., 1994[444]; Rubens, 1985[447]; Rode et al., 1992[448]; Vallar et al., 1990[449]; Oliveri et al., 1999[450]; Fleet et al., 1987[451]; Grujic et al., 1998[457]; Simon et al., 1995[512]; Smania et al., 1997[512]; Tham and Tegner, 1997[514]; Serfaty et al., 1995[515]; Pizzamiglio et al., 1990[516]; Perennou et al., 2001[517]; Gray et al., 1992.[518]

with hemineglect, however, use an environmental, rather than body-centered frame of reference.[433]

One of the traditional inpatient rehabilitation approaches has been to orient the bed so that the patient's neglected hemispace is toward the door entrance or a visitor's seat. The expectation is to draw the patient to visually search the more stimulating field. A study that compared bed orientation toward and away from the field showed no difference in functional outcome.[434] No single isolated strategy, however, is likely to improve visual tracking toward neglected hemispace.

A few logical approaches to enhance visual scanning to the left have not led to functional improvements. Many training devices, particularly computers, have been tried to decrease visual neglect. One study attempted to retrain visual searching to the left hemienvironment by providing audio feedback from eye movement recording glasses whenever the patients failed to look to the left for 15 seconds.[435] Although some patients increased their spontaneous scanning, other tests showed no change in left hemi-inattention. An electronic apparatus that flashed a fixation point and a stimulus point at another position on a screen was designed to train saccadic and exploratory eye movements.[436] It did improve visual exploration during the test, but did not reduce the size of the hemianopic field as the investigators had hoped. Prisms may be used to shift spatial and sensorimotor coordinates. A randomized trial with 15-diopter Fresnel prisms applied over the affected hemifield to shift a peripheral image towards the central retinal meridian improved scores on standard tests of visuoperception, but did not generalize to improvement in ADL and mobility over 4 weeks of inpatient use.[437] The prisms may have drawn attention to the neglected visual field by bringing images to the fore. Tabletop activities, such as finding food on a tray, may be expected to improve while the prisms are worn, but visual blurring may limit their use during ADLs. The approach may benefit from better lens materials or from training paradigms that would generalize to activities when subjects no longer wore the prisms.

Prisms have also been used to transform sensorimotor coordinates, rather than as passive prosthetics.[438] A 10° prism that shifts objects to the right causes the subject to reach to the left when the glasses are removed. The subject's internal visual and proprioceptive map, after adaptation to wearing the prism for 5 minutes, apparently realigns in the direction opposite to the optical deviation. The aftereffects of wearing the prism, in one study, included significant improvement in drawing objects and performing cancellation tasks in left hemispace for at least 2 hours after removal, and for up to 4 days.[438] The prism, then, induced short-term plasticity driven, perhaps, by a retinotopic and ocular exploration mechanism. A similar strategy of adaptation by prismatic shift compared seven subjects with left visuospatial neglect who were treated twice a day for 2 weeks (20 sessions) to six matched subjects who received only cognitive remediation.[439a] Six of the experimental subjects improved in pencil-and-paper and behavioral tests of ADLs from the Behavioral Inattention Test. The benefit persisted at a 5-week followup, and at 17 weeks when some subjects were retested. The subjects who improved exhibited an immediate after-effect when the prisms were removed by 1 week of practice, showing a 2° leftward deviation for pointing. Thus, short-term plasticity led to long-term visuospatial network plasticity and behavioral gains.

Many software programs have been designed to improve attention in patients with spatial hemineglect. A randomized trial of microcomputer-based scanning and attentional tasks showed no benefit.[439] Benefit for a specifically trained activity, wheelchair mobility, was significant in a case-control study when subjects practiced on a wheelchair simulator over a computer-generated 6 × 8 foot obstacle course.[440] This approach suggests the impact of the specificity of the practice, but may not carry over *in vivo* for some patients with a brain injury who cannot grasp a virtual world.

Transient, moving visual stimuli activate the superior colliculus to help generate a saccade. By decreasing input to the right eye or right hemifield, input to the contralateral left superior colliculus is reduced, which decreases its tendency to program saccades to the right. This concept provides a rationale for another therapeutic strategy for visual hemi-inattention. The right eye in patients with a right cerebral infarct was patched or visual stimuli were presented in the left field during a line bisection task.[441] Both procedures improved tests of left attention. In another study, however, a monocular patch over the right eye did not produce the gains in visual attention to the left or in ADLs that was acccomplished by binocular patches that created a relative right hemianopsia.[442] Hemipatches placed on a pair of glasses on the right side of the midline in patients who do not have a left hemianopsia may also behaviorally force the use of the left visual field. The effect may last beyond the time of long-term training, but needs further study.

Visual Field Expansion

Therapeutic strategies for visual field impairments are often attached to those for visual hemi-inattention. Some interventions have been proposed that reduce hemianopic defects that arise without visual neglect. This approach has been driven, in part, by the finding that spontaneous recovery of visual field defects has been reported in less than 20% of patients within 3 months of stroke.[443] One compensatory procedure systematically trained ocular saccadic scanning within the scotoma on a computer screen and in daily activities.[444] This training led to an increase in the field of search by a mean of 30°, reduced the size of the scotoma in some patients, and led to a transfer of the gains to some relevant ADLs. A similar approach that employed a large training board with four rows and eight columns of lights improved the perception of visual stimuli and the reaction time to identify a stimulus pattern of lights by moving the eyes, but not the head.[445] Related strategies may activate spared bilateral extrastriate cortex that can contribute to partial recovery of a hemianopic field.[446] Some instances of blindsight probably involve sparing of a portion of the visual cortices.

Vestibular Stimulation

Stimulation with cold water in the left ear or warm water in the right to evoke a slow phase of nystagmus and past pointing to the left produced transient improvement in tests of left neglect.[447] These results have been reproduced in a few reports, but without any lasting benefit on the neglect. Similar transient improvements have been reported in neglect and other associated signs, including somatophrenia, anosognosia, and sensory and motor deficits.[448,449] Stimulation of subcortical structures that play a role in attentional pathways may be the mechanism that caused these surprising findings. Vestibular input may also change the perception of the midline of peripersonal space. The findings suggest that one mechanism of spatial neglect is related to a defect in systems that combine visual and vestibular information for spatial orientation.[433] These sensory inputs are probably integrated in the inferior parietal lobule. Vestibular studies need replication. A longer lasting vestibulo-ocular reflex stimulus, such as electrical stimulation over the mastoid, may allow time for combining the technique with visuospatial training.

Cortical Stimulation

Visual scanning combined with cortical stimulation may help some patients overcome hemineglect. Transcranial magnetic stimulation delivered in single pulses to the left frontal cortex in relation to a bimanual tactile discrimination task significantly reduced contralateral extinction to tactile stimulation in patients with right brain lesions.[450] No effect was found in patients with left hemiphere lesions. Transient dysfunction of the left frontal region (in or near BA 9 and 46) by TMS apparently ameliorated the extinction by removal of left frontal-right parietal transcallosal inhibition or, perhaps, by a subcortical mechanism. This technique may be combined with training paradigms to increase hemiattention. In profound cases of neglect, it is imaginable that patients who responded to TMS could have epidural electrodes implanted and electrically stimulate themselves as needed during ADLs and instrumental ADL tasks.

Pharmacotherapy

Medications that affect neurotransmitters and neuromodulators may have positive or negative effects on dimensions of attention. Some drugs may affect general processes, others such as stimulants of the noradrenergic projections from the locus ceruleus may modulate the signal-to-noise ratio for attended stimuli. Others drugs may enable gains when combined with task-oriented practice. Case reports also describe trials of noradrenergic and dopaminergic agents, including amphetamine, methyl-

pram, was effective within 3 to 6 weeks in 65% of patients who had become depressed 7 or more weeks after a stroke, compared to recovery in 15% who received a placebo.[486] Fluoxetine produced a similar response rate in 4 to 6 weeks.[483] Drugs that raise serotonin also diminish outbursts of crying in patients with emotional incontinence[487] or apathy after a stroke.

Drug dosages, especially for the elderly, should be gradually increased. Rather low dosages may be effective, such as 10 mg of fluoxetine or 25 mg to 50 mg of desipramine (see Chapter 8).

SUMMARY

Impairments and disabilities tend to improve for at least 3 to 6 months after stroke. Inpatient rehabilitation allows patients to have close medical and nursing supervision, heads off complications of immobility and comorbid diseases, and attempts to shift the curve of recovery over time to the left to give more patients greater functional independence. Inpatient rehabilitation allows the patient and family to begin to adjust to new disability and to be educated about risk factors for recurrent stroke. The rehabilitation team uses subsequent outpatient care and, even later, adds intermittent pulses of therapy to solve ongoing problems that limit home and community activities and quality of life.

Many interventions draw upon neuroscientific mechanisms of plasticity, learning theories, and the social sciences. These strategies must take into account the special biologic and psychosocial adaptations of the elderly, as well as a cost-benefit analysis. Stroke rehabilitation can look forward to better strategies for task-oriented practice, biologic interventions with neural precursors or neurotrophins, drugs that enhance molecular mechanisms of learning and memory, and the benefits of neuroprostheses. Testing by well-designed clinical trials will place rehabilitationists beyond the boundaries of today's *Imaginot Line*.

REFERENCES

1. Bonita R, Solomon N, Broad J. Prevalence of stroke and stroke-related disability. Estimates from the Auckland Stroke Studies. Stroke 1997; 28:1898–1902.
2. Hartmann A, Rundek T, Mast H, Paik C, Mohr J, Sacco R. Mortality and causes of death after first ischemic stroke: The Northern Manhattan Stroke Study. Neurology 2001; 57:2000–2005.
3. Hankey G, Jamrozik K, Broadhurst R, Forbes S, Burvill PW, Anderson C, Stewart-Wynne E. Five-year survival after first-ever stroke and related prognostic factors in the Perth community stroke study. Stroke 2000; 31:2080–2086.
4. Dennis M, Burn J, Sandercock P, Wade D, Warlow C. Long-term survival after first-ever stroke: The Oxfordshire community stroke project. Stroke 1993; 24: 796–800.
5. Bronnum-Hansen H, Davidsen M, Thorvaldsen P. Long-term survival and causes of death after stroke. Stroke 2001; 32:2131–2136.
6. Sacco R. Risk factors and outcomes for ischemic stroke. Neurology 1995; 45(Suppl1):S10–S14.
7. Sacco R, Wolf P, Kannel W, McNamara P. Survival and recurrence following stroke: The Framingham study. Stroke 1982; 13:290–296.
8. Stroke Unit Trialists' Collaboration. How do stroke units improve patient outcomes? A collaborative systematic review of the randomized trials. Stroke 1997; 28:2139–2144.
9. Hankey G. Stroke: How large a public health problem, and how can the neurologist help? Arch Neurol 1999; 56:748–754.
10. Matchar D, Duncan P. Cost of stroke. Stroke Clinical Updates. National Stroke Association 1994; 5:9–12.
11. Taylor T, Davis P, Torner J, Holmes J, Meyer J, Jacobsen M. Lifetime cost of stroke in the United States. Stroke 1996; 27:1459–1466.
12. Rubin R, Gold W, Kelley D, Sher J. The cost of disorders of the brain: National Foundation for Brain Research, 1992.
13. Dobkin B. The economic impact of stroke. Neurology 1995; 45(Suppl 1):S6–S9.
14. Foulkes M, Wolf P, Price T, Mohr J, Hier D. The Stroke Data Bank. Stroke 1988; 19:547–554.
15. Burn J, Dennis M, Bamford J, Wade D, Sandercock P, Warlau C. Long-term risk of recurrent stroke after a first-ever stroke. Stroke 1994; 25:333–337.
16. Kobayashi S, Okada K, Koide H, Bokura H, Yamaguchi S. Subcortical silent brain infarction as a risk factor for clinical stroke. Stroke 1997; 28:1932–1939.
17. Jongbloed L. Prediction of function after stroke: A critical review. Stroke 1986; 17:765–776.
18. Dobkin B. Neuromedical complications in stroke patients transferred for rehabilitation before and after DRGs. J Neurol Rehabil 1987; 1:3–8.
19. Davenport R, Dennis M, Wellwood I, Warlow C. Complications after acute stroke. Stroke 1996; 27: 415–420.
20. Kalra L, Yu G, Wilson K, Roots P. Medical complications during stroke rehabilitation. Stroke 1995; 26: 990–994.
21. Dromerick A, Reding M. Medical and neurological complications during inpatient stroke rehabilitation. Stroke 1994; 25:358–361.
22. Langhorne P, Stott D, Robertson L, MacDonald J, Jones L, McAlpine C, Dick F, Taylor G, Murray G. Medical complications after stroke: A multicenter study. Stroke 2000; 31:1223–1229.
23. Roth E, Lovell L, Harvey R, Heinemann A, Semik

P, Diaz S. Incidence of and risk factors for medical complications during stroke rehabilitation. Stroke 2001; 32:523–529.

24. Roth E, Mueller K, Green D. Cardiovascular response to physical therapy in stroke rehabilitation. Neurorehabil 1992; 2:7–15.

25. Dobkin B, Starkman S. Chapter 4: The patient with stroke. In: Herr R, Cydulka R, eds. Emergency Care of the Compromised Patient. Philadelphia: J. B. Lippincott, 1994:67–78.

26. Zuccala G, Onder G, Pedone C, Carosella L, Pahor M, Bernabei R, Cocchi A. Hypotension and cognitive impairment. Neurology 2001; 57:1986–1992.

27. Reith J, Jorgensen H, Nakayama H, Olsen T. Seizures in acute stroke: Predictors and prognostic significance. The Copenhagen Stroke Study. Stroke 1997; 28:1585–1589.

28. Bladin C, Alexandrov A, Bellavance A, Bornstein N, Chambers B, Cote R, Lebrun L, Pirisi A, Norris J. Seizures after stroke: A prospective multicenter study. Arch Neurol 2000; 57:1617–1622.

29. Faught E, Peters D, Bartolucci A, Moore L, Miller P. Seizures after primary intracerebral hemorrhage. Neurology 1989; 39:1089–1093.

30. Broderick J, Adams H, Barsan W, Feinberg W, Feldmann E, Grotta J, Kase C, Krieger D, Mayberg M, Tilley B, Zabramski J, Zuccarello M. Guidelines for the management of spontaneous intracerebral hemorrhage. Stroke 1999; 30:905–915.

31. Gupta S, Naheedy M, Elias D, Rubino F. Postinfarction seizures. Stroke 1988; 19:1477–1481.

32. Kilpatrick C, Davis S, Hopper J, Rossiter S. Early seizures after acute stroke. Arch Neurol 1992; 49: 509–511.

33. Goldstein L. Potential effects of common drugs on stroke recovery. Arch Neurol 1998; 55:454–456.

34. Goldstein L, Dromerick A, Good D, et al. Possible time window for the detrimental effects of drugs on poststroke recovery. Neurology (suppl 3) 2002; 58:A5.

35. Greenlund K, Giles W, Keenan N, Croft J, Mensah G. Physician advice, patient actions, anhd health-related quality of life in secondary prevention of stroke through diet and exercise. Stroke 2002; 33:565–571.

36. Sacco R. Newer risk factors for stroke. Neurology 2001; 57(Suppl 2):S31–S34.

37. Wolf P, Clagett G, Easton J. Preventing ischemic stroke in patients with prior stroke and transient ischemic attack. Stroke 1999; 30:1991–1994.

38. Wolf P, D'Agostino R, Kannel W, Bonita R, Belanger A. Cigarette smoking as a risk factor for stroke. JAMA 1988; 259:1025–1029.

39. D'Agostino R, Wolf P, Belanger A, Kannel W. Stroke risk profile: Adjustment for antihypertensive medication. Stroke 1994; 25:40–43.

40. May M, CMcCarron P, Stansfeld S, Ben-Shlomo Y, Gallacher J, Yarnell J, Davey Smith G. Does psychological distress predict the risk of ischemic stroke and transient ischemic attack? Stroke 2002; 33:7–12.

41. Hess D, Demchuk A, Brass L, Yatsu F. HMG-CoA reductase inhibitors (statins): A promising approach to stroke prevention. Neurology 2000; 54:790–796.

42. Clarke R, Daly L, Robinson K, Naughten E, Cahalane S, Fowler B, Graham I. Hyperhomocystinemia: an independent risk factor for vascular disease. N Engl J Med 1991; 324:1149–1155.

43. Schnyder G, Roffi M, Pin R, Flammer Y, Lange H, Eberli F, Meier B, Turi Z, Hess O. Decreased rate of coronary restenosis after lowering of plasma homocysteine levels. New Engl J Med 2001; 345:1593–1600.

44. Homocysteine Lowering Trialists' Collaboration. Lowering blood homocysteine with folic acid based supplements: Meta-analysis of randomised trials. BMJ 1998; 316:894–898.

45. Levine S, Jacobs B. A prospective, seasonal odyssey into antiphospholipid protein synthesis. Stroke 2001; 32:1699–1700.

46. Milhaud D, Bogousslavsky J, van Melle G, Liot P. Ischemic stroke and active migraine. Neurology 2001; 57: 1805–1811.

47. Bushnell C, Goldstein L. Diagnostic testing for coagulopathies in patients with ischemic stroke. Stroke 2000; 31:3067–3078.

48. Gillum L, Mamidipudi S, Johnston S. Ischemic stroke risk with oral contraceptives. JAMA 2000; 284:72–78.

49. Gorelick P, Sacco R, Smith D. Prevention of a first stroke. JAMA 1999; 281:1112–1120.

50. Kawachi I, Colditz G, Stampler M, Willett W, Manson J, Rosner B, Speizer F, Hennekens C. Smoking cessation and decreased risk of stroke in women. JAMA 1993; 269:232–236.

51. Tell G, Howard G, McKinney W, Toole J. Cigarette smoking cessation and extracranial carotid atherosclerosis. JAMA 1989; 261:1178–1180.

52. INDANA Project Collaborators, Gueyffier F, Boissel J-P, Boutitie F, Pocock S, Coope J, Cutler J, Ekbom T, Fagard R, Friedman L, Kerlikowske K, Perry M, Prineas R, Schron E. Effect of antihypertensive treatment in patients having already suffered from stroke. Stroke 1997; 28:2557–2562.

53. Alter M, Friday G, Lai S, O'Connell J, Sobel E. Hypertension and risk of stroke recurrence. Stroke 1994; 25:1605–1610.

54. Sobel E, Alter M, Davinipour Z. Control of hypertension, arrhythmia, and MI 4 months after stroke in a whole population. Neurology 1990; 40 (Suppl 1):421.

55. Perry H, Davis B, Price T, Applegate W, Fields W, Guralnik J, Kuller L, Pressel S, Stamler J, Probstfield J. Effect of treating isolated systolic hypertension on the risk of developing various types and subtypes of stroke. JAMA 2000; 284:465–471.

56. PROGRESS Collaborative Group. Randomised trial of a perindopril-based blood-pressure-lowering regimen among 6105 individuals with previous stroke or transient ischaemic attack. Lancet 2001; 358:1033–1041.

57. Applegate W, SHEP Investigators. Prevalence of postural hypotension at baseline in the Systolic Hypertension in the Elderly Program (SHEP) cohort. J Am Geriatr Soc 1991; 39:1057–1064.

58. Dobkin B. Orthostatic hypotension as a risk factor for symptomatic cerebrovascular disease. Neurology 1989; 38:30–34.

59. Klijn C, Kappelle L, van Huffelen A, Visser G, Algra A, Tulleken C, van Gijn J. Recurrent ischemia in symptomatic carotid occlusion. Neurology 2000; 55: 1806–1812.

60. Vasan R, Larson M, Leip E, Evans J, Kannel W, O'Donnell C, Levy D. Impact of high-normal blood pressure on the risk of cardiovascular disease. New Engl J Med 2001; 345:1291–1297.

61. Insura J, Sacks H, Lau T, Lau J, Reitman D, Pagano D, Chalmers T. Drug treatment of hypertension in the elderly: A meta-analysis. Ann Intern Med 1994; 121:355–362.

62. Catella-Lawson F, Reilly M, Kapoor S, Cucchiara A, DeMarco S, Tournier B, Vyas S, Fitzgerald G. Cyclooxygenase inhibitors and the antiplatelet effects of aspirin. New Engl J Med 2001; 345:1809–1817.

63. Gent M, Blakely JA, Easton J, Ellis D, Hachinski V, Harbison J, Panak E, Roberts R, Sicurella J, Turpie A. The Canadian-American Ticlopidine Study in thromboembolic stroke. Lancet 1989; 1:1215–1220.

64. CAPRIE Steering Committee. A randomised, blinded, trial of clopidogrel versus aspirin in patients at risk of ischaemic events. Lancet 1996; 348:1329–1339.

65. Yusuf S, Zhao F, Mehta S, Chrolavicius S, Tognoni G, Fox K. Effects of clopidogrel in addition to aspirin in patients with acute coronary syndroms without ST-segment elevation. N Engl J Med 2001; 345:494–502.

66. Albers G, Easton J, Sacco R, Teal P. Antithrombotic and thrombolytic therapy for ischemic stroke. Chest 1998; 114(suppl):S683–698.

67. Mohr J, Thompson J, Lazar R, Levin B, Sacco R, Furie K, Kistler J, Albers G, Pettigrew L, Adams H, Jackson C, Pullicino P. A comparison of warfarin and aspirin for the prevention of recurrent ischemic stroke. New Engl J Med 2001; 345:1444–1451.

68. Gresham C, Duncan P, Stason W. Post-Stroke Rehabilitation: Assessment, Referral, and Patient Management. Clinical Practice Guideline No. 16: U.S. Public Health Service, Agency for Health Care Policy and Research, 1995.

69. Johnston M, Wood K, Stason W, Beatty P. Rehabilitative placement of poststroke patients: Reliability of the clinical practice guideline of the Agency for Health Care Policy and Research. Arch Phys Med Rehabil 2000; 81:539–548.

70. Duncan P, Horner R, Reker D, Samsa G, Hoenig H. Adherence to postacute rehabilitation guidelines is associated with functional recovery in stroke. Stroke 2002; 33:167–178.

71. Alexander M. Stroke rehabilitation outcome: A potential use of predictive variables to establish levels of care. Stroke 1994; 25:128–134.

72. Oczkowski W, Barreca S. The Functional Independence Measure: Its use to identify rehabilitation needs in stroke survivors. Arch Phys Med Rehabil 1993; 74:1291–1294.

73. Bates B, Stineman M. Outcome indicators for stroke: application of an algorithm treatment across the continuum of postacute rehabilitation services. Arch Phys Med Rehabil 2000; 81:1468–1478.

74. Mokler P, Sandstrom R, Griffin M, Farris L, Jones C. Predicting discharge destination for patients with severe motor stroke: Important functional tasks. Neurorehabil Neural Repair 2000; 14:181–185.

75. Ancheta J, Husband M, Law D, Reding M. Initial Functional Independence Measure score and interval post stroke help assess outcome, length of hospitalization, and quality of care. Neurorehabil Neural Repair 2000; 14:127–34.

76. Gibson CJ. Patterns of care for stroke survivors. Stroke 1990; 21(suppl II):38–39.

77. Dombovy M, Basford J, Whisnant J, Bergstralh E. Disability and use of rehabilitation services following stroke in Rochester, Minnesota. Stroke 1987; 18:830–836.

78. Smith D, Goldenberg E, Ashburn A. Remedial therapy after stroke: A randomized controlled trial. Br Med J 1981; 282:517–520.

79. Kramer A, Steiner J, Schlenker R, Eilertsen TB, Hrincevich C, Tropea D, Ahmad L, Eckhoff D. Outcomes and costs after hip fracture and stroke: A comparison of rehabilitation settings. JAMA 1997; 277: 396–404.

80. Harrington C, Himmelstein D. Does investor ownership of nursing homes compromise the quality of care? Am J Pub Health 2001; 91:1452–1455.

81. Alberts M, Hademenos G, Latchaw R, Jagoda A, Marler J, Mayberg M, Starke R, Todd H, Viste K, Girgus M, Shephard T, Emr M, Shwayder P, Walker M. Recommendations for the establishment of primary stroke centers. JAMA 2000; 283:3102–3109.

82. The Stroke Unit Trialists' Collaboration. A collaborative systematic review of the randomised trials of organised inpatient (stroke unit) care after stroke. BMJ 1997; 314:1151–1159.

83. Jorgensen H, Reith J, Nakayama H, Raaschou H, Larsen K, Kammersgaard L, Olsen T. What determines good recovery in patients with the most severe strokes? Stroke 1999; 30:2008–2012.

84. Indredavik B, Slordahl S, Bakke F, Rokseth R, Haheim L. Stroke unit treatment. Stroke 1997; 28:1861–66.

85. Indredavik B, Bakke F, Stordahl S. Treatment in a combined acute and rehabilitation stroke unit. Stroke 1999; 30:917–923.

86. Kalra L, Eade J. Role of stroke rehabilitation units in managing severe disability after stroke. Stroke 1995; 26:2031–2034.

87. Kwakkel G, Wagenaar R, Koelman T, Lankhorst G, Koetsier J. Effects of intensity of rehabilitation after stroke: A research synthesis. Stroke 1997; 28:1550–1556.

88. Kwakkel G, Wagenaar R, Twisk J, Lankhorst G, Koetsier J. Intensity of leg and arm training after primary middle cerebral artery stroke: A randomised trial. Lancet 1999; 354:191–196.

89. Indredavik B, Fjaertoft H, Ekeberg G, Loge A, Morch B. Benefit of an extended stroke unit service with early supported discharge. Stroke 2000; 31: 2989–2994.

90. Kalra L, Dale P, Crome P. Improving stroke rehabilitation: A controlled trial. Stroke 1993; 24:1462–1467.

91. Kalra L. The influence of stroke unit rehabilitation on functional recovery from stroke. Stroke 1994; 25:821–825.

92. Glader E-L, Stegmayr B, Johansson L, Hulter-Asberg K, Wester P. Differences in long-term outcome between patients treated in stroke units and in general wards. Stroke 2001; 32:2124–2130.

93. Sulch D, Perez I, Melbourn A, Kalra L. Randomized controlled trial of integrated (managed) care pathway for stroke rehabilitation. Stroke 2000; 31:1929–1934.

94. Johnston M, Keister M. Early rehabilitation for stroke patients: a new look. Arch Phys Med Rehabil 1984; 65:437–441.

95. Ween J, Alexander M, D'Esposito M, Roberts M. Factors predictive of stroke outcome in a rehabilitation setting. Neurology 1996; 47:388–392.

96. Paolucci S, Antonucci G, Grasso M, Morelli D, Troisi

E, Coiro P, Bragoni M. Early versus delayed inpatient stroke rehabilitation: a matched comparison conducted in italy. Arch Phys Med Rehabil 2000; 81: 695–700.

97. Heinemann A, Roth E, Cichowski K, Betts H. Multivariate analysis of improvement and outcome following stroke rehabilitation. Arch Neurol 1987; 44: 1167–1172.

98. Anderson E, Anderson T, Kottke F. Stroke rehabilitation: Maintenance of achieved goals. Arch Phys Med Rehabil 1977; 58:345–352.

99. Ferrucci L, Bandinelli S, Guralnik J, Lamponi M, Bertini C, Falchini M, Baroni A. Recovery of functional status after stroke: A postrehabilitation follow-up study. Stroke 1993; 24:200–205.

100. Gladman J, Lincoln N, Barer D. A randomised controlled trial of domiciliary and hospital-based rehabilitation for stroke patients after discharge from hospital. J Neurol Neurosurg Psychiatry 1993; 56:960–966.

101. Roderick P, Low J, Day R, Peasgood T, Mullee M, Turnbull J, Villar T, Raftery J. Stroke rehabilitation after hospital ddischarge: A randomized trial comparing domiciliary and day-hospital care. Age Ageing 2001; 30:303–310.

102. Young J, Forster A. The Bradford community stroke trial: Results at six months. Br Med J 1992; 304:1085–1089.

103. Dekker R, Drost E, Goroothoff J, Arendzen J, van Gijn J, Eisma W. Effects of a day-hospital rehabilitation in stroke patients: A review of randomized clinical trials. Scand J Rehab Med 1998; 30:87–94.

104. Rudd A, Wolfe C, Tilling K, Beech R. The effectiveness of a package of community care on one year outcome of stroke patients. BMJ 1997; 315:1039–1044.

105. Ronning OM, Guldvog B. Outcome of subacute stroke rehabilitation: A randomized controlled trial. Stroke 1998; 29:779–784.

106. Widen Holmqvist L, von Koch L, Kostulas V, Holm M, Widsell G, Tegler H, Johansson K, Almazan J, de Pedro-Cuesta J. A randomized controlled trial of rehabilitation at home after stroke in southwest Stockholm. Stroke 1998; 29:591–597.

107. Mayo N, Wood-Dauphinee S, Cote R, Gayton D, Carlton J, Buttery J, Tamblyn R. There's no place like home: An evaluation of early supported discharge for stroke. Stroke 2000; 31:1016–1023.

108. Nilsson A, Aniansson A, Grimby G. Rehabilitation needs and disability in community living stroke survivors two years after stroke. Top Stroke Rehabil 2000; 6:30–47.

109. Grimby G, Andren E, Daving Y, Wright B. Dependence and perceived difficulty in daily activities in community-living stroke survivors 2 years after stroke: A study of instrumental structures. Stroke 1998; 29:1843–1849.

110. Dobkin B. Overview of treadmill locomotor training with partial body weight support: A neurophysiologically sound approach whose time has come for randomized clinical trials. Neurorehabilitation and Neural Repair 1999; 13:157–165.

111. Taub E, Uswatte G, Pidikiti R. Constraint-induced movement therapy: A new family of techniques with broad application to physical rehabilitation-a clinical review. Rehabil Res Dev 1999; 36:237–251.

112. Silver K, Macko R, Forrester L, Goldberg A, Smith G. Effects of aerobic treadmill training on gait velocity, cadence, and gait symmetry in chronic hemiparetic stroke: A preliminary report. Neurorehabil Neural Repair 2000; 14:65–71.

113. Dean C, Richards C, Malouin F. Task-related circuit training improves performance of locomotor tasks in chronic stroke: A randomized, controlled pilot trial. Arch Phys Med Rehabil 2000; 81:409–417.

114. Wade D, Collen F, Robb G, Warlow C. Physiotherapy intervention late after stroke and mobility. BMJ 1992; 304:609–613.

115. Teixeira-Salmela L, Olney S, Nadeau S. Muscle strengthening and physical conditioning to reduce impairment and disability in chronic stroke survivors. Arch Phys Med Rehabil 1999; 80:1211–1218.

116. van der Lee J, Wagenaar R, Lankhorst G, Vogelaar T, Deville W, Bouter L. Forced use of the upper extremity in chronic stroke patients: Results from a single-blind randomized clinical trial. Stroke 1999; 30:2369–2375.

117. Tangeman P, Banaitis D, Williams A. Rehabilitation of chronic stroke patients: Changes in functional performance. Arch Phys Med Rehabil 1990; 71:876–880.

118. Dam M, Tonin P, Casson S, Ermani M, Pizzolato G, Iaia V, Battistin L. The effects of long-term rehabilitation therapy on poststroke hemiplegic patients. Stroke 1993; 24:1886–1891.

119. Macko R, DeSouza C, Tretter L, Silver K, Smith G, Anderson P, Tomoyasu N, Gorman P, Dengel D. Treadmill aerobic exercise training reduces the energy expenditure and cardiovascular demands of hemiparetic gait in chronic stroke patients. Stroke 1997; 28:326–330.

120. Smith G, Silver K, Goldberg A, Macko R. "Task-oriented" exercise improves hamstring strength and spastic reflexes in chronic stroke patients. Stroke 1999; 30:2112–2118.

121. Mongra T, Lawson J, Inglis J. Sexual dysfunction in stroke patients. Arch Phys Med Rehabil 1986; 67:19–22.

122. Boldrini P, Basaglia N, Calanca M. Sexual changes in hemiparetic patients. Arch Phys Med Rehabil 1991; 72:202–207.

123. Evans R, Matlock A-L, Bishop D, Stranahan S, Pederson C. Family intervention after stroke: Does counseling or education help? Stroke 1988; 19:1243–1249.

124. Evans R, Bishop D, Matlock A-L, Stranahan S, Halar E, Noonan W. Prestroke family interaction as a predictor of stroke outcome. Arch Phys Med Rehabil 1987; 68:508–517.

125. Niemi M-L, Laaksonen R, Kotila M, Waltimo O. Quality of life 4 years after stroke. Stroke 1988; 19:1101–1107.

126. Saeki S, Ogata H, Okubo T, Takahashi K, Hoshuyama T. Return to work after stroke. Stroke 1995; 26:399–401.

127. Black-Schaffer R, Osberg J. Return to work after stroke: Development of a predictive model. Arch Phys Med Rehabil 1990; 71:285–290.

128. Bonita R, Beaglehole R. Recovery of motor function after stroke. Stroke 1988; 19:1497–1500.

129. Jorgensen H, Nakayama H, Raaschou H, Olsen T, Vive-Larson J, Stoier M. Outcome and time course of recovery in stroke. Part I: Outcome. The Copenhagen Stroke Study. Arch Phys Med Rehabil 1995; 76:399–405.

130. Jorgensen H, Nakayama H, Raaschou H, Olsen T, Vive-Larson J, Stoier M. Outcome and time course of recovery in stroke. Part II: Time course. The Copenhagen Stroke Study. Arch Phys Med Rehabil 1995; 76:406–412.

131. Wade D, Hewer R. Motor loss and swallowing difficulty after stroke: Frequency, recovery, and prognosis. Acta Neurol Scand 1987; 76:50–54.

132. Duncan P, Goldstein L, Horner R, Landsman P, Samsa G, Matchar D. Similar motor recovery of upper and lower extremities after stroke. Stroke 1994; 25:1181–1188.

133. Libman R, Sacco R, Shi M, Tatemichi T, Mohr J. Neurologic improvement in pure motor hemiparesis. Neurology 1992; 42:1713–1716.

134. Duke R, Bloch R, Turpie A, Trebilcock R, Bayer N. Intravenous heparin for the prevention of stroke progression in acute partial stable stroke: A randomized controlled trial. Ann Int Med 1986; 105:825–828.

135. Hier D, Mondlock J, Caplan L. Recovery of behavioral abnormalities after right hemisphere stroke. Neurology 1983; 33:337–350.

136. Colebatch J, Gandevia S. The distribution of muscular weakness in upper motor neuron lesions affecting the arm. Brain 1989; 112:749–763.

137. Jones R, Donaldson I, Parkin P. Impairment and recovery of ipsilateral sensory-motor function following unilateral cerebral infarction. Brain 1989; 112:113–132.

138. Jorgensen H, Nakayama H, Raaschou H, Pedersen P, Houth J, Olsen T. Functional and neurological outcome of stroke and the relation to stroke severity and type, stroke unit treatment, body temperature, age, and other risk factors: The Copenhagen Stroke Study. Top Stroke Rehabil 2000; 6:1–18.

139. Patel A, Duncan P, Lai S, Studenski S. The relation between impairments and functional outcomes poststroke. Arch Phys Med Rehabil 2000; 81:1357–1363.

140. Reding M, Potes E. Rehabilitation outcome following initial unilateral hemispheric stroke: Life table analysis approach. Stroke 1988; 19:1354–1364.

141. Olsen T. Arm and leg paresis as outcome predictors in stroke rehabilitation. Stroke 1990; 21:247–251.

142. Roth E, Heinemann A, Lovell L, Harvey R, McGuire J, Diaz S. Impairment and disability: Their relation during stroke rehabilitation. Arch Phys Med Rehabil 1998; 79:329–335.

143. Barer D, Mitchell J. Predicting the outcome of acute stroke: Do multivariate models help? Q J Med 1989; 261:27–39.

144. Galski T, Bruno R, Zorowitz R, Walker J. Predicting length of stay, functional outcome, and aftercare in the rehabilitation of stroke patients. Stroke 1993; 24:1794–1800.

145. Kalra L, Crome P. The role of prognostic scores in targeting stroke rehabilitation in elderly patients. J Am Geriatr Soc 1993; 41:396–400.

146. Novack T, Haban G, Graham K, Satterfield W. Prediction of stroke rehabilitation outcome from psychologic screening. Arch Phys Med Rehabil 1987; 68:729–734.

147. Paolucci S, Antononucci G, Pratesi L, Traballesi M, Lubich S, Grasso M. Functional outcome in stroke inpatient rehabilitation: Predicting no, low and high response patients. Cerebrovasc Dis 1998; 8:228–234.

148. Warabi T, Inoue K, Noda H, Murakami S. Recovery of voluntary movement in hemiplegic patients. Brain 1990; 113:177–189.

149. Miyai I, Suzuki T, Kii K. Wallerian degeneration of the pyramidal tract does not affect stroke rehabilitation outcome. Neurology 1998; 51:1613–1616.

150. Miyai I, Blau A, Reding M, Volpe B. Patients with stroke confined to basal ganglia have diminished response to rehabilitation efforts. Neurology 1997; 48:95–101.

151. Hochstenbach J, van Spaendonck K, Cools A, Horstink M, Mulder T. Cognitive deficits following stroke in the basal ganglia. Clin Rehabil 1998; 12:514–520.

152. Miyai I, Suzuki T, Kang J, Kubota K, Volpe B. Middle cerebral artery stroke that includes the premotor cortex reduces mobility outcome. Stroke 1999; 30:1380–1383.

153. Macdonell R, Donnan G, Bladin P. Serial changes in somatosensory evoked potentials following cerebral infarction. Electroencephalogr Clin Neurophysiol 1991; 80:276–280.

154. Chester C, McLaren C. Somatosensory evoked response and recovery from stroke. Arch Phys Med Rehabil 1989; 70:520–525.

155. Pavot A, Ignacia D, Kutavanish A, Lightfoote E. Prognostic value of somatosensory evoked potentials in cerebrovascular accidents. Electromyogr Clin Neurophysiol 1986; 26:333–340.

156. Gott P, Karnaze D, Fisher M. Assessment of median somatosensory evoked potentials in cerebral ischemia. Stroke 1990; 21:1167–1171.

157. Feys G, Van Hees J, Bruyninck F, Mercelis R, De Weerdt W. Value of somatosensory and motor evoked potentials in predicting arm recovery after a stroke. J Neurol Neurosurg Psychiatry 2000; 68:323–331.

158. Macdonell R, Donnan G, Bladin P. A comparison of somatosensory evoked and motor evoked potentials in stroke. Ann Neurol 1989; 25:68–73.

159. Pennisi G, Rapisarda G, Bella R, Calabrese V, de Noordhout A. Absence of response to early transcranial magnetic stimulation in ischemic stroke patients. Prognostic value for hand recovery. Stroke 1999; 30:2666–2670.

160. Dominkus M, Griswold W, Jelinck V. Transcranial electrical motor evoked potentials as a prognostic indicator for motor recovery in stroke patients. J Neurol Neurosurg Psychiatry 1990; 53:745–780.

161. Heald A, Bates D, Cartlidge N, French J, Miller S. Longitudinal study of central motor conduction time following stroke: 2. Central motor conduction measured within 73 h after stroke as a predictor of functional outcome at 12 months. Brain 1993; 116:1371–1385.

162. Vang C, Dunbabin D, Kilpatrick D. Correlation between functional and electrophysiological recovery in acute ischemic stroke. Stroke 1999; 30:2126–2130.

163. Alagona G, Delvaux V, Gerard P, DePasqua V, Pennisi G, DelWaide P, Nicoletti F, Maertens de Noordhout A. Ipsilateral motor responses to focal transcranial magnetic stimulation in healthy and acute stroke patients. Stroke 2001; 32:1304–1309.

164. Marchal G, Serrati C, Rioux P, Petit-Taboue M, Viader F, de la Sayette V, LeDoze F, Lochon P, Derlon J, Orgogozo J. PET imaging of cerebral perfusion and oxygen consumption in acute ischaemic stroke: Relation to outcome. Lancet 1993; 341:925–927.

165. Marchal G, Beaudouin V, Rioux P, de la Sayette, Le Doze F, Viader F, Derlon J, Baron J. Prolonged persistence of substantial volumes of potentially viable brain tissue after stroke: A correlative PET-CT study with voxel-based data analysis. Stroke 1996; 27:599–606.

166. Beaulieu C, de Crespigny A, Tong D, Mosely M, Albers G, Marks M. Longitudinal magnetic resonance imaging study of perfusion and diffusion in stroke: Evolution of lesion volume and correlation with clinical outcome. Ann Neurol 1999; 46:568–578.

167. Binkofski F, Seitz R, Arnold S, Classen J, Benecke R, Freund H-J. Thalamic metabolism and corticospinal tract integrity determine motor recovery in stroke. Ann Neurol 1996; 39:460–470.

168. Bowler J, Wade J, Jones B, Nijran K, Jewkes R, Cuming R, Steiner T. Contribution of diaschisis to the clinical deficit in human cerebral infarction. Stroke 1995; 26:1000–1006.

169. Federico F, Simone I, Lucivero V, Giannini P, Laddomada G, Mezzapesa D, Tortorella C. Prognostic value of proton magnetic resonance spectroscopy in ischemic stroke. Arch Neurol 1998; 55:489–494.

170. Bragoni M, Caltagirone C, Troisi E, Matteis M, Vernieri F, Silvestrini M. Correlation of cerebral hemodynamic changes during mental activity and recovery after stroke. Neurology 2000; 55:35–40.

171. Nelles G, Spiekermann G, Jueptner M, Leonhardt G, Diener H, Muller S, Gerhard H. Evolution of functional reorganization in hemiplegic stroke: A serial positron emission tomographic activation study. Ann Neurol 1999; 46:901–909.

172. Heiss W-D, Kessler J, Thiel A, Ghaemi M, Karbe H. Differential capacity of left and right hemispheric areas for compensation of poststroke aphasia. Ann Neurol 1999; 45:430–438.

173. Carel C, Loubinoux I, Albucher J-F, Pariente J, Manelfe C, Chollet F. Correlation between motor recovery and cerebral reorganization. Neurology 2001; 56(Suppl 3):A25–A26.

174. Dobkin B, Sullivan K. Sensorimotor cortex plasticity and locomotor and motor control gains induced by body weight-supported treadmill training after stroke. Neurorehabil Neural Repair 2001; 15:258.

175. Rowe JW. Health care of the elderly. N Eng J Med 1985; 312:827–835.

176. Granger C, Hamilton B. The Uniform Data System for Medical Rehabilitation report of first admissions for 1992. Am J Phys Med Rehabil 1994; 73:51–55.

177. Fiedler R, Granger C, Post L. The Uniform Data System for Medical Rehabilitation: Report of first admissions for 1998. Am J Phys Med Rehabil 2000; 79:87–92.

178. Stineman M, Fiedler R, Granger C, Maislin G. Functional task benchmarks for stroke rehabilitation. Arch Phys Med Rehabil 1998; 79:497–504.

179. Gresham GE, Phillips TF, Wolf PA. Epidemiologic profile of long-term stroke disability: The Framingham Study. Arch Phys Med Rehabil 1979; 60:487–491.

180. Kelly-Hayes M, Wolf P, Kannel W, Gresham G. Factors influencing survival and the need for institutionalization following stroke: The Framingham Study. Arch Phys Med Rehabil 1988; 69:415–419.

181. Wade D, Langton Hewer R. Functional abilities after stroke: Measurement, natural history and prog-nosis. J Neurol Neurosurg Psychiatry 1987; 50:177–182.

182. Shah S, Corones J. Volition following hemiplegia. Arch Phys Med Rehabil 1980; 61:523–528.

183. Moskowitz E, Lightbody F, Freitag N. Long-term follow-up of the poststroke patient. Arch Phys Med Rehabil 1972; 53:167–172.

184. Wade D, Langton-Hewer R, Wood V. The hemiplegic arm after stroke. J Neurol Neurosurg Psychiatry 1983; 46:521–524.

185. Sunderland A, Tinson D, Bradley L, Hewer R. Arm function after stroke. J Neurol Neurosurg Psychiatry 1989; 52:1267–1272.

186. Katrak P, Bowring G, Conroy P, Chilvers M, Poulos R, McNeil D. Predicting upper limb recovery after stroke: The place of early shoulder and hand movement. Arch Phys Med Rehabil 1998; 79:758–761.

187. Skilbeck C, Wade D, Langston Hewer R, Wood V. Recovery after stroke. J Neurol Neurosurg Psychiatry 1983; 46:5–8.

188. Banks G, Short P, Martinez J, Latchaw R, Ratcliff G, Boller F. The alien hand syndrome. Arch Neurol 1989; 46:456–459.

189. Goldberg G, Bloom K. The alien hand sign. Am J Phys Med Rehabil 1990; 69:228–238.

190. Jorgensen H, Nakayama H, Raaschou H, Olsen T. Recovery of walking function in stroke patients: The Copenhagen Stroke Study. Arch Phys Med Rehabil 1995; 76:27–32.

191. Wade D, Wood V, Heller A, Maggs J, Langton Hewer R. Walking after stroke. Scand J Rehab Med 1987; 19:25–30.

192. Baer G, Smith M. The recovery of walking ability and subclassification of stroke. Physiother Res Int 2001; 6:135–144.

193. Smith M, Baer G. Achievement of simple mobility milestones after stroke. Arch Phys Med Rehabil 1999; 80:442–447.

194. Perry J, Garrett M, Gromley J, Mulroy S. Classification of walking handicap in the stroke population. Stroke 1995; 26:982–989.

195. de Bruijn S, Budde M, Teunisse S, de Haan R, Stam J. Long-term outcome of cognition and functional health after cerebral venous sinus thrombosis. Neurology 2000; 54:1687–1689.

196. Westerkam W, Cifu D, Keyser L. Functional outcome after inpatient rehabilitation following aneurysmal subarachnoid hemorrhage: A prospective analysis. Top Stroke Rehabil 1997; 4:29–37.

197. Wade D, Wood V, Langton-Hewer R. Recovery after stroke-the first 3 months. J Neurol Neurosurg Psychiatry 1985; 48:7–13.

198. Falconer J, Naughton B, Dunlop D, Roth E, Strasser D, Sinacore J. Predicting stroke inpatient rehabilitation outcome using a classification tree approach. Arch Phys Med Rehabil 1994; 75:619–625.

199. Tilling K, Sterne J, Rudd A, Glass T, Wityk R, Wolfe D. A new method for predicting recovery after stroke. Arch Phys Med Rehabil 2001; 82:2867–2873.

200. de Haan R, Limburg M, van der Meulen J, Jacobs H, Aaronson N. Quality of life after stroke: Impact of stroke type and lesion location. Stroke 1995; 26:402–408.

201. Heiss W-D, Emunds H-G, Herbolz K. Cerebral glucose metabolism as a predictor of rehabilitation after ischemic stroke. Stroke 1993; 24:1784–1788.

202. Dobkin B. Focused stroke rehabilitation programs do not improve outcome. Arch Neurol 1989; 46:701–703.

203. Ottenbacher K, Jannell S. The results of clinical trials in stroke rehabilitation research. Arch Neurol 1993; 50:37–44.

204. Stern P, McDowell F, Miller J, Robinson M. Effects of facilitation exercise techniques in stroke rehabilitation. Arch Phys Med Rehabil 1970; 51:526–531.

205. Lord J, Hall K. Neuromuscular reeducation versus traditional programs for stroke rehabilitation. Arch Phys Med Rehabil 1986; 67:88–91.

206. Logigian M, Samuels M, Falconer J. Clinical exercise trial for stroke patients. Arch Phys Med Rehabil 1983; 64:364–367.

207. Dickstein R, Hockerman S, Pillar T, Shaham R. Stroke rehabilitation: Three exercise therapy approaches. Phys Ther 1986; 66:1233–1238.

208. Basmajian J, Gowland C, Finlayson A, Hall A, Swanson L, Stratford P, Trotter J, Brandstater M. Stroke treatment comparison of integrated behavioral therapy vs. traditional physical therapy programs. Arch Phys Med Rehabil 1987; 69:401–406.

209. Jongbloed L, Stacey S, Brighton C. Stroke rehabilitation: Sensorimotor integrative treatment versus functional treatment. Am J Occup Ther 1989; 43: 391–397.

210. Wagenaar R, Meijer O, Kuik D, van Wieringen P, Hazenberg G, Lindeboom J, Wichers F, Rijswijk H. The functional recovery of stroke: A comparison between neuro-developmental treatment and the Brunnstrom method. Scand J Rehab Med 1990; 22:1–8.

211. Feys H, De Weerdt W, Selz B, Cox Steck G, Spichiger G, Vereeck L, Putman K, Van Hoydonck G. Effect of a therapeutic intervention for the hemiplegic upper limb in the acute phase after stroke. Stroke 1998; 29:785–792.

212. Inuba M, Edberg E, Montgomery J, Gillis K. Effectiveness of functional training, active exercise and resistive exercise for patients with hemiplegia. Phys Ther 1973; 53:28–35.

213. Bohannon R. Measurement and nature of muscle strength in patients with stroke. J Neuro Rehab 1997; 11:115–25.

214. Engardt M, Knutsson E, Jonsson M, Sternhag M. Dynamic muscle strength training in stroke patients: Effects on knee extension torque, electromyographic activity, and motor function. Arch Phys Med Rehabil 1995; 76:419–425.

215. Sunderland A, Tinson D, Bradley E, Fletcher D, Langdon Hewer R, Wade D. Enhanced physical therapy improves recovery of function after stroke. A randomised controlled trial. J Neurol Neurosurg Psychiatry 1992; 55:530–535.

216. Ashburn A, Partridge C, De Souza L. Physiotherapy in the rehabilitation of stroke: A review. Clin Rehabil 1993; 7:337–345.

217. Ernst E. A review of stroke rehabilitation and physiotherapy. Stroke 1990; 21:1081–1085.

218. Keith R, Cowell K. Time use of stroke patients in three rehabilitation hospitals. Soc Sci Med 1987; 24:529–533.

219. Tinson D. How stroke patients spend their days. Int Disabil Studies 1989; 11:45–49.

220. Walker M, Gladman J, Lincoln N, Siemonsma P, Whitely T. Occupational therapy for stroke patients not admitted to hospital: A randomised controlled trial. Lancet 1999; 354:278–280.

221. Platz T, Winter T, Muller N, pinkowski C, Eickhof C, Mauritz K-H. Arm Ability Training for stroke and traumatic brain injury patients with mild arm paresis: A single-blind, randomized, controlled trial. Arch Phys Med Rehabil 2001; 82:961–968.

222. Hesse S, Jahnke M, Bertelt C, Schreiner C, Lucke D, Mauritz K. Gait outcome in ambulatory hemiparetic patients after a 4-week comprehensive rehabilitation program and prognostic factors. Stroke 1994; 25:1999–2004.

223. Richards C, Malouin F, Wood-Dauphinee S, Williams J, Bouchard J, Brunet D. Task-specific physical therapy for optimization of gait recovery in acute stroke patients. Arch Phys Med Rehabil 1993; 74:612–620.

224. Satta N, Benson S, Reding M, Sagullo C. Walking endurance is better than speed or FIM walking subscore for documenting ambulation recovery after stroke. Stroke 1995; 26(abstract):192.

225. Sirigu A, Duhamel J, Cohen L, Pillon B, Dubois B, Agid Y. The mental representation of hand movements after parietal cortex damage. Science 1996; 273:1564–1568.

226. Jackson P, Lafleur M, Malouin F, Richards C, Doyon J. Potential role of mental practice using motor imagery in neurologic rehabilitation. Arch Phys Med Rehabil 2001; 82:1133–1141.

227. Taub E, Wolf S. Constraint induced movement techniques to facilitate upper extremity use in stroke patients. Top Stroke Rehabil 1997; 3:38–61.

228. Wolf S, Lecraw D, Barton L, Jann B. Forced use of hemiplegic upper extremities to reverse the effect of learned nonuse among chronic stroke and head-injured patients. Exp Neurol 1989; 104:125–132.

229. Taub E, Miller N, Novack T, Cook EW 3rd, Fleming W, Nepomuceno C, Connell J, Crago J. Technique to improve chronic motor deficit after stroke. Arch Phys Med Rehabil 1993; 74:347–354.

230. Kunkel A, Kopp B, Muller G. Constraint-induced movement therapy for motor recovery in chronic stroke patients. Arch Phys Med Rehabil 1999; 80: 624–628.

231. Miltner W, Bauder H, Sommer M, Dettmers C, Taub E. Effects of constraint-induced movement therapy on patients with chronic motor deficits after stroke. Stroke 1999; 30:586–592.

232. van der Lee J, Lankhorst G. Constraint-induced movement therapy and massed practice: Letter to editor. Stroke 2000; 31:986–989.

233. Dromerick A, Edwards D, Hahn M. Does the application of constraint-induced movement therapy during acute rehabilitation reduce arm impairment after ischemic stroke? Stroke 2000; 31:2984–2988.

234. Page S, Sisto S, Levine P, Johnston M, Hughes M. Modified constraint induced therapy: A randomized feasibility and efficacy study. J Rehabil Res Dev 2001; 38:583–590.

235. Liepert J, Bauder H, Miltner W, Taub E, Weiller C. Treatment-induced cortical reorganization after stroke in humans. Stroke 2000; 31:1210–1216.

236. Levy C, Nichols D, Schmalbrock P, Keller P, Chakeres D. Functional MRI evidence of cortical reorganization in upper-limb stroke hemiplegia treated

with constraint-induced movement therapy. Am J Phys Med Rehabil 2001; 80:4–12.

237. Nelles G, Jentzen W, Jueptner M, Muller S, Diener H. Arm training induced brain plasticity in stroke studies with serial positron emission tomography. NeuroImage 2001; 13:1146–1154.

238. Butefisch C, Hummelsheim H, Denzler P, Mauritz K-H. Repetitive training of isolated movements improves the outcome of motor rehabilitation of the centrally paretic hand. J Neurol Sci 1995; 130:59–68.

239. Dean C, Shepherd R. Task-related training improves performance of seated reaching tasks after stroke. Stroke 1997; 28:722–28.

240. Winstein C, Merians A, Sullivan K. Motor learning after unilateral brain damage. Neuropsychologia 1999; 37:975–987.

241. Lincoln N, Parry R, Vass C. Randomized, controlled trial to evaluate increased intensity of physiotherapy treatment of arm function after stroke. Stroke 1999; 30:573–579.

242. Teixeira L. Timing and force components in bilateral transfer of learning. Brain Cogn 2000; 44:455–469.

243. Mudie M, Matyas T. Can simultaneous bilateral movement involve the undamaged hemisphere in reconstruction of neural networks damaged by stroke? Disabil Rehabil 2000; 22:23–37.

244. Whitall J, Waller S, Silver K, Macko R. Repetitive bilateral arm training with rhythmic auditory cueing improves motor function in chronic hemiparetic stroke. Stroke 2000; 31:2390–2395.

245. Mudie M, Matyas T. Responses of the densely hemiplegic upper extremity to bilateral training. Neurorehabil Neural Repair 2001; 15:129–140.

246. Pohl P, Winstein C. Practice effects on the less-affected upper extremity after stroke. Arch Phys Med Rehabil 1999; 80:668–675.

247. Kioski L, Iacoboni M, Mazziotta J. Deconstructing apraxia: Understanding disorders of intentional movement after stroke. Curr Opin Neurol 2002; 15: 71–77.

248. Roy E, Heath M, Westwood D, Schweizer T, Dixon M, Black S, Kalbfleisch L, Barbour K, Square P. Task demands and limb apraxia in stroke. Brain Cognition 2000; 44:253–79.

249. Goldenberg G. Defective imitation of gestures in patients with damage in the left or right hemispheres. J Neurol Neurosurg Psychiatry 1996; 61:176–180.

250. Basso A, Capitani E, Della Salla S, Laiacona M, Spinnler H. Recovery from ideomotor apraxia: A study on acute stroke patients. Brain 1987; 110:747–760.

251. van Heugten C, Dekker J, Deelman B, Van Dijk A, Stehmann-Saris J, Kinebanian A. Outcome of strategy training in stroke patients with apraxia: A phase II study. Clin Rehabil 1998; 12:294–303.

252. Goldenberg G, Hagmann S. Therapy of activities of daily living in patients with apraxia. Neuropsychol Rehabil 1998; 2:123–141.

253. Smania N, Girardi F, Domenicali C, Lora E, Aglioti S. The rehabilitation of limb apraxia: A study in left brain damaged patients. Arch Phys Med Rehabil 2000; 81:379–388.

254. Sonde L, Gip C, Fernaeus E, Nilsson C, Viitanen M. Stimulation with low frequency (1.7hz) transcutaneous electric nerve stimulation (low-tens) increases motor function of the post-stroke paretic arm. Scand J Rehabil Med. 1998; 30:95–99.

255. Conforto A, Kaelin-Lang A, Cohen L. Increase in hand muscle strength of stroke patients after somatosensory stimulation. Ann Neurol 2002; 51:122–125.

256. Dannenbaum R, Dykes R. Sensory loss in the hand after sensory stroke: Therapeutic rationale. Arch Phys Med Rehabil 1988; 69:833–839.

257. Carey L, Matyas T, Oke L. Sensory loss in stroke patients: Effective training of tactile and proprioceptive discrimination. Arch Phys Med Rehabil 1993; 74: 602–611.

258. Yekutiel M, Guttman E. A controlled trial of the retraining of the sensory function of the hand in stroke patients. J Neurol Neurosurg Psychiatry 1993; 56: 241–244.

259. Pavlides C, Miyashita E, Asanuma H. Projection from the sensory to the motor cortex is important in learning motor skills in the monkey. J Neurophysiol 1993; 70:733–741.

260. Brown D, Kautz S, Dairaghi C. Muscle activity adapts to anti-gravity posture during pedalling in persons with post-stroke hemiplegia. Brain 1997; 120:825–837.

261. Potempa K, Lopez M, Braun L, et al. Physiological outcomes of aerobic exercise training in hemiparetic stroke. Stroke 1995; 26:101–105.

262. Giuliani C. Strength training for patients with neurological disorders. Neurol Rep 1995; 19:29–34.

263. Nugent J, Schurr K, Adams R. A dose-response relationship between amount of weight-bearing exercise and walking outcome following cerebrovascular accident. Arch Phys Med Rehabil 1994; 75:399–402.

264. Winstein C, Gardner E, McNeal D. Standing balance training: Effect on balance and locomotion in hemiparetic adults. Arch Phys Med Rehab 1989; 70: 755–762.

265. Thaut M, Kenyon G, Schauer M, McIntosh G. The connection between rhythmicity and brain function. IEEE Engineering In Medicine and Biology 1999; March/April:101–108.

266. Macko R, Smith G, Dobrovolny C, Sorkin J, Goldberg A, Silver K. Treadmill training improves fitness reserve in chronic stroke patients. Arch Phys Med Rehabil 2001; 82:879–884.

267. Visintin M, Barbeau H, Korner-Bitensky N, Mayo N. A new approach to retrain gait in stroke patients through body weight support and treadmill stimulation. Stroke 1998; 29:1122–1128.

268. Dobkin B, Harkema S, Requejo P, Edgerton V. Modulation of locomotor-like EMG activity in subjects with complete and incomplete chronic spinal cord injury. J Neurol Rehabil 1995; 9:183–190.

269. Harkema S, Hurley S, Patel U, Dobkin B, Edgerton V. Human lumbosacral spinal cord interprets loading during stepping. J Neurophysiol 1997; 77:797–811.

270. Hesse S, Bertelt C, Schaffrin A, Malezic M, Mauritz K. Restoration of gait in nonambulatory hemiparetic patients by treadmill training with partial body-weight support. Arch Phys Med Rehabil 1994; 75: 1087–1093.

271. Hesse S, Bertelt C, Jahnke M, Baake P, Mauritz K. Treadmill training with partial body weight support compared with physiotherapy in nonambulatory hemiparetic patients. Stroke 1995; 26:976–981.

272. Barbeau H, Fung J. The role of rehabilitation in the recovery of walking in the neurological population. Curr Opin Neurol 2001; 14:735–740.

273. Kosak M, Reding M. Comparison of partial body

341. Nicholas M, Helm-Estabrooks N, Ward-Lonergan J, Morgan A. Evolution of severe aphasia in the first two years post onset. Arch Phys Med Rehabil 1993; 74:830–836.

342. Lendrem W, Lincoln N. Spontaneous recovery of language in patients with aphasia between 4 and 35 weeks after stroke. J Neurol Neurosurg Psychiatry 1985; 48:733–738.

343. Kertesz A, McCabe P. Recovery patterns and prognosis in aphasia. Brain 1977; 100:1–18.

344. Enderby P, Wood V, Wade D, Langton-Hewer R. Aphasia after stroke: A detailed study of recovery in the first 3 months. Int Rehabil Med 1987; 8:162–165.

345. Holland A, Greenhouse J, Fromm D, Swindel C. Predictors of language restitution following stroke: A multivariate analysis. J Speech Hear Res 1989; 32: 232–238.

346. Kertesz A. What do we learn from recovery from aphasia. In: Waxman S, ed. Functional Recovery in Neurological Disease. New York: Raven Press, 1988:277–292.

347. Shewan C, Kertesz A. Effects of speech and language treatment on recovery from aphasia. Brain Lang 1984; 23:272–299.

348. Naeser M, Gaddie A, Palumbo C, Stiassny-Eder D. Late recovery of auditory comprehension in global aphasia. Arch Neurol 1990; 47:425–432.

349. Naeser M, Helm-Estabrooks N, Haas G, Auerbach S, Srinivasan M. Relationship between lesion extent in 'Wernicke's' area on computed tomographic scan and predicting recovery of comprehension in Wernicke's aphasia. Arch Neurol 1987; 44:73–82.

350. Alexander M, Naeser M, Palumbo C. Broca's area aphasias. Neurology 1990; 40:353–362.

351. Naeser M, Baker E, Palumbo C, Nicholas M, Alexander M, Samaraweera R, Prete M, Hodge S, Weissman T. Lesion site patterns in severe, nonverbal aphasia to predict outcome with a computer-assisted treatment program. Arch Neurol 1998; 55:1438–1448.

352. Hillis A, Woityk R, Tuffiash E, Beauchamp N, Jacobs M, Barker P, Selnes O. Hypoperfusion of Wernicke's area predicts severity of semantic deficit in acute stroke. Ann Neurol 2001; 50:561–566.

353. Musso M, Weiller C, Kiebel S. Training-induced brain plasticity in aphasia. Brain 1999; 122:1781–1790.

354. Mimura M, Kato M, Kato M, Sano Y, Kojima T, Naeser M, Kashima H. Prospective and retrospective studies of recovery in aphasia. Brain 1998; 121:2083–2094.

355. Rosen H, Petersen S, Linenweber B, Snyder A, White D, Chapman L, Dromerick A, Fiez J, Corbetta M. Neural correlates of recovery from aphasia after damage to left inferior frontal cortex. Neurology 2000; 55:1883–1894.

356. Heiss W-D, Kessler J, Karbe H, Fink G, Pawlik G. Cerebral glucose metabolism as a predictor of recovery from aphasia in ischemic stroke. Arch Neurol 1993; 50:958–964.

357. Karbe H, Kessler J, Herholz K, Fink G, Heiss W. Long-term prognosis of poststroke aphasia studied with positron emission tomography. Arch Neurol 1995; 52:186–190.

358. Robey R. A meta-analysis of clinical outcomes in the treatment of aphasia. J Speech Lang Hear Res 1998; 41:172–187.

359. Greener J, Enderby P, Whurr R. Speech and language therapy for aphasia following stroke (Cochrane Review). The Cochrane Library 2000:Oxford: Update Software.

360. Pulvermuller F, Neininger B, Elbert T, Mohr B, Rockstroh B, Koebbel P, Taub E. Constraint-induced therapy of chronic aphasia after stroke. Stroke 2001; 32:1621–1626.

361. Carlomagno S, Pandolfi M, Labruna L, Colombo A, Razzano C. Recovery from moderate aphasia in the first year poststroke: Effect of type of therapy. Arch Phys Med Rehabil 2001; 82:1073–1080.

362. Aftonomos L, Steele R, Wertz R. Promoting recovery in chronic aphasia with an interactive technology. Arch Phys Med Rehabil 1997; 78:841–846.

363. Weinrich M, Boser K, McCall D, Bishop V. Training agrammatic subjects on passive sentences: Implications for syntactic deficit theories. Brain Lang 2001; 76:45–61.

364. Kessler J, Thiel A, Karbe H, Heiss W. Piracetam improves activated blood flow and facilitates rehabilitation of poststroke aphasic patients. Stroke 2000; 31:2112–2116.

365. Damasio H, Grabowski TJ, Tranel D, Ponto LLB, Hichwa RD, Damasio AR. Neural correlates of naming actions and of naming spatial relations. NeuroImage 2001; 13:1053–1064.

366. Walker-Batson D, Curtis S, Natarajan R, Ford J, Dronkers N, Salmeron E, Lai J, Unwin D. A double-blind placebo-controlled study of the use of amphetamine in the treatment of aphasia. Stroke 2001; 32:2093–2098.

367. Huber W, Willmes K, Poeck K, Vanvleymen B, Deberdt W. Piracetam as an adjuvant to language therapy for aphasia: A randomized double-blind placebo-controlled pilot study. Arch Phys Med Rehabil 1997; 78:245–50.

368. Tanaka Y, Albert M, Yokoyama E, Nonaka C. Cholinergic therapy for anomia in fluent aphasia. Ann Neurol 2001; 50 (Suppl 1):S61–62.

369. Micoch A, Gupta S, Scolaro C, Moritz T. Bromocriptine treatment of nonfluent aphasia, Annual Meeting of the American Speech and Hearing Association, 1994.

370. Gold M, VanDam D, Silliman E. An open-label trial of bromocriptine in nonfluent aphasia: A qualitative analysis of word storage and retrieval. Brain Lang 2000; 74:141–156.

371. Waelti P, Dickinson A, Schultz W. Dopamine responses comply with basic assumptions of formal learning theory. Nature 2001; 412:43–48.

372. Fried I, Wilson C, Morrow J, Cameron K, Behnke E, Fields T, MacDonald K. Increased dopamine release in the human amygdala during performance of cognitive tasks. Nature Neurosci 2001; 4:201–206.

373. Mattay V, Callicott J, Bertolino A, Heaton I, Frank J, Coppola R, Berman K, Goldberg T, Weinberger D. Effects of dextroamphetamine on cognitive performance and cortical activation. Neuroimage 2000; 12:268–275.

374. Sabe L, Leiguarda R, Starkstein S. An open-label trial of bromocriptine in nonfluent aphasia. Neurology 1992; 42:1637–1638.

375. Albert M, Bachman D, Morgan A, Helm-Estabrooks N. Pharmacotherapy for aphasia. Neurology 1988; 38:877–879.

376. Leiguarda R, Merello M, Sabe L, Starkstein S. Bromocriptine-induced dystonia in patients with aphasia and hemiparesis. Neurology 1993; 43:2319–2322.

377. De Deyn P, De Reuck J, Deberdt W, Vlietinck R, Orgogozo J. Treatment of acute ischemic stroke with piracetam. Stroke 1997; 28:2347–2352.

378. Tatemichi T, Desmond D, Stern Y, Paik M, Sano M, Bagiella E. Cognitive impairment after stroke: Frequency, patterns, and relationship to functional abilities. J Neurol Neurosurg Psychiatry 1994; 57:202–207.

379. Hochstenbach J, Anderson P, van Limbeek J, Mulder T. Is there a relation between neuropsychologic variables and quality of life after stroke. Arch Phys Med Rehabil 2001; 82:1360–1366.

380. Hoffman M. Higher cortical function deficits after stroke: An analysis of 1,000 patients from a dedicated cognitive stroke registry. Neurorehabil Neural Repair 2001; 15:113–127.

381. Rockwood K, Wentzel C, Hachinski V, Hogan D, MacKnight C, McDowell I. Prevalence and outcomes of vascular cognitive impairment. Neurology 2000; 54:447–451.

382. Desmond D, Tatemichi T, Paik M, Stern Y. Risk factors for cerebrovascular disease as correlates of cognitive function in a stroke-free cohort. Arch Neurol 1993; 50:162–166.

383. Bernick C, Kuller L, Dulberg C, Longstreth W, Manolio T, Beauchamp N, Price T. Silent MRI infarcts and the risk of future stroke: The cardiovascular health study. Neurology 2001; 57:1222–1229.

384. Moroney J, Bagiella E, Desmond D, Paik M, Y S, Tatemichi T. Risk factors for incident dementia after stroke. Stroke 1996; 27:1283–1289.

385. Gorelick P. Status of risk factors for dementia associated with stroke. Stroke 1997; 28:459–463.

386. Desmond D, Moroney J, Paik M, Sano M, Mohr J, Aboumatar S, Tseng C, Chan S, Williams J, Remien R, Hauser W, Stern Y. Frequency and clinical determinants of dementia after ischemic stroke. Neurology 2000; 54:1124–1131.

387. Kokmen E, Whisnant J, O'Fallon W, Beard C. Dementia after ischemic stroke: A population based study in Rochester, Minn. Neurology 1996; 46:154–159.

388. Pohjasvaara T, Erkinjuntti T, Vataja R, Kaste M. Dementia three months after stroke. Baseline frequency and effect of different definitions of dementia in the Helsinki Stroke Aging Memory Study (SAM) Cohort. Stroke 1997; 28:785–792.

389. Henon H, Pasquier F, Durieu I, Godefroy O, Lucas C, Lebert F, Leys D. Preexisting dementia in stroke patients. Stroke 1997; 28:2429–2436.

390. Henon H, Durieu I, Guerouaou D, Lebert F, Pasquier F, Leys D. Poststroke dementia: Incidence and relationship to prestroke cognitive decline. Neurology 2001; 57:1216–1222.

391. Wade D, Parker V, Langton-Hewer R. Memory disturbance after stroke: Frequency and associated losses. Int Rehabil Med 1987; 8:60–64.

392. Ween J, Verfaellie M, Alexander M. Verbal memory function in mild aphasia. Neurology 1996; 47:795–801.

393. Corbett A, Bennett H, Kos S. Cognitive dysfunction following subcortical infarction. Arch Neurol 1994; 51:999–1007.

394. Mungas D, Jagust W, Reed B, Kramer J, Chui H, Weiner M, Schuff N, Norman D, Mack W, Willis L. MRI predictors of cognition in subcortical ischemic vascular disease and Alzheimer's disease. Neurology 2001; 57:229–235.

395. Damasio A, Graff-Radford N, Damasio H, Kassell N. Amnesia following basal forebrain lesions. Arch Neurol 1985; 42:263–271.

396. Johnson M, O'Connor M, Cantor J. Confabulation, memory deficits, and frontal dysfunction. Brain Cognition 1997; 34:189–206.

397. Schnider A. Spontaneous confabulation, reality monitoring, and the limbic system—a review. Brain Res Rev 2001; 36:150–160.

398. Irle E, Wowra B, Kunert H, Hampl J, Kunze S. Memory disturbances following anterior communicating artery rupture. Ann Neurol 1992; 31:473–480.

399. Dobkin B, Hanlon R. Dopamine agonist treatment of antegrade amnesia from a mediobasal forebrain injury. Ann Neurol 1992; 33:313–316.

400. Hanlon R. Motor learning following unilateral stroke. Arch Phys Med Rehabil 1996; 77:811–815.

401. Wilson B, Baddeley A, Evans J, Shiel A. Errorless learning in the rehabilitation of memory impaired people. Neuropsychol Rehabil 1994; 4:307–326.

402. Chui H. Vascular dementia, a new beginning, shifting focus from clinical phenotype to ischemic brain injury. Neurol Clin 2000; 18:951–978.

403. Halligan P, Marshall J. Left neglect for near but not far space in man. Nature 1991; 350:498–500.

404. Ellis S, Small M. Denial of illness in stroke. Stroke 1993; 24:757–759.

405. Taylor D, Ashburn A, Ward C. Asymmetrical trunk posture, unilateral neglect and motor performance following stroke. Clin Rehabil 1994; 8:48–53.

406. Watson R, Valenstein E, Day A, Heilman K. Posterior neocortical systems subserving awareness and neglect. Arch Neurol 1994; 51:1014–1021.

407. Mesulam M-M. Principles of Behavioral and Cognitive Neurology. New York: Oxford University Press, 2000.

408. Starkstein S, Fedoroff J, Price T, Leiguarda R, Robinson R. Anosognosia in patients with cerebrovascular lesions. Stroke 1992; 23:1446–1453.

409. D'Esposito M, McGlinchey-Berroth R, Alexander M, Verfaellie M, Milberg W. Dissociable cognitive and neural mechanisms of unilateral visual neglect. Neurology 1993; 43:2636–2644.

410. Sunderland A, Wade D, Langton-Hewer R. The natural history of visual neglect after stroke. Int Disabil Studies 1987; 9:55–59.

411. Marshall R, Sacco R, Lee S, Mohr J. Hemineglect predicts functional outcome after stroke. Ann Neurol 1994; 36(abstr):298.

412. Kalra L, Perez I, Gupta S, Wittink M. The influence of visual neglect on stroke rehabilitation. Stroke 1997; 28:1386–1391.

413. Stone S, Patel P, Greenwood R, Halligan P. Measuring visual neglect in acute stroke and predicting its recovery: The Visual Neglect Recovery Index. J Neurol Neurosurg Psychiat 1992; 55:431–436.

414. Stone S, Patel P, Greenwood R. Selection of acute stroke patients for treatment of visual neglect. J Neurol Neurosurg Psychiatry 1993; 56:463–466.

415. Mattingley J, Bradshaw J, Bradshaw J, Nettleton N. Residual rightward attentional bias after apparent re-

covery from right hemisphere damage: Implications for a multicomponent model of neglect. J Neurol Neurosurg Psychiatry 1994; 57:597–604.

416. Katz N, Hartman-Maeir A, Ring H, Soroker N. Functional disability and rehabilitation outcome in right hemisphere damaged patients with and without unilateral spatial neglect. Arch Phys Med Rehabil 1999; 80:379–384.

417. Halligan P, Marshall J. Spatial neglect: Position papers on theory and practice. Neuropsychol Rehabil 1994; 4:103–230.

418. Robertson I, Murre J. Rehabilitation of brain damage: Brain plasticity and principles of guided recovery. Psychol Bull 1999; 125:544–575.

419. Bartolomeo P, Chokron S. Left unilateral neglect or right hyperattention? Neurology 1999; 53:2023–2027.

420. Doricchi F, Incoccia C. Seeing only the right half of the forest but cutting down all the trees? Nature 1998; 394:75–78.

421. Gordon W, Diller L, Lieberman A, Shaver M, Hibbard M, Egelko S, Ragnarsson K. Perceptual remediation in patients with right brain damage: A comprehensive program. Arch Phys Med Rehabil 1985; 66:353–359.

422. Ben-Yishay Y, Diller L. Cognitive remediation in traumatic brain injury: Update and issues. Arch Phys Med Rehabil 1993; 74:204–213.

423. Lincoln N, Whitting S, Cockburn J, Bhavnani G. An evaluation of perceptual training. Int Rehabil Med 1985; 7:90–101.

424. Pizzamiglio L, Antonucci G, Judica A, Montenero P, Razzano C, Zoccolotti P. Chronic rehabilitation of the hemineglect disorder in chronic patients with unilateral right brain damage. J Clin Exp Neuropsychol 1992; 14:901–923.

425. Pizzamiglio L, Perani D, Cappa S, Vallar G, Paolucci S, Grassi F, Paulesu E, Fazio F. Recovery of neglect after right hemisphere damage. Arch Neurol 1998; 55:561–568.

426. Paolucci S, Antonucci G, Grasso M, Pizzamiglio L. The role of unilateral spatial neglect in rehabilitation of right brain-damaged ischemic stroke patients: a matched comparison. Arch Phys Med Rehabil 2001; 82:743–749.

427. Hanlon R, Dobkin B. Effects of cognitive rehabilitation following a right thalamic infarct. J Clin Exp Neuropsychol 1992; 14:433–447.

428. Young G, Collins D, Hren M. Effect of pairing scanning training with block design training in the remediation of perceptual problems in left hemiplegics. J Clin Neuropsychol 1983; 5:201–212.

429. Wiart L, Come A, Debelleix X, Petit H, Joseph P, Mazaux J, Barat M. Unilateral neglect syndrome rehabilitation by trunk rotation and scanning training. Arch Phys Med Rehabil 1997; 78:424–429.

430. Robertson I, North N. Spatio-motor cueing in unilateral neglect: the role of hemispace, hand and motor activation. Neuropsychologia 1992; 30:553–563.

431. Robertson I, Mattingley J, Rorden C, Driver J. Phasic alerting of neglect patients overcomes their spatial deficit in visual awareness. Nature 1998; 395:169–172.

432. Karnath H, Schenkel P, Fischer B. Trunk orientation as the determining factor of the contralateral deficit in the neglect syndrome and as the physical anchor

of the internal representation of body orientation in space. Brain 1991; 114:1997–2014.

433. Mennemeier M, Chatterjee A, Heilman K. A comparison of the influences of body and environment centred reference frames on neglect. Brain 1994; 117:1013–1021.

434. Loverro J, Reding M. Bed orientation and rehabilitation outcome for patients with stroke and hemianopsia or visual neglect. J Neurol Rehabil 1988; 2:147–150.

435. Lincoln N, Sackley C. Biofeedback in stroke rehabilitation. Crit Rev Phys Rehabil Med 1992; 4:37–47.

436. Pommerenke K, Markowitsch H. Rehabilitation training of homonymous visual field defects in patients with postgeniculate damage of the visual system. Restor Neurol Neurosci 1989; 1:47–63.

437. Rossi P, Kheyfets S, Reding M. Fresnel prisms improve visual perception in stroke patients with homonymous hemianopia or unilateral visual neglect. Neurology 1990; 40:1597–1599.

438. Rossetti Y, Rode G, Pisella L, Farne A, Li L, Boisson D, Perenin M. Prism adaptation to a rightward optical deviation rehabilitates left hemispatial neglect. Nature 1998; 395:166–169.

439. Robertson I, Gray J, Pentland B, Waite L. Microcomputer-based rehabilitation for unilateral left visual neglect: A randomized controlled trial. Arch Phys Med Rehabil 1990; 71:663–668.

439a. Frassinetti F, Angeli V, Meneghello F, Avanzi S, Ladavas E. Long-lasting amelioration of visuospatial neglect by prism adaptation. Brain 2002; 125:608–623.

440. Webster J, McFarland P, Rapport L, Morrill B, Roades L, Abadee P. Computer-assisted training for improving wheelchair mobility in unilateral neglect patients. Arch Phys Med Rehabil 2001; 82:769–775.

441. Butter C, Kirsch N. Combined and separate effects of eye patching and visual stimulation on unilateral neglect following stroke. Arch Phys Med Rehabil 1992; 73:1133–1139.

442. Beis J-M, Andre J-M, Baumgarten A, Challier B. Eye patching in unilateral spatial neglect: Efficacy of two methods. Arch Phys Med Rehabil 1999; 80:71–76.

443. Zihl J, von Cramon D. Visual field recovery from scotoma in patients with postgeniculate damage. Brain 1985; 108:439–469.

444. Kerkhoff G, MunBinger U, Meier E. Neurovisual rehabilitation in cerebral blindness. Arch Neurol 1994; 51:474–481.

445. Nelles G, Esser J, Tiede A, Gerhard H, Diener C. Compensatory visual field training in recovery from hemianopia after stroke. Neurology 2000; 54 (Suppl 3):A9–A10.

446. Nelles G, Widman G, deGreiff A. Brain representation in poststroke visual field defects. Stroke 2002; 33:1286–1293.

447. Rubens A. Caloric stimulation and unilateral visual neglect. Neurology 1985; 35:1019–1024.

448. Rode G, Charles N, Perenin M-T, Vighetto A, Trillet M, Aimard G. Partial remission of hemiplegia and somatoparaphrenia through vestibular stimulation in a case of unilateral neglect. Cortex 1992; 28:203–208.

449. Vallar G, Sterzi R, Bottini G, Cappa S, Rusconi M. Temporary remission of left hemianesthesia after vestibular stimulation: A sensory neglect phenomenon. Cortex 1990; 26:123–131.

450. Oliveri M, Rossini P, Traversa R, Cicinelli P, Pasqualetti P, Filippi M, Tomaiuolo F, Caltagirone C. Left frontal transcranial magnetic stimulation reduces contralesional extinction in patients with unilateral right brain damage. Brain 1999; 122:1731–1739.

451. Fleet W, Valenstein E, Watson R, Heilman K. Dopamine agonist therapy for neglect in humans. Neurology 1987; 37:1765–1770.

452. McNeny R, Zasler N. Neuropharmacologic management of hemi-inattention after brain injury. Neuro Rehabil 1991; 1:72–78.

453. Mukand J, Guilmette T, Allen D, Brown L, Brown S, Tober K, Vandyck W. Dopaminergic therapy with carbidopa L-Dopa for left neglect after stroke: A case series. Arch Phys Med Rehabil 2001; 82:1279–1282.

454. Coull J, Nobre A, Frith C. The noradrenergic a2 agonist clonidine modulates behavioural and neuroanatomical correlates of human attentional orienting and alerting. Cereb Cortex 2001; 11:73–84.

455. Granon S, Passetti F, Thomas K, Dalley J, Everitt B, Robbins T. Enhanced and impaired attentional performance after infusion of D1 dopaminergic receptor agents into rat prefrontal cortex. Neuroscience 2000; 20:1208–1215.

456. Volkow N, Wang G-J, Fowler J, Logan J, Gerasimov M, Maynard L, Ding Y, Gatley S, Gifford A, Franceschi D. Therapeutic doses of oral methyl-phenidate significantly increase extracellular dopamine in the human brain. J Neurosci 2001; 21:RC121 (1–5).

457. Grujic Z, Mapstone M, Gitelman D, Johnson N, Weintraub S, Hayes A, Kwasnica C, Harvey R, Mesulam M. Dopamine agonists reorient visual exploration away from the neglected hemispace. Neurology 1998; 51:1395–1398.

458. Robinson R. Neuropsychiatric consequences of stroke. Annu Rev Med 1997; 48:217–229.

459. Pohjasvaara T, Leppavuori A, Siira I, Vataja R, Kaste M, Erkinjuntti T. Frequency and clinical determinants of poststroke depression. Stroke 1998; 29:2311–2317.

460. Gillen R, Tennen H, McKee T, Gernert-Dott P, Affleck G. Depressive symptoms and history of depression predict rehabilitation efficiency in stroke patients. Arch Phys Med Rehabil 2001; 82:1645–1649.

461. Kimura M, Robinson R, Kosier J. Treatment of cognitive impairment after poststroke depression. Stroke 2000; 31:1482–1486.

462. Robinson-Smith G, Johnston M, Allen J. Self-care self-efficacy, quality of life and depression after stroke. Arch Phys Med Rehabil 2000; 81:460–464.

463. Carota A, Rossetti A, Karapanayiotides T, Bogousslavsky J. Catastrophic reaction in acute stroke: A reflex behavior in aphasic patients. Neurology 2001; 57:1902–1905.

464. Ghika-Schmid F, van Melle G, Guex P, Bogousslavsky J. Subjective experience and behavior in acute stroke: The Lausanne emotion in acute stroke study. Neurology 1999; 52:22–28.

465. House A, Dennis M, Molyneux A, Warlow C, Hawton K. Emotionalism after stroke. Br Med J 1989; 298:991–994.

466. Starkstein S, Fedoroff J, Price T, Leiguarda R, Robinson R. Apathy following cerebrovascular lesions. Stroke 1993; 24:1625–1630.

467. Wade D, Smith J, Legh-Smith J, Langton-Hewer R. Depressed mood after stroke: A community study of its frequency. Br J Psychiatry 1987; 151:200–206.

468. Robinson R, Price T. Post-stroke depressive disorders: A follow up study of 103 outpatients. Stroke 1982; 13:635–640.

469. Kotila M, Numminen H, Waltimo O, Kaste M. Depression after stroke. Stroke 1998; 29:368–372.

470. Wolf P, Bachman D, Kelly-Hayes M. Stroke and depression in the community: The Framingham Study. Neurology 1990; 40(suppl1):416.

471. Astrom M, Adolfsson R, Asplund K. Major depression in stroke patients: A 3-year longitudinal study. Stroke 1993; 24:976–982.

472. Robinson R, Bolduc M, Price T. Two-year longitudinal study of poststroke mood disorders. Stroke 1987; 18:837–843.

473. Robinson R, Kubos K, Starr L, Rao K, Price T. Mood disorders in stroke patients: Importance of location of lesion. Brain 1984; 187:81–93.

474. Kim J, Choi-Kwon S. Poststroke depression and emotional incontinence. Neurology 2000; 54:1805–1810.

475. Okada K, Kobayashi S, Yamagata S, Takahashi K, Yamaguchi S. Poststroke apathy and regional cerebral blood flow. Stroke 1997; 28:2437–2441.

476. Gordon W, Hibbard M, Ross E. Issues in the diagnosis of post-stroke depression. Rehabil Psychol 1991; 36:71–87.

477. Sinyor D, Jacques P, Kaloupek D, Becker R, Goldenberg M, Coopersmith H. Poststroke depression and lesion location. Brain 1986; 109:537–546.

478. Parikh R, Robinson R, Lipsey J, Starkstein S, Fedoroff J, Price T. The impact of poststroke depression on recovery of activities of daily living over a 2-year follow-up. Stroke 1990; 47:785–789.

479. Angeleri F, Angereri V, Foschi N, Giaquinto S, Nolfe G. The influence of depression, social activity, and family stress on functional outcome after stroke. Stroke 1993; 24:1478–1483.

480. Lipsey J, Robinson R. Nortriptyline treatment of poststroke depression. Lancet 1984; 1:297–299.

481. Reding M, Orto L, Winter S, McDowell F. Antidepressant therapy after stroke. Arch Neurol 1986; 43:763–765.

482. Lazarus L, Moberg P, Langsley P, Lingam V. Methylphenidate and nortriptyline in the treatment of poststroke depression: A retrospective comparison. Arch Phys Med Rehabil 1994; 75:403–406.

483. Wiart L, Petit H, Joseph P, Mazaux J, Barat M. Fluoxetine in early poststroke depression; A double-blind placebo-controlled study. Stroke 2000; 31:1829–1832.

484. Finklestein S, Weintraub R, Karmouz N, Askinazi C, Davar G, Baldessarini R. Antidepressant drug treatment for poststroke depression: Retrospective study. Arch Phys Med Rehabil 1987; 68:772–776.

485. Starkstein S, Robinson R. Affective disorders and cerebral vascular disease. Br J Psychiatry 1989; 154:170–182.

486. Andersen G, Vsetergaard K, Lauritzen L. Effective treatment of poststroke depression with the selective serotonin reuptake inhibitor citalopram. Stroke 1994; 25:1099–1104.

487. Andersen G, Vestergaard K, Riis J. Poststroke pathological crying treated with the selective serotonin uptake inhibitor, citalopram. Lancet 1993; 342:837–839.

488. Hu F, Stampfer M, Colditz G, Ascherio A, Rexrode

K, Willett W, Manson J. Physical activity and risk of stroke in women. JAMA 2000; 283:2961–2967.

489. Kiely D, Wolf P, Cupples L, Beiser A, Kannel W. Physical activity and stroke risk. Am J Epidemiol 1994; 140:608–620.

490. Klungel O, Heckbert S, Longstreth W, Furberg C, Kaplan R, Smith N, Lemaitre R, Leufkens H, de Boer A, Psaty B. Antihypertensive drug therapies and the risk of ischemic stroke. Arch Intern Med 2001; 161:37–43.

491. Perindopril Group. Randomised trial of a perindopril-based blood-pressure-lowering regimen among 6105 individuals with previous stroke or transient ischaemic attack. Lancet 2001; 358:1033–1041.

492. Rogers A, Neal B, McMahon S. The effects of blood pressure lowering in cerebrovascular disease. Neurol Rev Int 1997; 2:12–15.

493. Mas J-L, Arquizan C, Lamy C, Zuber M, Cabanes L, Derumeaux G, Coste J. Recurrent cerebrovascular events associated with patent foramen ovale, atrial septal aneurysm, or both. N Engl J Med 2001; 345:1740–1746.

494. Burchfiel C, Curb J, Rodrigues B, Abbot R, Chiu D, Yano K. Glucose intolerance and 22-year stroke incidence: The Honolulu Heart Program. Stroke 1994; 25:951–957.

495. Wagner E, Sandhu N, Newton K, McCulloch D, Ramsey S, Grothaus L. Effect of improved glycemic control on health care costs and utilization. JAMA 2001; 285:182–189.

496. Boushey C, Beresford S, Omenn G, Motulsky A. A quantitative assessment of plasma homocysteine as a risk factor for vascular disease. JAMA 1995; 274:1049–1057.

497. Jorenby D. A controlled trial of sustained-release bupropion, a nicotine patch, or both for smoking cessation. N Engl J Med 1999; 340:685–691.

498. Sacco R, Elkind M, Boden-Albala B, Lin I-F, Kargman D, Hauser W, Shea S, Paik M. The protective effect of moderate alcohol consumption on ischemic stroke. JAMA 1999; 281:53–60.

499. Eigenbrodt M, Rose K, Couper D, Arnett D, Smith R, Jones D. Orthostatic hypotension as a risk factor for stroke. Stroke 2000; 31:2307–2313.

500. Mohsenin V. Sleep-related breathing disorders and risk of stroke. Stroke 2001; 32:1271–1278.

501. Shlipak M, Simon J, Vittinghoff E, Lin F, Barrett-Connor E, Knopp R, Levy R, Hulley S. Estrogen and progestin, lipoprotein(a), and the risk of recurrent coronary heart disease events after menopause. JAMA 2000; 283.

502. Viscoli C, Brass L, Kernan W, Sarrel P, Suissa S, Horwitz R. A clinical trial of estrogen replacement therapy after ischemic stroke. N Engl J Med 2001; 345:1243–1249.

503. Willett W, Stampfer M. What vitamins should I be taking, doctor? N Engl J Med 2001; 345:1819–1824.

504. Lawrence E, Coshall C, Dundas R, Stewart J, Rudd A, Howard R, Wolfe C. Estimates of the prevalence of acute stroke impairments and disability in a multiethnic population. Stroke 2001; 32:1279–1284.

505. Dobkin B. The rehabilitation of elderly stroke patients. Clin Geriatr Med 1991; 7:507–523.

506. Dombovy M. Stroke: clinical course and neurophysiologic mechanisms of recovery. Crit Rev Phys Med Rehabil 1991; 2:171–188.

507. Basso A, Capitani E, Vignolo L. Influence of rehabilitation on language skills in aphasic patients. Arch Neurol 1979; 36:190–196.

508. David R, Enderby P, Bainton D. Treatment of acquired aphasia: Speech therapists and volunteers compared. J Neurol Neurosurg Psychiatry 1982; 45:957–961.

509. Lincoln N, Mulley G, Jones A, McGuirk E, Lendrem W, Mitchell J. Effectiveness of speech therapy for aphasic stroke patients. Lancet 1984; 1:1197–1200.

510. Wertz R, Weiss D, Aten J, Brookshire R, Garcia-Bunuel L, Holland A, Kurtzke J, LaPointe L, Miliante F, Brannegan R. Comparison of clinic, home, and deferred language treatment for aphasia. Arch Neurol 1986; 43:653–658.

511. Hartman J, Landau W. Comparison of formal language therapy with supportive counseling for aphasia due to acute vascular accident. Arch Neurol 1987; 44:646–649.

512. Simon E, Hegarty A, Mehler M. Hemispatial and directional performance biases in motor neglect. Neurology 1995; 45:525–531.

513. Smania N, Bazoli F, Piva D, Guidetti G. Visuomotor imagery and rehabilitation of neglect. Arch Phys Med Rehabil 1997; 78:430–436.

514. Tham K, Tegner R. Video feedback in the rehabilitation of patients with unilateral neglect. Arch Phys Med Rehabil 1997; 78:410–413.

515. Serfaty C, Soroker N, Glicksohn J, Sepkuti J, Myslobodsky M. Does monocular viewing improve target detection in hemispatial neglect? Restor Neurol Neurosci 1995; 9:7–13.

516. Pizzamiglio L, Frasca R, Guariglia C, Inoccia C, Antonucci G. Effects of optokinetic stimulation in patients with visual neglect. Cortex 1990; 26:535–540.

517. Perennou D, Leblond C, Amblard B, Micallef J, Herisson C, Pelissier J. Transcutaneous electric nerve stimulation reduces neglect-related postural instability after stroke. Arch Phys Med Rehabil 2001; 82:440–448.

518. Gray J, Robertson I, Pentland B, Anderson S. Microcomputer-based attentional retraining after brain damage: A randomised group controlled trial. Neuropsychol Rehabil 1992; 2:97–115.

Chapter 10

Acute and Chronic Myelopathies

For young men and women, a traumatic spinal cord injury (SCI) may mean negotiating a life yet uncharted in a wheelchair. For older victims of falls and accidents, a charted path veers to a pace slowed by physical barriers, bladder catheters, and pain. At first, no patient succumbs to the notion of life without walking. No person can imagine a lifetime of not being able to scratch one's nose or feed oneself. The sound bytes from the media about an imminent cure for SCI leads to desperate searches for interventions that had modest success in rodents or to spending money in backstreet clinics for illusory healing through sham treatments. Biologic and training interventions may well moderate disability in the next 10–20 years (see Chapter 2).[1] Axonal regeneration over 1–3 spinal segments that improves reaching or grasping after a cervical SCI or walking after a low thoracic SCI seems feasible. For now, clinicians have much to offer patients with traumatic and nontraumatic SCI to improve the quality of life.

EPIDEMIOLOGY

Traumatic Spinal Cord Injury

Estimates of the prevalence of traumatic SCI in the United States range from 525–1124 cases per 1 million population,[2] up to approximately 230,000 survivors.[3] The yearly incidence of hospitalized patients is approximately 40 per 1 million persons or 11,000 additional victims each year. Serious nontraumatic SCI cases are about double this incidence. Valuable epidemiologic information regarding SCI in the United States comes from at least 3 prospectively collected sources. The *National Spinal Cord Injury Statistical Center* (NSCISC) (www.spinalcord.uab.edu) provides data collected by 24 rehabilitation sites of the *Model Spinal Cord Injury Systems Program*, funded since around 1974 by the National Institute on Disability and

451

Rehabilitation Research.[4,5] Its database includes over 20,000 patients and represents approximately 13% of all acute traumatic SCI cases.[3]

The Uniform Data System for Medical Rehabilitation (UDS$_{MR}$) in Buffalo, N.Y. reports each year on first rehabilitation admissions for approximately 5000 patients with traumatic and 10,000 with nontraumatic myelopathies.[6] These patients represent nearly half of all survivors of traumatic SCI. In recent years, Model Systems sites are included in UDS$_{MR}$ data and both employ the Functional Independence Measure (FIM) instrument. In contrast, 3 randomized clinical trials from the *National Acute Spinal Cord Injury Study* (NASCIS) offer a prospective view of 1500 patients primarily for the first 6 weeks and 6 months after a traumatic SCI.[7,8] These interventional studies excluded patients, however, who were not evaluated within 8 hours of SCI, people with gunshot wounds, pregnant women, people who weighed over 240 pounds, and those with serious comorbidities.

MEASURES OF IMPAIRMENT AND DISABILITY

The *American Spinal Injury Association*'s (ASIA) "Standards for Neurological and Functional Classification of Spinal Cord Injury, Revised 1992," has become the most widely used format for categorizing the motor and sensory examinations (Fig. 10–1). The motor score, which uses the British Medical Council scale for key muscles that each represent a root level, does not measure the strength of the abdominal muscles, which can act as hip flexors when the pelvis is tilted. The sensory scale specifies only appreciation of pin prick and light touch, not proprioception. The zone of partial preservation refers to the dermatomes and myotomes caudal to a complete injury that retain partial sensorimotor function. The zone is usually confined to several segments and in the region of the gray matter injury. The ASIA Impairment Scale describes the completeness of the level of injury (Table 10–1). The scale modifies the older Frankel classification by its emphasis on sparing or involvement of sacral dermatomal sensation. The ASIA motor level is the lowest key muscle that has a grade of at least 3, providing the key muscles of segments above that level are graded 5.

Studies of outcome after SCI have used a variety of functional assessments. The Modified Barthel Index (MBI), a 100-point scale (see Table 7–14), was shown to be valid, reliable, and sensitive to functional change over time in patients with SCI.[9] The ASIA has recommended the FIM (see Table 7–15), and most centers in the United States now incorporate this scale. The MBI and an adaptation of the FIM that eliminated the cognition, communication, and social adjustment subscales were found to correlate well, especially on the self-care subscores.[10]

A useful research tool to stratify outcomes after SCI has been used by Curt and Dietz and other investigators to assess hand function and ambulation.[11] For hand motor function, patients are classified as (1) being unable to make a voluntary grasp (no wrist extension or intrinsic muscle function); (2) having active hand function with wrist extension and passive grasp by a tenodesis effect; and (3) having active grasp with use of the intrinsic hand muscle, allowing lateral pinch. For ambulation, patients are classified as (1) unable to stand or walk; (2) able to stand or walk with physical help of 2 therapists or braces in parallel bars for therapeutic activity; (3) possessing functional ambulation with daily walking over short distances without physical help or braces other than an AFO; and (4) little or no disturbance in walking.

A new observational tool, the Walking Index for Spinal Cord Injury (WISCI) assesses the ability to ambulate using a 19-item hierarchical ranking.[12] Although still a work in progress, the descriptors may supplement other locomotor outcomes. The scale ranges from "ambulates in parallel bars, with braces and physical assistance of 2 persons, less than 10 meters (level 1)" to "ambulates with 1 cane or crutch, with braces and physical assistance of 1 person, 10 meters (level 10)" to "ambulates with no devices, no braces and no physical assistance, 10 meters (level 19)."

DEMOGRAPHIC COMPARISONS

Subjects from the 16 facilities that comprise the Model Systems Program survived more than 24 hours after hospital admission or were entered within 1 year of an injury sustained after 1973. The mean age at injury is 32 years with a trend toward a higher age over the past

Figure 10-1. Standard neurologic classification of spinal cord injury. (Source: American Spinal Cord Injury Association.)

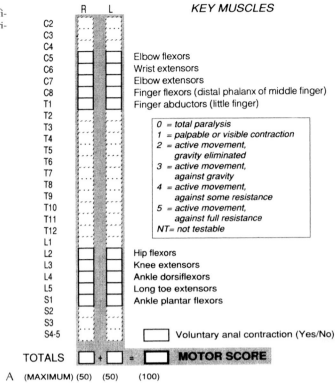

MOTOR

KEY MUSCLES

	R	L	
C2			
C3			
C4			
C5			Elbow flexors
C6			Wrist extensors
C7			Elbow extensors
C8			Finger flexors (distal phalanx of middle finger)
T1			Finger abductors (little finger)
T2			
T3			
T4			
T5			
T6			
T7			
T8			
T9			
T10			
T11			
T12			
L1			
L2			Hip flexors
L3			Knee extensors
L4			Ankle dorsiflexors
L5			Long toe extensors
S1			Ankle plantar flexors
S2			
S3			
S4-5			

0 = total paralysis
1 = palpable or visible contraction
2 = active movement,
   gravity eliminated
3 = active movement,
   against gravity
4 = active movement,
   against some resistance
5 = active movement,
   against full resistance
NT = not testable

☐ Voluntary anal contraction (Yes/No)

TOTALS ☐ + ☐ = ☐ **MOTOR SCORE**

A (MAXIMUM) (50) (50) (100)

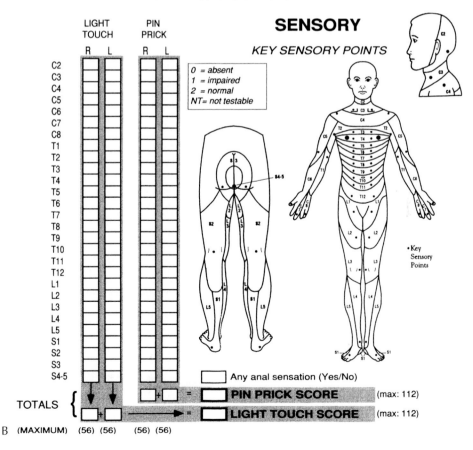

SENSORY

KEY SENSORY POINTS

LIGHT TOUCH · PIN PRICK

	R	L	R	L	
C2					
C3					
C4					
C5					
C6					
C7					
C8					
T1					
T2					
T3					
T4					
T5					
T6					
T7					
T8					
T9					
T10					
T11					
T12					
L1					
L2					
L3					
L4					
L5					
S1					
S2					
S3					
S4-5					

0 = absent
1 = impaired
2 = normal
NT = not testable

• Key Sensory Points

☐ Any anal sensation (Yes/No)

TOTALS { ☐ + ☐ = ☐ **PIN PRICK SCORE** (max: 112)

☐ + ☐ → = ☐ **LIGHT TOUCH SCORE** (max: 112)

B (MAXIMUM) (56) (56) (56) (56)

Table 10–1. **American Spinal Injury Association Impairment Scale**

A = Complete: No motor or sensory function is preserved in the sacral segments S-4–S-5.

B = Incomplete: Sensory but not motor function is preserved below the neurologic level and extends through the sacral segments S-4–S-5.

C = Incomplete: Motor function is preserved below the neurologic level, and the majority of key muscles below the neurologic level have a muscle grade less than 3.

D = Incomplete: Motor function is preserved below the neurologic level, and the majority of key muscles below the neurologic level have a muscle grade greater than or equal to 3.

E = Normal: Motor and sensory function is normal.

Clinical Syndromes
Central cord
Brown-Séquard
Anterior cord
Conus medullaris
Cauda equina

Source: American Spinal Injury Association.

10 years. The majority of patients are aged 16–30. Approximately 12% of patients are over the age of 60 years. The most frequently occurring age is 19 years. Males outnumber females by 4 to 1. In the NASCIS trials, 58% of acute traumatic SCI patients were also under 35 years of age and 12% were over 60 years old. The average age of UDS patients with traumatic SCI is 43 years old.

The causes of SCI vary with age, race, and economic status. Up until 1990, motor vehicle accidents (48%), falls (21%), sports (14%), and violent acts (14%) accounted for most cases of traumatic SCI. Over the past 10 years, automobile and motorcycle accidents have dropped to 38% as gunshot wounds have risen to the second most frequent cause at 26%. Sports injuries declined to 7%. Approximately 90% of sports-related injuries, such as surfing, football, and diving, result in complete or incomplete quadriplegia. Young white males are more apt to be injured in vehicular accidents and black males by acts of violence. In the NASCIS trials, which excluded gunshot wounds, automobile accidents accounted for 36% of SCI, motorcycle crashes for 8%, and falls for 26%. The average age for motorcycle accidents has been rising as more American baby boomers relive their youth on long motorcycle trips. Fall-induced fractures with SCI also appear to be rising in people over the age of 50 years. A Finnish study found an increase from 60 per 100,000 people in 1970 to 419 per 100,000 people in 1995.[13] The age-adjusted incidence rose 480% in women and 143% in men. No similar trend was found for people under the age of 40 years. Osteoporosis may play a role in the rise of fractures.

In Model Systems, a trend over the past 20 years is for more patients to have incomplete paraplegia and fewer with complete quadriplegia. Incomplete quadriplegia represents 30%, complete paraplegia 27%, incomplete paraplegia 21%, and complete quadriplegia 19% of patients. In the NASCIS patients, quadriplegia accounted for 35% of acute entries, paraplegia for 31%, quadriparesis for 13%, and paraparesis for 4%.

Overall mortality in the first year is 3.6%, but declines to 1.8% in the second year, and runs approximately 1% per year over the subsequent 10 years.[14] Table 10–2 shows the moderate decrease in longevity in relation to age at onset of injury and impairment. The most common causes of mortality in the Model Systems

Table 10–2. **Life Expectancy Beyond 1 Year After Spinal Cord Injury (Years)**

Age At Injury	Normal Subjects	With Motor Function At Any Level	Paraplegia	Quadriplegia C5–C8	Quadriplegia C1–C4	Ventilator-Dependent At Any Level
20	57	52	46	41	37	27
40	38	34	29	25	21	14
60	21	18	14	11	8	4

Source: National Spinal Cord Injury Statistical Center, 2001.[3]

cohort are respiratory (21%), cardiac (18%), septic (9%) and ill-defined (8%) complications, pulmonary emboli (8%), and suicide (6%).

FISCAL IMPACT

The direct costs for any year for new and chronic patients are approximately $14.5 billion with another $5.8 billion in indirect costs.[15] Indirect costs related to the value of expected wages in the absence of a SCI, minus the actual wages over the remaining work life of the patient, have been estimated. The analysis depends upon the year postinjury, age, race, level of independence in ADLs and mobility, education, marital status, employment status at the time of injury, inflation rates, and other variables. In 1992 dollars, Model Systems data estimated that a 25-year-old with a C-1–C-4 lesion and Frankel grade A, B, or C would incur a lifetime indirect cost of $1 million.[16] A patient at Frankel D at any level would lose $680,000.

Patients with paraplegia include those with myelopathies and conus/cauda equina lesions. From 1988 to 1998, one of the sites in Model Systems found that acute care costs for these patients were approximately $3200 per day and rehabilitation charges were $1200 daily.[17] The level of the injury was less important to length of stay and costs than the age of patients. Younger patients from 18 to 39 years old stayed 42 days, whereas those over 40 years stayed 60 days.

Table 10–3 shows the average direct costs of acute hospitalization, rehabilitation, and yearly health care and living expenses at 16 Model Systems sites. Costs for traumatic SCI rehabilitation are the same for men and women.[18] In 1997 inflation-adjusted dollars, the yearly av-erage charges for rehabilitation care and length of stay at Model Systems sites show interesting trends that seem related to cost controls instituted by Diagnostic-Related Groups payments by Medicare and by managed care groups.[19] Inpatient rehabilitation charges per patient were about the same in 1980 and 1990 at about $109,000, despite a decrease in length of stay of 35 days, down to 72 days. In 1997, charges dropped about $11,000 and the length of stay fell 21 days to 51 days. This trend of shorter stays and lower charges continues. The UDS database shows a decrease in mean length of inpatient rehabilitation stays from 48 days in 1990 to 33 days in 2000.

Rehospitalization

Hospital costs grow quickly for the treatment of complications of SCI. A mean length of stay of 28 days for pressure sore care in 1994 cost $24,000. Approximately one-third of the patients discharged from Model Systems were rehospitalized in the 1st and 2nd postinjury years. Subsequent readmissions occurred for the next 10 years at 25% per year for an average stay of 25 days.[20] In Model Systems, average readmission stays are 6 days.[19] Although no variables predict hospital admission, the number of days hospitalized correlates with greater age, fewer years of education, more days hospitalized in the previous year, and lower self-assessment of health. Education about skin, bladder and bowel care, self-monitoring for infections, and working with a physician familiar with the needs of people after SCI may reduce the rate of hospitalization. Given the extensive funding over the past quarter century provided by the U.S. Department of Education for the

Table 10–3. **Estimated Expenses and Lifetime Costs for Patients with Spinal Cord Injury Based on Severity (Year 2000 Dollars)**

Impairment	Year of Onset	Per Year	Lifetime Costs Age 25 Years	Lifetime Costs Age 50 years
Quadriplegia C-4	$572,000	$102,000	$2,186,000	$1,287,000
Quadriplegia C-5	$370,000	$42,000	$1,236,000	$783,000
Paraplegia	$209,000	$21,000	$730,000	$498,000
Motor Incomplete (any level)	$169,000	$12,000	$487,000	$353,000

Source: National Spinal Cord Injury Statistical Center, 2001.[3]

Model Systems Program, the reader of publications from the sites must wonder what the researchers have done to prevent rehospitalizations or to improve overall quality of care compared to nonfunded spinal cord centers. Few randomized clinical trials have been generated from the program.

PATHOPHYSIOLOGY

Acute management of traumatic SCI aims to reduce the amount of neurologic impairment and prevent additional injury.[21,22] The translation of pharmacologic neuroprotective interventions from animal models to humans has produced a steroid intervention that may reduce lipid peroxidation and inflammation. The second NSCIS trial established the efficacy of 24 hours of methylprednisolone with a 30 mg/kg intravenous bolus followed by 5.4 mg/kg when started within 8 hours of SCI.[23] The next trial showed greater efficacy if the drug is started within 3–8 hours of injury and continued for 48 hours.[8] Primary and secondary analyses found that the added effect on sensorimotor outcomes is modest at 6 weeks and 6 months postinjury, yielding significantly better sphincter control and ADLs for the upper extremities and a gain of 6 out of 70 points on an ASIA-like motor score. Subjects did not significantly change their neurologic category from, say, paraplegia to paraparesis. The efficacy of high-dose steroid, however, is based on the results of only 62 subjects who received this drug and 65 who received placebo. Some controversy has hounded the results of these trials, related to the questionable success of the randomizaton procedure and the use of subgroup analysis.[24] The effects of 48 hours of steroid may be mimicked by the addition of tirilizad. GM-1 ganglioside (Sygen) had an equivocal benefit for unoperated patients.[25]

The neuropathology of SCI offers insights into the types of neurologic deficits that follow cord trauma, the potential for sparing of fiber tracts that could contribute to clinical function, and factors associated with late recovery or decline.

Three SCI syndromes accounted for 31% of cases in the third NASCIS trial. An anterior syndrome was found in 5% of patients, a central cord syndrome in 18%, a Brown-Sequard syndrome in 7%, and no patients had a posterior syndrome. Clinically incomplete SCI oc-

curs more often than a complete lesion in people with cervical spondylosis who fall and from gunshot that does not penetrate the spinal canal. Complete injuries occur especially with bilateral cervical facet dislocations, flexion-rotation of the thoracolumbar spine, and from penetrating bullets.

Serious spinal column injuries are usually classified as follows:[26]

1. Flexion with anterior wedging of the vertebal body, especially at the T12 or L1 level
2. Flexion dislocation with anterior dislocation, especially at cervical levels
3. Extension with anterior disk rupture, sometimes with anterior spinal artery compromise
4. Axial compression with vertebral body fragmentation and fragment extrusion

Forces that displace the vertebral column also impart compressive forces on the cord and cause concussion, contusion, and sometimes laceration with partial or complete tissue disruption. These forces are tremendous. An 80-kg football player running to tackle another player develops 1000 newton-meters (Nm) of kinetic energy.[27] The musculoligamentous and bony elements at a cervical spine segment can absorb 3 Nm before failing. The cervical spine is by far the most frequently affected region in tacklers.

The earliest visible changes after severe cord injury include petechial hemorrhages, edema, and disruption of the parenchyma. Inflammatory responses and a cascade of secondary injury mechanisms, perhaps triggered or perpetuated by calcium ion fluxes into cells, lead to additional autodestruction (see Chapter 2). By 24 hours, central hemorrhagic myelomalacia is evident over at least several spinal cord segments. Bare axis cylinders are around the lesion, which involves central gray and white matter more than peripheral structures. By 5 days, glial cells replace the macrophages in the necrotic tissue and begin to form a cavity that will be crossed by gliovascular bundles.[26] By 6 months, secondary wallerian degeneration is found in the posterior columns above the lesion and in the descending tracts below.

Magnetic resonance imaging offers insights into likely cord pathology and may aid prognostication. In quadriplegic patients with an acute SCI, a high intensity T1 signal or low intensity T2-weighted image, indicating an intramedullary hemorrhage, is associated with complete SCI.[28,29] Improvement in sensori-motor function at 1-year follow-up is far more likely in patients without a hemorrhage. Magnetic resonance imaging also visualizes a cord transection. For patients with chronic SCI, a low T1-weighted and high T2-weighted signal intensity in gray matter points to necrosis and myelomalacia.[30]

Tissue sparing or regeneration is, of course, central to any possibility of significant recovery of function. Although nerve root atrophy at the level of central gray matter necrosis accompanies the chronic injury, regeneration of anterior and posterior roots, as in a posttraumatic neuroma, often develops. In addition, ascending and descending fiber tracts are found in the walls of the central cavity (see Chapter 2). Autopsy studies show a central cord syndrome at the segmental level of injury. Diffuse axonal disruption and demyelination at cervical levels, however, particularly of the medial dorsal columns, can be more prominent.[31] Animal models of SCI suggest that axonal destruction can be rather selective under experimental conditions. Greater injury occurs more deeply, relatively sparing axons near the pia mater, and involves larger-diameter myelinated axons.[32] What may be especially important for sensorimotor gains is the tendency for propriospinal tracts, an alternate slower-conducting pathway, to remain intact.[33] Spared axons, however, may not function normally.

One autopsy study revealed that 28% of 130 SCI patients who survived from 4 days to 14 years had no sensation or voluntary movement below the lesion, but had some anatomic continuity of cord parenchyma across the lesion.[26] These subjects may represent clinically incomplete cases in whom more careful or more sophisticated neurophysiologic testing would reveal the intact descending influences.[34] Experimental studies show that the conduction properties of axons that project through a SCI lesion can be abnormal; this block prevents recovery, for example, of hindlimb function in a cat cord contusion model.[35] Of interest, 4-aminopyridine in a related model sometimes improves conduction by its effect on potassium channel blockade.[36]

The minimum number of corticospinal fibers that permitted volitional movement with leg strength graded from muscle twitch to movement against gravity, but not against resistance, was 3.5%–10% of the total number of axons at the T4 level in a neuropathological study of people with complete and incomplete SCI and controls.[37] Another series of 20 subjects with traumatic cervical SCI found a general correlation between the degree of sparing of long motor and sensory tracts and the clinical examination of residual function, but four cases had clinically complete with neuropathologically incomplete lesions.[38] Kakulas related fiber counts in specific tracts to sensorimotor function.[39] Six chronic clinically incomplete and four complete SCI subjects were examined postmortem. At the T4 level, controls had approximately 41,000 nerve fibers in the lateral corticospinal tract. Sparing of approximately 3000 fibers on one side was associated with voluntary foot motion. Subjects with complete motor loss had approximately 2000 residual fibers. When touch and vibration were intact, approximately 117,000 of the 452,000 fibers found in the controls were spared. Lesions of the spinal cord that completely spare the lateral or ventral funiculi in nonhuman primates permit walking, and as little as approximately 25% of white matter tracts allow this.[40]

No studies have correlated morphologic changes with neurophysiologic and clinical changes in patients. The number and types of residual projecting axons will differentially modulate residual motor control, as well as reflex activity, phantom sensations, pain, spasms, and functional restitution as the plasticity of spinal circuits evolves. Causes of delayed pathoanatomic changes and neurologic deterioration include an enlarging neuroma, syringomyelia, and spinal stenosis or other degenerative changes of the vertebral column.

Nontraumatic Disorders

Patients admitted for rehabilitation for nontraumatic SCI, compared to patients with traumatic SCI, are significantly older (mean age approximately 60 years), married, retired, equally male and female, and have either paraplegia or an incomplete SCI.[41] The most common causes of nontraumatic SCI that lead to admission for rehabilitation are spinal stenosis and tumor, followed by ischemia, infection, and myelitis.[41] Specifically, MS is among the most common causes of a myelopathy to require inpatient therapy (see Chapter 12), followed by spinal cord infarction, epidural metastatic tumor, systemic diseases such as lupus, transverse myelitis from viral and postinfectious causes, delayed radiation necrosis, and uncertain causes.[42] Spinal cord swelling on MRI is most frequent in postinfectious and radiation-induced causes. Lesions wide in diameter tend to extend over more levels in a postinfectious transverse myelitis than in MS or trauma. The spinal fluid in MS is likely to reveal oligoclonal bands, whereas the fluid in patients with a postinfectious cause tends to reveal no bands but may contain more than 30 white cells. Gadolinium enhancement of lesions may occur MS and other causes. For spinal infarcts and systemic disease etiologies, the MRI lesions involve more than 2 vertebral levels and are centromedullary. The mean level of injury with spinal cord infarction is T-8 and the mean sensory level is T-12, associated with the cord's relative hypovascular zone from T-4 to T-8.[43]

A cervical myelopathy and cauda equina syndrome caused by spinal stenosis evolve gradually. Lumbar stenosis accounts for as many as 15% of SCI admissions.[44] Upper limb and truncal dysesthesias, a spastic paraparetic gait, and urinary urgency suggest cervical cord compression. Gluteal or thigh pain with standing and walking or extension of the back suggest a lumbar stenosis. Most reviews state that physical signs of weakness and sensory loss are rare,[45] but 20 of 22 patients managed for a lumbar stenosis at the University of California Los Angeles in the outpatient neurorehabilitation clinic had typical pain with a canal diameter of less than 10 mm and a readily demonstrable decline in leg strength in the distribution of 2 or more bilateral ventral roots immediately after walking a few hundred feet compared to sittng at rest. Multiroot compression and compression around a neural foramen causes a transient conduction block. Management by a wide lumbar laminectomy and brief rehabilitation that builds strength and endurance almost always stops the walking-induced pain and paresis in patients who had been declining in the distance they could walk.

MEDICAL REHABILITATIVE MANAGEMENT

Mortality and morbidity after SCI first began to fall and functional outcomes began to improve in 1944. This improvement accompanied the creation of specialized programs such as the British National Spinal Cord Injuries Center at Stoke Mandeville Hospital under Sir Ludwig Guttmann.

From 1973 to 1986, the American hospitals in the Model Systems Program found a 66% decrease in the risk of dying within 2 years of a traumatic SCI.[46] These investigators also reported a significant decline in the percentage of patients who required rehospitalization and the number of days hospitalized in the second year after SCI. The decline in mortality was also reflected in finding that, after adjusting for important covariants, the risk of dying during the first year after SCI was reduced by 67% in 1993–1998 compared to 1973–1977.[47] Respiratory (28%) and cardiac (32%) causes of death led sepsis (8%), digestive (7%), and urinary (4%) causes in the 1st year. Respiratory (22%) and cardiac (20%) complications are still the most frequent cause of death in the 2nd year.

Time of Onset to Start of Rehabilitation

The time from onset of SCI to transfer to rehabilitation has declined sharply over the past 20 years. The UDS database for 1992 reveals recent trends. Its 1719 traumatic SCI patients had a mean interval of 37 days until transfer for rehabilitation and the 2566 nontraumatic cases had a mean of 30 days, a fall from 1990 of 7 and 4 days, respectively, in just 2 years. In 1998, the time from onset of SCI to transfer declined to 22 and 14 days, respectively. In just 6 years, then, transfer time has dropped 15 days. In Model Systems, which incorporate acute SCI care, the yearly averages for time until transfer after traumatic SCI fell from 31 days in 1980 to 23 days in 1990 to 16 days in 1999.[19]

Economic pressures are likely to continue to shorten acute inpatient hospitalizations. This decline may have beneficial effects. Shorter intervals between injury and the start of a full rehabilitation program could prevent errors of omission and commission that lead to medical and psychologic complications. On the other hand, greater vigilance for lingering and previously unrecognized medical and psychosocial problems will be required by rehabilitationists. Shorter acute stays also mean that rehabilitation planning with patient and family should start within the 1st week after admission to the acute facility. Planning with insurers, visits to facilities by family or friends, a discussion of short-term training activities and goals, and giving the patient the benefit of an open-ended prognosis for gains in mobility and ADLs become more critical approaches as time wanes.

Specialty Units

Data from several of the participants in the Model Systems Program in the early 1980s suggest that initial care in a specialized unit for patients with acute SCI and early transfer to a spinal rehabilitation inpatient program may shorten total inpatient stays and reduce some medical complications. Patients treated in an acute SCI unit and then transferred to the inpatient rehabilitation program at the same facility after a mean of 27 days were compared with matched patients from a general hospital unit transferred at a mean of 60 days.[48] Both groups were admitted at similar functional levels. The number of pressure sores, long bone fractures, surgeries, internal injuries, and the incidence of deep vein thrombosis were similar at the time of transfer. Despite the 33-day difference in time from onset of SCI to transfer for rehabilitation, both groups were discharged with similar overall gains. They spent the same amount of time in rehabilitation, a mean of approximately 70 days for paraplegia and 86 days for quadriplegia. Thus, the specialty unit may have offered more efficient care, but not better medical care. In another retrospective study, quadriplegic patients who were quickly moved from an acute hospital bed to rehabilitation within 11 days had fewer pressure sores and respiratory complications compared to patients transferred later.[49] The number of medical complications in patients with paraplegia, however, did not differ.

The overall effectiveness of rehabilitation for SCI is rather clear,[50] but the specific elements of care and of interventions to improve functional and medical outcomes require more inquiry and experimental approaches.

Surgical Interventions

EARLY INTERVENTIONS

Surgical interventions during the acute hospital stay often affect a patient's rehabilitation.

Stabilization procedures and braces have become even more common concomitants of rehabilitation as the time from SCI to admission for rehabilitation shortens. Spinal surgery aims to restore alignment of the spine, reduce fractures, and although somewhat controversial, to remove all bone fragments.[51] The type and timing of decompressive and stabilizing spinal operations have an uncertain relationship to the prevention of additional cord dysfunction, to altering outcomes, and to affecting length of stay and long-term complications.[52–54] Retrospective studies suggest that surgery within several days of onset is safe. Up to one-third of patients will not need surgery.[55,56] Surgery does correct spinal column instability, especially in areas at greatest risk, such as the thoracolumbar junction and at the lumbar and midcervical regions. Stabilization procedures also correct angulation and displacement deformities. For example, one advantage of operative treatment of a lumbar fracture is to maintain enough of a lumbar lordosis to keep the patient's center of gravity behind the flexion/extension axis of rotation of the hips.[52] This stability assists ambulation with braces.

Immediate care of SCI and early rehabilitation efforts often include the use of external stabilization techniques. Devices include cervical stabilization with a halo vest, orthoses such as a *Philadelphia collar* for cervical injuries, and a thermoplastic, custom-molded body jacket that gives total thoracolumbar contact and 3-point fixation to allow healing after a fracture or operative fusion. A jacket limits spinal movement, but does not eliminate motion. Lower extremity fractures, especially of the femur, occur in up to 5% of acute SCI cases and lead to orthopedic interventions, casts, and appliances. Plastic jackets and casts, that might have to be worn for up to 4 months limit bed mobility, transfers, lower body ADLs, and flexibility for self-catheterization, which increases the assistance needed by patients during inpatient rehabilitation.

In the Model Systems Program, approximately 60% of patients had spine surgery and 45% of patients with SCI from motor vehicle accidents and falls underwent an anterior or posterior decompression or both.[51] A halo was worn by 40% of quadriplegic patients, of whom 68% had surgery. Complications such as deep vein thrombosis (14% of all patients), wound infections (4% of all), serious grade 3 and 4 pressure sores (5% of all), and pneumonia and atelectasis (42% of quadriplegic patients) did not differ between patients who did and did not undergo spine surgery.

Of the 1000 subjects who participated in the second and third NASCIS studies of acute pharmacologic interventions, only 14% of patients did not have a spinal fracture, dislocation, or both.[7,8] In the first 6 weeks after SCI in NASCIS 2, operative procedures by an anterior approach were performed in 12% and posteriorly in 51%, with a fusion in 46% and internal fixation in 43%.[23] A lateral approach for spinal cord decompression, along with hardware such as cages and rods for stabilization, depends on anatomic and clinical requirements.

In the near future, patients with root avulsions or tears or destruction of motoneurons in the ventral horn may benefit from reimplantation of ventral roots or autologous nerves into the cord at or above the SCI at the time of stabilization procedures. The goal is to reconnect limb muscles, the sphincters, and the bladder to viable motor and preganglionic neurons, followed by physical retraining (see Chapter 2). Perhaps further in the future, surgeons will have techniques to inject biologic promoters of axon regeneration within the cord and access to cell replacement strategies.

LATE INTERVENTIONS

Spinal stabilization procedures may need to be repeated for bony slipppage, infection, and removal of rods. Progression of neurologic symptoms and signs, especially within the first few years after a traumatic SCI, requires an evaluation for a syrinx. Nerve transfers have been proposed to enable walking, such as connecting the ulnar nerve to the gluteal and quadriceps muscles.[57]

Syringomyelia

One or more slit-like cavities centrally located in the cord and ranging from 1 mm to 5 mm wide are not infrequently seen on MRI. The slit may be a normal if unobliterated central canal, rather than a syrinx. If so, the openings produce no symptoms or neurologic signs. The slits do not expand the cord and never reach above the third cervical level the way a congenital or developmental syrinx may in people with a craniovertebral junction anomaly. A

follow-up MRI ought to be done 1 year after detection to confirm the benign nature of the cavity. In general, a cystic space, hydromyelia, and stable syrinx require no intervention unless new myelopathic symptoms are evolving. The diameter and length of a syrinx can be monitored by MRI.

Posttraumatic syringomyelia develops when subarachnoid adhesions or mechanical obstruction by a bony protuberance cause a block of CSF flow. The pressure of a Valsalva's maneuver with cough or sneeze, along with CSF pulsations, may increase the size of the central canal and the communicating posttraumatic cyst. An enlarging syrinx expands rostrocaudally along the path of least resistance. Symptoms include dysautonomia, central pain, greater spasticity and other new upper motor neuron or bladder symptoms, as well as new lower motor neuron findings in the limbs or loss of truncal strength as the syrinx damages motoneurons of the ventral horn.

Shunting the syrinx itself may not produce a lasting and physiologic solution. The filling mechanism must be inactivated.[58] Figure 10–2 demonstrates the MRI findings for a syrinx that required removal of bone and arachnoid adhesions. A careful assessment by a neuroradiologist and experienced neurosurgeon or orthopedic surgeon ought to reveal the location of arachnoid adhesions or a bony projection into the subarachnoid space at the level of a severe kyphosis that require repair. Sometimes, draining the subarachnoid space from above will collapse an enlarging syrinx.

Medical Interventions

Early rehabilitation efforts include measures to prevent and manage medical complications. The third NASCIS study prospectively monitored medical complications for 6 weeks after SCI. The rates have been similar for over 1400 patients in NASCIS trials. Table 10–4 shows the frequencies of the most common complications. Complications may differ in a patient population that includes victims of firearms. The NASCIS complication rates stand in some contrast to the medical comorbidities during rehabilitation (Table 10–5) and 2 years after a traumatic SCI (Table 10–6).

Patients with cervical and upper thoracic injuries and complete lesions have greater early morbidity than patients with lower spinal or in-

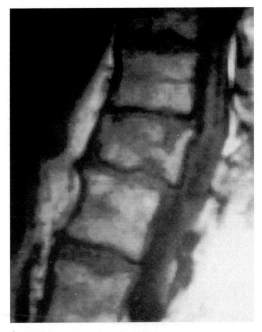

A

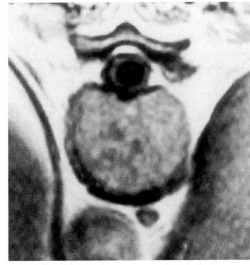

B

D

C

SP
SL

Figure 10–2. A 31-year-old woman slipped and fell down a flight of stairs, landed on her back, and was unable to move her legs. She recovered the ability to walk but had mild residual leg weakness, a drop foot, and dysesthesias of the feet. At age 42, she suddenly felt pain in the upper back and urinary incontinence while cheering at a basketball game. Upper thoracic, cervical, and right arm pain recurred with sneezing. At age 44, her left hand became dry and walking and urinary urgency and constipation worsened. The MRI scan shows a wide syringomyelia from T-12 to C-2 in the (A) sagittal and (B) axial planes. She had kyphotic angulation of the spine at T-12/L-1 and an L-1 fracture. A staged decompression of the subarachnoid space was carried out with an anterior spinal decompression and partial extradural vertebrectomy of L-1, followed by a T-12 and L-1 laminectomy with intradural lysis of adhesions and placement of a dural graft. The (C) sagittal and (D) axial scans a few months later reveal a marked decrease in the width of the syrinx. Her pain and ability to walk returned close to her level of function prior to age 40. (Courtesy of Ulrich Batzdorf, M.D., University of California Los Angeles.)

461

Table 10–4. Medical Complications in 500 Patients Within 6 Weeks of Acute Spinal Cord Injury

Complication	Percentage
Urinary tract infection	36
Musculoskeletal injury	20
Pneumonia	15
Decubiti	15
Respiratory failure	15
Head injury	10
Atelectasis	8
Sepsis	5
Phlebitis	5
Arrhythmia	4
Paralytic ileus	3
Incision, pin, halo infection	3
Gastrointestinal hemorrhage	2

Source: Adapted from Bracken et al., 1997.[8]

complete lesions. Ventilatory dysfunction, aspiration, dysautonomia with upright hypotension or paroxysmal hypertension, a neurogenic bowel with impactions, a neurogenic bladder with retention and infections, a catabolic state, and gastric atony are especially likely to complicate early management. Prophylaxis for deep vein thrombosis and management of decubiti, soft tissue pain, central pain, and other commmon complications are reviewed in Chapter 8.

Table 10–5. Medical Complications During Inpatient Rehabilitation for Traumatic Spinal Cord Injury

Complication	Percentage
Pressure sore	21
Abnormal renal tests	11
Atelectasis/pneumonia	9
Autonomic dysreflexia	7
Deep vein thrombosis	5
Pulmonary embolus	1
Renal stone	0.5
Gastrointestinal hemorrhage	0.4
Cardiac arrest	0.4

Source: Adapted from Model Systems Program, 1998 data in Chen et al., 1999.[244]

Table 10–6. Medical Complications in the 2nd Year after Traumatic Spinal Cord Injury

Complication	Percentage
Pressure ulcer	18
Autonomic dysreflexia	11
Abnormal renal tests	8
Atelectasis/pneumonia	4
Renal calculi	2
Deep vein thrombosis	1
Leg long bone fracture	1
Pulmonary embolus	0.2

Source: Adapted from Model Systems Program, 1998 data in McKinley et al., 1999.[61]

COGNITIVE DISORDERS

Up to half of patients with traumatic SCI have cognitive impairments from an associated traumatic brain injury, a prior TBI, or substance abuse.[59] Formal neuropsychologic testing demonstrates the coincidence of SCI with deficits often for attention, concentration, memory, mental flexibility, and problem solving. During inpatient rehabilitation and out-of-hospital living, these cognitive impairments could impede the patient's learning and execution of basic self-care skills, psychosocial adjustment, and vocational skills. Impaired thinking and judgment may increase the likelihood of hospital readmission for recurrent, avoidable medical complications. Routine screening of cognition and early intervention during inpatient rehabilitation could improve outcomes in these doubly disabled people.

RESPIRATORY COMPLICATIONS

Acute SCI carries a high risk of respiratory complications that impede rehabilitation. Model Systems data found that 67% of patients admitted within 48 hours of a C-1–T-12 SCI developed one or more complications.[60] The completeness of the injury had no clear impact on incidence. With levels at C-1–C-4, 84% of patients were affected, most often with pneumonia (63%), ventilatory failure (40%), and atelectasis (40%). At C-5–C-8, 60% had a complication with atelectasis (34%), pneumonia (28%), and ventilatory failure (23%). At T-1–

T-12, 65% had a complication, most often pleural effusion (38%), atelectasis (37%), and pneumothorax (32%). Ventilatory failure began on average 5 days after SCI, and pneumonia occurred on average at 25 days. Management includes standard respiratory prophylactic measures and vigilance, especially upon transfer of the patient for rehabilitation. Recently extubated patients and all patients with a cervical or upper thoracic SCI or recent atelectasis and pneumonia should have overnight oximetry measurements and a check for oxygen desaturation with physical activity. Weaning off a tracheostomy is an important milestone for patients once suctioning of secretions is minimal and oxygenation and swallowing no longer require the safety of a tube.

Patients with quadriplegia from complete lesions run a 4%–6% risk of pneumonia and atelectasis yearly for 15 years postinjury, compared to a 2%–3% risk for patients with incomplete quadriparesis and a 1% risk for patients with paraplegia.[61] Immune functions may be depressed in patients with SCI, especially if immobile.[62] High quadriplegic patients who require a tracheostomy and intermittent positive pressure ventilation have up to 40% mortality over 5 years from pulmonary complications.

Noninvasive methods have increasingly freed many patients from the communication and swallowing problems and altered quality of life imposed by a tracheostomy.[63] Advances include intermittent positive pressure ventilation (IPPV) by mouth, nose, and acrylic strapless oral–nasal interface (SONI), glossopharyngeal breathing, and chest shell ventilation, supplemented by respiratory muscle training and consistent pulmonary toilet. Speaking tracheostomy tubes and devices such as the *Venti-Voice* or one of the models of an artificial larynx allow oral communication despite a tracheostomy. In patients with high quadriplegia, phrenic nerve, diaphragm, and intercostal electrical pacing systems may eliminate tracheal complications, improve speech, and increase independence.[64] Functional magnetic stimulation of the expiratory muscles may offer a means to improve the force of a cough and increase expiratory muscle strength.[65]

On occasion, a patient with a high cervical lesion who requires ventilatory support refuses treatment. Although this is a moral and legal right in a competent person, the ethical procedures of informed consent and refusal always create uncertainty and dilemmas. Guidelines for discussion have been proposed.[66] This approach emphasizes a gradual, supportive process that provides information about long-term psychosocial function after SCI, demonstrates technological aids, and deals with misconceptions about depression, vocational possibilities, and quality of life.

BOWEL AND BLADDER

Neurogenic bowel and bladder dysfunction rank among the most life-limiting problems of people with SCI. No more than 15% regain normal control.[25] Fecal incontinence, constipation, and impaction affect most SCI patients until a practical bowel program is attained.[67] Digital stimulation with a lubricated and gloved finger in a gentle, circular motion will induce reflex peristalsis in patients with an intact conus medullaris. Glycerine suppositories and contact irritants, stool softeners, colonic stimulants, fiber in the diet, and bulk formers assist bowel evacuation that is timed to the convenience of the patient (see Chapter 8). Incontinence and autonomic dysreflexia can be helped by limiting the ingestion of gas-forming foods like beans, large amounts of dairy products, fruit juices, and berries. Hemorrhoids require immediate treatment.

The bladder is usually flaccid during the period of spinal shock. A detrusor reflex returns in 6 weeks to 12 months. Bladder drainage requires some combination of intermittent catheterization, an external collection system, reflexive emptying, and, occasionally, a urethral or suprapubic catheter. The paraplegic patient is trained to perform intermittent catheterization approximately 4 times a day, depending on the timing of fluid intake. If sensorimotor impairments persist, nearly all SCI patients with a lesion that spares the S-2–S-4 micturition center develop dyssynergia between the detrusor and the external sphincter. These uncoordinated contractions lead to incontinence and outlet obstruction. Urodynamic studies and an intravenous pyelogram are indicated as a baseline and to assist in therapy (see Chapter 8).

Bladder outlet obstruction in patients with a complete SCI above T-6 may cause dysautonomia. If untreated, patients with obstruction also develop recurrent infections, urosepsis, vesicourethral reflux, urolithiasis, and hydronephrosis. It is, of course, most important to optimize bladder emptying. Pharmacotherapy often helps in the management of detrusor, bladder outlet, and striated urethral sphincter dysfunction (see Table 8–1). Methicillin-resistant staph aureus and vancomycin-resistant enterococci have become the most commonly resistant organisms to colonize and infect patients at the time of admission to rehabilitation.[68] Infectious disease isolation procedures are necessary, but should not socially isolate the patient.

Model Systems data show that 34% of patients with incomplete quadriplegia and 41% with incomplete paraplegia void independently without a catheter or reflex stimulation in the first year after SCI. From 22% and 30%, respectively, do so 10 years later.[61] Approximately 1% of patients with complete lesions are free of catheters, however. Patients with complete quadriplegia are most likely to use an indwelling catheter or suprapubic tube, 24% in the 1st year and 20% at 10 years after the SCI. By 10 years, approximately 10% of patients with complete or incomplete quadriplegia and 22% with paraplegia carry out intermittent catheterization. Condom catheters are worn by nearly one-third of patients with complete SCI by 10 years after onset. Condom catheters with leg drainage bags are especially used by men to assure continence. For men with a small retractile penis that lets a condom slip off, a semirigid penile hinge prosthesis can help maintain continence and contribute to sexual function.

Urinary tract infections are associated with bladder overdistention, high pressure voiding, large postvoid residuals, vesicoureteral reflux, and stones or outlet obstruction. Urine culture criteria for the diagnosis of bacteriuria include $>10^2$ colony forming units per ml (cfu/ml) of urine from persons on intermittent catheterization, $>10^4$ cfu/ml from a clean void specimen in males using a condom collection device, and any bacteria from an indwelling catheter.[69] Prophylactic antimicrobials and attempts to change urine pH[70] are commonly used after repeated infections, but probably do not decrease bacterial colonization and symptomatic bacteriuria.[71]

In a study of over 100 women and 400 men with SCI who were followed for at least 10 years, no significantly different rates for urologic complications and renal dysfunction were related to the system of drainage.[72] The majority of women were managed with an in-dwelling catheter and the men with a condom catheter. Only quadriplegic men who used an ilioconduit had a significant decrease in one measure of renal perfusion. Renal dysfunction rises with age, especially over age 60 years, when 23% of patients in year 1 and 30% of patients in year 10 are affected, compared to 7% and 10% of patients, respectively, under the age of 40 years. Renal and ureter calculi occur in approximately 2%–4% of patients over the 15 years after SCI.[61]

An individual's clinical course best determines the frequency of urologic evaluations. General recommendations for maintnence care vary, but include a urinalysis at 4-month intervals, a urea nitrogen and creatinine twice a year, a renal scan yearly, renal ultrasound or MRI scan every 3 years, and urodynamic studies if storage and emptying problems arise.[73]

HETEROTOPIC OSSIFICATION

Ectopic bone may cause functional impairment or pain in up to 20% of patients, usually affecting the soft tissue below their neurologic level. Onset is usually in the first 4 months after injury. Patients with a complete lesion, pressure sores, spasticity, and age greater then 30 years may be at greatest risk.[74] Management is reviewed in Chapter 8.

PRESSURE SORES

Guidelines for the prevention of decubiti after SCI have been developed.[75] Model Systems data for patients admitted within 24 hours of traumatic SCI show that 4% subsequently develop pressure sores and 13% of these sores were graded as severe.[5] This data also show the prevalence of pressure sores to be 8% in the 1st year after SCI in incomplete patients and 24% in complete patients. At 10 years, the prevalence rises to 17% in incomplete and 27% in complete subjects.[61]

Sores mostly occur over the sacrum, heel, scapula, foot, and trochanter. Lower grade skin lesions develop over nearly any bony prominence and the genitals. A community study found 33% of chronic SCI persons to have one or more lesions graded Stages 1–4 (see Table 8–4).[76] Indeed, 28% of these lesions were Stages 3 and 4. Black patients had more high grade ulcers than whites. More severe lesions occur with late life injury and in patients with the poorest mobility. Men and women are equally affected. Prevention after SCI requires daily examination of the skin, good nutrition, intermittent wheelchair pushups, pressure relieving cushions for the wheelchair, attention to bed coverings, and for the immobile patient, occasional repositioning during sleep. Management is reviewed in Chapter 8.

DYSAUTONOMIA

Autonomic reflexes may fail in persons with SCI levels above T-6. Symptomatic postural hypotension is common in the first weeks after injury and may persist after quadriplegia. Plasma norepinephrine levels, which should at least double upon going from supine to standing, may not rise with upright posture and the stress of hypotension in these patients, although renin, vasopressin, and aldosterone levels often do reach normal levels.[77] Impaired norepinephrine release leads to denervation supersensitivity of alpha-1 and alpha-2 adrenoreceptors. Therapy is discussed in Chapter 8.

Episodic autonomic hyperreflexia related to uninhibited sympathetic outflow affects 30%–90% of people with high SCI, usually beginning several months after injury.[78] Hypertension, headache, diaphoresis, anxiety, reflexive bradycardia, nasal congestion, flushing above and pallor below the SCI level, extensor spasms, and piloerection can follow. Dysreflexia is instigated by visceral and joint pain, oropharyngeal suctioning (which can also cause bradyarrhythmias), pain from heterotopic ossification, pressure sores, bowel and bladder distention, fecal impaction, urinary infection and cystitis, ingrown toenails, pregnancy and labor, venous thrombosis, late development of a syrinx, tight clothing, a particular supine position, and sometimes by no evident cause. Suprapubic and indwelling Foley catheters cause dysreflexia about twice as often as intermittent catheterization.[61]

Treatment of sudden dysreflexia starts with removing the instigating cause. The patient is positioned upright and the bladder catheterized. Drug interventions are shown in Table 10–7. Some quadriplegic patients have very labile responses to antihypertensive drugs and suddenly become hypotensive, so short-acting agents such as nifedipine, labetolol, or nitropaste that can be removed are best. For frequent bouts of hypertension, maintenance therapy includes oral antihypertensive agents.

Table 10–7. **Regimen for Acute Autonomic Dysreflexia**

Sit patient up at 90°.

Monitor blood pressure every 3 minutes.

Check urine collection system or catheterize the bladder using lidocaine gel.

Look for source of noxious stimulation.

Examine rectum with topical anesthetic and remove feces.

If systolic blood pressure exceeds 170 mm Hg, apply 1 inch of nitropaste above spinal level.

If no change, give 10 mg nifedipine; repeat in 10 minutes as needed. Monitor for hypotension.

Start intravenous fluids if no change.

If hypertension and symptoms persist, give nitroglycerin 1/150 sublingual or hydralazine 10 mg intravenously.

If no change, give diazoxide, 100 mg, or labetalol, 20 mg intravenously for a longer effect.

Check blood pressure often.

For prophylaxis, give prazosin 5 mg orally up to 3 times daily.

For paroxysmal bradycardia, propantheline or a pacemaker may be needed. Glycopyrrolate, 0.5 mg to 1 mg several times a day, or scopolamine can prevent bouts of sweating.

ENDOCRINE DISORDERS

Immobilization and the effects of SCI cause the loss of calcium from bone at a rate of 3%–8% per month and rapid loss of trabecular bone by an average of 33% by 6 months after injury. Hypercalcemia may be evident from 2 weeks to 2 months after SCI and require treatment with intravenous saline, etidronate, or pamidronate.[79] This loss accounts for the 2%–6% incidence of long bone fractures in paraplegic persons.[80] Trabecular bone loss in patients with quadriplegia is evident in the radius by 6 months and cortical bone loss by 12 months after a SCI, with a similar evolution for the femur in persons with paraplegia and quadriplegia.[81] The fracture threshold of the proximal femur is reached by 1–5 years after SCI, but vertebral bone density may not decrease.[82]

Disuse osteoporosis results from an initial increase in osteoclastic resorption and especially decreased osteoblastic formation. Although osteoclastic activity returns to normal, the osteoporosis may not recover. Increased calcium release from bones of paralyzed limbs also suppresses parathormone and down-regulates calcitriol.[83] Pamidronate, one of the antiosteoclastic bisphosphonates, decreases the bone breakdown product N-telopeptide and decreases the loss of bone as measured by a dual energy X-ray absorptionmeter.[84] Functional electric stimulation of muscle, exposure to local electrical fields, weight-bearing, and trials of calcitonin and growth hormone have been tried with variable success to limit bone loss.

A variety of other endocrine abnormalities, particulary low triiodothyronine, high and low testosterone, hyperprolactinemia, and low growth hormone have been reported, although the relationship to the paralysis is often uncertain.[85]

CHRONIC PAIN

Pain after SCI arises from contractures, osteoporotic fractures, extensor spasms, soft tissue injury, musculoligamentous strain, myofascial pain, and inflammation of tendons and bursas, especially from overuse of the upper extremities. Current pain is reported by up to 80% of people with SCI. Common locations include the back (60%), hip and buttocks (60%), and legs and feet (58%).[86] In a community survey, pain limited participation in ADLs and IADLs for 2 weeks out of the previous 3 months. Chronic pain interferes with sleep in approximately 40% of people who experience it.[87] In another survey of 450 SCI patients, 72% reported chronic pain in the wrists or shoulders, especially during wheelchair propulsion and transfers.[88] Strain and cumulative trauma appeared to be the cause. Painful compression neuropathies like a carpal tunnel syndrome increase over time in patients with paraplegia who bear weight through the upper extremities for wheelchair propulsion. Wheelchair modifications such as reducing vibration from wheels that are out of line, using an ultralight chair, altering the grasping surface of the rim, or changing wheeling biomechanics may help. Home modifications, along with education about joint protection, may also reduce injuries.

Reflex sympathetic dystrophy after cervical SCI may be an underdiagnosed cause of pain (Table 8–8).[89] Visceral pain from the abdomen or pelvis below the cord lesion is often difficult

to localize, but especially arises from a distended bladder or bowel. Late onset of pain associated with changes in the neurologic examination suggests an expanding syringomyelia that may require venting.

Chronic at-level or below-level neuropathic pain evolves in up to one-third of patients with SCI, associated with gray or white matter damage, respectively (see Table 8–6).[90] Pain at the level of injury may be radicular or central with a sharp, burning, band-like, or electric quality. Similar discomfort may develop in patches of skin anywhere below the lesion, particularly in the perineum. Neuropathic pain can be diminished by transcutaneous stimulation, tricyclics, anticonvulsants, and other medications (see Table 8–9). Spinal cord stimulation has generally not been effective for pain below the sensory level,[91] but some pain management specialists report patients who do benefit. Intrathecal drugs such as baclofen and the combination of morphine and clonidine[92] benefit some patients.

Patients with refractory at-level pain after a SCI may be the best candidates for an ablation at the dorsal root entry zone (DREZ) by radiofrequency lesioning or by bipolar coagulation. The procedure aims to destroy nociceptive inputs to the most dorsal layers of the dorsal horn and the excitatory medial portion of Lissauer's tract. Combining the open surgical procedure with recordings of spontaneous dorsal horn activity at multiple segments and assessing for hyperexcitability during stimulation of cutaneous C fibers can guide the surgeon to ablate all of the unilateral or bilateral sources of deafferentation pain.[93] The most ideal candidate may be the patient with a conus/cauda equina lesion with dysesthetic pain at the level of the SCI.[94,95]

SENSORIMOTOR CHANGES AFTER PARTIAL AND COMPLETE INJURY

Acute surgical and neuromedical interventions are based upon the quest to diminish or reverse sensorimotor impairments. The natural history and causes of early and late changes associated with movement give clinicians some of the data trends that aid discussions about impairments and disabilities with patients and the rehabili-

Table 10–8. Change in Completeness of Traumatic Spinal Cord Injury During Inpatient Rehabilitation

Frankel Grade	% At Onset	% Improved	% No Change	% Worsened	% At Discharge
A	52	10	90	—	47
B	13	45	50	4	9
C	13	56	41	3	9
D	22	7	91	2	32
E	—	—	—	—	2

Source: Adapted from Model Systems Data in Stover, 1986.[5]

tation team. The following description of changes in completeness of the injury and in motor scores also offers insight into the design and statistical power requirements of interventional clinical research.

Neurologic Impairment Levels

In a Model Systems database of 4365 patients admitted for rehabilitation through 1997, 20% of patients have complete quadriplegia, 28% have incomplete quadriplegia, 30% have complete paraplegia, and 22% have incomplete quadriplegia. The most common neurologic levels are C-4 (15%), C-5 (15%), T-12 (8%), and L-1 (7%). Neurologic levels are symmetric in 85% of patients, within 1 level in 10%, and within 2 levels in 3%.[96] Sensory levels are symmetric in 79%, within 1 level in 13%, and within 2 levels in 3% of patients. Sensory and motor levels are the same in two-thirds of patients.

Model Systems data on nearly 5000 traumatic SCI patients admitted within 24 hours relate recovery in terms of the change in com-

pleteness of SCI by the Frankel grading system at acute hospitalization and at discharge from inpatient rehabilitation, a span of approximately 3–4 months.[20] Table 10–8 shows the percentage of patients who improved at least one Frankel grade. Similar rates of gain were identified in 1560 Model Systems patients subsequently graded on the ASIA Impairment Scale (Fig. 10–1).[96] The Frankel grade is defined the same as the ASIA impairment level (Fig. 10–1) except that the ASIA requires sacral sensation to be tested and found absent to call a patient ASIA A, sensorimotor complete.

Table 10–9 shows the overall Model Systems database of neurologic levels and Frankel grades for 9647 subjects admitted within 1 year of injury through 1985.[5] Patients with thoracic lesions tend to have complete sensorimotor impairments and patients with lumbosacral levels usually start with incomplete motor impairments. In this larger and more heterogenous group, discharge Frankel grades changed from admission in 7% of patients with Frankel A lesions, 37% with B lesions, 54% with C lesions, and 6% with D lesions. Approximately 40% of

Table 10–9. Distribution of Neurologic Levels and Frankel Grades on Admission for Rehabilitation of Traumatic Spinal Cord Injury

Frankel Grade	C-1– C-4 (%)	C-5– C-8 (%)	T-1– T-6 (%)	T-7– T-12(%)	L-1– L-5 (%)	S-1– S-5 (%)	All Levels (%)
A	45	45	80	66	17	0	51
B	8	14	6	7	7	0	10
C	13	9	4	6	11	4	8
D	34	32	9	20	64	96	30
E	0.2	0.1	0	0.1	0.1	0	1

Source: Adapted from Model Systems Data in Stover, 1986.[5]

the small number of patients graded Frankel A who improved reached grade B, and approximately 30% reached grades C and D. Of the patients graded Frankel B who improved, approximately 35% reached a grade C, 50% a D, and 0.7% recovered. Of those admitted at grade C who improved, most reached a D and 1.6% recovered. Lesser changes were described in a small number of patients for up to 18 months and, rarely, beyond that. Significantly fewer patients who were motor-complete with extended zones of sensation below the lesion, but without sacral sparing (13%), were likely to convert to motor-incomplete status compared to patients who had sacral sparing (54%).[96] Thus sacral sparing suggests relative preservation of posterolateral spinothalamic tracts and at least a rim of white matter sparing. The spinocerebellar pathway runs along the dorsolateral rim of spinal white matter, so it too may be spared by a central contusion. Conversion from complete to incomplete may take up to 12 weeks after a traumatic SCI.[25]

LATE CHANGES

Motor score changes at 1 year in Model Systems are smallest for patients with complete paraplegia at the time of onset and largest for admissions with grade C quadriplegia.[96] The level of preserved sensation in ASIA B patients contributes to the outcome. Although the standard deviations around the mean are large, the mean motor score (Fig. 10–1) changes from admission to 1 year after traumatic SCI for quadriplegic patients graded A is 10, B is 28, C is 43, and D is 26. For paraplegic patients, the change is 3 for ASIA A patients, 15 for B, 21 for C, and 14 for patients graded D.

Gains in sensorimotor function beyond the 1st year after traumatic SCI are unusual and follow several patterns. One study of 69 cases found an increase in the Frankel grade in approximately 35% of cases between the 1st and 5th years after injury and deterioration in 12%.[97] Between the 1-year and 3-year and the 3-year and 5-year examinations, these gains were generally from an A to a B or from a D to an E. No specific therapies were used over this time. Sensation did improve in some subjects and, as expected, patients with good motor function tend to continue to improve, although the measurement limitations of the

Frankel and ASIA scales may not detect all of the change. No patient with complete paralysis below the lesion 1 year after SCI subsequently developed any useful motor function.

Evolution of Strength and Sensation

The second NASCIS study provides some general information about sensorimotor changes over the 1st year after traumatic SCI.[7, 23] The investigators used a motor scale with gradations of 0–5 covering 14 unilateral upper and lower extremity root levels. The maximal score denoting normal strength of one arm and leg, then, is 70. The mean score on admission for patients in this trial was 16. Six weeks after entry, patients admitted with complete lesions who received methylprednisolone had increased their motor scores compared to the placebo group by 6.2 versus 1.3 points. At 6 months and 1 year, the difference was a statistically significant 17 versus 12 points. No correlation was attempted between this modest gain in strength and any functional recovery. The sensory evaluation of 29 segments from C-2 to S-5 on a scale of 1 (absent) to 3 (normal) revealed that pinprick improved in 33% receiving the drug and in 17% receiving placebo by 6 weeks, but nonsignificant changes were found at 6 months and 1 year to pinprick (11 vs. 8) and to touch (9 vs. 6).

Gains in strength by 1 year are fairly predictable by 1 month after injury, based upon the presence of any movement in the 1st month. Clinicians can anticipate these gains in making early decisions about upper extremity orthotics and lower extremity bracing and wheelchairs. The following sections review this neurologic recovery.

PREDICTIVE VALUE OF PHYSIOLOGIC TESTS

Transcranial magnetic stimulation assesses conduction along the corticospinal tracts (see Chapter 3). With nontraumatic SCI, latencies of MEPs may be prolonged with a low amplitude when injuries are incomplete. After traumatic SCI, the MEP is significantly related to the presence of residual motor function.[11] By 1 month after a SCI, and in patients with chronic posttraumatic SCI, the ASIA motor score is as predictive of the recovery of use of the hand and of walking as the presence or absence of elicitation of a MEP in the abductor digiti minimi and quadriceps, respectively. When a MEP is found, 90% of patients show abnormal latencies and amplitudes. No change in the MEP occurred in 36 patients between a median of 1 month and 6 months after a traumatic SCI.[11]

Somatosensory evoked potentials primarily assess intactness of the dorsal columns. Their presence in the hand or lower extremities beyond the first few days after an acute SCI helps predict functional use of the hand and functional walking 6 months later, although not as well as the ASIA motor score.[98] The combination of sensory evoked potentials and clinical assessments of pain and joint position sense had some predictive use for motor recovery after cervical SCI in one study.[113] Other investigators found little additional prognostic information from evoked potentials beyond the information offered by the early clinical examination.[114] The presence of a SSEP from the lower extremity shows dorsal column intactness, but its absence does not provide a measure of confidence about the potential for motor recovery. As is the case for MEPs, the SSEPs generally do not change over 6 months. These techniques are perhaps best utilized in patients who are unable to cooperate with the neurologic examination.

Other neurophysiologic tests that could help to determine the completeness and the caudal spread of a lesion would have great clinical value. Reinforcement of an H-reflex (Chapter 7) in an arm and leg muscle by a preceding loud auditory stimulus offers another approach to determining the presence of intact descending pathways.[115] This audiospinal reflex manipulates reticulospinal input to cervical and lumbosacral motoneurons. Testing for reflex modulation may provide information about the intactness of the anterolateral spinal white matter, which assists in the control of motor and, especially, locomotor activities. The corticospinal tract is necessary for modulating the H-reflex amplitude with a conditioning paradigm in rats (see Chapter 1),[115a] so the ability of patients to down-condition or up-condition this reflex may become a means to assess residual corticospinal and reticulospinal pathways.

A test battery was designed to look for an incomplete lesion, called discomplete by the investigators.[34] It examines muscle activity in response to tendon vibration, to reinforcement maneuvers using muscles above the lesion aimed at activating muscles below the lesion, and by attempts at voluntary suppression of plantar withdrawal reflexes. The developers of this potential clinical battery, however, probably allowed patients to increase their intraabdominal or intrathoracic pressure during a Jendrassik's maneuver, which was performed by the upper extremities above the cord lesion. The pressure rise may have stimulated afferents below the lesion, causing reflexive EMG activity in the legs. This activity may be misinterpreted as revealing intact pathways descending across the level of injury.

Changes in Patients with Paraplegia

In a longitudinal investigation, Waters and colleagues followed 148 patients who had complete traumatic paraplegia at 1 month after SCI, examining them again 1 year later to detect any change in strength and in sensation to pinprick and light touch.[99] Half the patients were victims of gunshot wounds. The sensory levels in these cases tended to improve by 1–3 dermatomes in the 1st year. No one with a neurologic level above T-9 regained any motor function and 142 remained complete. With a level at or below T-9, 38% improved by a mean of about 1 grade of strength in the hip flexors and knee extensors. With an initial level at or below T-12, 20% regained enough strength in the hip and knee muscles to walk with conventional orthoses and crutches. Only 2 of the entire group developed ankle or toe movements. Six patients converted to incomplete more than 4 months after injury, using a sacral sparing definition.

Thus, a patient with complete paraplegia 1 month after a traumatic SCI has no better than a 5% chance of evolving to incomplete paraplegia and becoming a community ambulator.[100] Some patients who do convert to incomplete will regain volitional bowel and bladder function, so the change is important. Patients with the most caudal SCI recover the most motor control. With a T-9 lesion, patients regain 2 points on the motor score by 1 year, at T-11 they gain 6.5 points, and at L-1 they gain 12 points. Several other observations by Waters and colleagues are of interest. Intact lower abdominal muscles in the 1st month after SCI predicted hip flexor recovery at 1 year. Early hip flexor function anticipated strengthening of the knee extensors. In the second year, a few patients with lesions below T-11 showed slight motor improvement. Consistent with studies of recovery of the upper extremities, increases in muscle strength in patients with complete paraplegia tend to occur in the lowest muscle that has any residual strength and in muscles just below that neurologic level.

The same investigators followed patients with incomplete paraplegia with these analyses.[101] Motor recovery was independent of the level of injury, although patients with levels above T-12 had less strength at 1 month than those with levels at or below T-12. Lower extremity ASIA motor scores increased an average of 12 (SD = 9) points between 1 month and 1 year. A plateau in motor recovery for most patients occurred at 6 months. For muscles graded 0/5 at 1 month, the chance of improving to 3/5 or better is 26%. If strength is 1/5 to 2/5 at 1 month, the chance of improving to 3/5 or better is 85%.[100] During early rehabilitation, patients may regain control of the toe extensors before the knee extensors, perhaps because of the more lateral location of the caudal leg fibers of the corticospinal tract in the thoracic cord.

Changes in Patients with Quadriplegia

The course of gains in motor function in the upper extremities in patients with traumatic quadriplegia is important to patients and to the rehabilitation team that plans for assistive devices and perhaps surgery such as a tendon transposition. In a study of 150 patients with acute C-4, C-5, and C-6 Frankel A and B SCI who were followed for 2 years by Ditunno and colleagues, many patients continued to improve from less than 3 out of 5 (3/5) strength in an upper extremity group to grade 3/5 or greater, beyond the time of their inpatient rehabilitation.[102] Patients with some power in muscles within the zone of partial preservation in the 1st week after SCI recovered earlier and to a greater degree than did those with muscles graded 0/5. For example, in 70%–80% of patients with C-4 levels who had some initial

biceps (C-5) power and patients with C-5 levels with any initial wrist extension (C-6), the median grade of strength in those muscles reached 4/5 at 6 months and plateaued at 12 months. Over 90% achieved at least 3/5 power within a year, whereas only 45% with no initial power improved to 3/5 strength by 1 year and 64% by 2 years.

Ditunno and colleagues[103] carried out another prospective study using sequential manual muscle testing at the time of onset of SCI and every week for 1 month, then monthly for 6 months, and then every 6 months until 2 years after the SCI. For patients with a C-4 level, the biceps improved to 3/5 or better in 70% of complete and 90% of incomplete SCI patients. At the C-5 level, the extensor carpi radialis improved in 75% of the complete and 90% of the incomplete quadriplegic patients. The triceps improved in almost 90% of complete and incomplete subjects who presented with a C-6 level. Over the first 3 months after SCI, patients with an incomplete lesion had more rapid gains in strength one level below the lesion than patients with a complete injury.

For a group of patients with incomplete quadriplegia, mean upper and lower extremity ASIA Motor Scores increased between 1 month and 1 year after SCI.[104] The rate of recovery rapidly declined over the first 6 months and plateaued. Upper and lower extremity motor scores increased from means of approximately 13 (SD = 12) at 1 month to 25 (SD = 12) at 1 year. All upper extremity and nearly all lower extremity muscles graded 1/5 to 2/5 at 30 days after traumatic SCI will recover to 3/5 strength or better by 1 year after injury. For muscle graded 0/5 at 1 month, the chance of achieving this gain is 20%.

Predictions about sensorimotor recovery for patients with complete quadriplegia is also most reliable 30 days after injury, past the time of acute medical and surgical complications that can interfere with testing. Strength and sensation were examined prospectively using ASIA scales in 61 patients after traumatic SCI during rehabilitation at 1 month, monthly for 6 months, and at 1 year after injury.[105] Six of these patients changed to an incomplete SCI by about 2 months, but one changed 30 months after SCI. Their functional motor recovery, however, was no greater than the rest of the cohort. Thus, quadriplegic patients who have complete injuries at 1 month have a 90% chance of continuing with no voluntary lower extremity movement. Although 10% improve to incomplete status, their leg strength does not increase enough to allow walking. Gains did evolve in the arms and hands. Upper extremity muscles graded 1/5 or 2/5 at 1 month had a 97% chance of improving to grade 3/5 by 1 year. Muscles graded 0/5, and located 1 neurologic level below the most caudal level that had any motor function, reached 3/5 or greater strength in 27% of cases by 1 year. Only 1% of subjects achieved this gain in muscles that were two levels below the lowest voluntarily active muscle and only 4% regained any measurable strength in those muscles. Motor Scores increased an average of 8.6 (SD = 4.7) points, with the rate of motor recovery rapidly declining by 6 months.

In these patients with quadriplegia, sensation often did not improve in dermatomes that were at the same cervical level as the muscles that improved from 0/5 to at least 3/5 strength. Another study of the recovery of sensation in Frankel A cases showed that approximately 80% of patients with C-5–C-8 SCI improved within 3 months within one sensory level to pin or touch, always in the zone of partial preservation.[106]

In summary, the clinical examination early after SCI provides the best handle on future sensorimotor gains. The ASIA Motor Score for the upper extremities is the most powerful predictor of outcomes for self-care skills, and the score for the lower extremities best predicts the ability to walk efficiently. Indeed, a multiple regression analysis revealed that the upper extremity score is three times more powerful in predicting self-care skills as the lower extremity score and the lower extremity score is twice as powerful as upper extremity strength scores at predicting ambulation.[116] These relationships can help stratify subjects in clinical trials of rehabilitation strategies.

Mechanisms of Sensorimotor Recovery

At least several mechanisms may contribute to improvements in sensation and motor control at and just below the level of SCI and explain improvements in muscles that can at least

twitch by 1 month after injury (see Table 2–1). Rapid recovery of sensation at 1–3 levels can be attributed to reversal of a conduction block at the root level, perhaps in concert with overlapping dermatomal innervation.[107] Rapid motor recovery in the zone of injury or in the zone of partial preservation may arise from reversal of local metabolic dysfunction or of a conduction block in spared central motor pathways and ventral roots.

A study attempted to assess conduction block using transcranial magnetic stimulation of MEPs in the first 6 hours after SCI. The results did not provide information about the likelihood of motor recovery in weak muscles near the injury or in paralyzed muscles just below the level of injury.[108] Impaired synchronization of descending excitatory volleys to motoneurons was found 6 weeks after injury in some of the muscles that had recovered.

Other biologic mechanisms for motor gains at the level of injury include peripheral sprouting of motor terminals from intact or metabolically recovered motoneurons and muscle fiber hypertrophy with exercise. A histopathological study of patients with a cervical central cord syndrome showed that hand weakness arises primarily from loss of fibers in the lateral corticospinal tracts and ventral tracts. Spinal motoneurons were spared.[109] Any residual pathways may need retraining over time to improve their function.

Mechanisms of representational neuroplasticity may play a role in gains and could be manipulated with drug and physical interventions. For example, transcranial magnetic stimulation enhanced the excitability of motor pathways that targeted the muscles just rostral to a SCI, and the technique evoked paresthesias in the anesthetic legs below a thoracic lesion.[110,111] Cortical reorganization was also suggested in patients who had dysesthetic pain below the level of injury. Patients with pain, compared to patients without pain, and in comparison to healthy controls, had better two-point discrimination above the lesion.[112] This sensory finding suggests an increase in the size of the somatosensory cortical areas allotted to the skin, induced by constant dysesthetic sensory input. Thus, cortical motor and sensory representations for the muscles and dermatomes around the level of the SCI can reorganize and enlarge their representational maps in a way that lessens

Table 10–10. **General Relationships Between Motor Level and Potential For Functional Skills**

Level of Injury	Feeding	Dressing	Bowel/Bladder Care	Transfers	Wheelchair Rolling	Vehicle Transport	Communication
C3–C4: bulbar, diaphragm, neck, and shoulder elevation action	Drink with straw; cough	Dependent	Dependent	Dependent; use lift or sliding board	Electric wheelchair, pneumatic or chin control; trunk support, abdominal binder	Dependent mouthstick/ microswitch;	Type at computer with mouthstick/ microswitch; use adapted phone; environmental control unit
C-5: shoulder and elbow flexor action	Assisted for setup, use hand cuff for utensils	Assisted for arms	Dependent	Assisted with sliding board	Electric wheelchair; manual wheel-chair with wheel lugs	Dependent or hand control system	As above
C-6: wrist extension, tenodesis grasp	Independent with universal cuff	Independent for arms	Independent bowel care; assist with self-catheterization	Independent with sliding board	Manual wheelchair with lugs	Drive adapted van	Write and type with cuff/device
C-7: elbow extension, wrist flexion, grasp	Independent	Independent with devices	Independent; use mirror; insert suppository	Independent by depression lift, except from floor	Manual wheelchair	Independent with hand controls	Independent with devices
C8: finger flexion and extension	Independent	Independent	Independent	Independent on all surfaces	Independent, standard wheel rims	As above	Independent
T-1: function as a paraplegic							

sensorimotor impairment. Task-oriented learning paradigms for training may enhance this reorganization (see Chapter 3).

FUNCTIONAL OUTCOMES

In prospective and retrospective reports of functional outcomes, patients with acute SCI improve substantially between onset of injury and discharge from inpatient rehabilitation. Patients maintain or improve their self-care skills and mobility in subsequent years, if medical and psychosocial complications are managed well. A general predictor of functional capabilities is based on the lowest level of intact neurologic motor activity, completeness of sensorimotor impairments, and age at onset. Table 10–10 shows the functional significance of the level of SCI and the mimimal goals for rehabilitation. In measuring functional goals based, for example, on the FIM, a comparison between patients with ASIA grades of A, B, and C to patients graded ASIA D is more relevant than comparisons between the A, B, and C categories. Patients either have or do not have functional motor control.

Cognitive function may play an important role in progress, especially given the high incidence of associated head injuries at the time of traumatic SCI. The cognitive subscale of the FIM does not identify the subtle impairments in these patients. Model Systems data revealed that only small changes are found in the cognitive subscale of the FIM between admission and discharge from inpatient rehabilitation; 80% of patients reach upper limit scores by discharge, suggesting a ceiling effect in the FIM.[117]

The yearly report of first admissions for SCI rehabilitation from hospital programs that subscribe to the UDS$_{MR}$ shows some interesting trends about functional gains after traumatic SCI.[6,118] In 1992, the mean time from onset of traumatic SCI to admission for rehabilitation was 37 days; in 1998, the mean fell to 23 days. In 1992, the mean length of stay was 45 days; in 1998, for 5000 reported cases in 1 year, this fell to 34 days. In 1992, the mean total FIM score was 75 on admission and 98 on discharge; in 1998, the scores were 61 and 89, respectively. These admission and discharge scores have held steady since 1996. About the same percentage of patients have returned home

over this time. Thus, the level of functional dependence has increased at the time of admission for rehabilitation, but the change in gain in FIM scores is similar, despite the significant decline of 25 days in the total time from onset of SCI to discharge from rehabilitation. In comparison to the UDS$_{MR}$ data, Model Systems hospitals report a decline from a total of 141 days of acute care and inpatient rehabilitation in 1974 to a total of 60 days in 1999.

Tables 10–11 and 10–12 show typical FIM subscores and demographic information reported by UDS for first hospital admissions for nontraumatic and traumatic SCI in the year 2000.

Self-Care Skills

The number of independent and assisted ADLs achieved with training depends on many interacting factors. These factors include the patient's residual strength and sensation, the ability to substitute muscles such as the shoulder abductors to produce elbow flexion, limitations imposed by joint immobility and musculoskeletal pain, presence of hypertonicity

Table 10–11. First Admission for Nontraumatic Spinal Cord Injury: Typical Yearly Results from Uniform Data System for Medical Rehabilitation

Average Score	Admission	Discharge
Self-Care	3.9	5.4
Sphincter	3.9	5.3
Mobility	2.9	4.8
Locomotion	1.9	4.0
Communication	6.5	6.6
Social Cognition	6.1	6.4
Total FIM	75	98
Age (years)	64	
Onset (days)	14	
Stay (days)	17	
Discharge (%)		
Community	82	
Long-term care	10	
Acute care	6	

FIM, Functional Independence Measure.
Source: Adapted from Fiedler et al., 1998.[6]

Table 10–12. First Admission for Traumatic Spinal Cord Injury: Typical Yearly Results from Uniform Data System for Medical Rehabilitation

Average Score	Admission	Discharge
Self-Care	4.0	5.4
Sphincter	3.9	5.2
Mobility	2.9	4.7
Locomotion	2.0	3.9
Communication	6.3	6.5
Social Cognition	5.8	6.2
Total FIM	63	89
Age (years)	43	
Onset (days)	22	
Stay (days)	33	
Discharge (%)		
Community	81	
Long-term care	10	
Acute care	5	

FIM, Functional Independence Measure.
Source: Adapted from Fiedler et al., 1998.[6]

and spasms, body weight, the availability of simple and high technology assistive devices, recurrent medical complications, psychosocial and vocational supports, how important carrying out the activity is to the individual, and how much time and energy it takes to accomplish a task, especially at home after discharge from inpatient therapy. For example, 10 subjects, ages 11–40 years, were tested for independence in dressing 2–10 months after rehabilitation for C-6 quadriplegia. All were able to do this within 1 hour, which is a common therapy goal.[119] All these patients, however, routinely asked for assistance from an attendant or the family at home, because dressing took too much time or effort. As in every rehabilitation setting, realistic goals for functioning depend on a patient's motivation and lifestyle choices.

Functional assessment tools describe overall gains after SCI. Using the Modified BI with 1382 patients, one of the Model Systems participants found that scores between admission and discharge improved from 42 to 80 (on a scale of 100) for patients with incomplete paraplegia, from 35 to 71 for complete paraplegia, from 19 to 60 for incomplete quadriplegia, and from 8 to 30 for complete quadriplegia.[120] At 3-year follow-up, at least 86% of each group maintained or improved its level of independence for specific skills.[121] Excluding ambulation and stair climbing, nearly all patients with paraplegia had become independent except for bowel and bladder management, of whom about 20% required assistance. For patients with incomplete quadriplegia, functional skills were independent in 50%–70%. For patients with complete quadriplegia, various ADLs were accomplished independently in 10%–25%.

Independence in ADLs was inversely related to increasing age in one study. Across all Frankel grades and neurologic levels, independence in ADLs at hospital discharge was found in 18% of patients younger than 15 years old, in 37% 16–45 years old, in 15% 46–60 years old, and in only 8% who were over the age of 60 years.[122]

In 1988, the Model Systems database began to collect the FIM at the time of admission and discharge from rehabilitation. In an analysis of 750 patients, the mean score upon admission to rehabilitation was 73 for patients with incomplete paraplegia, 68 for complete paraplegia, 59 for incomplete quadriplegia, and 47 for complete quadriplegia.[20] The mean length of hospital stay over this period was 92 days for patients with quadriplegia and 75 days for paraplegic persons. The mean gain was approximately 36 points for all but those with complete quadriplegia, who improved 15 points. These gains have persisted for patients evaluated in 1998.[18]

Table 10–11 and Table 10–12 list the gains on six subscores of the FIM for first admissions to rehabilitation for nontraumatic and traumatic SCI, respectively, at sites that report to UDS. These numbers provide some insight into the functional outcomes related to general rehabilitative interventions. Of interest, the FIM scores reveal greater disability and longer hospital stays for victims of trauma. Subgroup differences exist, however. Patients with nontraumatic SCI who are paraplegic have lower motor FIM scores and improve less than patients after traumatic injuries.[41] This finding may reflect the older age of people with nontraumatic SCI and lack of gains in people with thoracolumber tumor compression of the cord. Patients with incomplete quadriplegia from nontraumatic injuries are more functional than patients after traumatic injuries, reflecting incomplete cord injury from cervical spondylosis in the absence of trauma.

Table 10–13. **Relationship Between Motor Scores and Motor Functions for Each Injury Group at Discharge from Inpatient Rehabilitation for Traumatic Spinal Cord Injury**

Injury Group ASIA Impairment; Level	ASIA Motor Score	FIM Motor Score
A, B; C-1–C-4	9	23
A,B; C-5–C-8	26	38
C; C-1–C-4	57	48
C; C-5–C-8	63	61
D; C-1–C-4	69	67
D; C-5–C-8	79	74
A, B; T-1–T-8	51	64
A, B; T-9–T-12	52	71
A,B; L-1–L-5	60	71
C; T-1–T-8	77	75
C; T-9–T-12	76	71
C; L-1–L-5	75	78
D; T-1–T-8	83	82
D; T-9–T-12	74	77
D; L-1–L-5	83	74

ASIA, American Spinal Injury Association; FIM, Functional Independence Measure.

Source: Adapted from Greenwald et al., 2001.[18]

Table 10–13 lists FIM motor scores (maximum range, 13–91) in relation to ASIA Motor Scores (range 0–100) at discharge, based on 1070 traumatic SCI admissions of equal gender evaluated from 1988 to 1998.[18] The differences in scores between each block of ASIA injury groups (A vs. B vs. C vs. D) for patients with quadriplegia or paraplegia is statistically significant and, again, reflects the fact that greater motor control of the arms or the legs leads to greater independence for upper or lower extremity ADLs.

Ambulation

In general, ambulation as a form of exercise becomes a possibility for patients with complete lesions from T-2 to T-10. Physical assistance or guarding is necessary along with knee-ankle-foot orthoses (KAFOs) and forearm crutches or a walker. For patients with lesions at T-11 to L-2, independent ambulation with KAFOs or ankle-foot orthoses (AFOs) and forearm crutches is possible, but often limited to indoor activity and some stair climbing. In patients with lesions at L-3 and below, community ambulation can be independent with AFOs and forearm crutches or canes. For a given patient during rehabilitation, the ability to ambulate depends upon the completeness of the injury, residual strength, age, motivation, and, for some very impaired people, the ability to incorporate less commonly used techniques such as functional electrical stimulation.

Data that relate ASIA impairment levels and motor scores to subsequent ambulation have been difficult to retrieve from Model Systems and UDS, primarily because the FIM allows a score for either independence in wheelchair mobility or walking and the two are not readily separated in a retrospective analysis of the FIM motor score. This flaw is the sort researchers abut when they adopt standard functional assessments for a database without specific hypotheses in mind for the use of the tool.

NATURAL HISTORY OF RECOVERY

Prospective studies of the recovery of ambulation that enter patients soon after an acute SCI provide some working prognostic categories that help in discussions and planning with patients and their families.

A prospective study of 157 consecutive patients with SCI admitted through an emergency room found that 24% of patients who initially had quadriplegia and 38% of patients with paraplegia became functional ambulators with or without an orthosis 1 year later.[123] About half had complete lesions on admission and 20% of the cohort died by the time of follow-up. The greater their strength and sensation, the more likely it was that ambulation recovered. Using the Frankel Scale to study a series of quadriplegic patients, 39% of those graded Frankel B at 72 hours after SCI and 87% of patients graded Frankel C and D with cervical lesions on admission (those who died or were lost to follow-up were excluded) recovered a functional gait.[124] Other studies reveal less favorable outcomes, however.

Only 2%–7% of 190 patients with complete paraplegia and levels between T-1 and T-10 evolved partial motor recovery and only 1%–3% ambulated at 1 year.[125] Cases with complete lesions at T-11–L-1 recovered partial motor function in 9%–29%, perhaps doing better because the cauda equina was affected initially. Only 3% ambulated, however.

Patients with Frankel B lesions are an especially interesting group to follow. The Model Systems Program database included almost 1000 such patients. Forty percent improved their motor function after admission for acute care and 20% of the entire group eventually ambulated.[5] In another study, when 27 patients were classified within 72 hours of onset as Frankel B, 2/18 with intact touch and no pin sensation below the lesion recovered reciprocal ambulation for at least 200 feet with or without orthoses and assistive devices; however, 8/9 who retained partial or complete pinprick appreciation improved to Frankel D and E and walked.[126] Preserved sacral pin sensation in incomplete quadriplegia and paraplegia in the 1st month postinjury also significantly improved the prognosis for lower extremity motor recovery and subsequent ambulation in other studies.[104] Thus, a thorough sensorimotor examination has predictive value for the eventual ability to walk.

STRENGTH AND RECOVERY

The strength of the lower extremities determines the amount of work performed by the upper extremities for support, which, in turn, determines the rate of oxygen consumption and the practicality of ambulation.[127] Waters and colleagues studied patients with traumatic SCI-induced quadriparesis and paraparesis, most of whom ambulated with orthoses and assistive devices. The gait velocity, oxygen cost per meter walked, and peak axial load placed on assistive devices inversely correlated with lower limb strength. Patients usually became community ambulators when strength reached 60% or greater of normal in their hip flexors, abductors, and extensors and in their knee flexors and extensors. The investigators used the Ambulatory Motor Index (AMI), a 4-point scale in which 0 is absent movement, 1 is trace or poor, 2 is movement against gravity, 3 is fair strength, and 4 is movement against some or normal resistance. *Community ambulators had pelvic control with at least a 2 in the hip flexors and a 2 at one knee extensor*, so that they needed no more than one KAFO for a reciprocal gait pattern. To provide some perspective

on the effort required to ambulate, the oxygen cost was about 4 times higher to walk half as fast as normal controls, who used 0.15 mL/kg·m. As the AMI fell from a mean of 60% to 31% of normal, patients went from requiring no KAFO to needing 2 KAFOs, the load on the arms rose from a mean of 14% up to 79%, and the oxygen cost rose from a mean of 0.37–1.15, or nearly 10 times the energy cost of healthy subjects.

As noted earlier, many studies show that strength is an early predictor of the likelihood of ambulation.[128] A study using the ASIA Motor Score found that 20 of 23 incomplete tetraplegics who had an ASIA lower extremity motor score (LEMS) of 10 or more (the maximum normal score is 50) at 1 month after injury became community ambulators with crutches and orthoses by 1 year.[104] The patients subsequently achieved relatively effortless community ambulation if the LEMS improved to at least 30. In comparison, scores of 20 or less were associated with limited ambulation at slower average velocities, higher heart rates, greater energy expenditure, and greater peak axial loads on assistive devices.[129] Table 10–14 summarizes some of the contributions from Waters and colleagues on the likelihood of ambulation, based upon the ASIA LEMS at 1 month after SCI.[104]

REHABILITATION OUTCOMES FOR WALKING

Outcomes for ambulation after SCI vary with the cohort followed. In a study of 866 patients across all ages, Frankel grades and neurologic levels, approximately 18% were independent in ambulation at the time of discharge from inpatient rehabilitation.[122] In another series of patients with SCI admitted for rehabilitation, about half of the patients with incomplete paraplegia and quadriplegia ambulated 150 feet with assistive equipment at discharge.[130] In a study of 711 patients with acute SCI followed for 3 years after inpatient rehabilitation, only 10% of the incomplete paraparetic and 13% of the quadriparetic patients were independent enough to ambulate 50 meters or climb stairs.[121,131] No patients with complete lesions were independent.

Up to 95% of patients with symmetrical incomplete quadriplegia from a traumatic central cord syndrome recover functional ambulation between discharge and 1 year after injury, al-

Table 10–14. Relationship Between Strength at 1 Month After Traumatic Spinal Cord Injury and Likelihood of Achieving Community Ambulation 1 Year Later

Lower Extremity Motor Score*	Complete Paraplegia (%)	Incomplete Paraplegia (%)	Incomplete Tetraplegia (%)
0	<1	33	0
1–9	45	70	21
10–19	—	100	63
≥20	—	100	100
Percentage achieving ambulation	5	76	46

*Score based on 5 key muscles, maximum for the legs is 50 points.
Source: Adapted from Waters et al., 1994.[104]

though the rate may fall by half for patients over age 50 years.[132] Older patients often present with a chronic cervical spinal stenosis. The initial leg strength is usually better than upper limb strength in patients with a central cord syndrome. With sensory sparing of pinprick appreciation in sacral dermatomes, especially with an anterior cord syndrome, up to 90% of patients can ambulate by discharge from rehabilitation.

TRIALS OF SPECIFIC INTERVENTIONS

In addition to the level of SCI and motor score as key factors for functional gains, aspects of the rehabilitation process contribute to outcomes. The total amount of therapy was found to predict outcomes better than the amount of daily therapy or number of days in rehabilitation.[116] This suggests that well-timed, specific interventions that provide adequately supervised practice may lead to still better outcomes for patients.

Mobility

GENERAL STRATEGIES

Inpatient rehabilitation begins with therapies to improve trunk control, endurance for sitting and exercise, autonomic reflexes, and selective strength in normal and paretic muscles. Functional training emphasizes wheelchair mobility, repositioning to relieve pressure points, and sliding board transfers. No large randomized trials have compared therapy approaches for mobility. In a study of chronic SCI, patients were randomized to 8–16 weeks of three common rehabilitation strategies—physical exercise therapy, neuromuscular electrical stimulation, and EMG biofeedback.[133] The subjects made equal gains in muscle strength below the lesion, in self-care, and in mobility measures that did not include ambulation.

The patient with an incomplete lesion who has 3/5 strength or better at the hip flexors and knee extensors of at least one leg has a good chance to progress in standing and stepping in the parallel bars with assistance and temporary orthoses. As described previously, residual supraspinal input measured by upper and lower extremity strength, as well as the energy cost of locomotion, and the patient's level of conditioning and motivation tend to predict who may rehabilitate into a community ambulator using traditional orthoses and assistive devices. The patient with acute SCI who has any voluntary activity in the hip muscles is the ideal candidate for immediate selective arm and leg strengthening exercises and a conditioning program. This regimen aids progress toward ambulation and may limit any early regression related to disuse muscle atrophy. For most patients with incomplete quadriplegia and paraplegia, it is probably most cost-efficient to train for standing and stepping during outpatient care.

The rehabilitation team must educate the patient about the longer-term procedures and performance requirements needed to achieve any particular functional level of ambulation. Many people cling to the belief, for at least the first 6 months after a complete SCI, that they will recover and walk. As patients reintegrate into home and community, they can sensibly formulate their needs and desires. Most patients who cannot walk in an energy-efficient manner in the community eventually come to rely on their wheelchairs, rather than upon complex orthotics that allow a slow and effortful gait that does not fit into their lifestyle.

The patient can aim for one or, depending on circumstances, a combination of the following levels of activity with assistive devices as needed.

1. *Passive standing only.* Standing for 30 minutes a day may decrease the incidence of bed sores and bladder infections, improve knee extensor, range of motion, and add to quality of life of people with paraplegia.[134] Studies have shown no effect of passive standing on spasticity and bone loss.[135] Some patients report less hypotension and clonus and better trunk control with regular standing. A tilt-table, a stationary or power standing frame, or a stand-up wheelchair that stabilizes the knees may be used, depending on the amount of trunk and hip control. Some standing frames add exercise equipment for the arms. Bilateral KAFOs or hip-KAFOs may also be used.

2. *Short distance ambulation for exercise only.* This activity allows some cardiovascular conditioning. Persons at this level usually require help to don an orthosis, stand up, and achieve balance. They may be aided by some variation of a KAFO, including temporary use of an adjustable lower extremity telescopic orthosis (LETOR). The Vannini-Rizzoli Stabilizing Limb Orthosis plantarflexes the foot to stabilize the knee and lets the patient shift weight forward and to the side of the weighted foot to pendulum swing the unweighted foot.[136] A reciprocating-gait orthosis (RGO) is a hip-knee-ankle-foot orthotic that controls hip extension while assisting hip flexion. A person with paraplegia uses trunk extension to produce hip flexion in the swing limb for stepping with the support of a walker. Reciprocal stepping occurs on a mechanical basis by means of a cable between both hips of the device. A hip-guidance orthosis (HGO) is a rigid long leg brace interfaced to a rigid trunk and pelvic structure by low resistance hip joints. A swivel walker then assists stepping. Follow-up studies show that approximately one-half of people with paraplegia from a thoracic SCI give up use of a RGO for home ambulation within 1 year.[137]

3. *Functional indoor ambulation.* At this level, people tend to walk at home or work and use a wheelchair for longer distances in the community. They are independent in putting on and removing orthoses and in arising from the floor or a chair. The energy cost of walking tends to determine the practicality of activity.

4. *Independent community ambulation.* The patient must achieve a low energy cost for walking at a reasonable speed over typical community distances. An FNS, orthotic, or hybrid system for the ASIA A to C thoracic SCI subject has yet to be shown to allow practical community mobility. A variety of systems that take extensive training are marketed to people with SCI. Anecdotal endorsements find their way into advertisements. No data yet support the long-term satisfaction and use of these devices or their cost-effectiveness in, for example, the workplace. The minimal goals for designers are a safe and cosmetically acceptable system that permits arising from the floor, standing for at least an hour, stepping at a velocity in the range of 25 meters/minute for at least 1000 meters, and nonfatiguing mobility on uneven surfaces, ramps, and stairs.

Patients who do recover the ability to walk with a cane or rolling walker and no more than AFOs must practice their step pattern daily at casual and faster walking speeds to improve the pattern of gait and endurance. Marked hypertonicity that causes the legs to adduct or produces clonus or toe clawing that interfere with stepping may respond to oral antispasticity agents or local injection of botulinum toxin (Chapter 8). Some ambulatory patients have improved walking speed with 4-aminopyridine, which may improve axonal conduction.[138,139] Clinical trials are in progress.

EXPERIMENTAL STRATEGIES FOR STEPPING

As described in Chapter 1, the hindlimbs of adult animals that have had an experimentally induced thoracic spinal cord transection can be trained to step on a moving treadmill belt. This finding points to the interaction between central pattern generators in the lumbar cord that control automatic alternating flexion and extension of the hindlimbs with proprioceptive and cutaneous sensory inputs from the limbs and trunk. A growing number of investigators have built upon these findings to demonstrate the feasibility of training patients with chronic incomplete paraplegia to walk.[140–143]

Body Weight–Supported Treadmill Training

As an adjunct to traditional physical therapies, the suspension of a patient over a treadmill belt to control the level of weight bearing and cadence of stepping may serve as a safety measure to prevent falls and allow therapists to more easily assess and correct gait deviations. Ideally, BWSTT allows mass practice that is task-oriented (Chapter 6). With BWSTT for patients with SCI, up to 50% of body weight is suspended in a climbing harness connected to an overhead hydraulic lift (Fig. 10–3). Weight support is adjusted so that the knees neither buckle nor hyperextend during stance. Therapists manually assist the legs as needed so subjects can step with a kinematic pattern that approaches normal. The aim is make use of whatever residual motor control is elicited, provide the sensory inputs during the step cycle that approximate those ordinarily appreciated by the spinal cord and supraspinal networks, and gradually increase motor control of the trunk and legs until full weight bearing at treadmill speeds of 1.5–2.5 mph are reached. Although early training studies used very slow treadmill belt speeds, more therapists are trying to approach speeds of 2 mph, which among other variables enhances the contribution of hip extension leading to flexion at the critical onset of the swing phase. The intervention for patients with SCI often requires an assistant for each leg and another to help stabilize and rotate the hips and trunk from behind the patient. Another trainer observes the symmetries of the stance and swing phases and controls the level of weight support and treadmill speed.

Symptomatic hypotension and healing limb fractures are the primary contraindications to BWSTT. The technique appears safe in patients who wear a halo or thoracolumbar support or have had spinal surgery. The bowel and

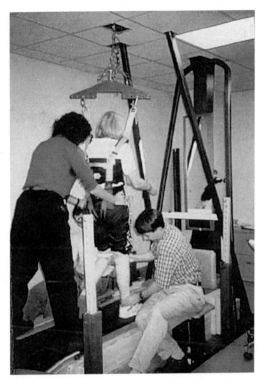

Figure 10–3. Body weight-supported treadmill training often requires the assistance of one trainer at each leg and one to assist pelvic and hip movements from behind the subject.

bladder ought to be emptied before a training session. The therapists must use great care in how they manipulate the subject, where they touch the legs, how they time each portion of the step cycle, and how tight the harness straps compress the skin, if they are to avoid inducing skin sores, spasms and clonus, and sensory feedback that is deleterious to locomotor signaling.

In many cases, sensory inputs related to loading and kinematics enhance motor output during BWSTT.[144,145] As in studies of the spinal transected cat, thigh pinching and electrical stimulation over the dorsum of the foot sometimes increases hip flexion when timed to the swing phase in patients with complete and incomplete SCI. These inputs may activate a motor pattern through spinal flexor reflex afferent pathways. Loading the leg that is in midstance at the time of double limb support as the other leg reaches the stage of toe-off, will elicit automatic hip flexion to initiate the swing phase. The angular velocity of the hip as it goes into extension is another critical element for the swing phase. These details have been appreciated in studies of spinal transected cats and patients with complete SCI (see Chapter 1 and Fig. 1–6). For all patients, practice in rhythmic, symmetrical stance and swing phases of stepping is engrained by the moving treadmill belt.

Patients with SCI who have some residual descending neural input, but are able to walk very little or not at all, may achieve independent walking on the treadmill.[141,146–149] The training allows selected subjects to walk overground for the first time and to improve the distance and velocity of their walking with assistive devices.[150] The strategy, combined with the 5-HT antagonist, cyproheptadine, and the alpha-2 noradrenergic agonist, clonidine, may improve aspects of stepping, but may also reduce EMG activity.[151,152]

Several theoretical benefits of an approach such as BWSTT are worth further study. In experiments with the cats after a low thoracic spinalization, locomotion was enhanced by treadmill training and adversely affected by a program of postural training for standing without stepping.[153,154] In neurologically impaired individuals, initial gait training, as a practical matter, is preceded by therapeutic exercise aimed at obtaining postural stability. This standing regimen could in theory depress locomotor capability. Typical physical therapy proceeds beyond standing only if the patient has the strength required for weight shifting and stepping.

Body weight–supported treadmill training facilitates a more rhythmic, reciprocal gait pattern without the requirements for good postural stability and full weight bearing. In addition, it is task-oriented therapy, which provides an opportunity for patients to repetitively practice their ability to find some greater level of motor control over the flexor and extensor muscles of the hip, knee, and ankle. This practice and problem solving may stimulate useful reorganization within residual descending pathways for locomotion. By providing a more typical locomotor pattern of cutaneous and proprioceptive input to the motor pathways during BWSTT, any residual cortical and subcortical representational maps within the distributed system for movement may be more effectively remodeled (see Fig. 3–8). The early initiation of supported stepping may also help

to prevent medical complications of immobility such as joint contractures, muscle atrophy, deconditioning, dysautonomia, pressure sores, osteoporosis, heterotopic ossification, depression, and spasticity (see Table 6–7). A multicenter randomized clinical trial that compares BWSTT to conventional mobility training for patients within 8 weeks of traumatic, incomplete SCI will be completed in 2004 and should provide insight about the efficacy and benefits of BWSTT.[143]

Body Weight–Supported Treadmill Training With Functional Neuromuscular Stimulation

A lift system combined with treadmill stepping offers opportunities to add other elements for locomotor retraining. Investigators could make use of peripheral nerve stimulation to drive one aspect of stepping such as flexion[155] (Fig. 1–6) or add a more sophisticated FNS component.[156–158] This combined approach can become expensive and weigh on the expertise required of clinicians. Investigators will need to develop an optimal training paradigm, patient selection criteria, and practical ways to stimulate as few muscles, nerves or cutaneous regions as possible. To prove the efficacy of the combined approach, a clinical trial will have to randomize patients to each component, BWSTT and FNS, as well as to the two in concert. This undertaking ought to await the results of studies that compare BWSTT to conventional treatment after SCI.[143] Robotic steppers continue to be developed to aid stepping on a treadmill[159] or to move the legs through the step cycle with force feedback from the patient.[160] These devices, too, ought to be tested in randomized clinical trials.

Strengthening and Conditioning

As already noted, the energy cost of locomotion may be too great for paraparetic people to take steps other than for exercise. The rate of oxygen consumption between ages 20 and 59 years averages 12 mL/kg per minute at the casual walking velocity of 80 meters/minute. The patient with paraplegia who wants to step may need KAFOs and crutches with a swing-through gait to reach an average speed of 30 meters/minute, but with an oxygen rate of 16 mL/kg per minute.[161] This oxygen consumption is 160% higher than normal subjects use at that speed and the oxygen cost per meter walked is 6 times normal. The energy cost for those with paraparesis who have adequate motor control and strength to take steps may be reduced by interventions that decrease hypertonicity in the legs, including antispasticity medications and physical therapies such as stretching spastic hip adductor muscles.[162] In addition, some hormonal and drug interventions show promise in increasing the strength of paretic muscles (see Chapter 2).[163] The ability to meet the demands of walking with assistive devices and FNS is enhanced by a program of strengthening and cardiovascular conditioning.

For those who cannot step, strengthening and fitness are potentially important goals to increase endurance for community tasks. For instance, routine wheelchair mobility utilizes 18% of the peak oxygen intake of paraplegic athletes in their mid-20's, approximately 30% less than that used by sedentary paraplegic people their age, whereas sedentary people with paraplegia in their 50s use over 50% of their peak oxygen intake for wheelchair activities. Fitness training can increase reserves for midlife activities.

REDUCTION OF CARDIOVASCULAR RISK

Risk factors for chronic disease can also be reduced by exercise. Several small group comparisons have suggested that persons with quadriplegia and paraplegia have significantly lower high-density lipoprotein (HDL) cholesterol levels than controls. In the first year after SCI, however, a prospective study of HDL levels in 100 patients found an increase of 26% in those with quadriplegia and 18% with paraplegia, but the levels are still low.[164] A regimen of 8 weeks of wheelchair ergometer training for subjects with SCI at the moderate intensity of approximately 60% of peak oxygen uptake for 20 minutes a day for 3 days a week increased HDL cholesterol levels by 20% and lowered low-density lipoprotein (LDL) levels by 15%.[165] This training could lower the long-term risk for coronary artery disease by 20%. Graded arm exercises 3 days a week for 3 months lowered LDL cholesterol by 26% and raised HDL cholesterol 10%, along with improving peak oxygen consumption by 30% and reducing cardiovascular risk by 25%.[166] Increased physical activity by able-bodied, sedentary people lowers blood pressure and reduces the risks for heart disease and noninsulin-dependent diabetes (see Chapter 9), so exercise ought to accomplish this in persons working out of wheelchairs.

EXERCISE

Inactive persons with paraplegia gained cardiorespiratory fitness by using arm crank training at 50% of peak oxygen intake on a schedule of 3 times a week for 40 minutes by 8–24 weeks.[167] In the able-bodied, workloads for the upper extremities should be approximately 50% of those used for leg training. The target heart rate should be 10 beats per minute lower than what is prescribed for leg training. At a given submaximal workload, exercise of the arms is done at a greater energy cost, but maximal physiological responses including cardiac output and stroke volume are lower.[168] Using these guidelines, a central conditioning effect can be achieved by able-bodied and neurologically impaired people, especially in those who are initially unfit. Freewheeling gamefield exercises that included propelling a wheelchair over a rising power ramp and a ramp of uneven platforms and by performing chin-ups from the chair produced heart rates and oxygen uptakes from arm exercise alone that were comparable to what is necessary for a training effect in able-bodied persons.[169] Vigorous, enjoyable wheelchair sports, recreational activities, or gadgets such as a wheelchair aerobic fitness trainer that adds ergometer resistance to wheeling[170] may accomplish the same for the person with SCI. The blood pressure, volume loss from sweating, and the ability to dissipate heat ought to be monitored at the start of a vigorous exercise program, especially for patients who may have reduced sympathetic tone.[171]

FUNCTIONAL ELECTRICAL STIMULATION

Among all the neurologic disabilities, the most scientific attention to the limitations and benefits of fitness training and testing has been given to paraplegia and tetraplegia.[172] After SCI, cardiovascular conditioning can be limited by exercising only the upper body's small muscle mass, by pooling of blood in the leg muscles that reduces cardiac preloading, and by impaired cardiovascular reflexes. Functional electrical stimulation-induced leg cycle ergometry can improve both peripheral muscular and central cardiovascular fitness.[173] Resistive voluntary arm activity has been combined with electrical stimulation of leg muscles to further enhance aerobic conditioning.[174]

The responses to FES depend on many variables. With commercial devices for FES-induced lower-extremity cycling such as the Regys I System (Therapeutic Alliances, OH), computer controlled stimulation of the quadriceps, gluteal, and hamstrings muscles reaches 50 rpm, approximately 300 contractions per minute. Stimulation starts at 0 watts and aims to build by 6-watt increments for 30 minutes of exercise to a rarely achieved maximum of approximately 42 watts. On that schedule, the steady state oxygen uptake would reach 2 L/minute, which is equivalent to approximately 50% of the maximum uptake of able-bodied joggers.[175] This effort is too great for most persons with SCI, however. They tend to reach uptake levels of 1 L/minute, which is equivalent to walking in able-bodied persons.

Muscular contractions evoked solely by electrical stimulation or superimposed on contractions by paretic muscles can increase muscle bulk and strength.[176] For example, FES training of the quadriceps, by stimulating full knee extension in sets of 5–15 repetitions against an increasing load resistance of 1 kg–15 kg, increases muscle bulk, improves strength, and reduces fatigability for the FES activity by 12 weeks.[175] In another study, cross-sectional area of most of the exercised leg muscles increased by approximately 30% over the course of 1 year of a gradual buildup of exercise tolerance 3 days a week for 30 minutes.[177] A 2-week trial of a beta$_2$-adrenergic agent such as salbutamol may increase muscle mass more when combined with FES-cycling compared to training alone,[178] but much more study of drug-induced muscle hypertrophy is needed (see Chapter 2). Functional electrical stimulation has also reduced the rate of loss of trabecular bone from the proximal tibia.[179]

During FES, muscle fibers are activated synchronously at high, fatiguing frequencies with an undesirable recruitment order from large-to-small motor units. The optimal combination of stimulation frequency, pulse shape, duration of stimuli, and overall training regimen are uncertain. Much of the research in FES and for FNS gait systems aims to develop a method of stimulation that can reproduce the nervous system's smooth, low fatiguing contractions. This type of contraction may require implanted arrays of electrodes with better controllers (see Chapter 4).

Although psychologic and physiologic benefits have been attributed to FES, long-term home programs require at least as much motivation as needed by able-bodied people who use a stationary bicycle for fitness. Exercise equipment is prone to become an expensive clothes tree unless motivation remains high. In a follow-up of 28 persons with SCI who trained for FES cycling for a median of 1 year before they purchased a home unit, one-third stopped using the device 1 month later.[180] Moreover, some studies of participants in an FES program show that depression and hostility increase in those who had unrealistic expectations for gains in function.[181]

Upper Extremity Function

In addition to the usual range of splints, orthotic devices, and strategies aimed at improving arm and hand function, selected patients with quadriplegia benefit from some specific adaptations. For example, patients with a partial C-4 lesion with preserved elbow flexion or a C-5 injury with a functional deltoid or biceps can improve hand placement for feeding, writing, and typing activities by using a balanced forearm orthosis. If some wrist extension at the C-6 level is intact, finger flexion for a grasp will accompany extension, and finger opening will follow passive wrist flexion when the long finger flexors are allowed to become a bit tight. A wrist-driven orthosis can assist this action. A well-designed elbow extension orthosis that corrects a torque imbalance between an active biceps and inactive triceps may improve flexion and extension functions with or without the addition of FNS.[182] Overhead and counterbalance slings and mobile arm supports eliminate or use the force of gravity to assist arm motion. Environmental controls, computers, and some simple robotic devices can enhance independence after more complete loss of upper extremity function.

Electromyographic biofeedback for upper extremity muscles within or near the zone of partial preservation, perhaps combined with other physical therapies and electrical stimulation, may improve strength and function. In one study of patients with quadriparesis, biofeedback increased the peak EMG of several intrinsic hand muscles by 2–5 times.[183] The mechanism postulated from the investigators' single unit recordings and measures of twitch tensions was an increase in the firing rates of motor units that were already active. The increase may be caused by the recruitment of previously unavailable units, the synchronization of additional units, a greater safety factor in neuromuscular transmission so that fibers fire longer or at higher rates, a sprouting of nerve terminals, or muscle fiber reinnervation. The subjects had large numbers of motor units that were activated or deactivated only after a latency of 10 seconds. A synergistic movement often elicited them. The findings suggest that a corticoreticulospinal or other slower pathway substituted for a faster corticospinal pathway. Studies that make these physiological distinctions may provide more specific and testable training methods. The addition of at least one EMG biofeedback strategy to supervised physical therapies for quadriparetic persons did not, however, clearly improve arm and hand strength or function for self-care.[184]

RECONSTRUCTIVE SURGERY

Upper extremity function can sometimes improve by one of the following measures:
1. A surgical transfer of a tendon from its normal insertion to another tendon or to the insertion point of another muscle
2. Tenodesis, the division or attachment of a tendon to a bone or ligament to help stabilize or passively tether a joint during movement
3. Arthrodesis to eliminate motion or realign a finger joint
4. Osteotomy to reshape a bone

These techniques have been used alone and in combination, along with orthotics, physical training, and electrical stimulation.[185] Specific procedures for C-5 and lower functional levels are most commonly used to increase elbow extension, pronation and supination of the forearm, wrist extension, finger flexion, key grip pinch between the thumb and flexed fingers, palmar prehension for the grasp of large ob-

jects, and for more subtle actions of the intrinsic hand muscles.[186] For example, active hand grasp may be achieved by a person with C-7 quadriplegia by means of surgical transfer of the brachioradialis to the flexor pollicus longus and transfer of the extensor pollicus longus to the flexor digitorum profundus. Surgeons prefer to wait at least 6 months postinjury and use muscles with at least 4/5 strength across joints that are free of contractures. Postoperative immobilization of the limb can last weeks. Activities such as wheelchair transfers and propulsion may be restricted for several months.

Neural Prostheses

Chapter 4 reviews the prospects for neuroprostheses that may soon enable cognitive control of movement through a variety of machine–brain interfaces. Recent commercial availability of FNS systems opens the door for hybrid brain–machine interfaces in which volitional EEG signals directly recorded from the brain control smart FNS outputs to paralyzed muscles (see Fig. 4–1).

HAND GRASP

Systems for FNS with visual and other sensory feedbacks are being developed especially to provide a hand grasp and release in patients with C-5 and C-6 quadriplegia (see Chapter 4). Some work also includes patients with C-4 and C-7 levels. The *NeuroControl FreeHand System* permits a key pinch and palmer grasp, using eight epimysial electrodes that are controlled by a shoulder position sensor that simulates an implanted electrical stimulator. In a prospective study of 51 patients with C-5 or C-6 complete SCI, 50 subjects were significantly more functional in ADLs and 90% used it regularly at home.[187] Computerized neuromuscular stimulation systems supplemented by splints have been triggered by voice and puff-and-suck commands to carry out hand and arm functions in a few C-4 subjects.[188] Systems for sensory feedback and for additional movements are the focus of research at a handful of bioengineering programs.

Remarkably few *FreeHand Systems* have been sold. Studies are needed to evaluate what factors, such as cost, medical complications, waiting for further upgrades, cosmetics, physician encouragement and knowledge, or other psychosocial issues may be deterring commercial sales. If this system does not find a market, other systems may not follow.

STANDING AND WALKING

Functional neuromuscular stimulation, alone and combined with an RGO, HGO, or other assistive and bracing devices, allows users to move from sit to stand, stand to sit, and step over modest distances.[189,190] The FNS systems may have 48 channels of fine wire electrodes to control the muscles of the trunk, hips, knees, and ankles (see Chapter 4).[191] A belt-mounted computer controls the sequence, frequency, and intensity of stimulation. Some paraplegic subjects have been able to step on even surfaces for approximately 1000 meters at speeds of up to 1 meter/second. Some can climb stairs. A study compared outcomes for walking with a custom-built Case Western Reserve University RGO, the RGO with FNS, and FNS alone in trained subjects. The hybrid system added stability and increased the distance walked, but reduced the speed over FNS alone because of a decrease in hip flexion.[192] The ideal design for a hybrid system is a work in progress.

Less complex systems place surface or implanted electrodes in the quadriceps to allow the subject to stand up and flex the hip. Depending on the system's design and the patient's strength, the hamstrings, gluteals, and ankle dorsiflexors are stimulated in a sequence for stepping. For example, the custom-designed Louisiana State University's RGO allows a paraplegic patient to stand fully balanced for long periods. Locomotion is achieved by simultaneous electrical stimulation of one quadriceps and the contralateral hamstrings to allow the swing of one leg and simultaneous push-off of the contralateral leg.[193] A thumb switch on the walker triggers a four-channel reciprocal stimulator. A lengthy strengthening and fitness program must precede the use of these devices. In patients who can stand or even take a few steps, simple 1- to 4-channel FES systems have not reduced energy costs or increased walking speed to a functionally useful degree.[194] One to 4-channel systems have also been tried in patients with incomplete SCI who walk slowly. An uncontrolled Canadian trial found a 40% increase, approximately 0.1 meters/second, in walking speed across subjects

with 1 year of training.[157] The largest relative gains were in subjects who initially walked without the FNS at less than 0.3 meters/second.

The Food and Drug Administration approved the *Parastep System* in 1994. It uses a 6-channel, microcomputer-controlled, battery-powered stimulator, surface electrodes, and a modified walking frame that coordinates signals to several leg muscles. In a multicenter trial, 129 subjects with paraplegia and incomplete quadriplegia were trained.[195] More than half did not finish. To ambulate a mean of 430 feet required about 35 training sessions over 100 days. A 2-year follow-up of trainees found that 78% still used the device at least 3 times a week for household ambulation. The device requires very good upper body strength, finger dexterity, and stamina. Patients should be free of significant cardiopulmonary disease, osteoporosis, and epilepsy. Falls from loss of balance or a power failure could cause serious injury. A study of ASIA A patients with T-4–T-11 levels showed that after three *Parastep* training sessions a week for 10 weeks, most subjects peaked at 20 minutes of standing and walking at a time and increased the girth of the thigh by a centimeter. Bone density did not increase. Wide variations among patients in walking distance, time spent upright, and stepping pace were found.[196] Modest improvements in cardiovascular responses[197] and self-concept[198] have accompanied use of the device.

BOWEL AND BLADDER STIMULATION

Implanted sacral anterior root stimulators, first developed by Brindley in England, have been in use for 2 decades for micturition on demand.[199] A device approved by the FDA, *NeuroControl's VOCARE* bladder system, uses electrodes implanted extradurally on the S-2–S-4 ventral roots. A receiver-stimulator is controlled by a radio transmitter operated with an external switch by the patient. Bilateral dorsal sacral rhizotomies are necessary. Patients with an upper motoneuron lesion, not a lower motoneuron injury, may benefit from the device. A preimplantation compared to 1-year after implantation study of 21 patients showed that 18 patients urinated much better with the stimulator, voiding more than 200 mL of urine with postvoid residuals of less than 50 mL.[200] Time for bowel evacuation was reduced by half and patients had fewer urinary tract infections and bouts of autonomic dysreflexia. The cost of the device (approximately $35,000) and its maintenance (approximately $465 per year) appears to be equal to the cumulative cost of supplies and medical care (approximately $8000 per year) needed for conventional intermittent catheterization and bowel management after 5 years of use.[201] This device, like the *Freehand*, appears not to be reaching the number of patients who may benefit.

Another approach in development is the use of transabdominal and sacral nerve magnetic stimulation to induce colonic and bladder contractions.[202,203] Early results point to full bladder emptying and a reduction in colonic transit time by 20%. A practical method for use by patients does not yet exist.

Spasticity

After the period of spinal shock from an acute SCI, a sequence of minimal reflex activity is often followed by flexor spasms, then flexor and extensor spasms, and then mostly extensor activity. Among 27 patients with a thoracic cord transection verified by laminectomy, however, 5 subjects with levels between T-3 and T-8 had flaccid, areflexic paralysis with marked muscular atrophy 2 years after injury.[204] Most other subjects had extensor spasms elicited by stretch of the iliopsoas. Flexor responses typically followed plantar and genital stimuli.

Medication for spasticity is often given to patients whose flexor withdrawal and extensor spasms cause pain, interrupt sleep, and interfere with ADLs such as wheelchair transfers or driving. Of 466 patients entered into the Model Systems, 26% were discharged on an antispasticity agent an average of 105 days after injury and 46% used medication by the 1-year follow-up.[205] Further analysis of this cohort revealed that spasticity was related to the time from onset of injury and most prominent with cervical and upper thoracic SCI (90% in the University of Michigan subcohort and 57% in the national cohort at follow-up). Patients with Frankel grades A and D were less likely to have been treated than those with grades B and C. The data did not relate the use of antispasticity medication to any positive or negative effects on mobility. This clinical report and others,[206,207] however, add to the impression that spasticity is most prominent after incomplete, rather than complete, motor and sensory lesions. Partial preservation of supraspinal input on neurons below the lesion may be necessary for many of the clinical and physiologic manifestations of severe hypertonicity.[208]

Supported standing several times a day can reduce spasms in nonambulators with a myelopathy.[209] Repetitive passive movement may decrease movement-provoked spasms,[210] but may not increase ankle mobility.[211] Variations in the excitability and patterns of muscle activation may be exaggerated by the stretch reflexes induced when ambulation loads a paretic limb at a dysfunctional angle, force, or point in the gait cycle. By controlling the magnitude of weight-bearing and optimizing the step pattern with, for example, BWSTT, one may reduce clonus and hypertonicity for a day or so after a session.

Although oral benzodiazepines, baclofen, and dantrolene can reduce extensor spasms, clonidine,[212] tizanidine,[213] and cyproheptadine[214] can be especially useful, since they may dampen noxious sensory input to the cord (see Table 8–10). For refractory severe spasms and pain, intrathecal baclofen given by an implanted, programmable pump infusion has generally replaced intrathecal morphine, electrical spinal cord stimulation, selective dorsal rhizotomy, and myelotomy. For perineal care, hip flexor phenol blocks and neurectomies are occasionally useful. Basic mechanisms of spasticity are discussed in Chapter 2 and management in Chapter 8.

LONG-TERM CARE

Health maintenence becomes a life-long challenge for people disabled by a myelopathy. Sensorimotor loss can mask awareness of infections, pressure sores, abdominal pain, and other medical and neurologic complications. Persons with SCI and their physicians have to pay attention to all organ systems. At the same time, physicians should be aware of how their interventions may affect the lifestyle and real-world functioning of the patient. Postrehabilitation outcomes for medical care, resource utilization, and handicap domains are greater in patients who have greater functional disability, less preinjury education, and frequent postinjury pain or abuse drugs.[215] Diabetes mellitus, hyperlipidemia, and cardiovascular disease rise

Table 10–15. **Common Medical Complications Postspinal Cord Injury**

1 Year Postinjury	(%)	30 Years Postinjury	(%)
Urinary tract infection	59	Pressure sore	17
Spasticity	38	Muscle and joint pain	16
Sepsis	19	Gastrointestinal disorder	14
Pressure sore	16	Cardiovascular disorder	14
Dysautonomia	8	Urinary tract infection	14
Contractures	6	Infection, tumor	11
Heterotopic ossification	3	Genitourinary dysfunction	8
Azotemia	2	Renal stone, renal failure	6
Wound infection	2		

Source: Adapted from Ditunno and Formal, 1994.[217]

in aging people with SCI, unless risk factors are identified and managed.[216] Table 10–15 lists the more common medical complications found 30 years after a SCI that require surveillance.[217]

Aging

The rather good health of the aging American and western European population may lead to a greater prevalence of people who suffer a traumatic or nontraumatic SCI after 65 years of age and to more persons with SCI who survive into old age. The elderly person with an acute SCI often brings different values and rehabilitation goals to therapy than younger patients who are beginning family life and careers. Like most elderly people, the more senior patient may be more concerned about not burdening family than success in walking again, which is usually the highest priority for young patients. In older patients, slower gains and lower levels of independence may be associated with easy fatigability, overuse of muscles and joints, depression, more medical problems, and greater susceptibility to the side-effects of medications. These factors complicate early therapy efforts and, as younger SCI patients age, will increasingly affect long-term management.

In one study, patients who were over the age of 61 at onset of SCI were compared to patients 16–30 years old.[122] Older patients were over twice as likely to suffer pneumonia or a gastrointestinal hemorrhage, 5 times more likely to develop a pulmonary embolus, and 17 times more likely to have renal stones. During the 2nd year after SCI, older patients were 4 times as likely to be rehospitalized, 72 times as likely to be living in a nursing home, and 7 times more likely to have hired an attendant. The 2-year survival rate of these older patients was only 59%, compared with an expected rate of 94%.

One-fourth of patients who had sustained their injuries 20–40 years ago evolved a greater need for physical assistance over the years, especially for help with transfers.[218] Patients reported shoulder pain, fatigue, weakness, weight gain, and a decline in the quality of life more often than patients who did not require more assistance.

A study of veterans with traumatic SCI found that those who survived at least 3 months had an additional 39-year survival, which is 85% of that of similarly aged American males.[219] Life expectancy for the first 20 years after injury was comparable to that of disabled veterans who did not have a SCI, but then it declined. By 20 years, the causes of death were similar for both groups of veterans, with a fall-off in SCI-related problems such as septicemia and renal failure. Complete quadriplegia was less predictive of poorer long-term survival than was older age at onset.

Sexual Function

Sexual relationships may be physical, emotional, or both. Sexual activity may be lower for single men and women than for married people. Although SCI is often accompanied by sexual dysfunction, most patients can be sexually active. Approximately 40% of men with quadriplegia and 60% of those with paraplegia graded Frankel A–C reported having intercourse in the prior 12 months.[220] Satisfaction with their sex lives ranked at the bottom of 12 life pursuits, although it was ranked as the fifth most important activity. A community-based sampling of women with SCI rated their sex lives 10th of 11 items in importance and satisfaction.[221] Approximately 60% had had sexual intercourse in the previous year. In another sample of women after SCI, 76% engaged in kissing, 68% in intercourse, 56% in oral sex, 40% in manual stimulation, 24% in vibratory stimulation, and 12% in anal intercourse.[222] Sexual satsifaction decreased with age, a trend opposite to able-bodied women. Counseling, education, and medical assistance are often necessary. In both men and women, pain, spasms, dysautonomia, incontinence, feelings of unattractiveness, the effort of preparation, and concerns about satisfying a partner or oneself can interfere with foreplay and intercourse.

Reflexogenic erections occur in over 90% of men with complete and incomplete SCI, but ejaculation may be functional in only 10% of those with complete SCI and one-third of those with incomplete SCI.[223] Severe headache may accompany ejaculation. Reflexive suboccipital and paraspinal muscle spasm, dysautonomia with hypertension, and migraine may account for the paroxysmal pain.

Erectile function and seminal ejaculation can be aided by many techniques. Sildenafil and newer orally taken drugs enable an erection that permits penetration for 80% of patients.[224] Intracavernous injections of papaverine and other substances work for some, but priapism is a more common adverse reaction in the person with SCI. Vacuum techniques are often useful for maintaining an erection. Implanted, semirigid penile prostheses benefitted 52 of 63 veterans with sexual dysfunction, some of whom had skin lacerations from external appliances, but they carried an initial 33% complication rate.[225] Infections occurred in 7% and skin erosions evolved in 11% after 6 months. Penile vibration, subcutaneous physostigmine with masturbation, and surgical vasal-epididymal sperm retrieval elicit semen for insemination. Infertility may be related to the poor quality of semen. Some causes are treatable.[226] In addition to the technique of anterior sacral root stimulation, erectile function and ejaculation can be controlled by electrical stimulation of the hypogastric plexus or via a rectal probe.[227]

Married women with a SCI are as satsified with sexual activities as those without a SCI.[228] Approximately 50% of women after SCI achieve orgasm. Medications such as sildenafil may improve arousal. Preservation of sensation in T-11–L-2 dermatomes is associated with psychogenically mediated genital vasocongestion.[229] In a controlled study, women after a SCI were less likely to achieve orgasm than women without SCI, especially women with lesions that disrupt the S-2–S-5 reflex arc after a complete lower motoneuron injury. A vaginal lubricating jelly can aid intercourse. Micturition or catheterization immediately after intercourse helps prevent bladder infections. Women remain fertile after SCI. Pregnancy can be complicated by hypertension and autonomic dysreflexia, pressure sores, urinary infections, central and dysesthetic pain, and failure to progress in labor. Term deliveries are common with close medical supervision, especially for women with complete lesions below T-10. The SCI, however, may not allow them to sense onset of labor.

Employment

Data from Model Systems showed employment rates 5 years after SCI at 28% for persons with paraplegia and 14% for those with quadriplegia; patients with incomplete lesions have somewhat higher work rates in each category.[5] Although 64% of patients were employed at the time of injury, 13% were working 2 years later and 38% had jobs 12 years later. In the first year, previously employed patients often return to their prior jobs. After that time, they tend to find new employers or, having completed their education, join the labor force. Approximately 6% in the data set were Department of Vocational Rehabilitation clients before injury, 38% became clients at the time of rehabilitation discharge, and 8% were clients 13 years after SCI.[20] In another sample of 286 people with SCI who were interviewed an average of 18 years postinjury, 48% were still working and 75% had worked at some point.[230] Aside from level of injury, the most critical predictor of employment was education. People with at least 16 years of education had employment rates since injury of 95%, compared with 63% for those who had completed high school and 38% for those who had not. Predictors of employment, then, include Caucasian race (approximately 3 times more likely to work than minority groups), a less severe injury especially with paraplegia, college and doctoral education, employment at the time of injury, and an injury unrelated to a violent act.[231,232]

Marital Status

Five years after injury, 90% of unmarried SCI subjects followed in the Model Systems program remained single compared to 64% of noninjured subjects of the same age. Of those already married, 78% remained so, compared to an expected rate of 89%. The risk of divorce was greater than in matched uninjured people, primarily in the 2nd and 3rd years after injury, but similar in the 1st, 4th, and 5th years.[20]

Adjustment and Quality of Life

An increasing amount of study has gone into the gradual process by which patients with SCI psychologically assimilate changes in their bodies, their self-concepts, and their interactions with their environment.[233] Life satisfaction, on average, tends to be lower for those with SCI compared to the general population of age-matched community dwellers. It is better in those who have less handicap in social integration, occupation, and mobility, regardless of the degree of neurologic impairment and disability.[234] Subjective ratings of QOL are strongly associated with perceived control, self-assessed health, and social support. The best QOL is experienced by married white females who are currently employed, have more than a high school education, and are more than a few years past the SCI.[235]

Depression is not an inevitable effect of SCI.[236] Suicide rates, however, were 2–4 times that of the general population within 5 years of SCI[237] and range from 6% to 13% or about 5 times higher than the general population.[238] Measures of despondency both before and after the SCI were higher in persons who died of suicide compared to a control group that did not commit suicide. Feelings of shame and apathy were documented during the rehabilitation hospitalization. This information poses an opportunity for intervention. Depressed or distressed patients with SCI reported spending more hours in bed, fewer days out of the house, and received more personal care assistance compared to persons who had adjusted to the SCI by 2–7 years after injury.[239] Depressed people also perceived having greater handicap with limitations, for example, in getting transportation. Again, by obtaining this information from the patient, clinicians can propose psychosocial interventions and possibly drug therapy for depression.

Anxiety and depression can also arise from a PTSD associated with the event that led to the SCI (see Chapter 8). In pediatric patients with SCI, the incidence of PTSD is approximately 30%.[240] Its presence is associated with poorer functional independence. The symptoms and signs of PTSD, such as environmental cues that set off anxiety attacks, intrusive recollections, hyperarousal, nightmares, and pananxiety should be sought in every patient in the first months after injury and treated with counseling and medications such as sertraline or a benzodiazepine.[241]

Psychological and social adjustment after SCI appear to be stronger predictors for long-term survival than antecedent medical complications. Using the Life Situation Questionnaire, one prospective study found that boredom, depression, loneliness, lack of transportation, conflicts with attendants, inability to control their lives, and alcohol and drug abuse characterized those who died in the last 4 years of a 15-year follow-up.[242] Personality and mood disorders associated with self-destructive behaviors such as getting little exercise, letting bladder infections and skin sores go without attention, and abusing tobacco, alcohol, narcotics, and sedatives contributes to this mortality. In one survey, 70% of people with traumatic SCI reported substance abuse before or after injury. Although 16% believed they needed treatment, only 7% received specific help.[243]

Families, the rehabilitation team, and the physicians who provide chronic care must monitor the psychosocial adjustments, mood, and behavior of SCI-disabled persons and provide assistance as soon as a problem is identified. Over the long run, clues about potential problems may be brought to light by periodically giving patients a standard QOL questionnaire.

SUMMARY

The early and long-term rehabilitation assessment and management of patients with traumatic SCI or a myelopathy of any cause closely follow residual sensorimotor function, the potential for more independent function, and the practical goals set by patients. The emphasis of training is on strengthening and conditioning, as well as employing adaptive devices and strategies to regain control of personal care and the home and work environment. Given near-normal upper extremity function, ambulation improves in relation to truncal and lower extremity strength and the energy cost of mobility. Most of the gains in functional independence and community reintegration continue to be made through improved technologies for assistive devices and efforts to limit environmental handicaps. Assistive devices, such as crutches and walkers, leg braces, orthoses, and mechanical and electrical stimulation systems, foster stepping and grasping in highly motivated people. Computer-interfaced devices increase functional independence across daily activities.

These innovations raise the quality of life for people with SCI, in concert with better approaches to manage central and peripheral pain, bowel and bladder control, muscle spasms, dysreflexia, skin care, and psychosocial supports for work and play. People with SCI are waiting for successful translation of biologic interventions from animal models to patients. In the interim, task-oriented training that makes use of activity-dependent plasticity within the motoneuron pools of the cord and in supraspinal networks may lessen impairments and disabilities.

REFERENCES

1. Ramer M, Harper G, Bradbury E. Progress in spinal cord research. Spinal Cord 2000; 38:449–472.
2. Harvey C, Rothschild B, Asmann A, Stripling T. New estimates of traumatic SCI prevalence: A survey based approach. Paraplegia 1990; 28:537–544.
3. National Spinal Cord Injury Statistical Center. Spinal cord injury: Facts and figures. J Spinal Cord Med 2001; 24:212–213.
4. Stover S, DeVivo M, Go B. History, implementation, and current status of the national spinal cord injury database. Arch Phys Med Rehabil 1999; 80:1365–1371.
5. Stover S. Spinal Cord Injury: The Facts and Figures. Birmingham, AL: University of Alabama, 1986.

6. Fiedler R, Granger C, Post L. The Uniform Data System for Medical Rehabilitation: report of first admissions for 1998. Am J Phys Med Rehabil 2000; 79:87–92.
7. Bracken M, Shepard M, Collins W, Holford T, Young W, Baskin D, Eisenberg H, Flamm E, Leo-Summers L, Maroon J. A randomized, controlled trial of methylprednisolone or naloxone in the treatment of acute spinal-cord injury. N Engl J Med 1990; 322:1405–1411.
8. Bracken M, Shepard M, Holford T, Leo-Summers L, Aldrich E, Fazi M, Fehlings M, Herr D, Hitchon P, Marshall L, Nockels R, Pascale V, Perot P, Piepmeir J, Sonntag V, Wagner F, Wilberger J, Winn H, Young W. Administration of methylprednisolone for 24 or 48 hours or tirilazad mesylate for 48 hours in the treatment of acute spinal cord injury. JAMA 1997; 277:1597–1604.
9. Granger C, Albrecht G, Hamilton B. Outcome of comprehensive rehabilitation: Measurement by PULSES and Barthel Index. Arch Phys Med Rehabil 1979; 60:145–154.
10. Roth E, Davidoff G, Haughton J, Ardner M. Functional assessment in spinal cord injury: A comparison of the Modified Barthel Index and the 'adapted' Functional Independence Measure. Clin Rehabil 1990; 4:277–285.
11. Curt A, Keck ME, Dietz V. Functional outcome following spinal cord injury: significance of motor evoked potentials and ASIA scores. Arch Phys Med Rehabil 1998; 79:81–86.
12. Ditunno J, Ditunno P, Graziani V, Scivoletto G, Bernardi M, Castellano V, Marchetti M, Barbeau H, Frankel H, D'Andrea Greve J, Ko H, Marshall R, Nance P. Walking index for spinal cord injury (WISCI): An international multicenter validity and reliability study. Spinal Cord 2000; 38:234–243.
13. Kannus P, Niemi S, Palvanen M, Parkkari J. Continuously increasing number and incidence of fall-induced, fracture-associated, spinal cord injuries in elderly persons. Arch Intern Med 2000; 160:2145–2149.
14. DeVivo M, Stover S, Black K. Prognostic factors for 12-year survival after SCI. Arch Phys Med Rehabil 1992; 73:156–162.
15. Berkowitz M, O'Leary P, Krusee D, Harvey C. Spinal cord injury—an analysis of medical and social costs. New York: Demos, 1998.
16. DeVivo M, Whiteneck G, Stover S, Charles E. Indirect costs of spinal cord injury. J Am Para Soc 1993; 16:92.
17. Seel R, Huang M, Cifu D, Kolakowsky-Hayner A, McKinley W. Age-related differences in length of stays, hospitalization costs, and outcomes for an injury-matched sample of adults with paraplegia. J Spinal Cord Med 2001; 24:241–250.
18. Greenwald B, Seel R, Cifu D, Shah A. Gender-related differences in acute rehabilitation lengths of stay, charges, and functional outcomes for a matched sample with spinal cord injury: a multicenter investigation. Arch Phys Med Rehabil 2001; 82:1181–1187.
19. Fiedler I, Laud P, Maiman D, Apple D. Economies of managed care in spinal cord injury. Arch Phys Med Rehabil 1999; 80:1441–1449.
20. DeVivo M, Richards J, Stover S, Go B. Spinal cord

injury: Rehabilitation adds life to years. West J Med 1991; 154:602–606.

21. Hall E. Pharmacological treatment of acute spinal cord injury: How do we build on past success? J Spinal Cord Med 2001; 24:142–146.

22. Chiles B, Cooper P. Acute spinal injury. N Engl J Med 1996; 334:514–520.

23. Bracken M. National Acute Spinal Cord Injury Study Group: Methylpredisone or naloxone treatment after acute spinal cord injury: 1-year follow-up data. J Neurosurg 1992; 76:23–31.

24. Short D. Is the role of steroids in acute spinal cord injury now resolved? Curr Opin Neurol 2001; 14: 759–763.

25. Geisler F, Coleman W, Grieco G, Poonian D. The Sygen Multicenter acute spinal cord injury study. Spine 2001; 26:S58–S98.

26. Kakulas B, Taylor J. Pathology of injuries of the vertebral column and spinal cord. In: Frankel H, ed. Spinal Cord Trauma. Vol. 61. Amsterdam: Elsevier, 1992:21–51.

27. Otis J. Biomechanics of spine injuries. In: Cantu R, ed. Neurologic Athletic Head and Spine Injuries. Philadelphia: WB Saunders, 2000.

28. Marciello M, Flanders A, Herbison G, Schaefer D, Friedman D, Lane J. Magnetic resonance imaging related to neurologic outcome in cervical spinal cord injury. Arch Ohys Med Rehabil 1993; 74:940–946.

29. Ramon S, Dominguez R, Ramirez L. Clinical and magnetic resonance imaging correlation in acute spinal cord injury. Spinal Cord 1997; 35:664–673.

30. Ohshio I, Hatayama A, Kaneda K, Takahara M, Nagashima K. Correlation between histopathologic features and magnetic resonance images of spinal cord lesions. Spine 1993; 18:1140–1149.

31. Bunge R, Puckett W, Becerra J, Marcillo A, Quencer R. Observations on the pathology of human spinal cord injury. In: Seil F, ed. Spinal Cord Injury. Vol. 59. New York: Raven Press, 1993:75–89.

32. Blight A. Cellular morphology of chronic spinal cord injury in the cat: Analysis of myelinated axons by line-sampling. Neuroscience 1983; 10:521–543.

33. Alstermark B, Lundberg A, Pinter M, Sasaki S. Subpopulations and functions of long C3–C5 propriospinal neurones. Brain Res 1987; 404:395–400.

34. Sherwood A, Dimitrijevic M, McKay W. Evidence of subclinical brain influence in clinically complete spinal cord injury: Discomplete SCI. J Neurol Sci 1992; 110:90–98.

35. Blight A. Axonal physiology of chronic spinal cord injury in the cat: Intracellular recording in vitro. Neurosci 1983; 10:1471–1486.

36. Blight A, Toombs J, Bauer M, Widmer W. The effects of 4-aminopyridine on neurological deficits in chronic cases of traumatic spinal cord injury in dogs. J Neurotrauma 1991; 8:103–119.

37. Kaelan C, Jacobsen P, Morling P, Kakulas B. A quantitative study of motoneurons and corticospinal fibres related to function in human spinal cord injury (abstract). Paraplegia 1989; 27:148–149.

38. Hayes K, Kakulas B. Neuropathology of human spinal cord injury sustained in sports-related activities. J Neurotrauma 1997; 14:235–248.

39. Kakulas B. A review of the neuropathology of human spinal cord injury with emphasis on special features. J Spinal Cord Med 1999; 22:119–124.

40. Vilensky J, Moore A, Eidelberg E, Walden J. Recovery of locomotion in monkeys with spinal cord lesions. J Mot Behav 1992; 24:288–296.

41. McKinley W, Seel R, Hardman J. Nontraumatic spinal cord injury: Incidence, epidemiology, and functional outcome. Arch Phys Med Rehabil 1999; 80:619–623.

42. de Seze J, Stojkovic T, Breteau G, Hachulla E, Michon-Pasturel U, Mounier-Vehier F, Hatron P, Vermersch P. Acute myelopathies: clinical, laboratory and outcome profiles in 79 cases. Brain 2001; 124: 1509–1521.

43. Cheshire W, Santos C, Massey E, Howard J. Spinal cord infarction: Etiology and outcome. Neurology 1996; 47:321–330.

44. McKinley W, Tellis A, Cifu D, Johnson M, Kubal W, Keyser-Marcus L, Musgrove J. Rehabilitation outcome of individuals with nontraumatic myelopathy resulting from spinal stenosis. J Spinal Cord Med 1997; 21:131–136.

45. Fritz J, Delito A, Welch W, Erhard R. Lumbar spinal stenosis: A review of current concepts in evaluation, management, and outcome measurements. Arch Phys Med Rehabil 1998; 79:700–708.

46. DeVivo M, Rutt R, Black K, Go B, Stover S. Trends in spinal cord injury demographics and treatment outcomes between 1973 and 1986. Arch Phys Med Rehabil 1992; 73:424–430.

47. DeVivo M, Krause J, Lammertse D. Recent trends in mortality and causes of death among persons with spinal cord injury. Arch Phys Med Rehabil 1999; 80: 1411–1419.

48. Heinemann A, Yarkony G, Roth E, Lovell L, Hamilton B, Ginsburg K, Brown J, Meyer P. Functional outcome following spinal cord injury. Arch Neurol 1989; 46:1098–1102.

49. Oakes D, Wilmot C, Hall K, Sherck J. Benefits of early admission to a comprehensive trauma center for patients with SCI. Arch Phys Med Rehabil 1990; 71: 637–643.

50. Inman C. Effectiveness of spinal cord rehabilitation. Clin Rehabil 1999; 13 (suppl 1):25–31.

51. Waters R, Meyer P, Adkins R, Felton D. Emergency, acute, and surgical management of spine trauma. Arch Phys Med Rehabil 1999; 80:1383–1390.

52. Donovan W. Operative and nonoperative management of spinal cord injury: A review. Paraplegia 1994; 32:375–388.

53. Wilmot C, Hall K. Evaluation of acute surgical intervention in traumatic paraplegia. Paraplegia 1986; 24:71–76.

54. Wilmot C, Hall K. Evaluation of the acute management of tetraplegia: Conservative versus surgical treatment. Paraplegia 1986; 24:148–53.

55. Fehlings M, Tator C. An evidence-based review of decompressive surgery in acute spinal cord injury: Rationale, indications, and timing based on experimental and clinical studies. J Neurosurg 1999; 91 (Spine 1):1–11.

56. Tator C, Fehlings M, Thorpe K, Math M, Taylor W. Current use and timing of spinal surgery for management of acute spinal cord injury in North America: Results of a retrospective multicenter study. J Neurosurg 1999; 91 (Spine 1):12–18.

57. Brunelli G, Brunelli G. Restoration of walking in paraplegia by transferring the ulnar nerve to the hip: a report on the first patient. Microsurgery 1999; 19:223–226.
58. Klekamp J, Batzdorf U, Samii M, Boethe H. Treatment of syringomyelia with arachnoid scarring caused by arachnoiditis or trauma. J Neurosurg 1997; 86: 233–240.
59. Davidoff G, Roth E, Richards J. Cognitive deficits in SCI: Epidemiology and outcome. Arch Phys Med Rehabil 1992; 73:275–284.
60. Jackson A, Groomes T. Incidence of respiratory complications following spinal cord injury. Arch Phys Med Rehabil 1994; 75:270–275.
61. McKinley W, Jackson A, Cardenas D, DeVivo M. Long-term medical complications after traumatic spinal cord injury: A regional Model Systems analysis. Arch Phys Med Rehabil 1999; 80:1402–1410.
62. Nash M. Known and plausible modulators of depressed immune functions following spinal cord injury. J Spinal Cord Med 2000; 23:111–120.
63. Bach J. New approaches in the rehabilitation of the traumatic high level quadriplegic. Am J Phys Med Rehabil 1991; 70:13–19.
64. Creasey G, Elefteriades J, DiMarco A, Talonen P, Bijak M, Girsch W, Kantor C. Electrical stimulation to restore respiration. J Rehabil Res Dev 1996; 33:123–32.
65. Lin V, Hsiao I, Zhu E, Perkash I. Functional magnetic stimulation for conditioning of expiratory muscles in patients with spinal cord injury. Arch Phys Med Rehabil 2001; 82:162–166.
66. Patterson D, Miller-Perrin C, McCormick T, Hudson L. When life support is questioned early in the care of patients with cervical-level quadriplegia. N Eng J Med 1994; 328:506–509.
67. Stiens S, Bergman S, Goetz L. Neurogenic bowel dysfunction after spinal cord injury: Clinical evaluation and rehabilitative management. Arch Phys Med Rehabil 1997; 78:S86–S102.
68. Mylotte J, Kahler L, Graham R, Young L, Goodnough S. Prospective surveillance for antibiotic-resistant organisms in patients with spinal cord injury admitted to an acute rehabilitation unit. Am J Infect Control 2000; 28:291–297.
69. National Institute on Disability and Rehabilitation Research Consensus Statement. The prevention and management of urinary tract infections among people with spinal cord injuries. J Am Para Soc 1992; 15:194–204.
70. Stover S, Lloyd K, Waites K, Jackson A. Urinary tract infection in SCI. Arch Phys Med Rehabil 1989; 70:47–54.
71. Morton S, Shekelle P, Dobkin B, Adams J, Vickrey B, Bennett C, Montgomerie J. Antimicrobial prophylaxis for urinary tract infection in persons with spinal cord dysfunction. Arch Phys Med Rehabil 2002; 83:129–138.
72. Jackson A, DeVivo M. Urological long-term follow-up in women with spinal cord injury. Arch Phys Med Rehabil 1992; 73:1029–1035.
73. Consortium for Spinal Cord Medicine. Outcomes following traumatic spinal cord injury: Clinical practices guidelines for health-care professionals. Washington, DC: Paralyzed Veterans of America, 1999:30.
74. Lal S, Hamilton B, Heinemann A, Betts H. Risk factors for heterotopic ossification in spinal cord injury. Arch Phys Med Rehabil 1989; 70:387–390.
75. Frost F. APS recommendations for skin care of hospitalized patients with acute spinal cord injury. J Spinal Cord Med 1999; 22:133–138.
76. Fuhrer M, Garber S, Rintala D, Clearman R, Hart K. Pressure ulcers in community-resident persons with spinal cord injury: Prevalence and risk factors. Arch Phys Med Rehabil 1993; 74:1172–1177.
77. Groomes T, Huang C. Orthostatic hypotension after SCI: Treatment with fludrocortisone and ergotamine. Arch Phy Med Rehabil 1991; 72:56–58.
78. Colachis S. Autonomic hyperreflexia with spinal cord injury. J Am Para Soc 1992; 15:171–186.
79. Massagli T, Cardenas D. Immobilization hypercalcemia treatment with pamidronate disodium after spinal cord injury. Arch Phys Med Rehabil 1999; 80:998–1000.
80. Elias A, Gwinup G. Immobilization osteoporosis in paraplegia. J Am Para Soc 1992; 15:163–170.
81. Frey-Rindova P, de Bruin E, Stussi E, Dambacher M, Dietz V. Bone mineral density in upper and lower extremities during 12 months after spinal cord injury measured by peripheral quantitative computed tomography. Spinal Cord 2000; 38:26–32.
82. Szollar S, Martin E, Sartoris D, Parthemore J, Deftos L. Bone mineral density and indexes of bone metabolism in spinal cord injury. Am J Phys Med Rehabil 1998; 77:28–35.
83. Vaziri N, Panadian M, Segal J, Winer R, Eltorai I, Brunnemann S. Vitamin D, parathormone, and calcitonin profiles in persons with long-standing spinal cord injury. Arch Phys Med Rehabil 1994; 75:766–769.
84. Nance P, Schryvers O, Leslie W. Intravenous pamidronate attenuates bone density loss after acute spinal cord injury. Arch Phys Med Rehabil 1999; 80:243–251.
85. Wang Y-H, Huang T-S, Lien I-N. Hormone changes in men with spinal cord injuries. Am J Phys Med Rehabil 1992; 71:328–332.
86. Turner J, Cardenas D, Warms C, McClellan C. Chronic pain associated with spinal cord injuries: a community survey. Arch Phys Med Rehabil 2001; 82:501–508.
87. Widerstrom-Noga E, Felipe-Cuervo E, Yerzierski R. Chronic pain after spinal injury: interference with sleep and daily activities. Arch Phys Med Rehabil 2001; 82:1571–1577.
88. Subbarao J, Klopfstein J, Turpin R. Prevalence and impact of wrist and shoulder pain in patients with spinal injury. J Spinal Cord Med 1995; 18:9–13.
89. Aisen M, Aisen P. Shoulder-hand syndrome in patients with cervical spinal cord injury. Neurology 1992; 42(suppl3):207.
90. Vierck C, Siddal P, Yezierski R. Pain following spinal cord injury: Animal models and mechanistic studies. Pain 2000; 89:1–5.
91. Cole J, Illis L, Sedgwick E. Intractable central pain in spinal cord injury is not relieved by spinal cord stimulation. Paraplegia 1991; 29:167–172.
92. Siddall P, Molloy A, Walker S, Mather L, Rutkowski S, Cousins M. the efficacy of intrathecal morphine and clonidine in the treatment of pain after spinal cord injury. Anesth Analg 2000; 91:1493–1498.
93. Edgar R, Best S, Quail P, Obert A. Computer-

assisted DREZ microcoagulation: Posttraumatic spinal deafferentation pain. J Spinal Disord 1993; 6:48–56.

94. Mertens P, Sindou M. Surgery in the dorsal root entry zone for treatment of chronic pain. Neurochirurgie 2000; 46:429–446.

95. Sampson J, Cashman R, Nashold B, Friedman A. Dorsal root entry zone lesions for intractable pain after trauma to the conus medullaris and cauda equina. J Neurosurg 1995; 82:28–34.

96. Marino R, Ditunno J, Donovan W, Maynard F. Neurologic recovery after traumatic spinal cord injury: Data from the model spinal cord injury systems. Arch Phys Med Rehabil 1999; 80:1391–1396.

97. Piepmeier J, Jenkins N. Late neurological changes following traumatic SCI. J Neurosurg 1988; 69:399–402.

98. Curt A, Dietz V. Ambulatory capacity in spinal cord injury: Significance of somatosensory evoked potentials and ASIA protocol in predicting outcome. Arch Phys Med Rehabil 1997; 78:39–43.

99. Waters R, Yakura J, Adkins R, Sie I. Recovery following paraplegia. Arch Phys Med Rehabil 1992; 73:784–789.

100. Waters R, Adkins R, Yakura J, Sie L. Functional and neurologic recovery following acute SCI. J Spinal Cord Med 1998; 21:195–198.

101. Waters R, Adkins R, Yakura J, Sie I. Motor and sensory recovery following incomplete paraplegia. Arch Phys Med Rehabil 1994; 75:67–72.

102. Ditunno J, Stover S, Freed M, Ahn J. Motor recovery of the upper extremities in traumatic quadriplegia. Arch Phys Med Rehabil 1992; 73:431–436.

103. Ditunno J, Cohen M, Hauck W, Jackson A, Sipski M. Recovery of upper extremity strength in complete and incomplete tetraplegia: A multicenter study. Arch Phys Med Rehabil 2000; 81:389–393.

104. Waters R, Adkins R, Yakura J, Sie I. Motor and sensory recovery following incomplete tetraplegia. Arch Phys Med Rehabil 1994; 75:306–311.

105. Waters R, Adkins R, Yakura J, Sie I. Motor and sensory recovery following complete tetraplegia. Arch Phys Med Rehabil 1993; 74:242–247.

106. Eschbach K, Herbison G, Ditunno J. Sensory root level recovery in patients with Frankel A quadriplegia. Arch Phys Med Rehabil 1992; 73:618–622.

107. Little J, Ditunno J, Stiens S, Harris R. Incomplete spinal cord injury: Neuronal mechanisms of motor recovery and hyperreflexia. Arch Phys Med Rehabil 1999; 80:587–599.

108. Macdonnell R, Donnan G. Magnetic cortical stimulation in acute spinal cord injury. Neurology 1995; 45:303–306.

109. Jimenez O, Marcillo A, Levi A. A histopathological analysis of the human cervical spinal cord in patients with acute traumatic central cord syndrome. Spinal Cord 2000; 38:532–37.

110. Cohen L, Topka H, Cole R, Hallett M. Paresthesias induced by magnetic brain stimulation in patients with thoracic spinal cord injury. Neurology 1991; 41:1283–1288.

111. Topka H, Cohen L, Cole R, Hallett M. Reorganization of corticospinal pathways following spinal cord injury. Neurology 1991; 41:1276–1283.

112. Song Z, Cohen M, Vulpe M, Ament P, Ho W, Schandler S. Two-point discrimination thresholds in spinal cord injured patients with dysesthetic pain. Paraplegia 1993; 31:485–493.

113. Li C, Houlden D, Rowed D. Somatosensory evoked potentials and neurological grades as predictors of outcome in acute SCI. J Neurosurg 1990; 72:600–604.

114. Jacobs S, Yeaney N, Herbison G, Ditunno J. Future ambulation prognosis as predicted by somatosensory evoked potentials in motor complete and incomplete quadriplegia. Arch Phys Med Rehabil 1995; 76:635–641.

115. Dobkin B, Taly A, Su G. Use of the audiospinal reflex to test for completeness of spinal cord injury. J Neurologic Rehabil 1994; 8:187–192.

115a. Chen XY, Carp J, Chen L, Wolpaw J. Corticospinal tract transection prevents operantly conditioned H-reflex increase in rats. Exp Brain Res 2002; 144:88–94.

116. Graves D, Rrankiewicz R, Carter E. Gain in functional ability during medical rehabilitation as related to rehabilitation process indices and neurologic measures. Arch Phys Med Rehabil 1999; 80:1464–1470.

117. Hall K, Cohen M, Wright J, Call M, Werner P. Characteristics of the Functional Independence Measure in traumatic spinal cord injury. Arch Phys Med Rehabil 1999; 80:1471–1476.

118. Granger C, Hamilton B. The Uniform Data System for Medical Rehabilitation report of first admissions for 1992. Am J Phys Med Rehabil 1994; 73:51–55.

119. Weingarden S, Martin C. Independent dressing after spinal cord injury: A functional time evaluation. Arch Phys Med Rehabil 1989; 70:518–519.

120. Yarkony G, Roth E, Meyer J, PR, Lovell L, Heinemann A, Betts H. Spinal cord injury care system: Fifteen-year experience at the Rehabilitation Institute of Chicago. Paraplegia 1990; 28:321–329.

121. Yarkony G, Roth E, Heinemann A, Lovell A, Wu Y. Functional skills after spinal cord injury rehabilitation: Three-year longitudinal follow-up. Arch Phys Med Rehabil 1988; 69:111–114.

122. DeVivo M, Kartus P, Stover S, Fine P. The influence of age at time of spinal cord injury on rehabilitation outcome. Arch Neurol 1990; 47:687–691.

123. Daverat P, Sibrac M, Dartigues J, Barat M. Early prognostic factors for walking in spinal cord injuries. Paraplegia 1988; 26:255–261.

124. Maynard F, Reynolds G, Fountain S. Neurological progress after traumatic quadriplegia. J Neurosurg 1979; 50:611–616.

125. Ducker T, Lucas J, Wallace C. Recovery from spinal cord injury. Clin Neurosurg 1983; 30:495–513.

126. Crozier K, Graziani V, Ditunno Jr. J, Herbison G. Spinal cord injury: Prognosis for ambulation based on sensory examination in patients who are initially motor complete. Arch Phys Med Rehabil 1991; 72:119–121.

127. Waters R, Yakura J, Adkins R, Barnes G. Determinants of gait performance following spinal cord injury. Arch Phys Med Rehabil 1989; 70:811–818.

128. Lazar R, Yarkony G, Ortolano D, Heinemann A. Prediction of functional outcome by motor capability after spinal cord injury. Arch Phys Med Rehabil 1989; 70:819–822.

129. Waters R, Adkins R, Yakura J, Vogil D. Prediction of ambulatory performance based on motor scores derived from standards of the American Spinal Injury Association. Arch Phys Med Rehabil 1994; 75:756–760.

130. Woolsey R. Rehabilitation outcome following spinal cord injury. Arch Neurol 1985; 42:116–119.

131. Yarkony G, Roth E, Heinemann A, Wu Y, Katz R, Lovell L. Benefits of rehabilitation for traumatic spinal cord injury. Arch Neurol 1987; 44:93–96.

132. Penrod L, Hegde S, Ditunno J. Age effect on prognosis for functional recovery in acute, traumatic central cord syndrome. Arch Phys Med Rehabil 1990; 71:963–968.

133. Klose K, Schmidt D, Needham B, Brucker B, Green B, Ayyar D. Rehabilitation therapy for patients with long-term spinal cord injuries. Arch Phys Med Rehabil 1990; 71:659–662.

134. Walter J, Sola P, Sacks J, Lucero Y, Weaver F. Indication for a home standing program for individuals with spinal cord injury. J Spinal Cord Med 1999; 22:152–158.

135. Kunkel C, Scremin E, Eisenberg B, Garcia J, Roberts S, Martinez S. Effect of "standing" on spasticity, contracture, and osteoporosis in paralyzed males. Arch Phys Med Rehabil 1993; 74:73–78.

136. Lyles M, Munday J. Report on the evaluation of the Vannini-Rizzoli stabilizing limb orthosis. J Rehabil Res 1992; 29:77–104.

137. Scivoletto G, Petrelli A, Lucente L, Giannantoni A, Fuoco U, D'Ambrosio F, Filippini V. One year follow up of spinal cord injury patients using a reciprocating gait orthosis: preliminary report. Spinal Cord 2000; 38:555–558.

138. Segal J, Brunnemann S. 4-aminopyridine alter gait characteristics and enhances locomotion in spinal cord injured humans. J Spinal Cord Med 1998; 21:200–204.

139. Segal J, Pathak M, Hernandez J. Safety and efficacy of 4-aminopyridine in humans with spinal cord injury: A long-term, controlled trial. Pharmacotherapy 1999; 19:713–723.

140. Barbeau H, Ladouceur M, Norman K, Pepin A, Leroux A. Walking after spinal cord injury: evaluation, treatment and functional recovery. Arch Phys Med Rehabil 1999; 80:225–235.

141. Wernig A, Muller S, Nanassy A, Cagol E. Laufband therapy based on "Rules of Spinal Locomotion" is effective in spinal cord injured persons. Europ J Neurosci 1995; 7:823–829.

142. Dietz V, Wirz M, Curt A, Colombo G. Locomotor patterns in paraplegic patients: Training effects and recovery of spinal cord function. Spinal Cord 1998; 36:380–390.

143. Dobkin B. Overview of treadmill locomotor training with partial body weight support: A neurophysiologically sound approach whose time has come for randomized clinical trials. Neurorehabil Neural Repair 1999; 13:157–165.

144. Dobkin B, Edgerton V, Fowler E. Sensory input during treadmill training alters rhythmic locomotor EMG output in subjects with complete spinal cord injury. Soc For Neurosci Abstr 1992; 18:1043.

145. Harkema S, Hurley S, Patel U, Dobkin B, Edgerton V. Human lumbosacral spinal cord interprets loading during stepping. J Neurophysiol 1997; 77:797–811.

146. Wernig A, Muller S. Laufband locomotion with body weight support improved walking in persons with severe spinal cord injuries. Paraplegia 1992; 30:229–238.

147. Barbeau H, Fung J. New experimental approaches in the treatment of spastic gait disorders. Med Sport Sci 1992; 36:234–246.

148. Dietz V, Colombo G, Jensen L. Locomotor activity in spinal man. Lancet 1994; 344:1260–1263.

149. Dobkin B, Harkema S, Requejo P, Edgerton V. Modulation of locomotor-like EMG activity in subjects with complete and incomplete chronic spinal cord injury. J Neurol Rehabil 1995; 9:183–190.

150. Wernig A, Nanassy A, Miller S. Maintenance of locomotor abilities following Laufband (treadmill) therapy in para- and tetraplegic persons: Follow-up studies. Spinal Cord 1998; 36:744–749.

151. Norman K, Pepin A, Barbeau H. Effects of drugs on walking after spinal cord injury. Spinal Cord 1998; 36:699–715.

152. Neris O, Barbeau H, Daniel O. Effects of intrathecal clonidine injection on spinal reflexes and human locomotion in incomplete paraplegic subjects. Exp Brain Res 1999; 129:433–440.

153. Hodgson J, Roy R, Dobkin B, Edgerton V. Can the mammalian spinal cord learn a motor task? Med Sci Sports Exerc 1994; 26:1491–1497.

154. Harkema S, Dobkin B, Edgerton V. Pattern generators in locomotion: Implications for recovery of walking after spinal cord injury. Top Spinal Cord Inj Rehabil 2000; 6:82–96.

155. Muir G, Steeves J. Sensorimotor stimulation to improve locomotor recovery after spinal cord injury. Trends Neurosci 1997; 20:72–77.

156. Ladouceur M, Barbeau H. Functional electrical stimulation-assisted walking for persons with incomplete spinal injuries: Changes in the kinematics and physiological cost of overground walking. Scand J Rehab Med 2000; 32:72–79.

157. Wieler M, Stein R, Ladouceur M, Whittaker M, Barbeau H, Smith A, Naaman S, Bugaresti J, Aimone E. Multicenter evaluation of electrical stimulation systems for walking. Arch Phys Med Rehabil 1999; 80:495–500.

158. Field-Fote E. Combined use of body weight support, functional electrical stimulation, and treadmill training to improve walking ability in individuals with chronic incomplete spinal cord injury. Arch Phys Med Rehabil 2001; 82:818–824.

159. Colombo G, Joerg M, Schreier R, Dietz V. Treadmill training of paraplegic patients using a robotic orthosis. J Rehab Res Dev 2000; 37:693–700.

160. Hesse S, Uhlenbrock D. A mechanized gait trainer for restoration of gait. J Rehabil Res Develop 2000; 37:701–708.

161. Waters R, Yakura J. The energy expenditure of normal and pathological gait. Crit Rev in Phys Rehabil Med 1989; 1:183–209.

162. Mattson E, Brostrom L, Karlsson J. Walking efficiency before and after long-term muscle stretch in patients with spastic paraparesis. Scand J Rehab Med 1990; 22:55–59.

163. Signorile J, Banovac K, Gomez M, Flipse D, Caruso J, Lowensteyn I. Increased muscle strength in paralyzed patients after spinal cord injury: Effect of beta-2 adrenergic agonist. Arch Phys Med Rehabil 1995; 76:55–58.

164. Apstein M, George B. Serum lipids during the first year following acute spinal cord injury. Metabolism 1998; 47:367–370.

165. Hooker S, Wells C. Effects of low and moderate intensity training in spinal cord injured persons. Med Sci Sports Exerc 1989; 21:18–22.

166. Nash MS, Jacobs PL, Mendez AJ, Goldberg RB. Circuit resistance training improves the atherogenic lipid profiles of persons with chronic paraplegia. J Spinal Cord Med 2001; 24:2–8.

167. Davis G, Plyley M, Shephard R. Gains of cardiorespiratory fitness with arm-crank training in spinally disabled men. Can J Sports Sci 1991; 16:64–72.

168. Franklin B. Aerobic exercise training programs for the upper body. Med Sci Sports Exerc 1989; 21:S141–S148.

169. Cardius D, McTaggart W, Donovan W. Energy requirements of gamefield exercises designed for wheelchair-bound persons. Arch Phys Med Rehabil 1989; 70:124–127.

170. Midha M, Schmitt J, Sclater M. Exercise effect with the wheelchair aerobic fitness training on conditioning and metabolic function in disabled persons: a pilot. Arch Phys Med Rehabil 1999; 80:258–261.

171. Teasell R, Arnold J, Krassioukov A, Delaney G. Cardiovascular consequences of loss of supraspinal control of the sympathetic nervous system after spinal cord injury. Arch Phys Med Rehabil 2000; 81:506–516.

172. Glaser R, Davis G. Wheelchair-dependent individuals. In: Franklin B, Gordon S, Timmis G, eds. Exercise in Modern Medicine. Baltimore: Williams & Wilkins, 1989:237–267.

173. Faghri P, Glaser R, Figoni S. Functional electrical stimulation leg cycle ergometer exercise: Training effects on cardiorespiratory responses of SCI subjects at rest and during submaximal exercise. Arch Phys Med Rehabil 1992; 73:1085–1093.

174. Figoni S. Perspectives on cardiovascular fitness and SCI. J Am Paraplegia Soc 1990; 13:63–71.

175. Glaser R. Physiology of functional electrical stimulation-induced exercise: Basic science perspective. J Neuro Rehab 1991; 5:49–61.

176. Kramer J. Muscle strengthening via electrical stimulation. Crit Rev Phys Rehabil Med 1989; 1:97–133.

177. Scremin A, Kurta L, Gentili A, Wiseman B, Perell K, Kunkel C, Scremin O. Increasing muscle mass in spinal cord injured persons with a functional electrical stimulation exercise program. Arch Phys Med Rehabil 2000; 80:1531–1536.

178. Murphy R, Kartkopp A, Gardiner P, Kjaer M, Beliveau L. Salbutamol effect in spinal cord injured individuals undergoing functional electrical stimulation training. Arch Phys Med Rehabil 1999; 80:1264–1267.

179. Hangartner T, Rodgers M, Glaser R, Barre P. Tibial bone density loss in spinal cord injured patients: Effects of FES exercise. J Rehabil Res 1994; 31:50–61.

180. Sipski M, Alexander C, Harris M. Long-term use of computerized bicycle ergometry for SCI subjects. Arch Phys Med Rehabil 1993; 74:238–241.

181. Bradley M. The effect of participating in a functional electrical stimulation exercse program on affect in people with spinal cord injuries. Arch Phys Med Rehabil 1994; 75:676–679.

182. Wiegner A. Can basic science help improve arm function in C5 tetraplegia? J Am Para Soc 1993; 16:75.

183. Stein R, Brucker B, Ayyar D. Motor units in incomplete spinal cord injury: Electrical acitivity, contractile properties and the effects of biofeedback. J Neurol Neurosurg Psychiat 1990; 53:880–885.

184. Klose E, Needham B, Schmidt D, Broton J, Green B. An assessment of the contribution of electromyographic biofeedback as an adjunct in the physical training of spinal cord injured persons. Arch Phys Med Rehabil 1993; 74:453–456.

185. VandenBerghe A, VanLaere M, Hellings S, Vercauteren M. Reconstruction of the upper extremity in tetraplegia: Functional assessment, surgical procedures and rehabilitation. Paraplegia 1991; 29:103–112.

186. Keith M, Lacey S. Surgical rehabilitation of the tetraplegic upper extremity. J Neurol Rehabil 1991; 5:75–87.

187. Peckham P, Keith M, Kilgore K, Grill J, Wuolle K, Thrope G, Gorman P, Hobby J, Mulcahey M, Carroll S, Hentz V, Wiegner A. Efficacy of an implanted neuroprosthesis for restoring grasp in tetraplegia: a multicenter study. Arch Phys Med Rehabil 2001; 82:1380–1388.

188. Nathan R, Ohry A. Upper limb functions regained in quadriplegia: A hybrid computerized neuromuscular stimulation system. Arch Phys Med Rehabil 1990; 71:415–421.

189. Sipski M, DeLisa J. Functional electrical stimulation in SCI rehabilitation: A review of the literature. NeuroRehabil 1991; 1:46–57.

190. Marsolais E, Kobetic R, Chizeck H, Jacobs J. Orthoses and electrical stimulation for walking in complete paraplegia. J Neurol Rehabil 1991; 5:13–22.

191. Marsolais E, Kobetic R, Miller P. Status of paraplegic FNS-assisted walking. J Am Paraplegia Soc 1994; 17:213.

192. Marsolais E, Kobetic R, Polando G, Ferguson K, Tashman S, Gaudio R, Nandurkar S, Lehneis H. The Case Western Reserve University hybrid gait orthosis. Spinal Cord Med 2000; 23:100–108.

193. Hirokawa S, Grimm M, Le T, Solomonow M, Baratta R, Shoji H, D'Ambrosia R. Energy consumption in paraplegic ambulation using the RGO and electric stimulation of the thigh muscles. Arch Phys Med Rehabil 1990; 71:687–694.

194. Stein R, Belanger M, Wheeler G, Weiler M, Popovic D, Prochazka A, Davis L. Electrical systems for improving locomotion after incomplete spinal cord injury. Arch Phys Med Rehabil 1993; 74:954–959.

195. Chaplin E, Winchester P, Habasevich R. FNS synthesized gait restoration following SCI. J Neurol Rehabil 1994; 8:84(abstr).

196. Klose K, Jacobs P, Broton J, Guest R, Needham-Shropshire B, Lebwohl N, Nash M, Green B. Evaluation of a training program for persons with SCI paraplegia using the Parastep®1 ambulation system: Part 1. Ambulation performance and anthropometric measures. Arch Phys Med Rehabil 1997; 78:789–793.

197. Jacobs P, Nash M, Klose K, Guest R, Needham-Shropshire B, Green B. Evaluation of a training program for persons with SCI paraplegia using the Parastep®1 ambulation system: Part 2. Effects of physiological responses to peak arm ergometry. Arch Phys Med Rehabil 1997; 78:794–798.

198. Guest R, Klose K, Needham-Shropshire B, Jacobs

P. Evaluation of training program for persons with SCI paraplegia using the Parastep®1 ambulation system: Part 4. Effect on physical self-concept and depression. Arch Phys Med Rehabil 1997; 78:804–807.

199. Brindley G, Rushton D. Long term follow-up of patients with sacral anterior root stimulator implants. Paraplegia 1990; 28:469–475.

200. Creasey G, Grill J, Korsten J, Betz R, Anderson R, Walter J. An implantable neuroprosthesis for restoring bladder and bowel control to patients with spinal cord injuries: A multicenter trial. Arch Phys Med Rehabil 2001; 82:1512–1519.

201. Creasey G, Dahlberg J. Economic consequences of an implanted neuroprosthesis for bladder and bowel management. Arch Phys Med Rehabil 2001; 82: 1520–1525.

202. Lin V, Nino-Murcia M, Frost F, Wolfe V, Hsiao I, Perkash I. Functional magnetic stimulation of the colon in persons with spinal cord injury. Arch Phys Med Rehabil 2001; 82:167–173.

203. Lin V, Wolfe V, Perkash I. Micturition by functional magnetic stimulation. J Spinal Cord Med 1997; 20: 218–226.

204. Kuhn R. Functional capacity of the isolated human spinal cord. Brain 1950; 73:1–51.

205. Maynard F, Karunas R, Waring W. Epidemiology of spasticity following traumatic spinal cord injury. Arch Phys Med Rehabil 1990; 71:566–570.

206. Riddoch G. The reflex functions of the completely divided spinal cord in man, compared with those associated with less severe lesions. Brain 1917; 40: 264–402.

207. Little J, Micklesen P, Umlauf R, Britell C. Lower extremity manifestations of spasticity in chronic spinal cord injury. Am J Phys Med Rehabil 1989; 68:32–36.

208. Dimitrijevic M. Residual motor functions in spinal cord injury. In: Waxman S, ed. Functional Recovery in Neurological Disease. Vol. 47. New York: Raven Press, 1988:139–155.

209. Bohannon R. Tilt table standing for reducing spasticity after spinal cord injury. Arch Phys Med Rehabil 1993; 74:1121–1122.

210. Skold C. Spasticity in spinal cord injury: Self- and clinically rated intrinsic fluctuations and intervention-induced changes. Arch Phys Med Rehabil 2000; 81:144–149.

211. Harvey L, Batty J, Crosbie J, Poulter S, Herbert R. A randomized trial assessing the effects of 4 weeks of daily stretching on ankle mobility in patients with spinal cord injuries. Arch Phys Med Rehabil 2000; 81:1340–1347.

212. Donovan W, Carter R, Rossi C, Wilkerson M. Clonidine effect on spasticity: A clinical trial. Arch Phys Med Rehabil 1988; 69:193–194.

213. Nance P, Bugaresti J, Shellenberger K, Sheremata W, Martinez-Arizala A. Efficacy and safety of tizanidine in the treatment of spasticity in patients with spinal cord injury. Neurology 1994; 44(Suppl 9): S44–S52.

214. Wainberg M, Barbeau H, Gauthier S. Quantitative assessment of the effect of cyproheptadine on spastic paretic gait: A preliminary study. J Neurol 1986; 233:311–314.

215. Waters R, Adkins R, Sie L, Cressy J. Postrehabilitation outcomes after spinal cord injury caused by firearms and motor vehicle crash among ethnically diverse groups. Arch Phys Med Rehabil 1998; 79: 1237–1243.

216. Bauman W, Spungen A. Carbohydrate and lipid metabolism in chronic spinal cord injury. J Spinal Cord Med 2001; 24:266–277.

217. Ditunno J, Formal C. Chronic spinal cord injury. N Engl J Med 1994; 330:550–556.

218. Gerhart K, Bergstrom E, Charlifue S, Menter R, Whiteneck G. Long-term spinal cord injury: Functional changes over time. Arch Phys Med Rehabil 1993; 74:1030–1034.

219. Samsa G, Patrick C, Feussner J. Long-term survival of veterans with traumatic spinal cord injury. Arch Neurol 1993; 50:909–914.

220. White M, Rintala D, Hart K, Fuhrer M. Sexual activities, concerns and interests of men with SCI. Am J Phys Med Rehabil 1992; 71:225–231.

221. White M, Rintala D, Hart K, Fuhrer M. Sexual activities, concerns and interests of women with SCI living in the community. Am J Phys Med Rehabil 1993; 72:372–378.

222. Black K, Sipski M, Strauss S. Sexual satisfaction and sexual drive in spinal cord injured women. J Spinal Cord Med 1998; 21:240–244.

223. Yarkony G. Enhancement of sexual function and fertility in spinal cord injured males. Am J PMR 1990; 69:81–87.

224. Giuliano F, Hulding C, El Masry W. Randomized trial of sildenafil for the treatment of erectile dysfunction in spinal cord injury. Ann Neurol 1999; 46: 15–21.

225. Collins K, Hackler R. Complications of penile prostheses in the spinal cord injury population. J Urol 1988; 140:984–985.

226. Linsenmeyer T, Perkash I. Infertility in men with SCI. Arch Phys Med Rehabil 1991; 72:747–754.

227. Peckham P, Creasey G. Neural prostheses: Clinical applications of functional electrical stimulation in SCI. Paraplegia 1992; 30:96–101.

228. Sipski M. Sexual response in women with spinal cord injury. J Spinal Cord Med 2001; 24:155–158.

229. Sipski M, Alexander C, Rosen R. Sexual arousal and orgasm in women: Effects of spinal cord injury. Ann Neurol 2001; 49:35–44.

230. Krause J. Employment after spinal cord injury. Arch Phys Med Rehabil 1992; 73:163–169.

231. Krause J, Kewman D, DeVivo M, Maynard F, Coker J, Roach M, Ducharme S. employment after spinal cord injury: An analysis of cases from the Model Spinal Cord Injury Systems. Arch Phys Med Rehabil 1999; 80:1492–1500.

232. Krause J, Sternberg M, Maides J, Lottes S. Employment after spinal cord injury: Differences related to geographic region, gender, and race. Arch Phys Med Rehabil 1998; 79:615–624.

233. Livneh H, Antonak R. Psychosocial reactions to disability: A review and critique of the literature. Crit Rev Phys Rehabil Med 1994; 6:1–100.

234. Fuhrer M, Rintala D, Hart K, Clearman R, Young M. Relationship of life satisfaction to impairment, disability, and handicap among persons with SCI living in the community. Arch Phys Med Rehabil 1992; 73:552–557.

235. Dowler R, Richards J, Putzke J, Gordon W, Tate D.

Impact of demographic and medical factors on satisfaction with life after spinal cord injury. J Spinal Cord Med 2001; 24:87–91.

236. Buckelew S, Baumstark K, Frank R, Hewitt J. Adjustment after SCI. Rehabil Psychol 1990; 35:101–109.

237. Charlifue S, Gerhart K. Behavioral and demographic predictors of suicide after traumatic SCI. Arch Phys Med Rehabil 1991; 72:488–492.

238. Hartkopp A, Bronnum-Hansen H, Seidenschnur A-M, BieringSorensen F. Suicide in a spinal cord injured population: Its relation to functional status. Arch Phys Med Rehabil 1998; 79:1356–1361.

239. Tate D, Forchheimer M, Maynard F, Dijkers M. Predicting depression and psychological distress in persons with spinal cord injury based on indicators of handicap. Am J Phys Med Rehabil 1994; 73:175–183.

240. Boyer B, Knolls M, Kafkalas C, Tollen L. Prevalence of posttraumatic stress disorder in patients with pediatric spinal cord injury: Relationship to functional independence. Top Spinal Cord Inj Rehabil 2000; 6(suppl):125–133.

241. Solomon S, Gerrity E, Muff A. Efficacy of treatments for posttraumatic stress disorder. JAMA 1992; 268:633–638.

242. Krause J, Kjorsvig J. Mortality after SCI: A four-year prospective study. Arch Phys Med Rehabil 1992; 73:558–63.

243. Heinemann A, Doll M, Armstrong M, Schnoll S, Yarkony G. Substance use and receipt of treatment by persons with long-term SCI. Arch Phys Med Rehabil 1991; 72:482–87.

244. Chen D, Apple D, Hudson L, Bode R. Medical complications during acute rehabilitation following spinal cord injury-current experience of the Model Systems. Arch Phys Med Rehabil 1999; 80:1397–1401.

Chapter 11

Traumatic Brain Injury

Patients with serious traumatic brain injury (TBI) test the mettle of clinicians, families, and community health, educational, social, and vocational providers. The rehabilitation team must engage the ebb and flow of a patient's cognition, motivation, and behavior within the undertow of myriad interacting impairments. The disabilities and residual abilities that follow a moderate to severe TBI differ quite a bit across patients, perhaps more than for any other acute neurologic disease. Early gains evolve from coma followed by confusion and agitation, before more appropriate behaviors can be trained. Even then, poor attention, limited recall, and lack of insight challenge the therapeutic strategies of the rehabilitation team. Postinjury gains from inpairments arise from the intrinsic and extrinsic mechanisms of restitution, substitution, and compensation discussed in Chapter 2.

This chapter deals primarily with patients who suffer from a moderate to severe closed head injury (CHI). It touches upon issues related to mild TBI and penetrating head trauma as well. Many of the interventions described are also appropriate for managing the moderate to severe cognitive and behavioral sequelae found in 50% of 1-year survivors of a cardiac arrest and in survivors of a subarachnoid hemorrhage associated with diffuse vasospasm or subfrontal ischemia.[1,2] Unfortunately, good clinical trials of defined approaches to manage the sequela of TBI are few in number.[3] Clini-

497

cians need to develop and test rehabilitative interventions for the cognitive, behavioral, and psychosocial burdens carried by patients.

EPIDEMIOLOGY

For 1992 to 1995, the U.S. National Hospital Survey of the Centers for Disease Control and Prevention estimated an annual rate of 394 per 100,000 people visiting emergency rooms for evaluation of TBI.[4] The rates of hospitalization declined by 50% between 1980 and 1995, from about 200 to 100 per 100,000 people per year. Mild TBI rates of hospitalization declined by 60%, especially for youngsters, suggesting more confidence in the results of brain imaging and outpatient care. Of course, not being hospitalized does not imply that a person's TBI leaves no residual cognitive impairment. Rates of hospitalization per 100,000 Americans are 51 for mild TBI, 21 for moderate TBI, and 19 for severe TBI. In Great Britain, between 200 and 300 persons per 100,000 population are hospitalized each year with TBI.[5]

Of the over 300,000 Americans who receive hospital treatment for TBI yearly out of approximately 1 million people with a TBI, 52,000 die, and up to 90,000 have long-term impairments and disabilities.[4] Traumatic brain injury-associated rates of death declined from 25 per 100,000 in 1980 to 19 per 100,000 in 1995, in part from preventative safety measures in cars and the use of helmets in bicyclers and motor bikers. The unadjusted rate for deaths from TBI in the elderly secondary to falls is approximately 31 per 100,000 people over 80 years old, which may reflect greater disability as a predisposing cause. Mortality for nonmilitary gunshot wounds to the brain that cause coma at onset runs up to 90%.[6] Traumatic brain injury also causes at least 5000 new

Table 11–1. **Causes of Traumatic Brain Injury with Hospitalization**

Cause	Percentage (%)
Vehicular accidents	50
Falls	20
Assaults and violence	20
Sports and recreation	10

Table 11–2. **Estimated Need for Rehabilitation Services After Traumatic Brain Injury**

Severity	Incidence per Million Population	Residual Disability (%)
Mild	1360	10
Moderate	158	67
Severe	71	100

Source: Adapted from Sorenson and Kraus, 1991.[7]

cases of epilepsy and 2000 cases of persistent vegetative state (PVS) in the United States yearly.

Penetrating head injuries (PHI) from bullet wounds account for 10% of all brain injuries and CHI for 90%. Significant factors causing TBI include motor vehicle accidents, lower socioeconomic class, and alcohol or drug abuse. Specific causes are listed in Table 11–1. Approximately 25% of TBI in children younger than 2 years old is caused by nonaccidental trauma, mostly from the shaken impact syndrome.

From 2.5 to 6 million Americans currently live with TBI-induced disabilities.[3] The peak incidences for TBI occur in males aged 16 to 25 years and in people over 65 years old.[7] The ratio of males-to-females is 8:1. These young and old disabled groups pose quite different challenges for rehabilitation efforts to reintegrate patients into the community. Residual disability in newly hospitalized persons who survive a TBI is likely to require inpatient or outpatient rehabilitation in approximately 313 per million persons in a community each year (Table 11–2).[7]

Economic Impact

The economic impact of TBI is stunning. The annual cost of acute care and rehabilitation in the United States is estimated at $10 billion.[3] Lifetime care for a person with severe TBI ranges from $600,000 to $1.9 million, not including the burden of lost income for the caregiving family and the injured person.

In 1983 dollars, a Maryland study found that the mean 1-year charge for a severe head-injured patient 16–45 years old was $106,000 with 18% going to rehabilitation care.[8] Serious to moderate TBI charges were approximately $57,000. Traumatic brain injury accounted for 19% of all hospital trauma discharges, but it contributed 26% to total charges. Based on a national study of estimated charges for all head-injured persons admitted to a hospital in 1 year,[9] the average direct and indirect lifetime cost in 1991 dollars for survivors was $111,600, whereas those with fatal outcomes cost $454,700.[10] The total national cost was $48.25 billion; $31.7 billion supported the survivors. Inpatient rehabilitation accounted for $1.15 billion, nursing home care for $350 million, home modifications for $62 million, and vocational rehabilitation for $4 million. By the year 2002, these costs likely increased by 30%.

Prevention

Rehabilitationists can appreciate the potential for preventing TBI. For example, the use of helmets has reduced deaths caused by motorcycle accidents by 18%, has lowered acute care costs by 40%, and has lessened disability.[11,12] National efforts could mandate seat belts, air bags, and other highway safety measures, require sturdy helmets for bicyclists and skaters, regulate guns, promote programs to decrease alcohol and drug abuse, and continue to identify and manage predisposing causes for falls in the elderly. For some injuries, such as motorcycle-related TBI, 60% or more of costs are borne by public funding.[13] Prevention, then, can have an impact on city, county, state, and federal shares of the economic burden of brain injury. A balance must be found between the personal freedom of individuals to choose whether or not to wear protective gear and the public responsibility of individuals and lawmakers.

PATHOPHYSIOLOGY

In patients with TBI, both immediate and delayed focal and diffuse injuries can unfold from a spectrum of interrelated pathophysiologic processes (Table 11–3). Expectations for neurorestoration are guided by the location and combination of these lesions, the severity of clinical consequences, and clinicopathologic changes over time after onset of TBI. Thus, it is valuable to review the spectrum of pathologies in some detail.

Table 11–3. **Primary and Secondary Pathophysiologic Consequences of Traumatic Brain Injury**

FOCAL INJURY
Contusion
Orbitofrontal, anterior temporal, basal ganglia
Edema
Hematoma
Intracerebral, subdural, epidural
Hygroma

DIFFUSE AXONAL INJURY
Petechial hemorrhages; edema; axotomy
Subcortical white matter, corpus callosum, dorsal brainstem
Cytoskeletal damage
Impaired axonal transport
Delayed demyelination
Retrograde neuronal death

HYPOXIC-ISCHEMIC INJURY
Systemic anoxia, hypotension
Laminar cortical necrosis
Arterial borderzone
Vulnerable neurons, e.g., hippocampus, basal ganglia
Microvascular injury
Loss of cerebrovascular autoregulation
Compression
Mass-induced larger arterial and venous occlusion
Vasospasm

INCREASED INTRACRANIAL PRESSURE
Focal and diffuse mass effect
Hyperemia
Obstructive hydrocephalus
Herniation

SECONDARY INJURY
Excitotoxin release, e.g., glutamate
Lactic acidosis
Arachidonic cascade and free radicals
Cytokines
Inflammatory cells
Apoptosis

In CHI, acceleration and deceleration of the brain relative to the skull causes compressive and tensile strains and displacements. Tensile forces act opposite to compressive forces. Both are translational linear forces generated especially when the moving body and head strike a solid object. Rotational or shearing forces occur parallel to the surface of the brain. If great enough, they lead to diffuse axonal injury and coma. A blow to the side of the head or chin, not uncommon in boxers, causes a rotational injury. Forces are greater when the neck muscles are limp compared to when they are tensed. A contrecoup injury results when the head accelerates before impact, causing the brain to lag toward the trailing surface. This lag squeezes away cerebrospinal fluid (CSF) and causes shearing where the CSF is the thinnest cushion, opposite to the coup injury.

The damage from a PHI depends especially upon the amount of energy imparted to the brain.[14] High-velocity bullets cause larger cavitations, more diffuse injuries, and higher mortality than low-velocity bullets. Missile fragments, such as shrapnel, tend to produce focal injuries.

A cascade of cellular events can follow either CHI or PHI, including intracellular edema, calcium and other ionic fluxes, glutamate neurotoxicity, glial cell compromise, lipid peroxidation, cytokine production,[15] failure of protein synthesis, neurofilament degradation,[16] and other effects of early and delayed ischemia and mechanical injury.[17] Managing increased intracranial pressure with pressure monitors and drug and surgical interventions has led to improved outcomes. Compared to acute interventions for ischemic stroke, which must be put into place within 6 hours of onset or, better, within 3 hours of onset, the cascade of biologic events that follow TBI probably offers a longer window of opportunity. Some drug interventions being developed for acute TBI may prolong the therapeutic window. The period of compromise of biologic plasticity may also have a longer duration after TBI compared to stroke. Certain types of pathology have particular consequences for rehabilitation care.

Diffuse Axonal Injury

Acceleration and rotational forces, which often occur in a motor vehicle accident, produce diffuse axonal injury (DAI). This disorder is characterized by swelling and retraction of the damaged ends of axons over days, followed by microglial infiltration and axonal degeneration over subsequent weeks. Axonal changes are related to axolemmal permeability, perturbations of the cytoskeleton with primary and secondary changes in the composition and alignment of neurofilaments, and other metabolic disturbances.[18] This micropathology leads to impaired axonal transport, continued axonal swelling, and, over a course that can take more than 12 hours, to disconnection of axons from their soma.[19] Diffuse axonal injury is often accompanied by focal and diffuse edema and petechial hemorrhages with secondary loss of vascular autoregulation and increased intracranial pressure. Thus, complex subsets of pathobiology follow trauma-induced axonal injury. Because this evolves over the time, interventions to reverse axonal injury may be possible.[20]

More severe trauma in a primate TBI model produces denser DAI in deeper and more diffuse regions of the cerebrum and focal damage in the corpus callosum and dorsolateral brain stem near the superior cerebellar peduncles. These lesions correlate with longer duration of coma and less clinical recovery.[20] Diffuse axonal injury in patients tends to be a midline process with the rostral upper brain stem and corpus callosum involved in 90% of serious cases. The callosal lesion is often just 5 mm wide, but several centimeters long rostrocaudally. The patient whose MRI scan is shown in Figure 11–1 suffered this distribution of lesions and had permanent cognitive impairments.

Mortality, the duration of unconsciousness, the degree of posttraumatic amnesia (PTA), and the persistence of confusion appear to correlate best, although not linearly, with the severity of DAI. A poor outcome for functional recovery is especially associated with rostral brain stem lesions. The dorsal pons and midbrain are the repositories for serotonergic, cholinergic, and noradrenergic neurons (see Chapter 1). Damage to these projection systems can have widespread consequences for thalamocortical and frontal lobe function. For example, cholinergic neurons act upon the reticular nucleus of the thalamus, which gates the inputs and outputs from the dorsal thalamic nuclei and prefrontal cortex.[21] Dysfunction in this area may account for some of the attentional and other cognitive sequelae of

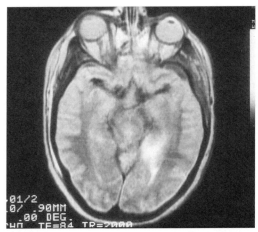

Figure 11–1. T$_2$-weighted magnetic resonance imaging scan at the level of the pons reveals hyperintensity of the dorsal pons, vermis of the cerebellum, and left medial temporal lobe (to the right of the brain stem) in a 40-year-old who survived a closed head injury in a motor vehicle accident. The subcortical white matter had multiple petechial hemorrhages. The patient emerged from a Glasgow Coma Scale score of 6, but 3 years later, had permanent, debilitating cognitive and motor impairments.

DAI. Pharmacologic replacement of neuromodulators may benefit some patients.

Diffuse axonal injury is of special interest, because it results in diffuse deafferentation of target sites. Positron emission tomography often reveals global cerebral hypometabolism soon after severe TBI. Over time, partial deafferentation of target neurons may lead to denervation hypersensitivity and to the ingrowth of spared axonal inputs (Chapter 2). Considerable focal DAI leads to a more concentrated amount of target denervation, to less reinnervation by axons of the same pathway, and to more input from neighboring, but functionally different axons. Adaptive or maladaptive plasticity may result. Potential rehabilitative biologic interventions for DAI include strategies that remyelinate axons, block molecules that inhibit the axonal growth cone, and use trophic factors to increase axonal extension to targets (see Chapter 2).

Hypoxic-Ischemic Injury

Other pathologic processes contribute to the effects of severe TBI. Systemic hypoxia and hypotension at onset of TBI add to the insult up to the point of causing cortical laminar necrosis or damaging especially vulnerable neuronal populations, such as those of the hippocampus, cerebellum, and basal ganglia. Hypoxic-ischemic injury decreases cerebral blood flow and increases cortical hyperemia and intracranial pressure. These sequelae generally correlate with poorer cognitive and overall outcomes.[22,23] Both hypoxic-ischemic injury and high intracranial pressure that cannot be medically and surgically managed lead to the greater likelihood of morbidity, a vegetative state, and mortality. For example, the National Traumatic Data Bank found that intracranial pressure above 30 mm Hg was associated with a poor outcome regardless of the initial score on the *Glasgow Coma Scale* (GCS) (see Table 7–3). Hypoxia on admission led to a 20% increase in mortality and the vegetative state. Hypoperfusion when the systolic blood pressure fell to less than 90 mm Hg was associated with a 30% increase in these negative outcomes.[24]

Focal Injury

Direct forces at the point of impact can produce focal coup and remote contracoup hematomas and contusions. Other focal contusions commonly occur within the anteroinferior temporal lobes and the orbitofrontal cortex, sites close to the bony skull, as shown in the CT scan in Figure 11–2. Damage and dis-

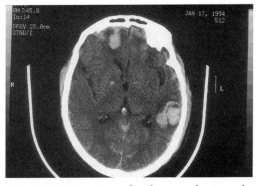

Figure 11–2. Computerized axial tomography scan at the level of the internal capsule and thalamus of a 70-year-old woman who was knocked to the floor by a bookcase that fell upon her during the 1994 California Northridge earthquake. Her initial Glasgow Coma Scale score was 8. Right frontal, right mesial globus pallidus, and left temporal lobe hematomas are shown. On higher cuts, a left subdural hematoma and cerebral edema were evident. She regained full motor function, but was left with profound impairments in memory and behavior.

ruption of connections to and from these sites account for impairments in executive functions, drives, mutimodal processing of information, mood, and memory. Hemorrhages develop in the distribution of sheared penetrating arteries, such as the lenticulostriates to the basal ganglia. Focal ischemia follows occlusion of small vessels by edema and of mid-sized posterior and anterior cerebral arteries if herniation ensues.

A PHI also tends to cause focal tissue destruction, hematoma, and edema. Vietnam War veterans with penetrating wounds, mostly from shrapnel, were followed in the Vietnam Head Injury Study. They were found to have lower global cognitive scores on the Wechsler Adult Intelligence Scale IQ test in relationship to greater lossses of brain volume.[25] Specific cognitive impairments developed more often with localized structural lesions. The study revealed the limitations of anatomic-functional correlations, however. Preinjury intelligence or education played a larger role than total volume loss or lesion location in predicting the persistence of cognitive deficits.

Neuroimaging

Neuroimaging with CT and MRI correlate moderately with the pathologies and outcomes of TBI. Computerized tomography may reveal transient hemorrhagic petechial foci, but over 80% of DAI lesions include microscopic blood not visible on scans. After mild to moderate TBI, 60% of patients have CT scan abnormalities; MRI reveals approximately twice the number of lesions. Focal injuries with and without blood in typical regions for DAI are better seen by MRI. Diffuse axonal injury may be better appreciated by diffusion-weighted MRI, but few studies have been reported. Perfusion-weighted MRI has revealed reduced blood volume in regions of contusions and in normal-appearing brains soon after TBI. The hemodynamic impairment was associated with poorer outcomes.[26] Proton magnetic resonance spectroscopy carried out within 2 weeks of TBI reveals neuroaxonal loss by a fall in N-acetylaspartate when conventional imaging appears normal. This evidence of injury in frontal white matter was associated with greater disability in adults[27] and in children.[28]

Visible hemorrhages in the central white matter and at gray-white junctions, along with white matter edema, best define DAI and greatly increase the risk for PVS and mortality. On the *Glasgow Outcome Scale* (GOS) (see Table 7–21), good recovery occurs more often with visible focal lesions such as a contusion than after DAI. In patients referred for inpatient rehabilitation after TBI, the GOS at 6 and 12 months correlates significantly with the duration of posttraumatic amnesia in patients with DAI, but does not correlate with a focal brain injury.[29] Scores on neuropsychologic tests of memory, learning, and visuomotor speed were higher in patients with diffuse cerebral edema, although gains over the next 6 months were less than for those with DAI. Deeper parenchymal lesions were associated with greater severity and duration of impaired consciousness; outcome at 6 months on the GOS was better with more superficial lesions.[30] Thus, the wider the distribution of axonal disconnections visible on imaging, the worse the prognosis.

In patients with a GCS of 13 to 15, the CT finding of an intracerebral contusion or hematoma alters the 6-month outcome from that found after mild CHI to a picture more like the consequences of a moderate TBI.[31] Indeed, approximately 30% of patients with an initial, so-called mild TBI have abnormalities on CT scan and only 45% of these patients have a good recovery by the GOS.[32] Cortical lesions are especially likely to correlate with specific neuropsychologic impairments, but focal cortical dysfunction is usually part of a heterogeneous group of lesions and may contribute only modestly to the clinical picture.[33] Aside from clinicopathologic relationships for focal injuries, anatomic imaging has not correlated tightly with neuropsychologic performance.[34] This lack of correlation reflects the limitations of anatomic imaging and the distributed representations for common TBI impairments, such as memory, executive functions, and attention.

Imaging during the period of inpatient and outpatient rehabilitation can uncover treatable structural causes of deterioration or of failure to improve in attention and cognition. For example, hydrocephalus, a cerebral hygroma, or an abcess may limit or reverse progress. Late imaging can also yield prognostic indicators associated with underlying pathology. For example, poor cognition at 1 year correlates with a wider third ventricle 3 months after severe

TBI, suggesting the impact of diencephalic atrophy associated with DAI and hypoxia.[35] Atrophy of the corpus callosum has been associated with DAI after severe TBI and with hemispheric disconnection syndromes.[36] Over the first few months after a TBI, enlarging ventricles from loss of subcortical white matter and an increase in the volume of the frontal horns of the lateral ventricles and the third ventricle may predict a poorer response to rehabilitation.[37] After mild to moderate TBI, focal atrophy in the frontal lobes found within 3 months and frontotemporal atrophy at 6 to 12 months were associated with poorer outcomes.[38] Focal areas of encephalomalacia associated with persisting motor and cognitive impairments tends to anticipate fewer functional gains related to those impairments.

Functional neuroimaging at rest with PET and with activation paradigms by PET or fMRI offer insights into cerebral structure and function after TBI. As reviewed in Chapter 3, functional neuroimaging can reveal the neuropsychologic effects of TBI in the absence of contusions by revealing patterns of cortical hypometabolism[39] and unusual patterns of activation related to the effort needed to accomplish a task that requires working memory,[40] an alternating strategy,[41] or verbal recall.[42] Cerebral activation studies carry great promise for testing cognitive and drug interventions during fMRI or PET. Functional imaging can serve as a physiologic marker for how well the interventions engage or reorganize networks for specific cognitive tasks.

NEUROMEDICAL COMPLICATIONS

Many neurologic, general medical, and orthopedic derangements can complicate and interfere with the early and late rehabilitation of patients after a moderate to severe head injury. Traumatic brain injury is often accompanied by injuries to bone, soft tissues, viscera, and to the spinal cord and peripheral nerves. Deep vein thrombosis has been detected by serial testing in over 50% of patients after major TBI within 3 weeks of onset.[43] This incidence rose to over 75% with associated femoral or tibial fractures. In a study of 180 TBI patients admitted for rehabilitation, 56% had neurologic complications, 50% developed gastrointestinal complications, 45% had urinary complications, 34% had respiratory disorders, and 21% had dermatologic disorders.[44] Potential complications are outlined in Table 11–4 to remind clinicians to be vigilant with patients who often cannot express their symptoms. We review the incidence and management of several of the more vexing problems that are unique to serious TBI. Pressure sores, bowel and bladder function, spasticity, contractures, and other complications are reviewed in Chapter 8.

Annual rehospitalization rates for the first 3 years after TBI are 20% for patients in the Model Systems Traumatic Brain Injury Program.[45] Seizures and psychiatric disorders each rose to 15% of causes for years 2 and 3. Orthopedic surgery accounted for 44% in year 1 and 24% in years 2 and 3. Infections accounted for 12% of admissions.

Nutrition

Multiple interacting factors account for indices of malnutrition in about 60% of patients with TBI who are transferred to a rehabilitation unit.[46] Acute trauma increases energy expenditure by an average of 40%. The highest metabolic energy expenditures and urinary nitrogen excretions affect patients with the lowest GCS, especially in the first several weeks after TBI.[47] Decerebration, spasms, seizures, agitation, and fever add to the hypermetabolic state. Mechanisms of hypercatabolism include acute-phase responses that also release cytokines, as well as autonomic hyperactivity and increases in blood catecholamines, glucagon, and cortisol. Renal and liver failure exacerbate protein loss. The likelihood of malnutrition increases when feedings are limited by gastric hypomotility, ileus, diarrhea, emesis, aspiration pneumonia, and a tracheal fistula. Swallowing disorders occur in the majority of patients who have a low GCS or tracheostomy.[48] Aphagia accompanies coma and poor attention, jaw and dental injuries, and central and peripheral causes of bulbar dysfunction, such as a vocal cord paralysis. Later, during rehabilitation, cognitive and behavioral function and side effects of medications affect the safety and quantity of oral intake and absorption. Better nutrition may improve functional outcomes.[47]

Several studies suggest that early parenteral hyperalimentation is better than nasogastric

Table 11–4. Potential Systemic Complications of Traumatic Brain Injury

SKIN

Decubitus ulcers	Infections
Acne, seborrhea, folliculitis	Edema
Sweating disorders	Cosmetic deformity
Drug reactions	

EYE

Corneal ulcer secondary to lid paralysis
Infection
Orbital fracture with diplopia
Visual acuity loss, blindness

EAR

Infection	Otorrhea	Hearing deficit

NOSE

Trauma with obstruction	Infection	Anosmia

MOUTH

Wired jaw after fracture
Bruxism
Loss of teeth
Oral infections—candidiasis
Dysphagia from oromotor impairment

LARYNX

Vocal cord trauma with dysphonia or aspiration

TRACHEA

With intubation—stenosis, erosion, fistula, excess
  secretions
Tracheostomy dependence
Infection

LUNGS

Emboli
Pneumonia—methicillin resistent staph aureus
Atelectasis
Flail chest and lung trauma
Restrictive defects
Recurrent pneumothorax
Broncho-pleural-cutaneous fistula
Adult respiratory distress syndrome
Pulmonary edema

GASTROINTESTINAL

Bowel ischemia
Gastroparesis
Reflux esophagitis
Peptic ulcer
Hepatitis, elevated liver function tests
Drug reactions
Diarrhea
Infection—Clostridia difficile
Impaction
Incontinence
Complications of feeding tubes

Malnutrition
Inadequate caloric intake for metabolic state
Bulimia and hyperphagia
Pancreatitis

CARDIAC

Trauma, pericardial effusion
Heart failure
Arrhythmias

PERIPHERAL VASCULAR SYSTEM

Thrombophlebitis
Hypotension
Hypertension
Limb ischemia

GENITOURINARY SYSTEM

Infection
Neurogenic bladder
Catheter complication
Trauma of bladder or kidney
Incontinence
Sexual dysfunction

FEMALE REPRODUCTIVE SYSTEM

Infection
Amenorrhea and oligomenorrhea
Organ trauma

METABOLIC-ENDOCRINE SYSTEM

Hypothalamic-pituitary failure
Inappropriate antidiuretic hormone syndrome

Continued on following page

Table 11–4.— continued

Salt-wasting
Hypothyroidism
Uremia
Electrolyte-fluid disorders
Malignant hyperthermia
Defective thermoregulation, central fever

BLOOD

Anemia of chronic disease
Clotting defect
Sepsis

MUSCULOSKELETAL SYSTEM

Weakness from medication or disuse atrophy
Contracture
Heterotopic ossification
Osteomyelitis
Fractures
Soft-tissue injury with pain
Osteoporosis

CENTRAL NERVOUS SYSTEM

Encephalopathy
  Drug reaction
  Metabolic disorder
  Systemic infection

Primary brain complications
  Recurrent or developing hematoma or hygroma

Infection, meningitis, ventriculitis from a shunt
Seizures
Communicating or noncommunicating
  hydrocephalus
Cerebrospinal otorrhea, rhinorrhea
Traumatic aneurysm or fistula
Spasticity
Occult spinal cord injury

Pain syndromes
  Complex regional pain syndrome
  Headache
    Cervical musculoligamentous source
    Migraine, hemiplegic migraine
  Radiculopathy
  Cutaneous neuroma
Decerebration with autonomic "storm"
Movement disorder

Cranial neuropathy
  Vertigo, dysarthria, dysphagia, drooling,
    diplopia, hearing loss, delayed optic neuropathy

PERIPHERAL NERVOUS SYSTEM

Neuropathy
  Drug reaction
  Metabolic
  Local injury (peroneal, sciatic, ulnar nerves)
  Compartment compression syndrome
Brachial or lumbar plexopathy

---

feeding for supplying calories, vitamins, and minerals including zinc. Regardless of the route, the Quetelet Index of weight (in Kg) over height (in M^2) should be brought into the range of 20–25. The serum albumin should be kept well within the normal range and attention should be given to providing a protein calorie contribution of 20% in the face of persistent hypercatabolism. Further general management issues are discussed in Chapter 8.

Hypothalamic-Pituitary Dysfunction

Severe TBI may raise serum catecholamines, aldosterone, and cortisol, lower thyroid hormone release, produce diabetes insipidus or inappropriate secretion of antidiuretic hormone, and cause hypofunctioning of any component of the hypothalamic-pituitary axis caused by direct injury. The incidence varies from approximately 4% in patients presenting with symptoms during rehabilitation to 60% in an autopsy series.[44] Just how common occult and late endocrinopathies may be is uncertain. A self-limited salt-wasting syndrome is one of the most frequent complications of TBI. The hyponatremia often persists at the time of admission for rehabilitation, especially in patients who required a craniotomy. Salt wasting must be managed with salt tablets, 4–8 grams daily, and fludrocortisone, 0.1–0.2 mg twice a day, then tapered over a week to see if the syndrome has abated. Hypothyroidism can contibute to hyponatremia.

Pain

Head trauma is commonly associated with headache, perhaps most often after minor injuries. Cervical musculoligamentous and myofascial sources are common causes of pain and must be distinguished from intracranial causes. During rehabilitation of less responsive and cognitively impaired or aphasic patients, pain caused by undetected musculoskeletal and visceral injuries and heterotopic ossification augments agitation and limits participation. For children, total body bone scans may detect a source of skeletal pain.[49] Management is covered in Chapter 8.

Seizures

Traumatic brain injury accounts for approximately 4% of causes of focal epilepsy and is the most common cause of epilepsy in young people 15–25 years old. Posttraumatic epilepsy may affect up to 30% of patients with severe TBI and 5%–10% with a moderate injury. Traumatic brain injury was the primary risk factor for refractory epilepsy in 10% of patients at the University of California, Los Angeles who had an anterior temporal lobectomy.[50] Half of these patients had hippocampal sclerosis. Despite the belief that the mesial temporal lobes are not usually directly injured by trauma, another series also found that 35% of refractory epileptic patients had hippocampal sclerosis after a TBI.[51] At onset of TBI, all of the affected patients had loss of consciousness for more than 30 minutes or coma for 1 week.

The incidence of seizures within the first week and later varies with the population reported. After PHI, mostly due to shrapnel, 53% of veterans had a seizure and one-half of them had ongoing epilepsy 15 years after the head injury.[52] In 18%, the first seizure happened more than 5 years after the PHI. Larger total brain volume loss detected by CT, a hematoma, retained metal fragments, aphasia, hemiparesis, and an organic mental disorder each increased the likelihood of a seizure. These risk factors, however, did not necessarily lead to epilepsy. Phenytoin therapy for the first year after PHI had no prophylactic effect on the incidence of seizures.

In a population study of over 2700 patients with mostly CHI, 2% had a seizure in the first 2 weeks after injury. Patients with brain contusions, hematomas, or 24 hours of unconsciousness or amnesia had a 7% 1-year and 11.5% 5-year risk of seizures.[53] Within the first 2 weeks in these severe cases, children under age 15 had a rate of 30%, compared to 10% in adults. After a moderate injury defined as a skull fracture or 30 minutes to 24 hours of unconsciousness or amnesia, 0.7% of patients at 1 year and 1.6% at 5 years had a seizure. The risk after a mild injury with brief unconsciousness or amnesia was 0.1% and 0.6%, the same as for the general population.

Some of the best data on natural history derive from a controlled trial of 400 patients admitted to one trauma center who were randomized to prophylactic phenytoin or placebo within 24 hours of injury.[54] Entry into the trial required a score of 10 or less on the GCS, a hematoma on CT scan, a penetrating skull wound, or a seizure within the first 24 hours. By day 7, 3.6% assigned to phenytoin had a seizure compared to 14% on placebo. Between day 8 and 1 year, 21.5% of patients on phenytoin had a seizure, compared to 15.7% who took placebo. By year 2, 27.5% on phenytoin and 21% on placebo had seizures. Phenytoin levels were in a therapeutic range in 70% of patients. Thus, epilepsy is common after a serious TBI and prophylaxis with phenytoin can reduce the incidence by about 70% in the first week, but not beyond that. The incidence of rash and fever from phenytoin in the first 2 weeks of use was 0.6%.[55]

In another randomized clinical trial that compared phenytoin and valproate, the rate of seizures within 2 weeks of TBI in hospitalized patients was not significantly different; 1.5% in patients who received phenytoin and 4.5% in patients who received valproate within 24 hours of the CHI.[56] In addition, continuing valproate for 1 month or 6 months did not significantly alter the rates of subsequent seizures, which were 15% and 24% respectively. These findings are consistent with the results of a randomized trial that compared phenytoin, carbamazepine, and placebo for seizure prophylaxis after a craniotomy for pathologies other than malignant tumors.[57] Seizures were most frequent in the first month after surgery, but early and late seizures occurred at the same frequency, 37%, in all groups.

With a 25% rate of first seizures regardless of anticonvulsant prophylaxis, the automatic use of antiseizure medications is not productive beyond the first 2 weeks after a serious TBI. This conclusion has special impact for those with brain injuries, because phenytoin,[55,58] phenobarbital, and carbamazepine, perhaps more than valproate[59] and newer drugs such as gabapentin, can modestly impair motor and cognitive function. In patients after TBI who were treated prophylactically with either phenytoin or carbamazepine and tested on and off the drugs, modest negative effects were apparent during drug use on tests that require rapid motor and cognitive responses.[60] Some patients show much greater slowing than others. Such individual variation may have an especially negative impact during rehabilitation, academic work, and job training. Anticonvulsant management for at least 2 seizure-free years is a common practice, however, when a seizure occurs beyond the first 2 weeks following an injury.

Delayed-Onset Hydrocephalus

Acute obstructive hydrocephalus is a relatively straightforward complication to recognize, arising from cerebral edema and blood or infection within the ventricles and subarachnoid space. A ventricular shunt is indicated. After a subarachnoid hemorrhage, the development of symptomatic hydrocephalus is predicted by finding cisternal and ventricular blood or hydrocephalus on the initial CT scan.[61]

Recognizing symptomatic nonobstructive or normal pressure hydrocephalus (NPH) is a challenge for clinicians. The condition can develop insidiously over months, even years, after TBI. Its incidence is probably no more than 5%.[62] Ventricular enlargement, however, develops in from 30% to 70% of patients with severe TBI.[63,64] Most patients have hydrocephalus ex vacuo, a passive enlargement from the loss of gray and white matter. For the patient who does not continue to improve or who declines modestly over the first weeks to a few months after a serious TBI, the clinician must weigh the possibility that delayed-onset hydrocephalus, not an ex vacuo change, is the culprit.

No test clearly points to the presence of NPH. Monitoring the intracranial pressure or trying several days of lumbar drainage of CSF helps predict the response to a shunting procedure.[65,66] Indium cisternography and fea-

tures of the MRI scan, such as periventricular white matter fluid or slow flow in the ventricles, and a clinical response to drainage of CSF by a single lumbar tap may offer some insight.[67] Focal and diffuse brain pathology can account for all of a patient's impairments or limit gains even after a shunt is placed for symptomatic hydrocephalus. As with other surgically accessible intracranial abnormalities that follow TBI, such as small residual subdural hematomas and hygromas, clinical acumen and the willingness of physicians, patient, and family to accept the risk for potential complications, such as an infection or shunt malfunction, guide decisions about the intervention.

Enlarging ventricles with the triad of increasing gait apraxia, cognitive dysfunction, and incontinence are the strongest indications for a ventricular shunt. The best clinical marker for NPH may be the serial observations by the family and physician regarding an unexplained decline in communication and walking. Excessively low ventricular pressures after placement of a ventriculoperitoneal shunt can also impair attention, alertness, and other cognitive processes, as well as produce headache.

In some patients, the ventricles are only modestly enlarged in the presence of increased intracranial pressure (ICP) after a shunt malfunction. Brain elasticity is thought to be elevated, allowing the intracranial pressure to be high or to rise precipitously with CSF pressure waves, which may cause acute fluctuations in a patient's cognition and mobility or progressive deterioration. Blood pressures in the low normal range may diminish cerebral perfusion pressure in this circumstance and cause more prominent symptoms. In another variation, some patients will have a low ventricular pressure after shunting, but the ventricular volume is not reduced and symptoms persist or later worsen. To deal with this, external ventricular drainage at subzero pressures has been used to decompress the ventricles over weeks.[68] In one patient, we drained from 200 to 400 mL of fluid daily for 35 days at pressures of -10 to -25 cm H_2O. The ventricles diminished in size without inducing a subdural hematoma or hygroma, and symptoms lessened. Drainage is followed by implanting a valveless shunt and maintaining the patient slightly upright, even in bed. The proposed mechanism of this low pressure hydrocephalic state is decreased viscoelasticity of the brain from expulsion of extracellular water and distortion and ischemia of brain tissue from the radial compressive stresses of the large ventricles.[68] Slow drainage presumably allows rehydration and restores elasticity.

Although no data are available to suggest the incidence of low-pressure hydrocephalus, clinicians should consider the possibility that motor and cognitive deterioration, even after a low-pressure shunt produces smaller ventricles, may mean that the shunt is blocked or the intervention has not optimally altered CSF pressure. When a programmable valve was used to test the effects of different intraventricular pressures in hydrocephalic subjects, great sensitivity to small pressure changes was found.[69] Thus, clinicians may have been too conservative in suggesting a shunt for patients who fail to improve during rehabilitation or whose condition deteriorates only modestly. In addition, shunts that are put into place may perform less than optimally, so if improvement after shunting is not found, the clinician needs to readdress the adequacy of the procedure. A programmable valve has the advantage of allowing the clinician to test for under-drainage or overdrainage, which have been found in from 45 to 75% of patients.[70] In the face of a decline in function after a shunt, patients must be evaluated for a subdural hematoma or infectious ventriculitis.

Acquired Movement Disorders

Movement disorders may follow serious TBI or repetitive concussions. Problems include rubral and other tremors, myoclonic jerks, and parkinsonism, particularly the punch-drunk syndrome of boxers. Less often, patients develop akinetic-rigid syndromes, chorea and ballismus, focal and more generalized dystonia, tics, psychogenic jerks, and other unwilled movements.[71] These disorders can develop within weeks, months, or as long as 10 years after injury. Late evolution raises the possibility of ongoing changes within the basal ganglia and their connections, such as denervation hypersensitivity, dendritic sprouting onto partially denervated target cells, and an accelerated decline in the number of striatal neurons as the patient ages.

Both peripheral and central injuries are associated with dystonia. An initial focal finger or foot dystonia or a hemidystonia can progress to a multifocal dystonia, a hemidystonia, or generalized dystonia.[72] Lesions in the contralateral basal ganglia and thalamus have been imaged by CT and MRI in most instances of hemidystonia. Several cases have been reported in which the scans were normal, but PET revealed metabolic abnormalities.[71] Metabolic imaging has also revealed reorganization as a contributing cause. Contralateral to a hemidystonia of the arm, frontal lobe overactivation was found during movement. The investigators suggested that the acquired dystonia arose from thalamofrontal disinhibition caused by structural disruption of inhibitory control by the basal ganglia.[73]

Therapy for movement disorders associated with TBI does not differ from drug interventions for the same disorders from other causes.[74] Patients with TBI may be especially susceptible to the cognitive side-effects of anticholinergic, dopaminergic, or dopamine receptor blocking agents, however. Stereotactic thalamotomy or deep brain stimulation may be necessary in a minority of patients with severe hemidystonia or tremor. Antispasticity agents, including intrathecal baclofen infusion, may be needed for spastic dystonia.[75]

Persistent Vegetative State

Patients in a persistent vegetative state (PVS) have no meaningful cognitive and motor responses. Ethical and medical–legal controversy often surround these helpless patients and their families. Persistent vegetative state is defined as no ability to follow a command, no intelligible verbal response, no verbal or gestural attempts to communicate, and no localizing or automatic motor response. A minimally conscious state, by consensus definition, implies partial consciousness with reproducible but inconsistent responses to localize sound and follow a command, to offer intelligible verbalization and discernable verbal or gestural communication, to fixate vision, and to make automatic responses.[76] Both emerge from severe TBI with coma at onset. The clinical outcome for a patient in a minimally responsive state 1 month after TBI is much better than for patients still in a PVS.

Persistent vegetative state follows TBI with coma in 1%–14% of 1-month survivors and follows nontraumatic coma in approximately 12%.[77] Nontraumatic causes in adults are mostly from hypoxic-ischemic injury, but they include cerebral hemorrhages, infections, and degenerative diseases. In children, metabolic disorders and developmental anomalies are additional causes, and tend to have an even worse prognosis than anoxia from drowning and cardiac arrest.

In an autopsy series of patients who survived for at least 1 month with PVS, the primary structural abnormalities in traumatic and nontraumatic causes were subcortical, involving the white matter and thalamus, which disconnect the cortex from afferent inputs.[78] Diffuse ischemic damage to the neocortex occurred in 10% of traumatic and 64% of nontraumatic cases. Diffuse axonal injury and structural damage to the thalamus were less common in patients who were severely disabled by TBI compared to those in a PVS at the time of death.

In patients with PVS, the electroencephalogram usually reveals diffuse slowing and PET reveals a marked reduction in global glucose utilization.[79] In patients who are most likely to die or remain vegetative, sensory evoked potentials are absent.

Rehabilitation specialists are often called upon to help in prognostication, to provide maintenance care, and to try interventions to improve the patient's awareness. The natural history of PVS, however, is dismal. Tables 11–5 and 11–6 summarize outcomes from several studies.[77] Families and coma-stimulation therapists often find hope for recovery in the inconsistent, nonpurposeful movements that are derived from reflex responses to stimulation and the patterned, innate responses related to internally driven, subcortical activity. With their intact brain stem functions, some patients have inconsistent auditory or visual orienting reflexes, but no clear-cut visual pursuit or fixation. Some grunt, cry, moan, and grimace to internal and, on occasion, to external stimuli. Persistent vegetative state means, however, that patients are unaware of self or environment and cannot interact in any purposeful way. Victims are awake but unaware, because the reticular activating system is disconnected from the thalami and cerebral hemispheres.

A careful evaluation will distinguish patients who can respond to their environs. By 1 year after onset, the real dilemma in patients with PVS is how much medical and nutritional support to continue. Mortality rates for these patients are 70% at 3 years and 84% at 5 years.[77]

Table 11–5. Glasgow Outcome Scale Classification for Recovery of Consciousness and Function in Adults in a Persistent Vegetative State Beyond 1 Month

Outcomes	3 Months (%)	6 Months (%)	12 Months (%)
TRAUMATIC BRAIN INJURY			
Death	15	24	33
Persistent vegetative state	52	30	15
Conscious	33	46	52
Severe disability			28
Moderate disability			17
Good recovery			7
NONTRAUMATIC BRAIN INJURY			
Death	24	40	53
Persistent vegetative state	65	45	32
Conscious	11	15	15
Severe disability			11
Moderate disability			3
Good recovery			1

Source: Adapted from Multi-Society Task Force on PVS, 1994.[77]

Table 11–6. Glasgow Outcome Scale Classification for Recovery of Consciousness and Function in Children in a Persistent Vegetative State Beyond 1 Month

Outcomes	3 Months (%)	6 Months (%)	12 Months (%)
TRAUMATIC BRAIN INJURY			
Death	4	9	9
Persistent vegetative state	72	40	29
Conscious	24	51	62
Severe disability			35
Moderate disability			16
Good recovery			11
NONTRAUMATIC BRAIN INJURY			
Death	20	22	21
Persistent vegetative state	69	67	65
Conscious	11	11	13
Severe disability			7
Moderate disability			1
Good recovery			6

Source: Adapted from Multi-Society Task Force on PVS, 1994.[77]

Rare case reports describe patients who recovered spontaneously several years after onset of PVS, but these patients were probably at least minimally conscious.

INTERVENTIONS

Interventions to reverse coma or PVS either early or late after onset have generally not been successful. A few reports have claimed recovery of consciousness using bromocriptine, amphetamine, electrical stimulation of the reticular formation and its connections, and in association with sensory stimulation programs. Families and clinicians often try sensory stimulation employing tasks from the Western Neurosensory Stimulation measure.[80] Bromocriptine, 2.5 mg twice a day, was associated anecdotally with greater gains than the investigators expected in five patients with PVS during inpatient rehabilitation.[81]

Programs for coma stimulation aim for input to the reticular activating system and try to enrich the environment for the sensory deprived patient. Electrical stimulation of the nonspecific thalamic nuclei and of the high cervical spinal cord with implanted electrodes was used in six patients for 12 hours a day at 30% of the threshold that elicited eye opening and pupil dilation.[82] Although the details are unclear, two patients who had a GCS of less than 6 for approximately 10 months, became able to handle oral feedings, and made simple responses to verbal commands over 10 months of stimulation. Less invasively, therapists have tried vestibular, tactile, auditory, olfactory, visual, and gustatory stimuli.[83] Sensory stimulation for periods up to 3 months has had no apparent effect on arousal or recovery.[84] Even in those extraordinary instances where coma stimulation seemed to shorten the time to arousal relatively early after onset of coma,[85] the affect on lessening subsequent disability is unknown. Although some investigators have begun to define the level of dysfunction of patients by more reliable scales[86] and monitor for specific physiologic or behavioral responses, reports of sensory stimulation do not yet offer evidence that promote its efficacy.

ASSESSMENTS AND OUTCOME MEASURES

For purposes of early and ongoing assessment, prognostication, and outcome, a number of measurement tools and descriptors can be recommended.[87] The range of physical, behavioral, and cognitive disabilities is so great in patients with moderate to severe TBI that it is worth elaborating on the usefulness of relevant measurement tools described in Chapter 7. Most of these scales are used almost exclusively in studies of TBI or hypoxic-ischemic injury to describe the stage of recovery and level of disability, and to categorize behavior.

Stages of Recovery

The GCS (see Table 7–3) defines the depth and duration of coma.[88] The GCS has been used in most outcome studies of TBI and allows distinctions regarding severity that have some prognostic meaning when given 6 hours after onset. The GCS is routinely used in emergency rooms and by acute trauma clinicians. It should be collected daily if the score is less than 15, until the patient is discharged from the hospital. On the GCS, the sum score of 13–15 is defined as a mild injury, 9–12 is a moderate TBI, and 8 or less is severe. The Extended GCS (GCS-E) was developed to include patients with mild concussion, adding an Amnesia Scale with eight categories for the duration of PTA.[89]

The Galveston Orientation and Amnesia Test (GOAT) is a simple, reliable assessment of PTA that separates patients into normal, borderline, and impaired groups (see Table 7–4). This 100-point scale is given as soon as the patient is alert and then daily until the score is normal. A score of 75 or higher on 2 consecutive days suggests normal functioning,[90] although the GOAT does not measure the consolidation of memory in that time.

Stages of recovery beyond coma are often described by the subjectively defined Rancho Los Amigos Levels of Cognitive Functioning (Table 11–7).[91] These levels take into account early, middle, and late stages in the evolution of recovery from DAI.[92,93] The initial stages go from coma to an unresponsive vigilant or vegetative state with sleep–wake cycles. Purposeful wakefulness with limited nonverbal or brief, hypophonic responses to commands often evolves in patients who do not remain in a vegetative state. Simple yes–no answers may be possible to elicit. A confusional stage follows with PTA, limited attention, and easy distractability. Agitation, hostility, perseveration,

and confabulation are often found. Behavioral interventions are more likely to be of value at this stage compared to approaches that deal with specific cognitive processes. The middle period, which can last from 3 to 12 months, takes the patient from the end of PTA to gradually increasing awareness of deficits and greater independence in ADLs with self-initiation. Patients work on specific cognitive dysfunctions, goal-setting, and resocialization. Neuropsychologic and language testing batteries for monitoring and planning interventions become more valuable at this stage than in previous ones. The last stage can subsume many behavioral, cognitive, and mood problems of serious or subtle severity that last years. Structured assessments produce different results than may be found in real-life situations. For example, disturbances in personality, in the ability to attend to multiple environmental stimuli, and to shift logically from one concept to another may not be brought out by routine pencil-and-paper tests.

Disability

The Disability Rating Scale (DRS) (Chapter 7) and the Functional Asessment Measure (Table 7–18), a 12-item addendum to the FIM that reflects community-based activities, and the GOS are the most frequently employed tools for functional outcomes in studies of TBI. A structured approach to use of the GOS improves its reliability and lessens subjective application.[94] The DRS, FIM, and FAM correlate highly with each other and with duration of coma, length of PTA, and the Rancho Los Amigos Scale.

On the DRS, scores > 15 on admission to rehabilitation, > 7 on discharge, and > 4 at follow-up 3 months after discharge predict the likely inability to return to work.[95] Thus, scores give an indication of employability. The DRS is so quick to use that it may also serve as a way to stratify rehabilitation inpatients for clinical trials and help track changes in outpatients. The Mayo-Portland Adaptability Inventory, which was developed for TBI, has also been correlated with the DRS and Rancho Scale. The Mayo-Portland Inventory adds useful ratings of emotional behavior to those of functional abilities and physical disabilities.[96] The Community Outcome Scale, which rates real-

Table 11–7. **Rancho Los Amigos Scale of Cognitive Functioning**

I. NO RESPONSE

Completely unresponsive to any stimuli.

II. GENERALIZED RESPONSE

Reaction to stimuli inconsistent and nonpurposeful. Responses often the same regardless of stimuli. Responses may include physiological changes, gross body movements, and/or vocalization. Delayed responses likely.

III. LOCALIZED RESPONSE

Reaction to stimuli is specific, but inconstant, and directionally related to the stimulus, e.g., turning head toward sound. May follow simple commands such as closing eyes, squeezing/extending extremity in an inconsistent, delayed manner. May show vague awareness of self and body by responding to discomfort. May respond to some persons, but not to others.

IV. CONFUSED, AGITATED

Heightened state of activity with severely decreased ability to process information. Behavior frequently bizarre and nonpurposeful. Verbalization frequently incoherent/inappropriate. Possible confabulation. May be hostile or euphoric. Gross attention to environment very short. Selective attention often nonexistent. Unable to perform self-care without maximum assistance.

V. CONFUSED, INAPPROPRIATE, NONAGITATED

Appears alert and responds to simple commands. Responses nonpurposeful to more complex commands. May show agitated behavior. Gross attention to environment, but highly distractible. Lacks ability to focus on specific tasks. Inappropriate verbalization. Severe memory impairment with confusion of past and present. Lacks initiation of functional tasks and often shows inappropriate use of objects without external direction. May perform previously learned tasks when structured, but unable to learn new information. Responds best to self, body, comfort, and sometimes family members. Can usually perform self-care activities with assistance. May wander.

VI. CONFUSED, APPROPRIATE

Shows goal-directed behavior, but dependent on external input for direction. Responds appropriately to discomfort. Consistently follows simple directions and remembers relearned tasks such as self-care. Responses are appropriate to situation.

VII. AUTOMATIC, APPROPRIATE

More goal-directed and self-initiated everyday behavior.

VIII. PURPOSEFUL, APPROPRIATE

Self-directed behavior that accomplishes basic and more skilled tasks. Might still need supervision.

world mobility, occupation, social integration, and engagement in the community, each by a score from 0 to 6, offers dimensions not found in the other scales for patients with TBI.[97]

Other measures used by the rehabilitation team and in studies of patients with TBI include the Katz Adjustment Scale—Relatives Form, a tool with somewhat uncertain validity used to assess how the family perceives the patient in the home, the Neurobehavioral Rating Scale (see Table 7–12), which is sensitive to the severity and chronicity of CHI,[98] and the Agitated Behavior Scale, 14-item instrument for documenting agitated behaviors.[99] The Katz Adjustment Scale includes 13 categories and 127 items. Scores have correlated with severity of TBI and social functioning when completed by patients.[100] The Neurobehavioral

Rating Scale-Revised was formulated to better reflect neuropsychologic impairments after TBI.[101] Instead of the four factors that subsume items of behavior shown in Table 7–12, the revised scale factors items under intentional behavior, emotional state, survival-oriented behavior and emotion, arousal state, and language. The Barrow Neurological Institute Screen for Higher Cerebral Functions (BNIS) measures seven domains, including awareness and affect, along with speech and language, orientation, attention/concentration, visual spatial and visual problem-solving, and memory. Subscores and total scores have correlated with the FIM plus FAM and gains during inpatient rehabilitation correlate with attaining inpatient goals.[102]

No specific battery of neuropsychologic tests has been put into general use for patients with TBI. In addition to the Wechsler Adult Intelligence Scale-Revised (WAIS-R) (see Chapter 7), the Halstead-Reitan,[103] and the Luria-Nebraska, tests often serve as core batteries. Four sites in the Traumatic Brain Injury Model Systems project adopted a group of 15 standard measures with established norms, all of which are included in Table 7–2.[104] The average rate of impairment on these tests for patients admitted for rehabilitation after CHI is 56%. Timed tasks in real-world settings such as the Rivermead Behavioral Memory Test[105] and the Multiple Errands and the Six Elements Tests[106] are especially useful for assessing memory, initiation, and planning in this population. The Rivermead Test is easily administered at the bedside and in the clinic.

PREDICTORS OF FUNCTIONAL OUTCOME

Predictors and measures of functional outcome continue to undergo methodologic refinements. Global and specific measures of functional disability, neurobehaviors, and physical and cognitive impairments are likely to vary in their reliability, validity, and sensitivity to change across the spectrum of initial severity of TBI and across subsequent curves of recovery. Other factors that contribute especially to the behavioral effects of TBI include premorbid education and psychiatric and behavioral disorders, age, socioeconomic factors, and the variety of pathologies characterized by neuroimaging.

The Glasgow head injury outcome prediction program correctly anticipated outcomes after severe TBI for 84% of patients with good or moderate outcomes, for 84% who died or had vegetative survival, and for 12% who had severe disability at 6–24 months after injury.[107] Predictions were based on variables collected during the first 7 days of hospitalization. For the 324 patients in the study, 15% of predictions were too pessimistic and 10% were overly optimistic about the late GOS, which is about as good as the best available predictor algorithms.

For example, a multivariate path analysis was carried out on over 100 acutely injured patients admitted for rehabilitation and followed up prospectively at 6 and 12 months after TBI.[108] Seventy percent of patients had an initial GCS of 3–8 and 63% had PTA lasting beyond 4 weeks. A comprehensive battery of evaluations assessed severity of TBI, premorbid traits and experience, neuropsychologic abilities, emotional state, and outcomes by the DRS, Community Integration Questionnaire, and level of employment or ongoing schooling. Premorbid functioning was associated with better functional skills and outcome. A significant direct relationship was found between severity of injury and both functional skills and cognition. Another significant relationship existed between cognition at 6 months and outcome at 12 months. No relationship was found between emotional status and either premorbid factors, severity of injury, or outcomes.

Level of Consciousness

The Traumatic Coma Data Bank (TCDB) related the GCS taken following nonsurgical resuscitation to the GOS at hospital discharge.[109] For mortality, lower scores combined with pupillary abnormalities and age over 40 accounted for most of the variance. With an initial GCS of 3, 78% died, compared to a mortality of 18% with a score of 6–8. Higher scores increase the likelihood of a viable rehabilitation effort. With a GCS of less than 6, 16% reached a level of good recovery or moderate disability by the GOS. Between 6 and 8, 64% did so. Only 4% of patients over age 45 with scores below 9 had a good recovery by 6 months compared to 29% of younger patients. The lowest early GCS and absent pupil reactivity were much more predictive of a poor outcome than high intracranial pressure or, by CT scan, the presence of diffuse cerebral swelling or mass lesion.[24] Consistent with the TCDB study, the International Coma Data Bank of acute neurosurgical patients found that only 11% of patients with a best GCS of 5 by 3 days after injury reached the levels of good recovery or moderate disability.[110] The GCS has become the most widely used acute prediction measure, with a precision of over 75% for the GOS at 6 months after CHI.[111] Of course, alcohol, drugs, and neurosurgical and medical complications may affect scoring the tasks.

Duration of Coma and Amnesia

Duration of coma and time to recovery have a rather linear relationship, especially when neuroimaging suggests DAI as the primary pathology.[112] As coma extends from 1 month to beyond 2 months, recovery to moderate disability or better falls to approximately 40%.[113] After an anoxic injury, coma that lasts beyond 1 week leaves almost no chance of recovery to better than severe disability.[114] Duration of PTA also has a telling effect, although measures of the inability to acquire and retrieve information vary among studies. In the International Coma Data Bank, duration of less than 2 weeks was associated with good recovery in over 80% and left no patient with severe disability, whereas PTA lasting more than 4 weeks was associated with a good recovery in only 25% and severe disability in 30% of patients.[110]

Katz and Alexander found similar relationships for patients referred to one rehabilitation unit.[29] In a group of 243 consecutive admissions, a significant inverse relationship was found between GCS and length of coma (LOC), and a strong positive relationship was observed between LOC and PTA. For patients with DAI, a regression analysis showed that duration of PTA (in weeks) was equal to $(0.4 \times LOC \text{ (in days)}) + 3.6$. Of 119 patients with likely DAI, no one in a coma for more than 2 weeks or with PTA for over 12 weeks had a good recovery by the GOS at 1 year postinjury. Two-thirds of the small subgroup with LOC for more than 2 weeks improved to moderate disability when LOC was 2–4 weeks duration. Only one-third achieved this level if coma persisted for more than 4 weeks. Half of the rehabilitation patients with PTA lasting 2–8 weeks reached the level of moderate disability

and 80% of those with PTA for less than 2 weeks had a good recovery. Posttraumatic amnesia was longer with advancing age. Outcomes were worse in subjects over age 60.[115]

Several studies provide other useful information using the length of PTA.[116] As PTA diminishes, orientation tends to recover in the sequence of person, place, and then time. Retrograde amnesia tends to recede from more remote to more recent chronological information after moderate and severe CHI. During PTA, memory decays rapidly. Procedural memory, however, is better (see Chapter 1). During rehabilitation, patients with severe CHI were able to acquire motor and pattern analyzing skills, even when they recalled little about how they came to learn the skills. In children, the duration of PTA correlated with impairment in verbal learning and memory skills at the time of resolution of amnesia, as well as 12 months after TBI.

Neuropsychologic Tests

Stuss and colleagues carried out a prospective study of 94 patients with acute TBI without hypoxic-ischemic complications to test the predictive value of a 24-hour continuous memory task.[117] Patients were given three words and asked to recall the set the next day. If free recall failed, three target words and six distractor words were given as a test of retrieval. Daily testing continued until the patients had perfect free recall on 2 consecutive days or were discharged. The GCS and duration of loss of consciousness correlated rather strongly, but the 24-hour recall task provided additional information. Severity of TBI was redefined as mild for a median of 6 days to recover word recall, moderate for a median of 15 days, severe for a median of 22 days, and extremely severe for a median of 42 days. Multiple bedside measures, then, including the GCS, LOC, duration of PTA, and 1-day verbal recall tasks, may improve predictions about overall functional gains after TBI.

A formal battery of 15 neuropsychologic tests adopted by the Traumatic Brain Injury Model Systems[118] tested 293 adults with CHI at a mean of 42 days after injury during inpatient rehabilitation.[104] Scoring in the normal range on any 1 of 10 standard tests was a significant predictor of return to work or to fulltime academic pursuit 1 year later. The Trail-Making Test B, which is easy to administer at the bedside, is one of the predictor tests. Of patients who completed at least 1 of the 10 tests during inpatient care, 38% became productive, compared with 6% of those who could not complete any tests. Studies of patients undergoing inpatient rehabilitation who recover from PTA find that less impaired subjects, those who score above the 75th percentile on neuropsychologic tests, are 1.6 times as likely to be productive as patients who score at the 25th percentile 1 year after injury.[119]

Population Outcomes

Most population studies of TBI carry inherent biases from the mix of patients, success of follow-up, and reliability of measurements. A recent study of adults from Glasgow offers a solid foundation for outcomes in patients who, for the most part, did not have access to rehabilitation resources.[32] Five hospitals contributed 2962 patients, 90% with mild, 5% with moderate, and 3% with severe TBI by the GCS. From this group, 769 patients were stratified by GCS on admission and 71% were available for follow-up 1 year later. The cohort included 66% with mild, 18% with moderate, and 13% with severe TBI. The mean age was 38 years and 19% were over age 65, of whom 90% had a mild injury. A structured GOS was used. Remarkably, 35% of subjects who had a mild head injury and were under age 40 and previously healthy failed to reach a good recovery. Table 11–8 shows the outcomes at 1 year for each stratified group. At 1 year, cognitive complaints about memory, concentration, and decision-making persisted in 43% of the mild, 49% of the moderate, and 76% of the severe TBI patients. A similar percentage in each group had mood-related symptoms such as anxiety, depression, and irritability. Problems in ADLs affected approximately one-third of patients with mild or moderate TBI and two-thirds of the severe group. The study estimates the annual incidence of disability in adults with TBI admitted to the hospital to be 100–150 per 100,000 persons, which is considerably higher than previously reported, less well-designed studies. This disability may be reduced by formal programs of rehabilitation that target the specific problems of such patients.

LEVELS OF REHABILITATIVE CARE

Locus of Rehabilitation

Rehabilitation programs for TBI rely on a continuum of treatment options built upon medical, neurobehavioral, social, educational, and vocational models.[120] Medically stable patients who remain in a coma are usually placed in nursing facilities where techniques such as coma stimulation may be tried. Patients who are emerging from coma and those who are disabled by problems in mobility and ADLs, or by confusion, agitation, and cognitive dysfunction are appropriate for interdisciplinary inpatient rehabilitation efforts. Table 11–9 lists some of the interventions typically provided by the inpatient team. Cognitively impaired patients who become mobile and wander may require therapy on a locked unit. Patients often graduate to one of several therapy options other than routine outpatient rehabilitation services (Figure 11–3).

A day treatment program helps to relieve the family of full-time care. Along with therapies

Table 11–8. Outcomes at 1 Year Based on Hospital Admission Glasgow Coma Score

Glasgow Coma Score	Good Recovery (%)	Moderate Disability (%)	Severe Disability (%)	Dead or Vegetative (%)
13–15	45	28	20	8
9–12	38	24	22	16
3–8	14	19	29	38
Uncertain	29	24	24	24

Source: Adapted from Thornhill et al., 2000.[32]

ACUTE   POSTACUTE

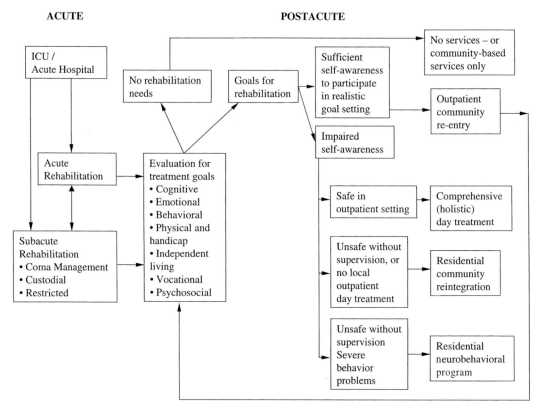

Figure 11–3. Algorithm of levels of rehabilitative care after traumatic brain injury.

for physical disabilities and cognitive impairments, patients are trained in skills for independent living, socialization, and vocational or school reentry. If behavioral and cognitive dysfunction dominate, a neurobehavioral residential program designed especially for behavioral modification aims for better socialization and more independence. A supervised, home-like transitional living setting or community reentry program trains skills for independent living, community activity, and employment. Insurers and case managers may not be obligated contractually to provide a particular service setting.

Milieu or therapeutic community settings can provide the structure to resolve psychosocial and behavioral problems. Programs emphasize social competence and dealing with the limitations imposed by brain injury. Group interactions, counseling, psychotherapy, and behavioral modification are provided within the context of ADLs and leisure activities. Vocational rehabilitation centers and school programs, which are often government efforts, provide useful resources, but may not be able

to cater to the needs of young patients with brain injury. In a supported employment program[121] or protected work trial, the patient works under the supervision of a therapist and job supervisor or coach. The setting tolerates the cognitive and behavioral impairments that would ordinarily not be permitted at a workplace. Task-oriented skills are reinforced. Supportive counseling and behavior modification techniques help ease the patient into volunteer, protected, or competitive work.

Efficacy of Programs

After a moderate to severe TBI, most patients who meet criteria for inpatient rehabilitation (Fig. 11–3) improve in their skills and become less disabled as they move through nonhospital-based programs.[122] No studies have been done that allow clinicians to know which settings and services are most efficacious and which are of little value. Type, intensity, and duration of services at any of these levels of

Table 11–9. General Sequence of Approaches to Therapy During Inpatient Rehabilitation for Traumatic Brain Injury

Adapt subject to a day and night wake–sleep cycle.

Provide brief therapies during periods of greater arousal and responsiveness.

Eliminate the use of centrally-acting drugs for sleep, agitation, and pain.

Eliminate sources of pain.

Stimulate awareness of environs and sustained attention.

Reorient subject with cues.

Find cues and strategies that increase selective and divided attention.

Compare the efficacy of massed practice and errorless learning strategies to the efficacy of distributed practice and practice with fading cues for best learning. Use positive reinforcements.

Shape and reinforce acceptable behaviors and lessen disinhibited behaviors.

Encourage self-awareness and responsibility for aspects of care.

Encourage repetition and practice of attentional, visuospatial, sensorimotor, and task-specific skills. Do not overload attentional and working memory capacity.

Develop compensatory strategies for memory and executive functions.

Address speed and accuracy in tasks.

Encourage and monitor social interactions with staff, family, and friends.

care depend on judgements about needs and whether a plateau in gains appears to have been reached. Moreover, any study of postacute rehabilitation faces problems in sampling, defining outcomes, showing how a treatment outcome generalizes to the real world, and in calculating cost-effectiveness.[123] Most importantly, the form and day-to-day content of programs tend not to be fully explained when trials are carried out.

Methodologic flaws hamper the interpretation of most studies of programs of inpatient and outpatient rehabilitation.[124] Many investigators use quasi-experimental designs, stating that it is not ethical to withhold the favored treatment approach.[125] Although this concern is debatable, investigators should have no qualms about studying key components of a program in a randomized trial that employs blinded outcome measures.

ACUTE INPATIENT PROGRAMS

A few studies have been invoked as presumptive evidence that programs do benefit patients. One small trial, oft quoted, suggests that patients admitted to rehabilitation within 35 days of TBI spend half the number of days in therapy as those admitted later.[126] The subjects were matched for age and length of coma, but not for GCS or PTA. The late admission group

included more patients with a tracheostomy, bowel and bladder dysfunction, and greater cognitve dysfunction, so these patients may have been more impaired. Outcomes on a scale of social function did not differ at the 2-year follow-up.

A retrospective study from 10 facilities found that a formal program of rehabilitation assessment and intervention beginning within a few days after acute hospitalization was associated with one-third the duration of coma and length of rehabilitation stay, compared with patients who were not provided an early program.[127] The level of cognition and number of discharges home were also significantly higher in the early-therapy group. Aside from physical, occupational, and speech therapies, the formalized program provided family support and sensory stimulation for coma patients. Coma stimulation, however, is not of proven value. This study is likely flawed by the initial severity of TBI in the groups. The length of coma was 20 days for the early-intervention group versus 54 days for the late-intervention group.

Other inpatient studies suggest that by increasing the number of hours of organized daily therapy by 25% to 50%, patients reach a level of function that allows earlier discharge to the home.[128] A comparison between providing 2 and 4 hours per day of therapy for 36 randomized patients with moderate to severe

TBI showed a trend toward higher FIM scores and a good outcome by the GOS after 2–3 months of treatment at the higher intensity.[129] The group getting less therapy was catching up by 6 months. Across nearly all studies of therapy in general and therapy for a specific skill, greater intensity and duration of treatment correlate with better immediate outcomes.

Two prospective trials compared formal inpatient rehabilitation to another setting of care. A nonrandomized, prospective comparative trial by Barnes and colleagues assessed (1) the efficacy of coordinated multidisciplinary inpatient therapy on a TBI service for 33 subjects to (2) the efficacy of management at local hospitals with single therapies provided much less frequently for 18 subjects.[130] All subjects had a GCS of 8 or less for at least 6 hours at onset. Treatment began a mean of 49 days after onset for the group on the TBI service and continued for a mean of 200 days; the intervention began 18 days after onset for the patients in the unorganized service and continued for 111 days. The group that received coordinated care made significantly greater gains for up to 6 months on the FIM and maintained the treatment effect on a range of functional skills when reassessed at 1 and 2 years. Caregiver stress was greater for the patients treated without an organized approach.

Salazar and colleagues randomly assigned 120 active-duty military personnel to (1) a standardized, inpatient milieu-based cognitive rehabilitation program or (2) to a home program with weekly phone support from a nurse and mental and physical exercises carried out on their own for approximately 30 minutes a day.[131] The inpatient program used both didactic cognitive and functional experiential approaches. Treatment lasted 8 weeks. The mean GCS of the subjects was 9.5, mean duration of PTA was 41 days, and mean time postinjury was 38 days. By 12 weeks after injury, most recovered to a Rancho level 7. Outcomes did not differ 1 year later in standard cognitive tests, social adaptation, mood, behavior, or fitness for military duty. Over 90% returned to work. Aggression increased in both groups, suggesting the need for ongoing support. This trial should be replicated in a nonmilitary population with moderate CHI that may not have the same high level of education and community support. Similar results to the study by Salazar and colleagues could have a strong impact on a cost-benefit analysis of inpatient treatment and day care for this subgroup of patients.

POSTACUTE PROGRAMS

A review of 25 uncontrolled studies of residential community, outpatient, and day treatment programs for TBI showed that most patients appear to benefit.[132] Approximately 60% of these selected patients returned to work or school. The data are important, but trials without control subjects who receive a lesser intervention cannot be compelling. For example, a day treatment program for approximately 100 patients who were unable to work 1 to 2 years after TBI provided a range of interventions in group therapy for a mean of 190 days. The investigator found a significant reduction in physical disability, increased self-awareness and emotional self-regulation, and more effective participation in interpersonal activities.[133] One year after completion, 72% lived independently and 57% were employed.

Other comparison trials suggest that a program with more hours of formal therapy improves outcomes. Wade and colleagues randomized 314 hospitalized patients within 10 days of a TBI to receive services by a specialist team or to receive standard services.[134] The experimental group was given advice and education, and 46% received additional outpatient treatment or telephone support. Fifty subjects dropped out of each group. Social disability and postconcussion symptoms were reduced by the specialized intervention at follow-up 6 months later.

A quasi-experimental matched-groups study compared the efficacy of treatment in a residential setting to home care after inpatient discharge.[135] The average duration of therapy was 8 months for the 46 severely disabled subjects. Residential services were highly organized with trained staff. One-third of subjects at home received no therapy and others received some rehabilitation care. Both groups improved at 1 to 2 years. By 1 year, the residential group improved significantly more in motor and cognitive functions and community integration.

Late interventions may also take the form of a pulse of therapy for a specific disability or a form of education. A randomized trial entered 110 patients with mostly chronic TBI (1) to an outreach program in the community or (2) to provision of written material about resources for patients and families.[136] The outreach group met approximately twice a week for a mean of 27 weeks. The outreach group made modest, but significant gains in scores on the Barthel Index and a brain injury outcomes measure at 2 years, assessed by a blinded observer. No differences were found between the groups for socialization, employment, anxiety, or depression.

REHABILITATION INTERVENTIONS AND THEIR EFFICACY

Survivors of a serious TBI tend to make their greatest gains in mobility, functional skills, and language over the first 3 to 6 months, much like patients after stroke. Performance measures, such as the ability to do a timed or novel task, recover more slowly. Some patients continue to improve for several years in distinct cognitive and behavioral measures. Indeed, young patients with fixed impairments probably learn new skills and make adaptations with supervised help and on their own indefinitely, as the need arises.

Overview of Functional Outcomes

Organized inpatient rehabilitation services provided within the first months after injury are likely to benefit patients and families who actively participate. Overall, patients clearly make functional gains during inpatient care. Table 11–10 shows outcomes from the Traumatic Brain Injury Model Systems Project. Table 11–11 shows data from recent yearly reports of the Uniform Data System for Medical Rehabilitation (UDS$_{MR}$) for changes between admission and discharge on the FIM across approximately 400 hundred inpatient rehabilitation programs. In 1992, UDS reported that the

Table 11–10. **Traumatic Brain Injury Model Systems Project, 1989–2000 (2553 Cases)**

Variable	Onset	Rehabilitation Discharge	1 Year Postinjury
Mean Age (years)	36		
Male (%)	75		
Married (%)	29		
High School Diploma(%)	68		
Vehicle-related(%)	52		
Alcohol-related(%)	41		
Employed(%)	59		24
Living Home(%)	97		85
Loss of Consciousness(%)	94		
Posttraumatic Amnesia(%)	98		
>30 days(%)	34		
8–29 days(%)	34		
1–7 days(%)	8		
Mean Lowest Glasgow Coma Score	7		
Duration of Coma (days)	3.8		
Acute Hospital Stay (days)	22		
Rehabilitation Inpatient Stay (days)		32	
Total FIM Score	56	97	115
Disability Rating Scale	12.6	6	2.9
Community Integration Questionnaire			15.5

FIM, Functional Independence Score.
Source. Traumatic Brain Injury National Data Center (www.tbims.org).

Table 11–11. **First Admission for Cerebral Trauma: Typical Yearly Results from Uniform Data Systems for Medical Rehabilitation**

	AVERAGE SCORES	
	Admission	**Discharge**
Self-Care	3.5	5.2
Sphincter	3.7	5.4
Mobility	3.0	5.0
Locomotion	2.1	4.3
Communication	4.2	5.2
Social Cognition	3.5	4.6
Total FIM	58	92
Age (years)	47	
Onset (days)	21	
Stay (days)		23
Discharge Status (%)		
Community		81
Long-term care		9
Acute care		5

FIM, Functional Independence Measure.

mean time from onset of TBI to admission for rehabilitation was 34 days and the length of stay was 40 days.[137] By 2000, time to admission fell by 13 days and inpatient stay declined by 17 days, but the admission and discharge total FIM scores and placement in the community remained the same. This trend parallels the decline in duration of inpatient care for patients with stroke and SCI, yet outcomes based on the FIM remain stable.

After a TBI, patients may perceive themselves to have recovered more than their clinicians and families believe. A longitudinal study of 157 patients admitted to a Seattle hospital found that half the subjects reported 65%, 80%, and 85% or greater return to their normal state at 1, 6, and 12 months, respectively.[138] Approximately 25% of the participants reported a return of less than 50%, 60%, and 68% at 1, 6, and 12 months. At 6 and 12 months after injury, self-reported good and poor outcomes did correlate with scores on the GOS. Less than 20% of patients who perceived a poor recovery had GOS scores indicating good recovery. Overall, patients believed that physical problems were the greatest barrier to recovery, but their concerns about physical dif-

ficulties decreased and concerns about cognition increased over the year. Physical difficulties in speech, balance, dizziness, and functional limitations may be more noticeable and important to young people and deserve the attention of rehabilitationists.

Most clinical studies report on a particular type of program or on a specific type of problem, such as cognitive or behavioral dysfunction. Most often, the interventions are carried out beyond the usual time of inpatient care. Sensorimotor interventions and approaches to facilitate ADLs are similar to those for stroke and other neurologic diseases already described (Chapters 5, 6, and 9). Here, we emphasize TBI rehabilitation for cognitive, behavioral, and vocational function.

Physical Impairment and Disability

Although physical impairments that cause disability are common after a moderate to severe CHI at the time of transfer into a rehabilitation program (Table 11–12), these impairments most often improve within 6 months. Cognitive and behavioral sequelae linger. The Vietnam Head Injury Study examined 420 veterans who suffered PHI, mostly from low-velocity shrapnel that caused a preponderance of focal brain injuries. One week after injury, 21% had a hemiparesis and 11% had a hemisensory impairment.[52] Fifteen years later, 10% were hemiparetic and 21% had a residual

Table 11–12. **Impairments in 1-Month Survivors of Severe Traumatic Brain Injury**

Impairment	Percentage (%)
Cognitive	60–90
Hemiparesis, diparesis	40–60
Dysarthria	50
Cranial neuropathy	30
Dysphagia	30
Ataxia	10
Aphasia	10
Hemianopia	5
Optic neuropathy	1
No neurologic signs	25

Source: Adapted from Levin H et al., 1990.[36]

sensory loss, a greater number because the exam became more reliable.

Upper extremity paresis was present in 30% and moderate to severe paresis of an arm was found in 17% of 264 consecutive patients admitted for inpatient rehabilitation after TBI.[139] By 6 months, 82% with moderate or greater paresis had recovered. If paresis were present 2 months aftet injury, only 56% recovered useful motor function. Time to recover, a mean of 7 weeks, depended on initial level of weakness, as is typical of other diseases such as stroke.

Contractures and spasticity associated with flexor and extensor posturing and traumatic injuries to the limbs require special attention during the acute medical and rehabilitation inpatient stays. Early interventions include proper positioning, range of motion for joints, orthoses, serial casting, and even temporary motor point blocks. These interventions may prevent later complications and the need for surgical management when the patient has regained enough cognitive and motor function to participate in movement therapies.

In addition to the spectrum of physical therapy approaches, many TBI patients need ongoing encouragement and a structured program to maintain general fitness. An individualized aerobic training program can improve motor skills, decrease fatiguability, and improve mood.[140] A randomized trial compared the addition of 3 months of aerobic exercise or of relaxation training to an outpatient therapy program that 142 patients entered a mean of 24 weeks after TBI. The investigators found a significant increase in exercise capacity for the exercise group, but no differences betweeen the two augmented interventions in FIM scores, walking speed or balance, or in report of depression, anxiety, or fatigue.[141]

Most patients admitted for inpatient rehabilitation after TBI improve in their self-care and community reintegration skills over time. Studies have generally not been designed to distinguish a specific treatment effect from the effects of a patient's milieu or the natural history of recovery. In general, after moderate to severe TBI, self-care and mobility improve from admission to discharge and gains are maintained or continue to increase for approximately 6 months.[142] Approximately 50% of patients return to work by 6 months. Socialization and leisure activities generally do not return to premorbid levels.

Brain injury often interferes with the ability to generalize a functional skill from one situation to another. Functional training in the face of cognitive dysfunction requires an approach that is skill-specific and often context-specific. Adaptations are often required by the family, by the school and workplace, and by other people in the patient's social system.

Psychosocial Disability

Problems in social, leisure, work, and family role performances are related more to the cognitive, behavioral, and emotional sequelae of TBI than to physical impairments. The nature and severity of postinjury psychosocial difficulties varies with measures of the severity of TBI and time from injury to observation. Problems tend to improve over the first year.[143] The Sickness Index Profile has been a useful assessment tool, along with measures of social networks and checklists of physical and psychological symptoms. Negative symptoms and poor socialization increase the stress felt by patients and caregivers.[144] Counseling, education, and psychotherapy can assist families.

A return to residence and work or school are important goals for therapy and serve as key outcome measures. Successful vocational outcomes need to be considered in terms of premorbid work abilities and postinjury hours of supervision and level of productivity.

General predictors of employability after CHI are shown in Table 11–13. After PHI, 56% of the veterans studied were employed 15 years after injury, compared to 82% of healthy control subjects.[145] The researchers found a linear association between work status and the

Table 11–13. **Predictors of Successful Employment**

Favorable preinjury intellectual and work status

Shorter duration of coma and posttrauamtic amnesia

Improving cognition, especially for verbal memory, speed of information processing, and pragmatic communication

Behavioral self-control

Coachability

No clinically significant anxiety or depression

Family and employer support

number of residual impairments. These problems include epilepsy, paresis, visual field loss, verbal memory and learning, visual memory, psychologic difficulties, and self-reported violent behavior. In other studies, impaired verbal memory and slow information processing strongly relate to unemployment 7 years after a severe CHI.[146] Better DRS and FIM scores during inpatient rehabilitation predict greater likelihood of returning to work.[147] Other factors include greater community reintegration, social needs, drug abuse, economic conditions, and social supports.[148,149] After severe TBI, most follow-ups beyond 2 years reveal that approximately 10% return to former jobs and fewer than 30% are employed.[121] With supported employment services in the workplace, which are provided under the Rehabilitation Act Amendments of 1992, more patients are able to gain permanent work in warehouse, clerical, and service-related occupations. The cost can be considerable, however. In one well-organized interventional study, a mean of 250 hours of supportive staff time was necessary to return 67% of patients to work at a mean of 6 years after severe TBI.[121] The supportive employment approach, which may include a therapist helping the patient to solve problems in the workplace, seems to be the most successful intervention available.[150]

Cognitive Impairments

The more common and disabling cognitive problems after TBI include a mix of impairments in attention, concentration, memory, executive functions, and self-awareness (Table 11–14). The structures that network these cognitive processes are described in Chapters 1 and 3. Impairments may overlap to confound tests of specific neuropsychologic processes. Approaches to therapy for any one impairment often overlap and successful remediation often depends on influencing more than one process.[151,152]

The amount and rate of recovery of neuropsychologic functions depends mostly on location and severity of focal and disconnecting cerebral lesions. For example, CHI may compromise the ability to make cohesive discourse. A left prefrontal injury may cause sentences to become disorganized with an impoverished narrative, whereas a right prefrontal lesion may

Table 11–14. Cognitive Processes Commonly Impaired After Traumatic Brain Injury

ATTENTION
Alertness
Slow mental processing
Selective attention during distraction
Divided attention
Sustained attention
Awareness of disability and impairment

PERCEPTION		
Visual	Auditory	Visuospatial

MEMORY
Retrograde and antegrade amnesia
Immediate, delayed, cued, and recognition recall
Visual and verbal learning; acquisition worse than retrieval
Maintenance and manipulation in working memory

EXECUTIVE
Planning
Initiation
Maintain goal or intention
Conceptual and relational reasoning
Hypothesis testing and shifting response
Self appraisal
Self regulation

INTELLIGENCE
Verbal and performance
Problem-solving
Abstract reasoning

LANGUAGE
Aphasia
Discourse (vague, tangential, confabulatory communication; verbose or impoverished speech; no affective expression)

cause tangential, socially inappropriate expression.[153] These impairments interact with dysfunction in other frontal executive processes and have a negative impact on socialization. Recovery also is influenced by the patient's age, by premorbid intellect and education, and by the initial and early rate of recovery of cognitive and affective function. Patients whose cognition improves during inpatient rehabilitation, especially for memory, affect, and visuospatial functions, and who become aware of deficits are most likely to achieve important rehabilitation goals.[102] In general, measured functions improve over the first year. Gains in the second year are limited to fewer functions, and mostly in those patients with the most severe injuries.[154] As noted earlier, impairments tend to plateau faster with focal lesions than with DAI.

A thorough neuropsychologic evaluation helps describe the loci of cognitive impairments within the neurocognitive architecture. The details of an analysis are combined with the bag of available treatments and the goals for treatment set by patients and therapists. Test scores help define what is right and what is wrong with a patient in a systematic way, so that techniques can be applied in a fashion as appropriate as the state of knowledge allows. Progress in cognitive rehabilitation, like any aspect of rehabilitation, follows what is learned as therapy proceeds from the initial assessment, from the generation of hypotheses, and by monitoring the consequences of interventions.

Although clinical services for cognitive rehabilitation are in high demand for patients with TBI, they are delivered without much empirical support. Services are provided by physical, occupational, speech, and vocational therapists and psychologists within the context of mobility and spatial orientation, self-care and community activities, communication, and work or schooling.

OVERVIEW OF INTERVENTIONS

A few general approaches have been taken to ameliorate the cognitive difficulties of head-injured patients. These styles of care include (1) functional adaptation and compensatory techniques, (2) general cognitive stimulation, (3) training specific cognitive processes, and (4) behavioral conditioning. In practice, a range of approaches are taken. Counseling about strengths and weaknesses, providing emotional and social support, and compensatory problem solving are standard team interventions. Multimodal programs stress learning task-specific skills by remediative techniques, in addition to teaching self-awareness about

impairments, and building toward independent living and return to work.[155] The contribution of remediation of particular cognitive domains is difficult to cull out, because many interventions go on simultaneously in a program of care and outcome measures often reflect broad functional categories, rather than those specific domains.

The Brain Injury-Interdisciplinary Special Interest Group of the American Congress of Rehabilitation Medicine reviewed the literature prior to 2000 that supports particular approaches for cognitive rehabilitation.[156] For patients with TBI, the group recommended, as practice standards, interventions for functional communication such as pragmatic conversational skills training and compensatory memory strategy training, at least for patients with mild memory impairment. As practice guidelines, the group recommended training for attention, visual scanning, specific language impairments, and problem-solving strategies applied to everyday situations. As practice options, the group recommended memory notebooks and other external aids applied to daily activities for patients with moderate to severe memory impairment; systematic training of visuospatial and organizational skills for patients with hemispatial inattention; verbal self-instruction and self-monitoring techniques building upon a patient's strengths; the combination of cognitive and interpersonal therapies during a structured rehabilitation program; and computer-based interventions as part of a multimodal program to develop compensatory skills and foster insight into cognitive strengths and weaknesses. Computer-based practice without frequent involvement by a therapist was not recommended.

COMPENSATORY APPROACH

Compensation involves overcoming impairments and disabilities by recognizable behaviors (see Chapter 2). With an adaptive approach, therapy takes place in a real or simulated functional setting, such as the home, place of work, or school. These programs try to lessen or circumvent the effects of cognitive impairments on daily activities. The underlying notion is that addressing specific cognitive impairments is unlikely to improve functional outcomes more than specifically training the desired functions. Instead of treating impairments, therapists manage the more important disabilities and handicaps that impairments impose. Adaptive techniques tend to rely upon repetition, cues, overlearning, and cognitive assistive devices, much like the routine compensatory interventions for ADLs training. In addition, the environment is structured so that it is predictable and cues the patient.

Functional remediation, as well as specific cognitive process remediation, should try to employ learning principles (see Chapter 5). Ideally, the therapist provides an optimal schedule of feedback during performance and about results. Overlap of the elements and the organization of a task, as well as practice in a variable context, can increase the likelihood that the subject will learn a skill. The diverse cognitive sequelae of TBI may counteract this reinforcement, however. Errorless learning may be a better approach for patients with greater memory impairment. For other patients, learning one strategy to perform a task may not generalize to novel circumstances or even transfer to another related task or setting. Careful attention to the components of a task and to the cues where practice takes place may lead to the patient's ability to transfer what has been learned to a related task or another setting.[157]

BEHAVIORAL TRAINING

Behavioral training targets discrete behaviors or tasks and reinforces them with rewards. Behavioral modification protocols must be structured and used by the entire team, especially when the goal is to eliminate disruptive behavior. For example, a token economy in which the patient earns chits that can be used to purchase candy and magazines can be used to reward patients during inpatient rehabilitation or in a transitional living setting. Rewards may be given immediately or with some delay, depending on the reinforcement schedule, for completing a self-care task or for reducing aggressive actions.[158] In an uncontrolled study, management of 24 patients on a specialized behavioral unit was associated with improved quality of life and living arrangements.[159]

COGNITIVE REMEDIATION

General cognitive stimulation training assumes that mental stimulation of all sorts may improve mentation. Therapists use workbooks, art, computer programs, and other stimuli to encourage cognitive processing. Mental jumping jacks, however, are not likely to recondition the brain for the acquisition and retention of skills and strategies that reduce disability. Cognitive remediation takes a more theoretic approach.

Cognitive remediation has many nuances, but usually includes a cognitive process-specific approach that articulates subroutines of a mental process. Therapists aim to ameliorate impairments in problem-solving, often use feedback, and consider that their methods reorganize the function of cognitive neural networks.[160,161] The approach targets distinct, if theoretic, components of separable cognitive processes. Repetition of a task at one level of difficulty or related to one subcomponent of the cognitive process continues until the goal is reached. Then the task is enlarged within its presumed hierarchic organization. For example, once 2-dimensional constructions are copied, 3-dimensional drawings are practiced. Once auditory attention is achieved, auditory encoding is practiced. Gains are expected to generalize to related tasks and to transfer into real-world activities.

In practice, when cognitive impairments are mapped by neuropsychologic testing, early interventions are often designed to boost the efficiency of a domain for which the patient has demonstrated some capacity, rather than tackle domains for which the patient's ability is poor. When possible, a relatively intact cognitive skill is emphasized to compensate for a severely impaired one. For example, impaired auditory encoding may be compensated for by writing what was said and by using a visual memory strategy.

Cognitive remediation techniques have been carried out for many of the common sequelae of TBI. The techniques are less successful as the severity of impairments increases. Specific approaches, based upon still inexact theories of cognitive processing, have been outlined for generic disorders of orientation, attention, memory, visuoperception, language, executive functions, and problem-solving.[151,155,162] For example, selective attention, which is the ability to focus on a particular stimulus or response, can be reinforced behaviorally, compensated for by placing the patient in a nondistracting environment, possibly improved by withdrawing medications that reduce arousal, attention, and the speed of mental processing, and possibly remediated by dealing individually with the still murky processes that reflect goal-directed controls by the frontal lobes.

Remediation of various attention-related skills has shown benefit in some small, prospective controlled studies of focused compared to less structured therapy after TBI,[163,164] but not in others.[165,166] Computer-assisted training is a favored approach. The actual amount of time spent carrying out the focused intervention in these studies ranged from $1/2$ hour to 1 hour a day for 4–9 weeks. A pilot trial of a strategy to improve tasks that require frontal lobe functions such as attention, self-regulation, and planning, called Goal Management Training, showed that this approach, compared to motor skills training, led to significantly better gains on everyday pencil-and-paper tasks that mimicked the goal-oriented problems of patients with TBI.[167] The approach directs a patient's awareness toward specific goals. The patient and therapist select specific goals and divide them into subgoals. Practice encodes and retains the goals. The patient compares the outcome of actions with the desired goals or subgoals. This top-down approach to goal management aims to maintain the intentions of goals in mind and monitor the steps of training. Patients must have some insight for the technique to work.

MULTIMODAL SKILLS TRAINING

Therapy programs usually offer interventions for multiple cognitive impairments either simultaneously or sequentially. Computer-assisted cognitive rehabilitation (CACR) is included in such programs. Computer software allows clinicians to make serial measurements of the patient's progress in what are usually repetitive tasks. The computer is rigid in its demands, which offers the consistency needed by many TBI patients. Partial and complete visual and auditory cues can be built in to aid declarative and nondeclarative learning. Reinforcement schedules for knowledge of performance and knowledge of results can be set. Pleasurable visual and auditory reinforcers are easy to create. In general, patients can work with intermittent supervision, which should lessen the expense of therapy.

Although computer technology provides environmental control systems and external aids, perhaps enough to be considered as a mental prosthesis, its value in cognitive remediation and skills training is less certain. Some patients have been trained in tasks such as data entry, database management, and word processing by taking advantage of preserved cognitive abilities, including the ability to respond to partial cues and acquire procedural information.[168] This knowledge is specific to the patient's training and does not readily generalize to even modest changes in requirements. Patients have been trained in verbal and visual mnemonic strategies to learn a computer graphics program.[169] Other subjects have been trained to do cooking and vocational tasks with an interactive guidance system that cues each subtask and builds up to the required task.[170] Computer-based cognitive remediation software programs also show promise for special education classes in a school setting.[171]

These limited, but interesting successes suggest that the computer can assist in skills training as a kind of learning or reminding prosthesis. Software programs may eventually serve to help remedy specific cognitive processes by allowing systematic practice on their subcomponents. Although some modest successes have been published in small group or single-case studies, clear gains by CACR in, for example, attentional deficits as noted earlier, have often failed.[164,166] A matched-comparison study of 40 patients evaluated the efficacy of Bracy's Process Approach, which identifies 25 basic processes associated with deficits in functional skills.[172] No significant differences were found between the group given CACR with the Bracy software compared to traditional cognitive therapies without CACR, despite greater duration of treatment for the CACR group. The groups were not well matched, however.

Even the most powerful computer has to await our knowledge of what these cognitive processes are and how to modulate them. With greater and inexpensive computing power, easier interfaces, voice recognition, and the growing ability of software to simulate real-world settings, the possibilities for computers in cognitive rehabilitation will require continuous reassessment and clever applications.

COMPREHENSIVE OR HOLISTIC APPROACH

Most acute and postacute rehabilitation programs combine cognitive remediation with other organized services. The content of training includes the skills that the patient needs for

ADLs, socialization, or work. These sometimes lengthy programs are generally associated with gains in some important outcomes, although the content and duration of therapy is moot.

In one interdisciplinary program, 18 highly selected patients received cognitive and psychologic therapies that emphasized awareness of deficits, along with skills training for social, work, and family activities.[173] The subjects had good family support, no premorbid psychiatric history, and had moderate to severe cognitive dysfunction. Mostly one-on-one therapies were given 6 hours a day for 4 days a week and lasted at least 6 months. In comparison to 17 matched patients who received a traditional approach, 50% of the intensively treated group and 36% of the control group were employed 6 to 26 months later. The intensive therapy group also tended to do better in some cognitive tests, including the Wechsler Memory Scale. The self-selection of these patients for participation in the experimental group may have been an uncontrolled factor that accounted for the modest findings.

A similar scheme of therapy was used in a larger group of patients who had completed traditional therapy and had failed to regain employment.[174] The patients received approximately 400 hours of cognitive remediation, instruction on interpersonal communication and social skills, and counseling to understand and accept their disability. The patients continued with 3 to 9 months of supervision in a work setting. Six months later, 84% were employed, about half in a competitive setting. At a 3-year follow-up of a subgroup of these patients, 76% were still employed, half in a competitive job. Other single institution reports of late rehabilitation have also found a positive effect on posttreatment work status, attendant care, and independent living that the authors believed were cost-effective.[122,175]

Much has been written about the confusing and poor methodologies of studies of multimodal programs of rehabilitation.[176,177] Publications from single institutions about their results in uncontrolled trials must be viewed with caution; however, the effects of programs that use multiple, simultaneous interventions can be evaluated systematically.

In one approach, three matched groups were assigned to three different mixes of remedial interventions.[178] All subjects received the same number of hours of therapy over 20 weeks, counseling, and interaction with peers in group activities. One group received cognitive remediation using a hierarchy of training procedures for constructional and visual analysis tasks and verbal reasoning. Another received this training, plus training in interpersonal skills that emphasized acceptance of disability and awareness of deficits. The other group received interpersonal skills training without cognitive remediation. Measures specific to each type of training improved in those who received the therapy. Cognitive training did lead to modest gains in neuropsychologic outcome measures related to the individualized therapy. Thus, gains may be attributed to more than the overall milieu of rehabilitation. Other comparisons of different packages of therapies would have ethical, scientific, and practical benefits while taking advantage of the supportive milieu.

Psychotherapy

Psychotherapy has been recommended for nonpsychotic symptoms and for general support as a part of TBI rehabilitation.[179,180] The practices of psychotherapeutic techniques differ widely and measures of efficacy are less than striking. Psychotherapy may help patients understand what has happened to them and improve self-awareness and insight. Problems in awareness and acceptance of disability can affect the patient's motivation for rehabilitation and impede progress on cognitive, social, and emotional fronts. At some stage of recovery, patients may underestimate their difficulties in memory and emotional control. Lack of insight, however, as best measured, does not necessarily correlate with failure to make rehabilitation gains.[181] Psychotherapy can also help patients control anger and other disruptive affective responses, achieve self-acceptance and find hope, make realistic commitments, and assess their changing role in the family. Spousal and family therapy can contribute to domestic tranquility, understanding, and the patient's reintegration. Although some patients after TBI may be too impaired cognitively to participate, patients who seem to need the intervention usually can work with a therapist.

PHARMACOLOGIC FACILITATION

Rehabilitation physicians have probably tried more neuropharmacologic agents in individual TBI patients to attempt to modify cognition and behavior than for any other disease. On occasion, a positive experience or single-case study design has led to a small randomized clinical trial, but not often enough to provide evidence for practices. Drugs for postinjury behavioral and psychiatric disorders have been more clearly efficacious and are discussed later in this chapter.

Table 11–15 lists some of the more commonly used classes of drugs used for cognitive disorders. Dosages are as idiosyncratic as the drugs themselves. A reasonable approach is to select several measurable impairments or behaviors, choose a class of drug that neuromod-

Table 11–15. Possibly Useful Drug Classes for Cognitive Disorders After Traumatic Brain Injury

CHOLINERGIC AGONISTS

Cholinesterase inhibitors
  Donepezil[185]
  Physostigmine[186]
  Galantamine
  Rivastigmine

Acetylcholine replacement
  CDP-choline

Cholinergic receptor agonists
  Xanomeline

CATECHOLAMINE AGONISTS

D-amphetamine
Methylphenidate,[188]
L-dopa
Amantadine
Bromocriptine[182,193]
L-deprenyl
Desipramine

SEROTONERGIC AGONISTS

Fluvoxamine

NOOTROPICS

Pramiracetam

NEUROPEPTIDES

Vasopressin

AMPAKINES

ulates a particular system (see Chapter 1), and start therapy at the lowest dose typically used for the agent. If the drug seems effective by report or by retesting as it is titrated upward, continue it for several months, add cognitive therapies and practice for the targeted problems, and test again. When the patient reaches a plateau, taper off the drug and reassess any loss of benefit a few weeks later. This approach may also be taken by alternating drug trials with placebo pills in an N-of-1 design (see Chapter 7).[182] As noted in Chapter 1, neuromodulators and other neurotransmitters interact to alter neural transmission and production of neurotrophins, so the precise locus of action may not be predictable.

After dorsal pontine or midbrain DAI, which may damage any of at least three neurotransmitter pools, replacement with agonists of serotonin, norepinephrine, and acetylcholine has considerable rationale. A pilot study of 96 patients in vegetative or minimally conscious states between 4 and 16 weeks after TBI found better outcomes when trazadone, a serotonergic agent, was given at any time in the 16-week study or when amantadine was given within the first 4 weeks.[183] Bromocriptine led to a decline in the outcome measure, the DRS.

Traumatic brain injury may cause memory deficits similar to those observed after experimental lesions of the septohippocampal cholinergic projections that are critical for memory.[184] The effects of disruption of the cholinergic pathway in Alzheimer's disease, the negative effect on recall by the cholinergic antagonist scopolamine, and the availability of cholinesterase inhibitors has made cholinergic agonists a favorite drug to try in patients with memory disorders. Positive results, however, have been less reproducible and of more limited consequence than the modest effects of these drugs on the dementia of Alzheimer's disease. An open-label trial of donepezil, a central acetylcholinesterase inhibitor, found modest gains in retrieval and consolidation in four subjects who had memory impairment lasting 3 or more years after a severe TBI.[185] Shorter-acting physostigmine improved sustained attention compared to placebo in a trial of 16 patients.[186]

Monaminergic agonists and vasopressin have occasionally benefited patients by increasing arousal, attention, and initiation. A vasopressin analogue studied in a double-blind, placebo-controlled, matched-pairs trial, had no effect, however, on cognitive recovery in the 3 months following a mild TBI.[187] Methylphenidate improved the speed of mental processing in a blinded, randomized, repeated crossover trial design, but did not affect distractability, sustained attention, or motor speed.[188] This drug has both dopaminergic and noradrenergic effects. Amphetamine also has more than an adrenergic effect and may improve aspects of working memory when it is impaired,[189] along with aspects of language, at least in some aphasic patients after stroke.[190]

Bromocriptine, a D-2 receptor agonist, and other dopamine receptor agonists have occasionally improved mutism, akinesia, a flat affect, goal-directed behavior, and aspects of memory[182] and motor function[191] in some patients with frontal lobe injuries. In an unblinded, dose-escalation, repeated measures design, 11 patients with brain injury of 2 months to 5 years duration were chosen to receive increments of 2.5 mg of bromocriptine weekly, because they were very passive and poorly motivated for daily activities.[192] At 5–10 mg, all subjects improved in ratings of spontaneity and participation and improved their scores in tasks of selective reminding task, digit span, and verbal fluency. Mood did not change. Eight subjects maintained these gains when the maximum dose of medication was withdrawn. The drug may enable a subject to learn a cognitive strategy[182] or may initiate the drive for network activity and eventually no longer be needed. A drug holiday is always worthwhile in individual experiments with patients to determine the ongoing value of the intervention.

Bromocriptine more clearly improved certain performance measures after 24 subjects were randomized in a double-blind, placebo-controlled crossover trial.[193] The patients had a subacute or chronic TBI. They were tested 90 minutes after receiving 2.5 mg of the agonist. The drug improved prefrontal executive functions, but not tasks that involve the maintenance of information in working memory. For example, patients improved significantly in completing dual tasks, the Trailmaking test, and the Wisconsin Card Sorting test. Dual-task paradigms, in which a subject performs a reaction-time task during a concurrent digit span task, are a practical way to evaluate the executive dysfunction often found in patients after TBI.[194] The effects of dopamine at a cellular level on rewarding novel learning and as a teaching signal for associative learning,[195] discussed in Chapters 1 and 2, place this neuromodulator in the thick of experimental approaches for the patient with TBI. Other dopamine agonists, as well as levodopa/carbidopa and amantadine, may work as well or may be used to augment each other.

Other drugs, such as modafinil to increase arousal and the ampakines and other potential memory molecules (see Chapter 2) are worthy of phase II clinical trials in patients with targeted symptoms, primarily of hippocampal and frontal dysfunction.

The effects of a drug intervention are not readily predictable. Clinicians may anticipate that positive effects on one aspect of cognition could have an adverse effect on another. For example, amphetamines may increase attention, but lead to hypervigilence to extraneous stimuli, stereotyped behavior, and paranoia. The design of drug trials must take into consideration that short-term crossover studies may mask an effect that lasts longer than the time allowed for withdrawal from the study medication. Also, the optimal dose, amount of time on a drug, and type of practice in cognitive tasks while on a drug all factor into assessing a measurable change. Centrally acting drugs may be as likely to cause a decline in cognition from an adverse reaction as they are apt to enhance an aspect of cognition.

APPROACHES FOR AMNESTIC DISORDERS

Cognitive disorders that affect memory are so pervasive after TBI that some specific therapy approaches need to be discussed. After TBI, tests may reveal impaired short-term memory, which is about capacity rather than time-related recall, and working memory, which is online, rehearsing recall, as well as impaired antegrade and retrograde long-term memory for verbal, visuospatial, and declarative information. Chapter 1 reviews the structure and function of cognitive processes. Particular stages in memory processing may be impaired. Some of the more easily described ones include attention, organizational strategy, registration, encoding, storage, and retrieval. The maintenance of stored memories and the ability to return to them for use depends on widespread interactions between primary sensorimotor cortex, association cortex, and frontal executive functions. The latter organize storage and an efficient, selective search at the time of retrieval. Prospective memory, which is the ability to remember to carry out a task in the future, often falters after a TBI. Patients may recall what they were supposed to do when cued or asked, but do not do so on their own, because the executive functions that maintain a goal state over time fail.[106]

As noted, the therapist may not easily separate other cognitive processes commonly affected by TBI from those that involve mechanisms of memory. Regional frontal lobe injuries produce myriad deficits that may interact with the acquisition and retrieval of new declarative and procedural learning.[196–198] The relevant and better definable components of attention include sustaining attention across time and a task, the capacity for holding and processing information, selecting targets and managing conflicts between targets, screening out nontargets and overcoming distractions, shifting attention from one task or thought to another, and multitasking. Executive functions are especially critical for managing new information and situations. Other functions that interact with memory processes include the voluntary initiation of thoughts and activities, the ability to persist in undertaking those thoughts and activities, the ability to inhibit responses and behaviors that are not appropriate to a task or interaction with people, the capacity to identify goals and plan how to carry them out in a framework of time and place, the ability to monitor and be aware of oneself, and the ability to think creatively, flexibly, and generate new ideas.

Natural History of Recovery

Residual memory disturbances are apparent in approximately 25% of patients after a moderate CHI and in approximately 50% of patients after severe CHI.[199] After mild TBI, memory usually recovers by 3 months.[200,201] The gains vary, however, with the test used to measure the severity of CHI, the amount of time from injury to testing, the indicator tests employed, and the comparison group.[202] One year after severe CHI, patients followed in the Traumatic Coma Data Bank had greater impairments in verbal and visual memory and in other cognitive tasks, such as naming to confrontation and block construction, compared with normative data.[24] Selective, rather than global cognitive impairments, were likely at 1 year. Memory was disproportionately impaired compared to overall intellectual functioning in 15% of moderate and 30% of severe CHI patients. In another group of patients, 25% of 1-year to 3-year survivors of moderate and severe CHI who could be tested showed defective memory on visual and auditory measures, despite normal verbal and performance IQs.[199]

A prospective study found that memory impairments were related to the time from injury to assessment, to the nature of the memory task, and to the severity of the injury. A group of 102 patients with TBI from ages 10–60 years were followed after hospitalization for any period of unconsciousness, PTA of more than 1 hour, or evidence of cerebral trauma. Dikmen and colleagues examined the subjects at 1 and 12 months postinjury.[203] At 1 month, the TBI group performed significantly worse on the Wechsler Memory Scale (WMS) and the Selective Reminding Test than did a control group. Patients who could not follow a command for the longest times beyond 24 hours postinjury had more subtests of the WMS below the control scores. Tests of orientation and short-term memory were inferior in their ability to reveal memory deficits compared to tests that required storage of new information for later use. At 1 year, patients performed better than they had at 1 month after onset. The group most severely impaired at 1 year initially had been unable to follow a command for more than a day, had PTA for over 14 days, and had a GCS score of 8 or less.

A long-term follow-up study of 26 patients who had a TBI and had undergone rehabilitation 5 to 10 years earlier found that 58% were unchanged, 31% performed better, and 11% did worse on the Rivermead Behavioral Memory Test and WMS.[204] Their mean length of coma had been 5 weeks, with a range of 1 hour to 24 weeks. Many patients still relied on memory aids.

Interventions for Amnestic Disorders

A compensatory approach to memory training teaches the use of verbal and written rehearsal, semantic elaboration, specific mnemonics, visual imagery, and memory notebooks. These techniques are useful if memory impairment is not too severe.

Therapists may teach skills through procedural memory processes, improve recall with priming techniques, and employ more specific semantic strategies to enhance episodic memory. These more sophisticated attempts at memory remediation cannot be isolated endeavors. For example, even when recovery is generally good, the memory performance of many patients declines in the face of a distracting task.[205] After severe CHI, patients tend to underestimate their memory and emotional impairments, even as they acknowledge physical and other cognitive problems. Without this insight or concern about their sense of knowing what they know, these patients may deny any impairment and may withdraw or become angry with attempts at rehabilitation. Lack of insight and loss of the sense of familiarity may lead to confabulation that interferes with therapy. During PTA, many patients show an increased rate of forgetting over the course of 30 hours on a visual recognition test compared to CHI patients who are past their PTA.[90] This finding suggests that therapy during PTA should emphasize skills learning and spend less effort on repetitive mental exercises that seek to improve the episodic and semantic components of declarative memory.

Previous exposure to verbal and especially to nonverbal information can, with cues and prompts, allow many amnestic patients after TBI to recall that information, a phenomenon called *priming*. Tests of recognition memory are especially sensitive methods to detect residual memory in patients with severe amnesia. Implicit memory can support the rapid acquisition of novel verbal and nonverbal material. Patients can be primed to learn automatic behavioral sequences for a motor, perceptual or cognitive skill, even though they may recall only nonspecific knowledge about having learned or having done the task. Techniques to acquire domain-specific knowledge include the method of vanishing cues. For example, patients were taught new computer terms by gradually reducing the number of letters in the new words and training them to complete the fragment.[162] Eventually, some patients were able to provide the word without any letter cues when given its definition. During the period of PTA, patients with TBI have learned motor and pattern analysis skills at the same time their memory for word lists and recent events was poor. The patients carried over some of this procedural memory into the period of recovery from PTA.[206]

After moderate to severe TBI, repetitive drills may have little impact on general recall or on enhancing memory outside of the training session.[173] Styles of practice and methods of optimal reinforcement of learning require further exploration in patients across the range of contributors to memory impairments. For example, severely amnestic patients learned more in one program when errors during training were minimized by the therapists; subjects performed worse when allowed to generate guesses that produced incorrect responses.[207]

External aids such as a calendar and appointment diary and internal strategies such as the mnemonic devices of rehearsal, visual imagery, and peg words help some patients to improve their ability to learn. Some of the most frequently deployed memory devices still used by TBI patients five or more years after being trained in their use are listed in Table 11–16.[204] Touch screen pocket computer devices with memory prompts and "help" software, pagers that receive typed messages, alarm wrist watches, calendars, and a place for phone numbers and notes can be adapted for some patients. Generalized use of a memory notebook depends heavily on sparing of procedural memory. Although internal aids may be of value within a structured task or setting, their postinjury use often does not generalize to real-world settings.[208] The person with TBI has to remember to invoke them and must hurdle past other impairments, such as concrete thinking that impedes the strategy.

A randomized, controlled trial of patients with CHI found that a group given memory strategy training and another given drill and repetitive practice training on memory tasks subjectively rated their everyday memory as improved, compared to a no-treatment group.[209] These patients were a mean of 5 years postinjury, half were employed, and they had experienced a mean of 30 days of PTA. Only the memory strategy training group showed objective gains in memory performance, which was more apparent at a 4-month follow-up than at the end of two 3-week sessions of training. This delayed gain suggests that the subjects were using the trained strategies. Thus, therapists can attempt to teach memory strategies to patients with residual cognitive dysfunction and determine if the

Table 11–16. **Aids and Strategies for Memory Impairment**

EXTERNAL

Reminders by others—voice, cell phone

Tape recorder

Notes written on cards or in a hand-held computer

Post-It notes

Time reminders

    Alarm clock/phone call

    Personal organizer/diary; calendar/wall planner

    Orientation board

    Electronic wristwatch

Place reminders

    Labels with words or coded by colors or symbols

    Electronic pictures with descriptors in a programmable hand-held computer

Person reminders

    Name tags

    Clothes that offer a cue

    Photographs in a hand-held computer

Organizers

    Lists; grouped items

    Electronic or written calendar organizer

    Post a trail of a numbered series of reminders

    Automatic phone number dialer

    Programmable wrist and hand-held computers

Alphanumeric radiopagers

INTERNAL

Mental retracing of events; rehearsal

Visual imagery

Alphabet searching; first-letter mnemonics

Associations with items already recalled

Chunking or grouping items

techniques will generalize to other material or to a novel context. If trained skills do not generalize, then therapy can concentrate on strategies that lead to a transfer of learning. In a successful transfer, the patient uses the same organizational approach to a task which is nearly the same as the trained-for task.

In summary, the approach to the cognitive remediation of amnestic disorders draws upon the various modules of memory networks that are being defined by neuroscientific studies. Techniques aim to train patients in the use of the subcomponent processes that underlie declarative and nondeclarative memory. Domain-specific knowledge and specific skills are trainable in patients with moderate to severe impairment. Compensatory strategies that can be employed under varying circumstances work for patients who are less impaired. The amount of time spent in practice in most studies is modest. Greater intensity or duration of treatment is a variable that needs clinical testing. Interventions for memory are, of course, not to be isolated from other components of brain injury rehabilitation.

OVERALL EFFICACY

Does cognitive rehabilitation work for patients with moderate and severe TBI? Although clinicians have argued about this from the point of view of theory, methodology, interventions, and measures of outcome, the studies that may answer this question have not been attempted. The methods and benefits of cognitive rehabilitation after TBI have not been questioned any more vigorously than other interventions for neurologic impairments and disabilities, however. Therapy programs seem worthwhile, because efforts protect patients from physical and emotional complications that may limit spontaneous gains and interfere with practice. Programs also promote adaptive functional gains, create compensatory strategies, retrain social skills, improve behavior, reduce psychosocial and neuropsychiatric problems, and help patients reintegrate into home, school, or work. The most efficacious and cost-effective approaches to these goals for most subjects are still uncertain. The most controversial issue for TBI rehabilitation is whether specific cognitive interventions can be identified and applied so that they change what they aim to treat, as well as improve related functional outcomes.

Cognitive remediation is one of the youngest of neurorehabilitation endeavors. It was once bounded by approaches borrowed from educational curricula and behavioral psychology. It now looks up at the constellations of experimental work related to neurocognitive networks and neuroplasticity. In this expanding universe of data, clinicians can hope to develop theory-driven practices that show efficacy upon rigorous testing. Informed clinicians who take a heuristic approach that leads to clinical trials will influence any future array of cognitive remediation innovations.

Table 11–17. **Common Changes in Behavior and Personality After Traumatic Brain Injury**

Disinhibition
Impulsivity
Aggressiveness
Irritability
Lability
Euphoria
Paranoia
Lack of self-criticism and insight
Irresponsibility, childishness
Egocentricity, selfishness
Sexual deviation or inappropriateness
Substance abuse
Self-abuse
Poor personal habits
Indecision
Lack of initiation
Blunted emotional responses
Poor self-worth
Apathy, inertia
Indifference
Passive dependency

Neurobehavioral Disorders

If cognitive dysfunction is the powerful undertow that threatens to pull down efforts at TBI rehabilitation, then behavioral and personality changes are the waves that crash against patients and their supporters. Some of these puzzling, demanding behaviors are listed in Table 11–17. The usual behavioral phenotypes of patients, which evolve from experience and gene expression, are perturbed by TBI. New, sometimes rapidly changing behaviors may follow. Tests and clinical descriptions define new phenotypes in subjects related to cerebral disconnections and tissue injury, medications, environmental influences, altered insight, and the expression of susceptibility genes for, say, mania or depression.

PATHOLOGY

Behavioral and mood dysfunction often accompany TBI, as well as stroke, multiple sclerosis, and the cortical and subcortical demen-

tias. As noted in Chapter 1, at least five parallel, segregated circuits link the frontal lobe and subcortical structures that include the sriatum and thalamus. Behavioral and mood syndromes caused by frontal lobe injury are recapitulated by lesions of the subcortical member structures of these circuits. Three distinct neurobehavioral syndromes have been described.[210]

1. The *dorsolateral prefrontal syndrome* includes deficits in motor programming, evident in alternating, reciprocal, and sequential motor tasks. Executive function impairments include the inability to generate hypotheses and show flexibility in maintaining or shifting sets required by changes in the demands of a task. Patients also exhibit poor organizational strategies for learning tasks and copying complex designs, as well as diminished verbal and drawing fluency. Lesions span the dorsolateral caudate, globus pallidus, and ventral anterior and dorsomedian thalamus (see Color Fig. 3–3 in separate color insert).

2. The *orbitofrontal syndrome* especially affects personality. The range of characteristics include altered interests, initiative, and conscientiousness, disinhibition, tactless words, irritability, lability, and euphoria. Patients tend to be enslaved by environmental cues. They might automatically imitate the gestures and actions of others. Lesions span the same structures as the dorsolateral syndrome, but in different sectors (see Color Fig. 3–4 in separate color insert).

3. The *anterior cingulate syndrome* includes profound apathy, even akinetic mutism. Lesions range from the cortex to the nucleus accumbens, globus pallidus, and dorsomedian thalamus. Both dorsolateral prefrontal and orbitofrontal subcortical circuits seem to have a role in depression. Mixed behavioral features suggest the involvement of more than one circuit.

CLINICAL SYMPTOMS

Changes in personality have been reported in up to 75% of patients from 1 to 15 years after TBI and tend not to improve beyond 2 years after onset.[211] A study of 196 patients assessed 1 year after a minor head injury found that 40% had 3 or more neurobehavioral symptoms, found more often in patients from a lower socioeconomic class and level of education.[212] Symptoms ranged from social disinhibition in 3%, lack of initiative in 15%, to irritability in 35%.

Frontolimbic injuries are associated with agitated, aggressive, out-of-control behavior that stresses the family, rocks relationships, and prevents acceptance into work and society. Agitated motor and verbal behaviors were found in 11% of patients during acute inpatient rehabilitation.[213] Another 35% of these patients were restless. Many patients quickly evolve away from the confused, agitated behavior of level IV on the Rancho Los Amigos Scale in the first weeks after they emerge from coma. As cognition improves, agitation declines.[214] Other patients exhibit directed and nondirected aggressive, impulsive behavior. Patients with frontal dysfunction may stand too close to others as they interact, show decreased empathy, seem tactless, exhibit emotionally colored perception, respond abnormally to a threat, acquire compulsive behaviors, and develop hyperorality.

Clinicians assume that the behavioral sequelae after TBI arise from brain trauma. A prospective study of 157 patients followed for 1 year found that patients with TBI did have significantly more symptoms than a normative matched-control group, but had similar emotional and behavioral symptoms as patients who suffered general trauma that spared the head.[100] The Katz Adjustment Scale was given at 1 month and 1 year after injury. On the GCS, 78% of patients had a mild, 10% had a moderate, and 12% had a severe TBI. Compared to the normative control group, patients after TBI were at least 1 standard deviation above the mean on subscales sensitive to anxiety, anger/impulsivity, sensory-perceptual distortions with bizarre ideation, confusion, cognitive problems, antisocial tendencies, suspiciousness, social or emotional withdrawal, and general adjustment difficulties. Patients ages 30–49 years old had the most problems. Both the patients after TBI and subjects after general trauma improved over the year on the Katz Scale. The TBI group, however, reported an increase in anger, antisocial behavior, and worse self-monitoring. Abnormalities in perceptual, behavioral, and cognitive items did not reflect a psychopathologic state. A potentially confounding problem for this excellent study is that patients with mild to moderate TBI and those suffering general trauma may overreport problems. More severe TBI is associated with decreased awareness and underreporting.

INTERVENTIONS

Interventions for neurobehavioral symptoms include a medical assessment for exacerbating problems such as pain and drug-induced confusion, behavioral modification, providing structure in the environment, individual and group psychotherapy, and trials of psychoactive medication.

Behavioral Modification

Behavioral modification of maladaptive conduct requires consistent and attentive care. Important target behaviors and their antecedent events or conditions are identified and counted. The team designs positive reinforcers and rewards and applies them on a consistent schedule of reinforcement. Rewards can be as simple as special foods, breaks from therapy, phone calls, passes, praise, and some time alone. A token economy, in which credits are earned for appropriate behaviors and exchanged for treats and privileges, can provide powerful incentives. The rehabilitation milieu for these patients should be supportive, peaceful, and not threatening. Negative reinforcement paradigms should be avoided.

Pharmacologic Interventions

Some centrally acting medications can alter neurotransmitter activity and, in turn, affect disorders of behavior and personality (Table 11–18). Hypoarousal sometimes improves with stimulants such as methylphenidate and amphetamine, as well as with dopamine agonists.

Table 11–18. **Drug Interventions for Neurobehavioral Disorders with Hypomania, Aggression, Restlesness, and Episodic Dyscontrol**

Anticonvulsants (carbamazepine, valproate)
Beta-blockers (propanolol, atenolol)
Lithium carbonate
Antidepressants (amitriptyline, fluoxetine)
Stimulants (methylphenidate, pemoline)
Neuroleptics (haloperidol, risperidol)
Benzodiazepines (long-acting)
Clonidine
Verapamil

Blocking dopaminergic and noradrenergic receptors and increasing cerebral serotonin levels may reduce aggressive behavior.[215] Most of the agents that have antimanic effects are worth trying in the difficult to control patient. Hypomanic behavior may respond to lithium, which is an especially effective agent for the mood-related symptoms of a bipolar, manic-depressive disorder.[216] The drug requires considerable monitoring for side-effects and for optimizing the dose. Anticonvulsants such as carbamazepine may prevent outbursts related to episodic dyscontrol. Lithium, carbamazepine, and valproate are titrated to their usual therapeutic serum levels. Beta-blockers can decrease feelings of irritability. A randomized trial of propanolol with a dose escalation to 420 mg a day showed a reduction in the intensity of agitation, but not the frequency of episodes, compared with a placebo.[217] In both treatment groups, the episodes dropped sharply by week 6 after admission for rehabilitation. Indeed, the frequency of symptoms and bouts of loss of control tend to decline over time. Premorbid personality and mood disorders may contribute to the persistence of symptoms and the need for drug therapy.

Neuropsychiatric Disorders

Premorbid psychopathologic features may be common in patients who suffer TBI. In one study of patients who suffered trauma without head injuries, 56% had this history, especially if alcohol and a violent act were associated with their injuries.[218] The prevalence of psychosis has been estimated at up to 5% after a moderate, and 10% after a severe, TBI.[219]

DEPRESSION

From 20% to 70% of patients with TBI may develop depression within 1 to 2 years.[220] The risk of depression may remain elevated for decades after TBI. A comparison of 520 World War II veterans hospitalized with TBI and 1200 veterans hospitalized for other wounds revealed a lifetime prevalence for major depression to be 18% in the TBI group and 13% in the control group.[221] Current major depression, 50 years after the war, was 11% versus 8%, respectively.

Depression has been related to lesion location in some correlative studies. Left anterior injuries, as in unilateral stroke, are associated with an early, transient depression.[222] Other focal and diffuse injuries make it difficult to relate mood disorders to specific sites, however. In the Vietnam Head Injury Study, anxiety and depression were associated with a right orbitofrontal lesion and anger and hostility were related to a left dorsofrontal penetrating injury.[223] Late-onset depression in CHI is more closely associated with premorbid psychiatric history and lower psychosocial function than with lesion location.[222] Long-term depression and anxiety relate more to problems in social adjustment.

A randomized trial comparing cognitive remediation to supportive day treatment for 8 weeks found that depression improved with both approaches.[224] Cognitive remediation, which tends to confront patients with their impairments, did not worsen their emotional state or psychosocial adjustment. The effectiveness of psychotherapy is uncertain in the face of memory or language dysfunction and limited awareness of deficits. Although no large randomized clinical trials have compared antidepressant medications for patients with TBI, clinical experience points to the usual effectiveness of especially the selective serotonin reuptake inhibitors (see Chapter 8).

PSYCHOSEXUAL DISORDERS

Psychosexual dysfunction evolves in up to 50% of patients after TBI. Infrequent intercourse is the most common problem.[225] Neuroendocrine dysfunction, pain, neurologic impairments, cognitive and behavioral dysfunction, alterations in libido, bowel and bladder incontinence, and psychosocial issues can often be managed.[226] Hypersexuality and disinhibition of sexual activity sometimes follow a medial basal-frontal or diencephalic injury. The Kluver-Bucy syndrome is associated with bitemporal injuries. Change in sexual preference has been related to limbic lesions.[227]

SLEEP DISORDERS

Sleep disturbances are common in the first few months and late after injury.[228] Up to half of persons after TBI have difficulty initiating and maintaining sleep, while about one-third complain of somnolence. Management of sleep dysfunction is an important part of any rehabilitation effort, especially for patients who have memory, attention, and mood disorders. An abnormal sleep cycle can prevent consolidation of newly learned information.

POSTTRAUMATIC STRESS DISORDER

Although the incidence of posttrauamtic stress disorder after TBI has not been reported, clinicians may expect that patients who suffer violent injuries and witness the injury or death of a companion are at risk. Antegrade and retrograde amnesia probably protect most patients with a moderate to severe TBI from this disorder. Management is discussed in Chapter 8.

SPECIAL POPULATIONS

Pediatric Patients

Children are especially susceptible to injuries of the frontal and anterior temporal lobes. They may also incur diffuse brain swelling, called the malignant edema syndrome, caused by hyperemia without a mass lesion. Some of these cases have been related to a mutation in a calcium channel subunit gene.[229] Related gene defects on chromosome 19 also predispose to familial hemiplegic migraine and posttraumatic migraine.

The severity of brain injury and neurobehavioral impairment have a dose-response relationship in children and adolescents, as they do in adults.[230] The duration of PTA, as measured by the Children's Orientation and Amnesia Test (COAT), time to reach a 75% score on the COAT, initial GCS, time to reach a GCS of 15, and duration of loss of consciousness are all directly proportional to neurobehavioral outcomes.[231] Long-term survival of children and adolescents beyond 6 months after serious TBI was estimated to be reduced by fewer than 5 years in higher-functioning persons after TBI, similar to the mortality rate of children with cerebral palsy.[232] Survival was reduced to a mean of 15 years, however, in those youngsters who were fed by tube or had no mobility for rolling, sitting, and ambulation.

Eight months after children ages 4 months to 5 years suffer a severe head injury, cognitive functions tend to recover more completely than motor skills.[233] Compared to a group of matched peers, however, children who were 6 to 15 years old at the time of a moderate to severe TBI, based on the GCS, showed significant neurocognitive, academic, and functional deficits at 1 and 3 years postinjury.[234] The head-injured youngsters scored lower in 40 out of 53 variables tested, including measures of intelligence, adaptive reasoning, memory, and psychomotor, motor, and academic performance. Their rate of improvement was strong in the first year after TBI, but it slowed markedly over the next 2 years, especially in the most severely injured youngsters.[235] The group with TBI also scored inferiorly on parent ratings of behavior and social competence. The ability to engage in abstract concept learning was seriously reduced and this impairment could, when combined with other impairments, disrupt the acquisition of cognitive skills. Discourse skills are often impaired for organizational processing and understanding the message of a story or cartoon in children who sustained a serious TBI before 8 years of age, even when language skills test normal.[236] These findings, along with the plateau reached by the more severely affected children, pose a major challenge for cognitive rehabilitation and schooling.

Mild TBI is as heterogenous in children as in adults. Residual morbidity in children who score 13–15 on the initial GCS is minimal, unless patients have neuroradiologic abnormalities on cerebral imaging.[237] Mild TBI causes more symptoms 1 week later than reported by children without TBI, but symptoms usually resolve by 3 months after injury.[238] Children who had premorbid difficulties with learning or behavioral control reported ongoing symptoms, however.

A study by Levin and colleagues showed how TBI affects normal maturation of the brain.[239] The investigators serially imaged the corpus callosum at 3 and 36 months after TBI in children who were a mean age of 10 years. Children who had severe TBI subsequently had reduced growth of this structure, whereas children with mild to moderate TBI and better functional outcomes recovered the normal enlargement of this structure over time to maturity. The corpus callosum and traversing white matter fibers are, of course, especially vulnerable to DAI. Of note, DAI is not an important mechanism of injury in nonaccidental TBI in abused infants (shaken baby syndrome), but focal axonal injury is common.[240] A secondary attention-deficit disorder after TBI in children aged 4 to 19 years old is associated with injury to the thalamus or basal ganglia.[241]

Rehabilitation for the pediatric age group must take into account age-specific neurologic, cognitive, and psychosocial development. Hyperactivity, poor attention, impulsivity, and apathy are common behavioral sequelae that may respond to behavioral strategies. Preinjury family and child functioning can explain many behavioral and academic outcomes.[242] Family adjustment and return to school require planning, support services, and long-term monitoring.[243,244] Attempts at early management of physical, intellectual, and emotional sequelae seem especially important in children. For example, after mild TBI, symptoms present 5 years postinjury tended to persist 18 years later. These symptoms correlate with diminished psychosocial adaptation.[245] Early intervention may mitigate this situation. A trial compared no intervention at 1 week after mild TBI to an assessment, information book about symptoms, and discussion about coping strategies in one visit. At 3 months, the group that did not receive the intervention reported more symptoms and stress.[238]

Geriatric Patients

The incidence of TBI rises beyond age 70, especially due to falls. Subdural hematomas, which are associated with the rapid acceleration of the brain during falls and with cerebral atrophy that allows greater stretch of bridging veins, accompany 25% of CHI in the elderly.[246] Few long-term studies of late middle-aged and elderly people have been carried out to assess the sequelae of TBI. A 5-year, prospective Finnish study of 588 people over 70 years of age found a significant decline in scores on the Mini-Mental Status Examination in participants who fell and had a major, but not minor, head injury.[247] Other studies suggest that greater disability and less likelihood of returning home follow equivalent severities of TBI in the elderly compared to younger patients.[248] Cognition may be at special risk. At a mean follow-up of 10 months postinjury, half of 70 consecutive hospitalized patients over age 50 had cognitive dysfunction not closely related to the initial severity of CHI.[249] Remarkably, 21%

had what appeared to be a dementia secondary to the trauma. An interaction between having early Alzheimer's disease or a vascular dementia and even mild TBI may manifest underlying cognitive impairments that had not previously been recognized by patients and families. It is not uncommon to find a greater decline than expected in elderly patients admitted for inpatient rehaiblitation or evaluated as outpatients after TBI. Some of that change is reversible, but the baseline dementia remains apparent.

Postdischarge support is especially necessary for many of the elderly who return home. Help is often needed for bathing, housework, shopping, and pain and medication management. With cognitive dysfunction, some elderly patients require full-time supervision.

Mild Head Injury

Commotio cerebri was described in the year 900. Its causes, symptoms, pathology, and sequelae continue to be defined.[250] The terms concussion and mild TBI are almost synonomous, as are the symptoms of the postconcussional or posttraumatic syndrome. Clinically, concussion implies a transient functional neuronal disturbance and the postconcussion syndrome implies symptoms that include both cerebral and peripheral vestibular and musculoskeletal etiologies. Persistent pathology leads clinicians to question the use of a term like minor or mild TBI. Much controversy, especially in medicolegal circles, surrounds the frequency of persistent symptoms of cognitive dysfunction.[251] Many of the disciplines of a rehabilitation team may become involved in the care of these patients, both as inpatients when mild TBI complicates a spinal or other traumatic injury and as outpatients for ongoing symptoms.

Mild TBI usually means injury severity measured by a GCS of 13 to 15, loss of consciousness for fewer than 20 minutes, and PTA for fewer than 24 hours. Patients may have some alteration of consciousness or mentation at the time of injury or persist with any memory, cognitive, or brain-related physical symptoms.[252]

Mild TBI accounts for approximately 5% of injuries in high school athletes. Two-thirds occur in football players.[253] Approximately 300,000 cases of mild TBI during sports and recreation are reported by American hospitals yearly. Many more occur. A variety of reasonable guidelines have been made about when to allow an athlete to return to play.[254] Most athletes recover by 10 days after the concussion. The combination of a learning disability and concussion in college football players appears to synergistically lower subsequent cognitive performance.[255] Amateur soccer players are also at greater risk compared to other athletes for impaired memory and plannning performance, especially after known concussion and probably associated with frequent headers to move the soccer ball.

The posttraumatic syndrome can include headache, vertigo and dysequilibrium, irritability, hypersensitivity to light or noise, malaise, insomnia, and impaired concentration and memory. Many clinicians believe that emotional factors and compensation through litigation play a role in aggravating or prolonging these symptoms. For example, a meta-analysis of mild TBI studies showed a much greater effect size for financial incentives on persistent symptoms and impairments than the effect size of injury on cognitive dysfunction.[256] Neuropsychologic testing of memory, attention, and speed of information processing at 1 week after injury, however, shows significant impairments compared to matched controls, although most patients improve by 1 month later.[200] Approximately 20% of patients will have some disability after mild TBI.[257] Although symptoms can interfere with vocational activity for an average of 3 months, some patients take 18 months or more to recover. Slowness in mental processing is less apparent after mild, compared to more severe TBI, but divided attention often suffers. For example, 1 week after a relatively mild TBI with a mean duration of PTA of 5 days, 89% of patients were impaired on the Paced Auditory Serial Addition Task (see Chapter 7) as compared to controls.[258] At 6 months, 56% were impaired. On the other hand, a matched-peer control study of mild head injury in children and adolescents did not reveal measurable differences in neuropsychologic and academic or social performance at 1 or 3 years postinjury.[259]

Cognitive dysfunction can also accompany a whiplash injury without a direct head injury.[260] Headache and neck pain are common symptoms. Neuropsychologic testing may be abnormal, especially for complex attentional tasks.

Cognitive symptoms tend to fade by 6 months after injury.

Management of mild TBI and the postconcussion syndrome includes protecting the patient from the emotional repercussions of memory impairment, inefficient information processing, and difficulty dealing with simultaneous and distracting stimuli. Education, reassurance, and stress management can reduce the time needed to be able to return to work.[257] For patients with memory dysfunction, compensatory strategies and aids limit adverse consequences on daily activities. Students with impaired divided attention may benefit from taping lectures, rather than trying to simultaneously take notes and listen in class. At home and at work, the patient should structure tasks so that only one is tackled at a time until completed. Physical therapies for headache related to soft tissue injury, antimigraine medications for posttraumatic vascular headache, and antidepressants are among the more frequently prescribed interventions. Persistence of symptoms may evolve from continuation of centrally acting medications, however.

Repeated concussions carry the potential for producing the malignant secondary impact syndrome when they occur within a short time frame. Cumulative brain injuries over years may lead to beta amyloid deposition[261] and dementia. Recurrent TBI may be the strongest environmental risk factor for Alzheimer's disease. Repeated concussion can lead to dementia pugilistica in career boxers. Indeed, a single moderate to severe TBI in young adults may at least double the risk for Alzheimer's disease later in life.[262] After a severe TBI, the risk for developing dementia later in life was four times that of the general population in one study.[219] Case-control and epidemiologic studies are inconsistent, however, in pointing to one episode of TBI with loss of consciousness as a risk factor for subsequent Alzheimer's disease.

ETHICAL ISSUES

Ethical issues arise often during rehabilitation of patients with TBI. The medicolegal demands related to a personal injury, assessment of competence of the patient to make small and large decisions,[263] the humane use of behavioral modification techniques, the application of interventions of borderline acceptance (such as coma stimulation and, recently, the absurd use of hyperbaric oxygen, and provision of appropriate postacute rehabilitation services are among the issues that draw controversy. Perhaps more so than in the rehabilitation of people with other neurological diseases, TBI brings out the issue of what constitutes a good or acceptable outcome.[264] Survivors of TBI who have persisting disabilities are also central to the social, economic, and political activities of the movement for independent living.

A pseudoethical dilemma is espoused by clinicians who want to study interventions in patients with TBI. European and North American studies of cognitive rehabilitation techniques too often state, "Given the constraint that in a rehabilitation setting it is, *for ethical reasons*, not acceptable to assign patients randomly to treatment groups or to control groups, . . . (we used a) quasi-experimental group studies . . . alternative design."[265] This constraint is iatrogenic nonsense. The process of obtaining informed consent from cognitively impaired subjects poses ethical issues, but these have been resolved in the design of clinical trials of interventions for dementia. Progress in developing cost-effective programs and specific interventions, whether functional, cognitive or neurobiologic, eventually depends on controlled, randomized comparison trials. Comparison trials of safe interventions cannot be unethical when clinicians do not know whether one approach is truly better than another.

SUMMARY

Brain injury rehabilitation must take an especially broad, holistic approach. The range of disabilities, many of them tied to cognitive and neurobehavioral impairments, along with the wide range of ages of patients, demand alternatives for therapy settings, styles of treatment, and functional goals. Many strategies can be taken by the rehabilitation team. Some attempt to build recovery from our present understanding of the architecture of neurocognitive networks. Neuropsychologic tests may unveil strengths and weaknesses for targeting interventions. Such process-specific cognitive rehabilitation has not been well supported, however, by clinical trials, especially when considering memory and executive impairments. Functional skills training, education, and compensatory strategies generally show efficacy. Structured learning using procedural and declarative memory mechanisms aids cognitive and psychosocial gains. Behavioral approaches that emphasize external cues and reinforcement may best serve problems such as poor self-awareness, disinhibition and agitation, inattention, limited initiation, and poor prospective recall. More prospecting is needed to reveal the critical features of multimodal interventions. Pharmacologic augmentation has a real, if still unsteady place in the treatment armamentarium. As in other diseases that leave residual functional, greater intensity of a rehabilitative intervention is a decisive variable.

A lot of art goes into managing individual patients. Insights into efficacy of a defined approach for an individual patient can be gained by N-of-1 experimental designs. New approaches to types and intensity of retraining may arise from insights provided during functional neuroimaging, especially in relation to activity-dependent plasticity during practice. Pharmacologic and training strategies that pass the test of clinical trials can be expected to return more patients with moderate to severe TBI to home, community, school, and work.

REFERENCES

1. Sonesson B, Ljunggren B, Saveland H, Brandt L. Cognition and adjustment after late and early operation for ruptured aneurysm. Neurosurg 1987; 21:279–287.
2. Roine R, Kajaste S, Kaste M. Neuropsychological sequelae of cardiac arrest. JAMA 1993; 269:237–242.
3. NIH Consensus Development Panel. Rehabilitation of persons with traumatic brain injury. JAMA 1999; 282:974–983.
4. Thurman D, Guerrero J. Trends in hospitalization associated with traumatic brain injury. JAMA 1999; 282:954–957.
5. Miller J. Head injury. J Neurol Neurosurg Psychiatry 1993; 56:440–447.
6. Zafonte R, Wood D, Harrison-Felix C, Millis S, Valena N. Severe penetrating head injury: A study of outcomes. Arch Phys Med Rehabil 2001; 82:306–310.
7. Sorenson S, Kraus J. Occurrence, severity, and outcomes of brain injury. J Head Trauma Rehabil 1991; 6:1–10.
8. MacKenzie E, Shapiro S, Siegel J. The economic impact of traumatic injuries. JAMA 1988; 260:3290–3296.
9. Max W, MacKenzie E, Rice D. Head injuries: Costs and consequences. J Head Trauma Rehabil 1991; 6:76–91.
10. Rubin R, Gold W, Kelley D, Sher J. The cost of disorders of the brain. National Foundation for Brain Research, 1992.

11. Murdock M, Waxman K. Helmet use improves outcomes after motorcycle accidents. West J Med 1991; 155:370–372.
12. Offner P. The impact of motorcycle helmet use. J Trauma 1992; 32:636–642.
13. Rivara F, Dicker B, Bergman A, Dacey R, Herman C. The public cost of motorcycle trauma. JAMA 1988; 260:221–223.
14. Grafman J, Salazar A. Methodological considerations relevant to the comparison of recovery from penetrating and closed head injuries. In: Levin H, Grafman J, Eisenberg H, eds. Neurobehavioral Recovery From head Injury. New York: Oxford University Press, 1987:43–54.
15. Ott L, McClain C, Gillespie M, Young B. Cytokines and metabolic dysfunction after severe head injury. J Neurotrauma 1994; 11:447–472.
16. Posmantur R, Hayes R, Dixon C, Taft W. Neurofilament 68 and neurofilament 200 protein levels decrease after traumatic brain injury. J Neurotrauma 1994; 11:533–545.
17. Reilly P. Brain injury: The pathophysiology of the first hours. J Clin Neurosci 2001; 8:220–226.
18. Pettus E, Christman C, Giebel M, Povlishock J. Traumatically induced altered membrane permeability: Its relationship to traumatically induced reactive axonal change. J Neurotrauma 1994; 11:507–522.
19. Povlishock J. Traumatically induced axonal injury: Pathogenesis and pathobiological implications. Brain Pathol 1992; 2:1–12.
20. Gennarelli T, Thibault L, Graham D. Diffuse axonal injury: An important form of traumatic brain damage. The Neuroscientist 1998; 4:202–215.
21. Brooks V. The Neural Basis of Motor Control. New York: Oxford University Press, 1986.
22. Robertson C, Contant C, Narayan R, Grossman R. Cerebral blood flow, AVDO2, and neurologic outcome in head-injured patients. J Neurotrauma 1992; 9(Suppl 1):S349–S358.
23. Uzzell B, Obrist W, Dolinskas C, Langfitt T. Relationship of acute CBF and ICP findings to neuropsychological outcome in severe head injury. J Neurosurg 1986; 65:630–635.
24. Levin H, Gary H, Eisenberg H, Ruff R, Barth J, Kreutzer J, High W, Portman S, Foulkes M, Jane J. Neurobehavioral outcome one year after severe head injury: Experience of the Traumatic Coma Data Bank. J Neurosurg 1990; 73:699–709.
25. Grafman J, Salazar A, Weingartner H, Vance S, Amin D. The relationship of brain-tissue loss volume and lesion location to cognitive deficit. J Neurosci 1986; 6:301–307.
26. Garnett M, Blamire A, Corkill R, Rajagopalan B, Young J, Cadoux-Hudson T, Styles P. Abnormal cerebral blood volume in regions of contused and normal appearing brain following traumatic brain injury using perfusion magnetic resonance imaging. J Neurotrauma 2001; 18:585–593.
27. Garnett M, Blamire A, Corkill R, Cadoux-Hudson K, Rajagopalan B, Styles P. Early proton magnetic resonance spectroscopy in normal-appearing brain correlates with outcome in patients following traumatic brain injury. Brain 2000; 123:2046–2054.
28. Ashwal S, Holshouser B, Shu S, Simmons P, Perkin R, Tomasi L, Knierim D, Sheridan C, Craig K, Andrews G, Hinshaw D. Predictive value of proton mag-

netic resonance spectroscopy in pediatric closed head injury. Pedriatr Neurol 2000; 23:114–125.
29. Katz D, Alexander M. Traumatic brain injury: Predicting course of recovery and outcome for patients admitted to rehabilitation. Arch Neurol 1994; 51: 661–670.
30. Levin H, Williams D, Crofford M, High W, Eisenberg H, Amparo E, Guinto F, Kalisky Z, Handel S, Goldman A. Relationship of depth of brain lesions to consciousness and outcome after closed head injury. J Neurosurg 1988; 69:861–866.
31. Williams D, Levin H, Eisenberg H. Mild head injury classification. Neurosurgery 1990; 27:422–428.
32. Thornhill S, Teasdale G, Murray G, McEwen J, Roy C, Penny K. Disability in young people and adults one year after head injury: Prospective cohort study. Brit Med J 2000; 320:1631–1635.
33. Wilson J, Wiedmann K, Hadley D, Condon B, Teasdale G, Brooks D. Early and late magnetic resonance imaging and neuropsychological outcome after head injury. J Neurol Neurosurg Psychiatry 1988; 51:391–396.
34. Wilson J, Wyper D. Neuroimaging and neuropsychological functioning following closed head injury: CT, MRI, and SPECT. J Head Trauma Rehabil 1992; 7:29–39.
35. Reider-Groswasser I, Cohen M, Costeff H, Groswasser Z. Late CT findings in brain trauma: Relationship to cognitive and behavioral sequelae and to vocational outcome. Am J Roentgenol 1993; 160: 147–152.
36. Levin H, Williams D, Valastro M, Eisenberg H, Crofford M, Handel S. Corpus callosum atrophy following closed head injury: Detection with magnetic resonance imaging. J Neurosurg 1990; 73:77–81.
37. Bigler E. Quantitative magnetic resonance imaging in traumatic brain injury. J Head Trauma Rehabil 2001; 16:117–134.
38. van der Naalt J, Hew J, van Zomeren A, Sluiter W, Minderhoud J. Computed tomography and magnetic resonance imaging in mild to moderate head injury: Early and late imaging related to outcome. Ann Neurol 1999; 46:70–78.
39. Fontaine A, Azouvi P, Remy P, Bussel B, Samson Y. Functional anatomy of neuropsychological deficits after severe traumatic brain injury. Neurology 1999; 53:1963–1968.
40. McAllister T, Saykin A, Flashman L, Sparling M, Johnson S, Guerin S, Mamourian A, Weaver J, Yanofsky N. Brain activation during working memory 1 month after mild traumatic brain injury. Neurology 1999; 53:1300–1308.
41. Lombardi W, Andreason P, Sirocco K, Rio D, Gross R, Umhau J, Hommer D. Wisconsin Card Sorting Test performance following head injury: Dorsolateral fronto-striatal circuit activity predicts perseveration. J Clin Exp Neuropsychol 1999; 21:2–16.
42. Ricker J, Muller R-A, Zafonte R, Black K, Millis S, Chugani H. Verbal recall and recognition following traumatic brain injury: A (O-15)-water positron emission tomography study. J Clin Exp Neuropsychol 2001; 23:196–206.
43. Geerts W, Code K, Jay R, Chen E, Szalai J. A prospective study of venous thromboembolism after major trauma. N Engl J Med 1994; 331:1601–1606.
44. Kalisky A. Medical problems encountered during re-

habilitation of patients with head injury. Arch Phys Med Rehabil 1985; 66:25–29.

45. Cifu D, Kreutzer J, Marwitz J. Etiology and incidence of rehospitalization after traumatic brain injury: A multicenter analysis. Arch Phys Med Rehabil 1999; 80:85–90.

46. Haynes M. Nutrition in the severely head-injured patient. Clin Rehabil 1992; 6:153–158.

47. Young B, Ott L, Yingling B, McClain C. Nutrition and brain injury. J Neurotrauma 1992; 9(Suppl 1): S375–S383.

48. Mackay L, Morgan A, Bernstein B. Swallowing disorder in severe brain injury: Risk factors affecting return to oral intake. Arch Phys Med Rehabil 1999; 80:365–371.

49. Sobus K, Alexander M, Harcke H. Undetected musculoskeletal trauma in children with TBI or spinal cord injury. Arch Phys Med Rehabil 1993; 74:902–904.

50. Mathern G, Babb T, Vickrey B, Melendez M, Pretorius J. Traumatic compared to non-traumatic clinical-pathologic associations in temporal lobe epilepsy. Epilepsy Res 1994; 19:129–139.

51. Diaz-Arrastia R, Agostini M, Frol A, Mickey B, Fleckenstein J, Bigio E, Van Ness P. Neurophysiologic and neuroradiologic features of intractable epilepsy after traumatic brain injury in adults. Arch Neurol 2000; 57:1611–1616.

52. Salazar A, Jabbari B, Vance S, Grafman J, Amin D, Dillon J. Epilepsy after penetrating head injury. Clinical correlates. Neurology 1985; 35:1406–1414.

53. Annegers J, Grabow J, Groover R, Laws E, Elveback L, Kurland L. Seizures after head trauma: A population study. Neurology 1980; 30:683–689.

54. Temkin N, Dikmen S, Wilensky A, Keihm J, Chabal S, Winn H. A randomized, double-blind study of phenytoin for the prevention of post-traumatic seizures. N Eng J Med 1990; 323:497–502.

55. Haltiner A, Newell D, Temkin N, Dikmen S, Winn R. Side effects and mortality associated with use of phenytoin for early posttraumatic seizure prophylaxis. J Neurosurg 1999; 91:588–592.

56. Temkin N, Dikmen S, Anderson G, Wilensky A, Holmes M, Cohen W, Newell D, Nelson P, Awan A, Winn H. Valproate therapy for prevention of posttraumatic seizures: A randomized trial. J Neurosurg 1999; 91:593–600.

57. Foy P. Do prophylactic anticonvulsant drugs alter the pattern of seizures after craniotomy? J Neurol Neurosurg Psychiatry 1992; 55:753–757.

58. Dikmen S, Temkin N, Miller B, Machamer J, Winn H. Neurobehavioral effects of phenytoin prophylaxis of posttraumatic seizures. JAMA 1991; 265:1271–1277.

59. Dikmen S, Machamer J, Winn H, Anderson G, Temkin N. Neuropsychological effects of valproate in traumatic brain injury. Neurology 2000; 54:895–902.

60. Smith K, Goulding P, Wilderman D, Goldfader P, Holterman-Hommes P, Wei F. Neurobehavioral effects of phenytoin and carbamazepine in patients recovering from brain trauma. Arch Neurol 1994; 51:653–660.

61. Vermeij F, Hasan D, Vermeulen M, Tanghe H, van Gijn J. Predictive factors for deterioration from hydrocephalus after subarachnoid hemorrhage. Neurology 1994; 44:1851–1855.

62. Gudeman S, Kishore P, Becker D, Lipper M, Girevendulis A, Jeffries B, Butterworth JF 4th. Computed tomography in the evaluation of incidence and significance of post-trauma hydrocephalus. Radiology 1981; 141:397–402.

63. Cope D, Date E, Mar E. Serial computed tomographic evaluations in TBI. Arch Phys Med Rehabil 1988; 69:483–486.

64. Levin H, Meyers C, Grossman R, Sanvar M, Meyers C. Ventricular enlargement after closed head injury. Arch Neurol 1981; 38:623–629.

65. Reilly P. In normal pressure hydrocephalus, intracranial pressure monitoring is the only useful test. J Clin Neurosci 2001; 8:66–69.

66. Bergsneider M. Management of hydrocephalus with programmable valves after traumatic brain injury and subarachnoid hemorrhage. Curr Opin Neurol 2000; 13:661–664.

67. Vanneste J. Three decades of normal pressure hydrocephalus: Are we wiser now? J Neurol Neurosurg Psychiatry 1994; 57:1021–1025.

68. Pang D, Altschuler E. Low-pressure hydrocephalic state and viscoelastic alterations in the brain. Neurosurg 1994; 35:643–656.

69. Black P, Hakim R, Bailey N. The use of the Codman-Medos programmable Hakim valve in the management of patients with hydrocephalus. Neurosurg 1994; 34:1110–1113.

70. Zemack G, Rommer B. Seven years of clinical experience with the programmable Codman Hakim valve: A retrospective study of 583 patients. J Neurosurg 2000; 92:941–948.

71. Koller W, Wong G, Lang A. Posttraumatic movement disorders: A review. Move Disord 1989; 4:20–36.

72. Lee M, Rinne J, Marsden C, Ceballos-Baumann A, Thompson P. Dystonia after head trauma. Neurology 1994; 44:1374–1378.

73. Ceballos-Baumann A, Passingham R, Marsden C, Brooks D. Motor reorganization in acquired hemidystonia. Ann Neurol 1995; 37:746–757.

74. Katz D. Movement disorders following traumatic head injury. J Head Trauma Rehabil 1990; 5:86–90.

75. Meythaler J, Renfroe S, Grabb P, Hadley M. Long-term continuously infused intrathecal baclofen for spastic-dystonic hypertonia in traumatic brain injury: 1-year experience. Arch Phys Med Rehabil 1999; 80:13–19.

76. Giacino J, Ashwal S, Childs N, Cranford R, Jennett B, Katz D, Kelly J, Rosenberg J, Whyte J, Zafonte R, Zasler N. The minimally conscious state. Neurology 2002; 58:349–353.

77. Multi-Society Task Force on PVS. Medical aspects of the persistent vegetative state. New Engl J Med 1994; 330:1572–1579.

78. Adams J, Graham D, Jennett B. The neuropathology of the vegetative state after an acute brain insult. Brain 2000; 123:101–112.

79. Laureys S, Goldman S, Phillips C, Van Bogaert P, Aerts J, Luxen A, Franck G, Maquet P. Impaired effective cortical connectivity in vegetative state: Preliminary investigation using PET. NeuroImage 1999; 9:377–382.

80. Ansell B, Keenan J. The Western Neurosensory Stimulation Profile: A tool for assessing slow to recover head-injured patients. Arch Phys Med Rehabil 1989; 70:104–108.

81. Passler M, Riggs R. Positive outcomes in traumatic brain injury-vegetative state: Patients treated with bromocriptine. Arch Phys Med Rehabil 2001; 82: 311–315.

82. Hosobuchi Y, Yingling C. The treatment of prolonged coma with neurostimulation. In: Devinsky O, Beric A, Dogali M, eds. Electrical and Magnetic Stimulation of the Brain and Spinal Cord. New York: Raven Press, 1993.

83. Freeman E. Coma arousal therapy. Clin Rehabil 1991; 5:241–249.

84. Radar M, Alston J, D E. Sensory stimulation of severely brain-injured patients. Brain Inj 1989; 3:141–148.

85. Mitchell S, Bradley V, Welch J, Britton P. Coma arousal procedure: A therapeutic intervention in the treatment of head injury. Brain Inj 1990; 4:273–279.

86. Rappaport M, Dougherty A, Kelting D. Evaluation of coma and vegetative states. Arch Phys Med Rehabil 1992; 73.628–634.

87. Hall K, Johnston M. Measurement tools for a nationwide data system. Arch Phys Med Rehabil 1994; 75(Suppl 12):SC10–18.

88. Jennett B, Teasdale G. Aspects of coma after severe head injury. Lancet 1977; 1:876–881.

89. Nell V, Yates D, Kruger J. An extended Glasgow Coma Scale (GCS-E) with enhanced sensitivity to mild brain injury. Arch Phys Med Rehabil 2000; 81:614–617.

90. Levin H, High W, Eisenberg H. Learning and forgetting during post-traumatic amnesia in head injured patients. J Neurol Neurosurg Psychiatry 1988; 51:14–20.

91. Hagen C, Malkmus D, Durham P. Levels of cognitive functioning. Rancho Los Amigos Hospital, Downey, CA 1972.

92. Katz D. Neuropathology and neurobehavioral recovery from closed head injury. J Head Trauma Rehabil 1992; 7:1–15.

93. Stuss D, Buckle L. Traumatic brain injury: Neuropsychological deficits and evaluatin at different stages of recovery and in different pathologic subtypes. J Head Trauma Rehabil 1992; 7:40–49.

94. Teasdale G, Pettigrew L, Wilson J, Murray G, Jennett B. Analyzing outcome of treatment of severe head injury. J Neurotrauma 1998; 15:587–597.

95. Hall K, Hamilton B, Gordon W, Zasler N. Characteristics and comparisons of functional assessment indices: Disability Rating Scale, Functional Independence measure, and Functional Assessment Measure. J Head Trauma Rehabil 1993; 8:60–74.

96. Malec J, Thompson J. Relationship of the Mayo-Portland Adaptability Inventory to functional outcome and cognitive performance measures. J Head Trauma Rehabil 1994; 9:1–15.

97. Stilwell P, Stilwell J, Hawley C, Davies C. Measuring outcome in community-based rehabilitation services for people who have suffered traumatic brain injury: The Community Outcome Scale. Clin Rehabil 1998; 12:521–531.

98. Levin H, High W, Goethe K, Sisson R, Overall J, Rhoades H, Eisenberg H, Kaliszky Z, Gary H. The neurobehavioral rating scale: Assessment of the behavioural sequelae of head injury by the clinician. J Neurol Neurosurg Psychiatry 1987; 50:183–193.

99. Corrigan J. Development of a scale for assessment of agitation following traumatic brain injury. J Clin Exp Neuropsychol 1989; 11:261–277.

100. Hanks R, Temkin N, Machamer J, Dikmen S. Emotional and behavioral adjustment after traumatic brain injury. Arch Phys Med Rehabil 1999; 80:991–997.

101. Vanier M, Mazaux J, Lambert J, Dassa C, Levin H. Assessment of neuropsychologic impairments after head injury: Interrater reliability and factorial and criterion validity of the Neurobehavioral Rating Scale-Revised. Arch Phys Med Rehabil 2000; 81:796–806.

102. Prigatano G, Wong J. Cognitive and affective improvement in brain dysfunctional patients who achieve inpatient rehabilitation goals. Arch Phys Med Rehabil 1999; 80:77–84.

103. Macciocchi S. Neuropsychological assessment following head trauma using the Halstead-Reitan Neuropsychological Battery. J Head Trauma Rehabil 1988; 3(1):1–11.

104. Boake C, Millis S, High W, Delmonico R, Kreutzer J, Rosenthal M, Sherer M, Ivanhoe C. Using early neuropsychologic testing to predict long-term productivity outcome from traumatic brain injury. Arch Phys Med Rehabil 2001; 82:761–768.

105. Malec J, Zweber B, Depompolo R. The Rivermead Behavioral Memory Test, laboratory neurocognitive measures, and everyday functioning. J Head Trauma Rehabil 1990; 5:60–68.

106. Shallice T, Burgess P. Deficits in strategy application following frontal lobe damage in man. Brain 1991; 114:727–741.

107. Nissen J, Jones P, Signorini D, Murray L, Teasdale G, Miller J. Glasgow head injury outcome prediction program: An independent assessment. J Neurol Neurosurg Psychiatry 1999; 67:796–799.

108. Novack T, Bush B, Meythaler J, Canupp K. Outcome after traumatic brain injury: Pathway analysis of contributions from premorbid, injury severity, and recovery variables. Arch Phys Med Rehabil 2001; 82:300–305.

109. Marshall L, Gautille T, Klauber M. The outcome of severe closed head injury. J Neurosurg 1991; 75:S28–S36.

110. Jennett B, Teasdale G, Braakman R, Fry J, Minderhoud J, Heiden J, Kurze T. Prognosis in a series of patients with severe head injury. Neurosurgery 1979; 4:283–289.

111. Ono J-I, Yamaura A, Kubota M, Okimura Y, Isobe K. Outcome prediction in severe head injury: Analyses of clinical prognostic factors. J Clin Neurosci 2001; 8:120–123.

112. Lobato R, Cordobes F, Rivas J, de la Fuente M, Montero A, Barcena A, Perez C, Cabrera A, Lamas E. Outcome from severe head injury related to the type of intracranial lesion: A computed tomography study. J Neurosurg 1983; 59:762–774.

113. Bricolo A, Turazzi S, Feriotti G. Prolonged post-traumatic unconsciousness. J Neurosurg 1980; 52:625–634.

114. Levy D, Carona J, Singer B. Predicting outcome from hypoxic-ischemic coma. JAMA 1985; 253:1420–1426.

115. Katz D, Kehs G, Alexander M. Prognosis and recovery from traumatic head injury: The influence of advancing age. Neurology 1990; 40(Suppl 1):276.

116. Levin H. Neurobehavioral recovery. J Neurotrauma 1992; 9(Suppl 1):S359–S373.

117. Stuss D, Binns M, Carruth F, Levine B, Brandys C, Moulton R, Snow W, Schwartz M. Prediction of recovery of continuous memory after traumatic brain injury. Neurology 2000; 54:1337–1344.
118. Caplan B. The National Institute on Disability and Rehabilitation Research TBI Model Systems program. J Head Trauma Rehabil 1996; 11:1–96.
119. Sherer M, Sander A, Nick T, Rosenthal M, High W, Malec J. Early cognitive status and productivity outcome after traumatic brain injury. Arch Phys Med Rehabil 2002; 83:183–192.
120. McMillan T, Greenwood R. Models of rehabilitation programmes for the brain-injured adult. Clin Rehabil 1993; 7:346–355.
121. Wehman P, Sherron P, Kregel J, Kreutzer J, Tran S, Cifu D. Return to work for persons following severe traumatic brain injury. Am J Phys Med Rehabil 1993; 72:355–363.
122. Cope D, Cole J, Hall K, Barrkan H. Brain injury: Analysis of outcome in a post-acute rehabilitation system. Brain Inj 1991; 5:111–139.
123. Brooks N. The effectiveness of post-acute rehabilitation. Brain Inj 1991; 5:103–109.
124. Hall K, Cope D. The benefit of rehabilitation in traumatic brain injury: A literature review. J Head Trauma Rehabil 1995; 10:1–13.
125. Gray D. Slow-to-recover severe traumatic brain injury: A review of outcomes and rehabilitation effectiveness. Brain Inj 2000; 14:1003–1014.
126. Cope D, Hall K. Head injury rehabilitation. Arch Phys Med Rehabil 1982; 63:433–437.
127. Mackay L, Bernstein B, Chapman P, Morgan A, Milazzo L. Early intervention in severe head injury: Long-term benefits of a formalized program. Arch Phys Med Rehabil 1992; 73:635–641.
128. Shiel A, Burn J, Henry D, Clark J, Wilson B, Burnett M, McLellan D. The effects of increased rehabilitation therapy after brain injury: Results of a prospective controlled trial. Clin Rehabil 2001; 15:501–515.
129. Zhu X, Poon W, Chan C, Chan S. Does intensive rehabilitation improve the functional outcome of patients with traumatic brain injury: Interim result of a randomized controlled trial. Br J Neurosurg 2001; 15:464–473.
130. Semlyen J, Summers S, Barnes M. Traumatic brain injury: Efficacy of multidisciplinary rehabilitation. Arch Phys Med Rehabil 1998; 79:678–683.
131. Salazar A, Warden D, Schwab K, Spector J, Braverman S, Walter J, Cole R, Rosner M, Martin E, Ecklund J, Ellenbogen R. Cognitive rehabilitation for traumatic brain injury: A randomized trial. JAMA 2000; 283:3075–3124.
132. Malec J, Basford J. Postacute brain injury rehabilitation. Arch Phys Med Rehabil 1996; 77:198–207.
133. Malec J. Impact of comprehensive day treatment on societal participation for persons with acquired brain injury. Arch Phys Med Rehabil 2001; 82:885–895.
134. Wade D, King N, Wenden F, Crawford S, Caldwell F. Routine follow-up after head injury: A second randomised, controlled trial. J Neurol Neurosurg Psychiat 1998; 65:177–183.
135. Willer B, Button J, Rempel R. Residential and home-based postacute rehabilitation of individuals with traumatic brain injury: A case control study. Arch Phys Med Rehabil 1999; 80:399–406.
136. Powell J, Heslin J, Greenwood R. Community based rehabilitation after severe traumatic brain injury: A randomised controlled trial. J Neurol Neurosurg Psychiat 2002; 72:193–202.
137. Granger C, Hamilton B. The Uniform Data System for Medical Rehabilitation report of first admissions for 1992. Am J Phys Med Rehabil 1994; 73:51–55.
138. Powell J, Machamer J, Temkin N, Dikmen S. Self-report of extent of recovery and barriers to recovery after traumatic brain injury: A longitudinal study. Arch Phys Med Rehabil 2001; 82:1025–1030.
139. Katz D, Alexander M, Klein R. Recovery of arm function in patients with paresis after traumatic brain injury. Arch Phys Med Rehabil 1998; 79:488–493.
140. Wolman R, Cornall C, Fulcher K, Greenwood R. Aerobic training in brain-injured patients. Clin Rehabil 1994; 8:253–257.
141. Bates E, Reilly J, Wulfeck B, Dronkers N, Opie M, Fenson J, Kriz S, Jeffries R, Miller L, Herbst K. Differential effects of unilateral lesions on language production in children and adults. Brain Lang 2001; 79:223–265.
142. Heinemann A, Sahgal V, Cichowski K. Functional outcome following traumatic brain injury rehabilitation. J Neuro Rehabil 1990; 4:27–37.
143. McLean A, Dikmen S, Temkin N. Psychosocial recovery after head injury. Arch Phys Med Rehabil 1993; 74:1041–1046.
144. Gray J, Shepherd M, McKinlay W. Negative symptoms in the traumatically brain-injured during the first year postdischarge. Clin Rehabil 1994; 8:188–197.
145. Schwab K, Grafman J, Salazar A, Kraft J. Residual impairments and work status after penetrating head injury. Neurology 1993; 43:95–105.
146. Brooks N, McKinlay W, Simington C, Beattie A, Campsie L. Return to work within the first 7 years of severe brain injury. Brain Inj 1987; 1:5–19.
147. Cifu D, Keyser-Marcus L, Lopez E, Wehman P, Kreutzer J, Englander J, High W. Acute predictors of successful return to work 1 year after traumatic brain injury: A multicenter analysis. Arch Phys Med Rehabil 1997; 78:125–131.
148. Rao N, Kilgore K. Predicting return to work in traumatic brain injury using assessment scales. Arch Phys Med Rehabil 1992; 73:911–916.
149. Wagner A, Hammond F, Sasser H, Wiercisiewski D. Return to productive activity after trauamtic brain injury: Relationship wiht measures of disability, handicap, and community reintegration. Arch Phys Med Rehabil 2002; 83:107–114.
150. Yasuda S, Wehman P, Targett P, Cifu D, West M. Return to work for persons with traumatic brain injury. Am J Phys Med Rehabil 2001; 80:852–864.
151. Sohlberg M, Mateer C. Cognitive Rehabilitation. New York: Guilford Press, 2001.
152. Stuss D, Winocur G, Robertson I. Cognitive neurorehabilitation. Cambridge: Cambridge University Press, 1999.
153. Alexander M, Benson D, Stuss D. Frontal lobes and language. Brain Lang 1989; 37:656–691.
154. Dikmen S, Machamer J, Temkin N, McLean A. Neuropsychological recovery in patients with moderate to severe head injury: Two years' follow-up. J Cin Exp Neuropsychol 1990; 12:507–517.
155. Ben-Yishay Y, Diller L. Cognitive remediation in

traumatic brain injury: Update and issues. Arch Phys Med Rehabil 1993; 74:204–213.

156. Cicerone K, Dahlberg C, Kalmar K, Langenbahn D, Malec J, Bergquist T, Felicetti T, Giacino J, Harley J, Harrington D, Herzog J, Kneipp S, Laatsch L, Morse P. Evidence-based cognitive rehabilitation: Recommendations for clinical practice. Arch Phys Med Rehabil 2000; 81:1596–615.

157. Parente R, Twum M, Zoltan B. Transfer and generalization of cognitive skill after traumatic brain injury. NeuroRehabil 1994; 4:25–35.

158. Parente R. Effect of monetary incentives on performance after traumatic brain injury. NeuroRehabil 1994; 4(3):198–203.

159. Eames P, Wood R. Rehabilitation after severe brain injury: A follow-up study of a behaviour modification approach. J Neurol Neurosurg Psychiatry 1985; 48:613–619.

160. Prigatano G. Neuropsychological Rehabilitation After Brain Injury. Baltimore: The Johns Hopkins University Press, 1986.

161. Luria A, Naydin V, Tsvetkova L, Vinarskaya E. Restoration of higher cortical function following local brain damage. In: Vinken P, Bruyn G, eds. Handbook of Clinical Neurology: Disorders of Higher Nervous Activity. Vol. 3. Amsterdam: North-Holland Publishers, 1969:368–433.

162. Glisky E, Schacter D. Extending the limits of complex learning in organic amnesia: Computer training in a vocational domain. Neuropsychologia 1989; 27:107–120.

163. Niemann H, Ruff R, Baser C. Computer-assisted attention retraining in head-injured individuals: A controlled efficacy study of an outpatient program. J Consult Clin Psychol 1990; 58:811–817.

164. Gray J, Robertson I, Pentland B, Anderson S. Microcomputer-based attentional retraining after brain damage: A randomised group controlled trial. Neuropsychol Rehabil 1992; 2:97–115.

165. Novack T, Caldwell S, Duke L, Berquist T, Gage R. Focused versus unstructured intervention for attention deficits after traumatic brain injury. J Head Trauma Rehabil 1996; 11:52–60.

166. Ponsford J, Kinsella G. Evaluation of a remedial programme for attentional deficits following closed head injury. J Clin Exp Neuropsychol 1988; 10:693–708.

167. Levine B, Robertson I, Clare L, Carter G, Hong J, Wilson B, Duncan J, Stuss DT. Rehabilitation of executive functioning: An experimental-clinical validation of Goal Management Training. J Int Neuropsychol Soc 2000; 6:299–312.

168. Glisky E. Computer-assisted instruction for patients with traumatic brain injury: Teaching of domain-specific knowledge. J Head Trauma Rehabil 1992; 7:1–12.

169. Prevey M, Delaney R, De l'Aune W, Mattson R. A method of assessing the efficacy of memory rehabilitation techniques using a "real-world" task. J Rehabil Res 1991; 28:53–60.

170. Kirsch N, Levine S, Lajiness-O'Neill R, Schnyder M. Computer-assisted interactive task guidance: Facilitating the performance of a simulated vocational task. J Head Trauma Rehabil 1992; 7(3):13–25.

171. Thomas-Stonell N, Johnson P, Schuller R, Jutai J. Evaluation of a computer-based program for remediation of cognitive-communication skills. J Head Trauma Rehabil 1994; 9:25–37.

172. Chen S, Thomas J, Glueckauf R, Bracy O. The effectiveness of computer-assisted cognitive rehabilitation for persons with traumatic brain injury. Brain Inj 1997; 11:197–209.

173. Prigatano G, Fordyce D, Zeiner H, Roueche J, Pepping M, Wood B. Neuropsychological rehabilitation after closed head injury in young adults. J Neurol Neurosurg Psychiatry 1984; 47:505–513.

174. Ben-Yishay J, Silver S, Plasetsky E, Rattock J. Relationship between employability and vocational outcome after intensive holistic cognitive rehabilitation. J Head Trauma Rehabil 1987; 2:35–48.

175. Johnston M. Outcomes of community reentry programmes for brain injury survivors. Brain Injury 1991; 5:141–168.

176. Bergquist T, Boll T, Harley J. Neuropsychological rehabilitation: Proceedings of a consensus conference. J Head Trauma Rehabil 1994; 9:50–61.

177. High W, Boake C, Lehmkuhl L. Critical analysis of studies evaluating the effectiveness of rehabilitation after traumatic brain injury. J Head Trauma Rehabil 1995; 10:14–26.

178. Rattok J, Ben-Yishay Y, Ezrachi O. Outcomes of different treatment mixes in a multidimensional neuropsychological rehabilitation program. Neuropsychology 1992; 6:395–415.

179. Christensen A-L, Rosenberg N. A critique of the role of psychotherapy in brain injury rehabilitation. J Head Trauma Rehabil 1991; 6:56–61.

180. Prigatano G. Disordered mind, wounded soul: The emereging role of psychotherapy in rehabilitation after brain injury. J Head Trauma Rehabil 1991; 6:1–10.

181. Maila K, Torode S, Powell G. Insight and progress in rehabilitation after brain injury. Clin Rehabil 1993; 7:23–29.

182. Dobkin B, Hanlon R. Dopamine agonist treatment of antegrade amnesia from a mediobasal forebrain injury. Ann Neurol 1992; 33:313–316.

183. Katz D, Whyte J, DiPasquale M. Prognosis and effects of medications on recovery from prolonged unconsciousness after traumatic brain injury. Neurology 2002; 58(suppl 3):A6.

184. Gorman L, Fu K, Hovda D, Murray M, Traystman R. Effects of traumatic brain injury on the cholinergic system in the rat. J Neurotrauma 1996; 13:457–463.

185. Masanic C, Bayley M, vanReekum R, Simard M. Open-label study of donepezil in traumatic brain injury. Arch Phys Med Rehabil 2001; 82:896–901.

186. Levin H, Peters B, Kalisky Z, High W, von Laufen A, Eisenberg H. Effects of oral physostigmine and lecithin in memory and attention in closed head injured patients. Cent Nerv Syst Trauma 1986; 3:333–342.

187. Bohnen N, Twijnstra A, Jolles J. A controlled trial with vasopressin analogue (DGAVP) on cognitive recovery immediately after head trauma. Neurology 1993; 43:103–106.

188. Whyte J, Hart T, Schuster K, Polansky M, Coslett H. Effects of methylphenidate on attentional function after traumatic brain injury. A randomized, placebo-controlled trial. Am J Phys Med Rehabil 1997; 76:440–450.

189. Mattay V, Callicott J, Bertolino A, Heaton I, Frank J, Coppola R, Berman K, Goldberg T, Weinberger

D. Effects of dextroamphetamine on cognitive performance and cortical activation. Neuroimage 2000; 12:268–275.

190. Walker-Batson D, Curtis S, Natarajan R, Ford J, Dronkers N, Salmeron E, Lai J, Unwin D. A double-blind placebo-controlled study of the use of amphetamine in the treatment of aphasia. Stroke 2001; 32:2093–2098.

191. Guidice M, LeWitt P, Berchou R, Holland M. Improvement in motor functioning with levodopa and bromocriptine following closed head injury. Neurology 1986; 36 (Suppl 1):198–199.

192. Powell J, Al-Adawi S, Morgan J, Greenwood R. Motivational deficits after brain injury: Effects of bromocriptine in 11 patients. J Neurol Neurosurg Psychiat 1996; 60:416–21.

193. McDowell S, Whyte J, D'Esposito M. Differential effect of a dopaminergic agonist on prefrontal function in traumatic brain injury patients. Brain 1998; 121: 1155–1164.

194. McDowell S, Whyte J, D'Esposito M. Working memory impairments in traumatic brain injury: Evidence from a dual-task paradigm. Neuropsychologia 1997; 35:1341–1353.

195. Waelti P, Dickinson A, Schultz W. Dopamine responses comply with basic assumptions of formal learning theory. Nature 2001; 412:43–48.

196. Spikman J, Deelman B, van Zomeren A. Executive functioning, attention and frontal lesions in patients with chronic CHI. Clin Exp Neuropsychol 2000; 22:325–338.

197. Bechara A, Tranel D, Damasio H. Characterization of the decision-making deficit of patients with ventromedial prefrontal cortex lesions. Brain 2000; 123: 2189–2202.

198. Leclercq M, Couillet J, Azouvi P, Marlier N, Martin Y, Strypstein E, Rousseaux M. Dual task performance after severe diffuse traumatic brain injury or vascular prefrontal damage. J Clin Exp Neuropsychol 2000; 22:339–350.

199. Levin H, Goldstein F, High W, Eisenberg H. Disproportionately severe memory deficit in relation to normal intellectual functioning after closed head injury. J Neurol Neurosurg Psychiatry 1988; 51:1294–1301.

200. Levin H, Mattis S, Ruff R, Eisenberg H, Marshall L, Tabaddork, High W Jr, Frankowski R. Neurobehavioral outcome following minor head injury: A three center study. J Neurosurg 1987; 66:234–243.

201. Dikmen S, McLean A, Temkin N. Neuropsychological and psychosocial consequences of minor head injury. J Neurol Neurosurg Psychiatry 1986; 49:1227–1232.

202. Dikmen S, McLean A, Temkin N, Wyler A. Neuropsychologic outcome at one-month postinjury. Arch Phys Med Rehabil 1986; 67:507–513.

203. Dikmen S, Temkin N, McLean A, Wyler A, Machamer J. Memory and head injury severity. J Neurol Neurosurg Psychiatry 1987; 50:1613–1618.

204. Wilson B. Recovery and compensatory strategies in head injured memory impaired people several years after insult. J Neurol Neurosurg Psychiatry 1992; 55:177–180.

205. Stuss D, Ely P, Hugenholtz H. Subtle neuropsychological deficits in patients with good recovery after closed head injury. Neurosurgery 1985; 17:41–47.

206. Ewert J, Levin H, Watson M, Kalisky Z. Procedural memory during posttraumatic amnesia in survivors of severe closed head injury. Arch Neurol 1989; 46:911–916.

207. Wilson B, Baddeley A, Evans J, Shiel A. Errorless learning in the rehabilitation of memory impaired people. Neuropsychol Rehabil 1994; 4:307–326.

208. Richardson J. Imagery mnemonics and memory remediation. Neurology 1992; 42:283–286.

209. Berg I, Koning-Haanstra M, Deelman B. Long-term effects of memory rehabilitation. Neuropsychol Rehabil 1991; 1:97–111.

210. Cummings J. Frontal-subcortical circuits and human behavior. Arch Neurol 1993; 50:873–880.

211. Van Zomeran A, Saan R. Psychological and social consequences of severe head injury. In: Braakman R, ed. Handbook of Clinical Neurology: Head Injury. Vol. 13. Amsterdam: Elsevier, 1990.

212. Deb S, Lyons I, Koutzoukis C. Neurobehavioural symptoms one year after a head injury. Br J Psychiatry 1999; 174:360–365.

213. Brooke M, Questad K, Patterson D, Bashak K. Agitation and restlessness after closed head injury: A prospective study of 100 consecutive admissions. Arch Phys Med Rehabil 1992; 73:320–323.

214. Corrigan J, Mysiw J. Agitation following traumatic head injury: Equivocal evidence for a discrete stage of cognitive recovery. Arch Phys Med Rehabil 1988; 69:487–492.

215. Davidson R, Putnam K, Larson C. Dysfunction in the neural circuitry of emotion regulation—a possible prelude to violence. Science 2000; 289:591–594.

216. Price L, Heninger G. Lithium in the treatment of mood disorders. N Engl J Med 1994; 331:591–598.

217. Brooke M, Patterson D, Questad K, Cardenas D, Farrel-Roberts L. Treatment of agitation during initial hospitalization after traumatic brain injury. Arch Phys Med Rehabil 1992; 73:917–921.

218. Whetsell K, Patterson C, Young D, Schiller W. Preinjury psychopathology in trauma patients. J Trauma 1989; 29:422–428.

219. Gualtieri T, Cox D. The delayed neurobehavioral sequelae of traumatic brain injury. Brain Inj 1991; 5:219–232.

220. Rosenthal M, Christensen B, Ross T. Depression following traumatic brain injury. Arch Phys Med Rehabil 1998; 79:90–103.

221. Hoslsinger T, Steffens D, Phillips C. Head injury in early adulthood and lifetime risk of depression. Arch Gen Psychiatry 2002; 59:17–22.

222. Jorje R, Robinson R, Arndt S, Strarkstein S. Comparison between acute and delayed onset depression following traumatic brain injury. J Neuropsychiatry Clin Neurosci 1993; 5:43–49.

223. Grafman J, Vance S, Weingartner H, Salazar A, Amin D. The effects of lateralized frontal lesions on mood regulation. Brain 1986; 109:1127–1148.

224. Ruff R, Niemann H. Cognitive rehabilitation versus day treatment in head-injured adults: Is there an impact on emotional and psychosocial adjustment? Brain Inj 1990; 4:339–347.

225. O'Carroll R, Woodrow J, Maroun F. Psychosexual and psychosocial sequelae of closed head injury. Brain Inj 1991; 5:303–313.

226. Zasler N, Horn L. Rehabilitative management of sexual dysfunction. J Head Trauma Rehabil 1990; 5(2): 14–24.

227. Miller B, Cummings J, McIntyre H, Ebers G. Hypersexuality or altered sexual preference following brain injury. J Neurol Neurosurg Psychiatry 1986; 49: 867–873.

228. Cohen M, Oksenberg A, Snir D, Stern M, Groswasser Z. Temporally related changes of sleep complaints in traumatic brain injured patients. J Neurol Neurosurg Psychiatry 1992; 55:313–315.

229. Kors E, Terwindt G, Vermeulen S, Fitzsimons R, Jardine P, Heywood P, Love S, van den Maagdenberg A, Haan J, Frants R, Ferrari M. Delayed cerebral edema and fatal coma after minor head trauma: Role of the CACNA1A calcium channel subunit gene and relationship with familial hemiplegic migraine. Neurology 2001; 49:753–760.

230. Levin H, Eisenberg H, Wigg N, Kobayashi K. Memory and intellectual ability after head injury in children and adolescents. Neurosurg 1982; 11:668–673.

231. McDonald C, Jaffe K, Fay G, Polissar N, Martin K, Liao S, Rivara J. Comparison of indices of traumatic brain injury severity as predictors of neurobehavioral outcome in children. Arch Phys Med Rehabil 1994; 75:328–337.

232. Strauss D, Shavelle R, Anderson T. Long-term survival of children and adolescents after traumatic brain injury. Arch Phys Med Rehabil 1998; 79:1095–1100.

233. Ewing-Cobbs L, Miner M, Fletcher J, Levin H. Intellectual, motor and language sequelae following head injury in infants and preschoolers. J Pediatr Psychol 1989; 14:531–547.

234. Fay G, Jaffe K, Polissar N, Liao S, Rivara J, Martin K. Outcome of pediatric traumatic brain injury at three years: A cohort study. Arch Phys Med Rehabil 1994; 75:733–741.

235. Jaffe K, Polissar N, Fay G, Liao S. Recovery trends over three years following pediatric traumatic brain injury. Arch Phys Med Rehabil 1995; 76:17–26.

236. Ewing-Cobbs L, Brookshire B, Scott M, Fletcher J. Children's narrative following traumatic brain injury: linguistic structure, cohesion, and thematic recall. Brain Lang 1998; 61:395–419.

237. Hsiang J, Yeung T, Yu A, Poon W. High-risk mild head injury. J Neurosurg 1997; 87:234–238.

238. Ponsford J, Willmott C, Rothwell A, Cameron P, Ayton G, Nelms R, Curran C, Ng K. Impact of early intervention on outcome after mild traumatic brain injury in children. Pediatrics 2001; 108:1297–1303.

239. Levin H, Benavidez D, Verger-Maestre K, Perachio N, Song J, Mendelsohn D, Fletcher J. Reduction of corpus callosum growth after severe traumatic brain injury in children. Neurology 2000; 54:647–653.

240. Geddes J, Hackshaw A, Vowles G, Nickols C, Whitwell H. Neuropathology of inflicted head injury in children. Brain 2001; 124:1290–1298.

241. Gerring J, Brady K, Chen A, Quinn C, Herskovits E, Bandeen-Roche K, Denckla M, Bryan R. Neuroimaging variables related to development of secondary attention deficit hyperactivity disorder after closed head injury in children and adolescents. Brain Inj 2000; 14:205–218.

242. Rivara J, Jaffe K, Polissar N, Fay G, Martin K, Shurtleff H, Liao S. Family functioning and children's academic performance and behavior problems in the year following traumatic brain injury. Arch Phys Med Rehabil 1994; 75:369–379.

243. Ylvisaker M, Hartwick P, Stevens M. School reentry following head injury: Managing the transition from hospital to school. J Head Trauma Rehabil 1991; 6:10–22.

244. Lash M, Scarpino C. School reintegration for children with traumatic brain injuries. NeuroRehabil 1993; 3(3):13–25.

245. Klonoff H, Clark C, Klonoff P. Long-term outcome of head injuries: A 23 year follow up study of children with head injuries. J Neurol Neurosurg Psychiatry 1993; 56:410–415.

246. Luerssen T, Klauber M, Marshall L. Outcome from head injury related to patient's age: A longitudinal prospective study. J Neurosurg 1988; 68:409–416.

247. Luukinen H, Viramo P, Koski K, Laippala P, Kivela S. Head injuries and cognitive decline among older adults: A population study. Neurology 1999; 52:557–562.

248. DeMaria E, Kenney P, Merriam M, Casanova L, Gann D. Aggressive trauma care benefits the elderly. J Trauma 1987; 27:1200–1206.

249. Mazzucchi A, Cattelani R, Misale G, Gugliotta M, Brianti R, Parma M. Head-injured subjects over age 50 years: Correlations between variables of trauma and neuropsychogical follow-up. J Neurol 1992; 239: 256–260.

250. McCrory P, Berkovic S. Concussion: The history of clinical and pathophysiological concepts and misconceptions. Neurology 2001; 57:2283–2289.

251. Satz P, Alfano MS, Light R, Morgenstern H, Zaucha K, Asarnow R, Newton S. Persistent post-concussive syndrome: A proposed methodology and literature review to determine the effects, if any, of mild head and other bodily injury. J Clin Experi Neuropsychol 1999; 21:620–628.

252. Report of the Quality Standards Subcommittee AAoN. Practice parameter: The management of concussion in sports. Neurology 1997; 48:581–585.

253. Powell J, Barber-Foss K. Traumatic brain injury in high school athletes. JAMA 1999; 282:958–963.

254. Collins M, Lovell M, Mckeag D. Current issues in managing sports-related concussion. JAMA 1999; 282:2283–2285.

255. Collins M, Grindel S, Lovell M, Dede D, Moser D, Phalin B, Nogle S, Wasik M, Cordry D, Daugherty K, Sears S, Nicolette G, Indelicato P, McKeag D. Relationship betwen concussion and neuropsychological performance in college football players. JAMA 1999; 282:964–970.

256. Binder L, Rohling M, Larrabee G. A review of mild traumatic head trauma. Part I: Meta-analytic review of neuropsychological studies. J Clin Experi Neuropsychol 1997; 19:421–431.

257. Levin H, Hamilton W, Grossman R. Outcome after head injury. In: Braakman R, ed. Handbook of Clinical Neurology. Vol. 13. Amsterdam: Elsevier, 1990: 367–395.

258. Gronwall D. Paced auditory serial-addition task: A measure of recovery from concussion. Percept Mot Skills 1977; 44:367–373.

259. Fay G, Jaffe K, Polissar N, Liao S, Martin K, Shurtleff H, Rivara J, Winn H. Mild pediatric trauma brain injury: A cohort study. Arch Phys Med Rehabil 1993; 74:895–901.

260. Ettlin T, Kischka U, Reichmann S, Benson D, Radii E, Heim S, Wengen D. Cerebral symptoms after whiplash injury of the neck: A prospective clinical

neuropsychological study. J Neurol Neurosurg Psychiatry 1993; 55:943–948.

261. Uryu K, Laurer H, McIntosh T, Pratico D, Martinez D, Leight S, Lee V, Trojanowski J. Repetitive mild brain trauma accelerates A-beta deposition, lipid peroxidation, and cognitive impairment in a transgenic mouse model of Alzheimer amyloidosis. J Neurosci 2002; 22:446–454.

262. Plassman B, Havlik R, Steffens D, Helms M, Newman T, Drosdick D, Phillips C, Gau B, Welsh-Bohmer K, Burke J, Guralnik J, Breitner J. Docu-mented head injury in early adulthood and risk of Alzheimer's disease and other dementias. Neurology 2000; 55:1158–1166.

263. Haffey W. The assessment of clinical competency to consent to medical rehabilitative interventions. J Head Trauma Rehabil 1989; 4:43–56.

264. Banja J, Johnston M. Ethical perspectives and social policy. Arch Phys Med Rehabil 1994; 75:SC19–SC26.

265. von Cramon D, von Cramon G, Mai N. Problem-solving deficits in brain-injured patients: A therapeutic approach. Neuropsychol Rehabil 1991; 1:45–64.

Chapter 12

Other Central and Peripheral Disorders

The rehabilitation team has opportunities to enhance the function of patients who are stricken with other monophasic illnesses, such as an acute inflammatory polyradiculoneuropathy, as well as progressive, fluctuating, or chronic diseases, such as Duchenne muscular dystrophy (DMD) and multiple sclerosis (MS).

Inpatient therapy can enable the patient with MS who suffers an exacerbation or the patient with Parkinson's disease whose mobility deteriorates during an intercurrent illness to return home. Ideally, a rehabilitation life management plan can be developed for patients whose course is not static. Impairments that increasingly interfere with activities in the home and workplace can be anticipated within the framework of long-term management of chronic diseases.

As impairments and disabilities increase, patients and families need a physician with expertise in neurologic disease and in rehabilitation to provide disease-related and disability-related information, interventions for specific problems, prophylactic measures, assistive devices, counseling, and advice for caregivers. Disability-oriented outpatient therapy provides guidance and physical approaches to maintain a feasible level of mobility, personal and community activities, nutrition, speech, and respiratory function.

Disease-specific organizations such as the National Multiple Sclerosis Society and government-affiliated regional and national organizations provide educational materials, funds for aspects of patient care, and Internet and newsletter updates on medical advances. Some, such as the Muscular Dystrophy Association, offer clinics, supportive services for equipment, and therapies. Members of the rehabilitation team often join or initiate support groups that offer activities to improve fitness, psychosocial interactions, and quality of life (QOL). Some hospitals and disease-specific organizations offer day programs and organized disability-oriented programs under Medicare in a comprehensive outpatient rehabilitation facility (CORF).

This chapter supplements earlier chapters as it touches on rehabilitative practices for disabilities not yet discussed. Few controlled trials of a system of care or of a particular intervention have been undertaken. Education, problem-solving, and pulse inteventions for specific disabling conditions, however, are clearly important to the welfare of patients and families.

DISORDERS OF THE MOTOR UNIT

The rehabilitation of patients with diseases of the anterior horn cell, peripheral nerve, neuromuscular junction, and muscle depends especially on the temporal course of the specific illness, its natural history, and the distribution of weakness. Approaches to neuromuscular rehabilitation have far more similarities than differences, whether the disease affects primarily muscle or nerve.[1,2] These approaches have not changed much over the past 25 years, but better evidence for their safety and efficacy has evolved. The prospects for gene therapies,[3] molecular approaches,[4] trophic factors,[5,6] immune therapies, and approaches to regeneration of muscle[7] have raised the hopes of physicians and patients for new interventions and cures for hereditary diseases (see Chapter 2).

Best care practices aim to prevent complications of immobilization, improve selective muscle strength and limb function, prevent disuse muscle atrophy and deconditioning, optimize ventilation and oral nutrition, provide orthoses and assistive and communication devices to make ADLs more independent, manage various sources of pain especially related to overuse, restore sensation in the case of neuropathies, educate and counsel, and solve problems that limit the patient's independence or add to the burdens of caregivers. Determining a strategy for exercise within the limitations of patients that does no harm is one of the more challenging goals. Chapter 2 describes fundamental mechanisms of plasticity of muscle, especially in response to nonuse and to resistance exercises. This section emphasizes clinical approaches and evidence for efficacy.

Muscle Strengthening

RESISTANCE EXERCISE

Resistance exercise induces the gene expression that prevents atrophy and increases muscle fiber volume and force. Properly executed exercise also improves aerobic fitness and may reduce the common symptom of fatigability in patients with neuromuscular disorders. Small group and case studies have shown that selective muscle strengthening and general conditioning can be achieved by modest levels of exercise, almost regardless of the pathophysiology of the neurologic disease.[8,9] The type, intensity, and duration of a muscle contraction and the frequency and duration of exercise sessions determine whether or not strength will increase. In healthy persons, strength improves significantly by isometric resistance against 60% of the person's maximum load for a single knee extension for example. Ten repetitions each done for 5 seconds must be performed 3 times a week for 6 weeks.[10] Strengthening of atrophic muscles can be accomplished, however, by training with forces of only 20%–30% of the patient's maximum resistance. The goal is to recruit a large percentage of the musculature at an intensity that stimulates morphologic, biochemical, and histochemical adaptations (see Chapter 2). For patients with neurologic diseases, the potential confounding problem is that impaired function along the motor unit can cause rapid fatigue or may overwhelm the muscle cell's metabolic and contractile functions.

At least 12 studies have reported the effects of exercise in patients with neuromuscular diseases at 20%–70% of the force of their maximum single voluntary contraction. For example, a program of moderate resistance exercise that started at from 10% to 30% of each subject's maximum resistance enabled a group of patients with myotonic dystrophy, hereditary sensorimotor neuropathies, spinal muscular atrophy, and limb-girdle syndromes to modestly increase strength for hand grip, knee extension, and elbow flexion.[11] Over 12 weeks, these patients gradually increased the amount of resistance and the number of repetitions during isotonic exercise of one side of the body. At follow-up, both the exercised and unexercised homologous muscles had improved, up to 20% for the knee extensors. Gains were a bit larger for healthy control subjects. A neural adaptation from focused exercise and greater functional activity may account for the improvement in the unexercised muscles. The same 10 patients joined 15 others who had a mix of 4 types of neuromuscular disorders for a high-resistance exercise program 3 days a week for 12 weeks.[12] The group worked out with the maximum weight each could lift 12 times and gradually increased the number of sets of 10 repetitions and the amount of weight. The patients had a mixed response, compared to the first regimen. A measure of exercise work increased more than it had from the moderate-resistance protocol, but the elbow flexors were weaker, perhaps from overuse. Exercise for strengthening and reconditioning is also feasible and imperative after organ transplantation procedures that produce disuse and chronic illness-related myopathy.[13]

Across diseases of muscle and nerve, the stronger muscles tend to improve more than weaker ones with resistance training, and patients with less severe weakness show greater improvement in cardiovascular conditioning.[14] This finding makes sense. Patients who have more power in the large leg muscles more easily reach a level of exertion that produces a conditioning effect.

At least 6 small trials show that walking or bicycling aerobically, to maintain a heart rate of approximately 60% of maximum (calculated as 220 minus age in years) for up to 30 minutes 3 times a week for 6 weeks, improves aerobic capacity and ADLs.[9] Even patients with respiratory chain defects from a mitochondrial myopathy can improve their peak work capacity and oxidative capacity, which is associated with the expected proliferation of mitochondria in muscle that accompanies exercise in deconditioned people.[15] Of interest, the mutant rather than wild-type mitochondrial DNA proliferates in these patients, which makes the value of such training uncertain.

Although the precise relationship between the effects of strengthening and conditioning on functional outcomes is not backed by much evidence for patients with motor unit and, especially, myopathic disorders, a few generalizations can be offered. For muscle groups that are functionally important, such as the proximal arm groups for reaching and the leg groups for arising and walking, patients should have a daily home program for resistance training. Pa-

tients with very weak muscles may have to initiate selective muscle strengthening against manual resistance. The family can help with this exercise. Patients may concentrate on the upper body and trunk one day alternating with the lower body the next day. Some very weak patients may generate their maximum force in daily activities, simply moving against gravity, so additional resistance training adds little and can overwork a particular muscle group.[16] Some form of aerobic training that at least causes mild dyspnea with exertion for 20 minutes a day should also be part of the daily regimen. Modestly disabled patients tend to prefer exercise that is more practical or pleasurable than resistance training. Walking, swimming, stationary bicycling, rowing, and resisting the tension of a stretchable rubber material such as a *Theraband* as part of a flexibility and conditioning program may be more motivating and lead to greater compliance.

Aging poses another challenge to patients with chronic diseases of the motor unit, as well as patients with upper motoneuron diseases. In the absence of neurologic disease, the number of motor and sensory axons falls by up to 50% by age 80; large, fast motor units especially decrease; cross-sectional area of muscle fibers progressively declines; and a longer delay in recovery follows fatiguing exercises.[17] As a consequence, strength reductions of up to 40% may affect the leg muscles by age 70, unless patients exercise. Indeed, despite these effects of aging, even frail elderly people can improve strength in a muscle group with resistance exercises.[18,19]

Respiratory Function

Respiratory dysfunction is a prominent feature of many diseases of the motor unit.[20] Acute respiratory failure caused by a neuromuscular disease occurs most often in myasthenia gravis and the Guillain-Barre syndrome. Symptoms may not develop until the vital capacity falls to 25% of predicted. Mechanical ventilation begins as the vital capacity falls to 15 mL/kg body weight. Chronic alveolar hypoventilation eventually affects most patients with DMD, amyotrophic lateral sclerosis (ALS), and other motor unit disorders.

In DMD, the vital capacity starts to fall by about age 15 years, when the child is wheelchair dependent. At that point, nighttime intermittent positive pressure ventilation (IPPV) can prevent the symptoms of hypercarbia.[21] During the day, customized adaptive seating can improve the vital capacity. A variety of respiratory aids can prolong independence before intubation and mechanical support become necessary. One specialty program reported that continuous ventilatory support allowed 86 patients with DMD and 800 other patients in need of ventilatory support to avoid tracheostomy.[22,23] Patients and families are trained to use a daytime mouthpiece and nighttime lipseal or nasal IPPV. Some also learn glossopharyngeal breathing.

Patients with ALS can also be managed with bilevel positive airway pressure (BiPAP) or nasal IPPV when nocturnal hypoventilation intervenes. Intermittent abdominal pressure ventilation or a negative pressure ventilator helps other patients. For the latter, air is removed from under a thoracic shell, which expands the chest and sucks air into the lungs. Exercises for the diaphragm or chest wall muscles are of equivocal benefit. Tracheostomy may not be needed until the peak cough expiratory flow falls below 3 liters/second and the maximum capacity for insufflation falls below the vital capacity.[24]

Four randomized trials of nocturnal mechanical ventilation in patients with neuromuscular diseases include just 51 patients.[25] A treatment effect over the short run was significant, if modest, for lessening hyercapnea and increasing oxygen saturation and for reducing the risk of death at 1 year. The optimal form of ventilation is controversial. No comparisons are available between intermittent positive pressure and negative pressure ventilation, between volume-cycled and pressure-cycled ventilation, and most importantly, between invasive and noninvasive mechanical means. Pressure controlled ventilation using a mini-tracheostomy tube and use of a small #4 tube (a 5 mm opening) both offer advantages and drawbacks related to training, cost, suctioning, and acceptance.[26,27]

Many reports show that severely disabled ventilator-assisted individuals with neuromuscular disease are satisfied with their lives.[28] Much of the satisfaction relates to social relations and the ability to communicate with computer-assistive devices. In one community study, however, only 10% of patients with ALS

chose intubation and home ventilation, but 90% said they would choose it again.[29] Family caregivers reported significant burdens. The yearly cost may exceed $150,000.

Motor Neuron Diseases

AMYOTROPHIC LATERAL SCLEROSIS

This neurodegenerative disease has an annual incidence of up to 3 per 100,000 persons and a prevalence rate of up to 6 per 100,000 persons. Ventilator dependence or death usually occurs by 4 years after onset, but up to 20% of patients survive 10 years.

By involving both upper and lower motoneurons and bulbar control, ALS requires strategies to try to prolong self-care and maintain QOL for its victims. As patients begin to become disabled, many of their needs can be anticipated. The maximal voluntary isometric contraction of each affected muscle appears to be the most reliable technique to monitor the progress of the disease.[30] The Tufts Quantitative Neuromuscular Exam (Chapter 7) is a useful tool to measure overall impairment over time.[31] The strength of the flexors and extensors of the lower extremities, when less than 25% of the predicted maximal isometric contraction, make it much less likely that patients will be able to walk in the community.[32] When all of the hip, knee, and ankle primary movers fall below 40% of predicted torque, patients with ALS probably cannot ambulate. Of interest, greater than 50% of predicted hip flexor strength was associated with ambulation in the home and greater than 75% knee flexor strength made it 395 times more likely that the patient would ambulate in the community.

In addition to range of motion and mild resistive and walking exercises, patients with ALS may need rehabilitative interventions for spasticity, foot-drop, hand paresis, dysarthia, and dysphagia. The inertia of a spastic paretic gait and spasms usually respond to baclofen, the benzodiazepines or other antispasticity agents (Table 8–10). All antispasticity medications can worsen bulbar function, however. Levodopa/carbidopa, 25/100 mg, may relieve nocturnal movements and sometimes lessens hypertonicity. Standing can reduce leg tone temporarily. Anticholinesterase medications such as pyridostigmine, 30–120 mg, may modestly increase strength and decrease muscle fatigue for a few hours. This effect may relate to structural and functional abnormalities of the neuromuscular junction.[33] Quinine gluconate or sulfate, 250–325 mg before bed or a few times a day, can relieve cramping.

Distal weakness of the hand and wrist occurs early; a wrist extensor orthotic may permit a better grip. Wrist and finger orthotics can prolong a useful grasp and pincer movement. An AFO for foot drop, a frequent early impairment, will improve the safety of gait. Many patients use a scooter before they require fulltime use of a wheelchair. Any residual movement can be used to run a computerized augmentative communication device and voice synthsizer. A neuroprosthesis may be valuable for patients who cannot move at all (see Chapter 4).[34]

Initial dysarthria may lessen if the patient learns to speak more slowly and to exaggerate articulatory sounds. A palatal lift can reduce hypernasal speech. Augmentative devices and computer software controlled by a simple microswitch are needed eventually. Dysphagia arises from a combination of a pseudobulbar palsy from bilateral upper motoneuron loss and from tongue and other muscle denervation. Symptoms and signs of dysphagia start with cough, drooling, and slow chewing and swallowing. Some gains are made for a short time with oromotor exercises and compensatory strategies after the onset of bulbar dysfunction. A modified barium swallow can suggest therapeutic approaches (Chapter 5). Head control and the safety of oral intake improves by using a cervical collar, a steel spring head support, or a high-back wheelchair with head rest. A suctioning machine in the home may be necessary. Glycopyrrolate, from 0.5 to 1 mg, or 2.5 mg of methscopolamine taken up to 3 times daily, or amitriptyline, 10–25 mg at night, can lessen drooling and a wet voice. Caregivers should learn the Heimlich maneuver in case food lodges over the airway and should assist the patient with oral hygiene.

Before they have to make a decision about using a ventilator, most patients must decide whether they will agree to a gastrostomy (PEG) feeding tube. Some controversy accompanies the placement of a PEG in people with ALS whose forced vital capacity is below 50% of predicted, because the procedure may lead to aspiration and respiratory depression.[35] Hospice care is most helpful for patients who decide against tracheostomy and mechanical ventilation.

POSTPOLIO SYNDROME

At least 300,000 American survivors of the polio epidemic of the 1950s, along with older victims that may add another one-half million people, are at risk for the postpolio syndrome (PPS). The World Health Organization estimates 20 million people survived the polio epidemics from 1940 to 1960. Based upon a community study, 30 or more years after the poliovirus attack, new symptoms evolve in approximately 65% of survivors, which changes the lifestyle of 20%.[36] Symptoms of PPS include fatigue, weakness, joint pain, muscle cramps, and a decline in mobility. New symptoms of weakness arise in muscles originally affected. For example, previously involved bulbar muscles can again cause oropharyngeal dysfunction and dysphagia.[37] Fractures are also more frequent than expected for a matched population and occur in a weak limb.[38]

Postpolio syndrome does not reproduce the level of disability that patients originally suffered. Indeed, the clinical examination and electrophysiologic studies may detect no change over 5 years, despite new symptoms possibly related to the sequelae of the disease.[39] The functional consequences are usually modest. New difficulties were, however, reported by 260 Dutch respondents who had polio in 1956. Symptoms put limitations on their work, housekeeping, and sports in 23%, 28%, and 29%, respectively.[40] Approximately 60% reported an increase in weakness and a decline in ambulation. Overall satisfaction with life is lower in people after polio than in healthy control subjects, mostly related to the sense of diminished health, but the level of satisfaction is significantly higher in people after polio than in persons after spinal cord injury.[41]

A neural cause of new motor dysfunction has been considered as a contributor to PPS.[42] New and ongoing denervation has been found in initially weak and in uninvolved or asymptomatic muscles. Equivocal evidence for immunologic abnormalities and perhaps a new viral offensive has been described. Ongoing reorganization and age-related dropout of normal or previously injured motor neurons and of reinnervated muscles may contribute. A regenerated terminal axon and neuromuscular junction may be chronically dysfunctional. The possible fragility of elements of the reinnervated neuromuscular junction cause some concern regarding the safety of exercise that stresses these structures.

One site of muscle fatigability in PPS is at the level of excitation–contraction coupling. Weakening with exertion seems less likely to be caused by energy depletion, an accumulation of metabolites such as hydrogen ion, central fatigue, fatigue at the nerve or neuromuscular junction, or impaired excitability of the muscle membrane.[43] Slow recovery after muscle contraction, rather than neuromuscular blockade, was found in one study of patients with polio.[44] Submaximal exercise capacity in persons with polio with and without PPS is markedly reduced in association with weakness.[45] Thus, the energy cost of activity may be low enough to predispose patients to premature fatigue.

Late decline in function can also be related to imbalances in muscle strength and musculotendon length across joints, overuse of compensatory muscle actions, faulty biomechanics, overstretch of ligaments, abnormal stresses on joints, joint pain and fibromyalgia, progression of scoliosis or a kyphosis, gain of weight, and increased energy expenditure caused, in part, by these impairments. These conditions are a good starting point for looking into reversible causes of PPS. For example, years of ambulation with gait deviations such as a hip hike to clear the foot or a genu recurvatum would be expected to result in mechanical dysfunction with back, hip, or knee joint pain and overuse weakness. Attention to the mechanics of movement, selective strengthening, and stretching exercises may prevent such declines once their origins are defined.

CLINICAL TRIALS

Even in subjects with PPS, in whom fatigue from overuse of muscles is a common complaint, leg ergometry with interval exercise training improved maximal oxygen uptake by 15% and increased knee extensor strength by 30%.[46] In another study of patients with PPS, resistance exercise led to muscle strengthening by a combination of neural and muscular adaptations.[47] A 12-week program of alternating daily isometric (3 sets of 4 contractions) and isokinetic (3 sets of 12 repetitions) strengthening exercises of moderate intensity for the weak quadriceps muscle led to a significant increase in strength

and endurance.[48] A more modest exercise program had previously not increased strength in the same subjects. Thus, exercise at a level that produces selective muscle strengthening is not associated with any adverse effects in patients who had polio. The choice of which muscles to try to preferentially strengthen is important. For example, the best predictor of fast and slow velocity of walking and cadence in these patients is the torque of the plantar flexors.[49] The combination of residual strength in the ankle plantar flexors and the hip abductors predicts stride length at fast speeds. These key muscles ought to be strengthened when feasible.

Physical therapies aim to improve postural alignment during gait and sitting to place muscles in an optimal position for contractions. Gait deviations are improved with orthotic and assistive devices that decrease the energy cost of ambulation. Therapists can also treat soft tissue and joint sources of pain. Assistive devices and splints can reduce pain and lessen overuse of the weak upper extremities. Pain from carpal tunnel syndrome associated with use of a cane or wheelchair can often be treated with a wrist splint. Work and home modifications and support groups are especially valued by persons with PPS.

Randomized trials of medications to increase strength or to decrease fatigue have shown no benefit. Prednisone for strengthening and amantadine for fatigue did not improve function.[50] Pyridostigmine, an anticholinesterase inhibitor, lessens jitter, the electrophysiologic correlate of neuromuscular fatigue, but 60 mg taken 3 times a day for 6 months did not improve muscle strength, lessen fatigue, or improve QOL over the placebo contol.[51] Diminished secretion of growth hormone and its relationship to the trophic factor insulin-like growth factor (IGF-1) are leading to trials with these substances, but results from preliminary studies are not optimistic. The nocturnal secretion of growth hormone was low in a group of polio survivors compared to healthy young men. Replacement therapy for 3 months, done without any exercise, did not improve strength.[52] Resistance exercises may be critical to augment the action of any drug intervention.

Neuropathies

Despite the enormous range of etiologies of the neuropathies, a few types of rehabilitative interventions apply to most disorders that produce sensory or motor impairments. Neuropathic pain with paresthesias, hyperalgesia, lancinating pain, and hyperpathia with repetitive skin stimulation accompanies many of the neuropathies. Management is reviewed in Chapter 8. Quality of life measures for treatment usually include a pain scale.[53] Some generalizations can be made using the acute polyneuropathy of the Guillain-Barre syndrome (GBS) and focal nerve injuries as clinical models.

GUILLAIN-BARRE SYNDROME

Rehabilitation efforts are supportive during the early stage of an acute inflammatory polyradiculoneuropathy (AIP). Hand and ankle splinting and proper positioning help avoid skin sores, contractures, and pain. Range of motion and light resistance exercises may be performed unless they worsen paresthesias or induce pain after completion. A need for mechanical ventilation is associated with greater risk for a poor outcome at 1 year. In one study, 39% of ventilated and 10% of nonventilated patients could not ambulate; 81% of patients with a poor outcome had required ventilation.[54] Paralysis of the upper extremities, peak median time to maximum impairment of 10 days compared to 5 days, inexcitable nerves, and mechanical support for a mean of 63 compared to 37 days also were associated with poor functional outcomes in ventilated patients. Residual motor impairments affect from 15% to 60% of patients and tend to be the primary limitation on ADLs and leisure and work activities.[55]

Once stable, particularly following a course of plasmapheresis or immunoglobulin, work on bed mobility and movement against gravity can begin. An exacerbation may occur during inpatient rehabilitation, so daily assessments of strength and function become a focus for the team. Failure to make progress is a relative indication to try a course of intravenous immunoglobulin, up to 2.4 g/kg/day for 5 days.

During inpatient rehabilitation, fatigue and dysautonomia can slow progress in mobility and ADLs for patients with AIP. Selective strengthening exercises must avoid overworking muscles and causing discomfort. The number of repetitions and sets of isometric exercises are tailored to the patient's tolerance. In the presence of orthostatic hypotension, tilt-table exercise can help reestablish postural cardiovascular reflexes and increase vascular volume. Chapter 8 reviews other measures for treating orthostatic hypotension. Anticholinesterase inhibitors such as pyridostigmine sometimes decrease muscle fatigability. The conduction block of AIP was not reversed, nor was clinical benefit found, when a group of patients was treated with 3,4-diaminopyridine (see Multiple Sclerosis in this chapter).[56]

OTHER NEUROPATHIES

Chronic motor and sensory impairments may lessen following a mononeuropathy or peripheral polyneuropathy by one of several mechanisms. Reinnervation of muscle and of sensory receptors can follow denervation. Mechanisms for reinnervation are discussed in Chapter 2. One important point to make to patients is that resistance exercises produce neurotrophins in muscle that participate in axonal regeneration by retrograde transport and in reinnervation. Centrally, the motor and sensory representational maps for movements and sensation can change at levels from the spinal cord to the thalamus and sensorimotor cortices with task-specific exercise (see Chapter 2). To improve functional movement, the patient relearns to accomplish the skill of a movement without the complete use of the affected muscle group. Successful substitution results from practice. An orthotic device that puts active muscles at a biomechanical advantage may enable that practice.

For sensory reeducation, various strategies have been used, primarily by hand therapists. For example, the patient practices manipulating blocks with and without visual input and builds up a tactile-visual image of the edges and sizes. Next, the patient works with various textures. All along, the therapist trains touch localization. Then, the patient slowly explores everyday objects with feedback regarding size, weight, texture, and shape. The approach depends heavily on the kinesthetic input of motor manipulation. Another approach stresses retraining specific sensory inputs via rapid and slow adapting mechanoreceptors.[57] The sequence of inputs goes from pinprick to vibration at 30 Hz, followed by moving touch, constant touch, and then vibration at 256 Hz. Visual inputs are also used to help in recognition. These tasks should be combined with the application of learning principles. Both techniques aim to train the somatosensory areas to recognize a new pattern of sensory coding. Case reports of improvement with these techniques are intriguing, especially in the way they support experimental notions of experience-induced neuroplasticity (see Chapters 1 and 2).

Magnetic resonance imaging of the nerves involved by a focal compressive or inflammatory lesion may provide insight into the best physical therapy approach based upon anatomic detail. Figure 12–1, for example, delineates the edema and demyelination affecting a femoral nerve and lumbar plexus caused by a postinfectious inflammatory neuropathy. Paresthesia and pain from a thoracic outlet syndrome or from compression of the sciatic nerve by the pyriformis muscle can be identified by similar imaging and aid the planning of a trial of stretching and exercise prior to more invasive management.

The most frequent chronic polyneuropathy

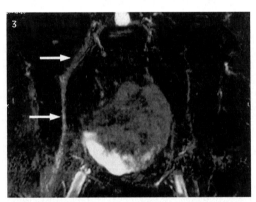

Figure 12–1. Magnetic resonance neurography shows patchy hyperintensities of the lumbar plexus (upper arrow) and especially within the femoral nerve (lower arrow). These regions were 30%–50% wider than the unaffected nerve in the other leg. The patient presented with severe right hip and thigh pain and fluctuating, progressive paralysis of the quadriceps group, sparing the iliopsoas and hip adductors, then involving the L-4 and L-5 components of the sciatic nerve as the inflammation spread a few millimeters to the junction of the lumbar plexus with the descending L-5 root. Only high dose steroids controlled and partially reversed the process. Rehabilitation efforts included pain management with gabapentin, sertraline, and an opiate analgesic; massage and stretching of thigh muscle groups that knotted with exertion; use of a scooter to protect the knee for distance mobility and crutches and then a cane for walking; fitness training using the arms and unaffected leg; and selective strengthening of affected muscle groups as they regained some function. Partial reinnervation proceeded slowly for a year. The quadriceps recovered well before the tibialis anterior and other ankle movers.

is caused by diabetes mellitus. Approximately 16 million Americans have diabetes and approximately 50% will develop one of the diabetic neuropathy syndromes. Although the distal symmetric sensorimotor polyneuropathy is most common, patients who need rehabilitation more often present with a mononeuritis multiplex or polyradiculopathy. Oxidative stress from hyperglycemia may lead to mitochondrial dysfunction and apoptosis of Schwann cells and dorsal root ganglia neurons as part of the neuropathic process.[58] Rehabilitative interventions include medications and transcutaneous stimulation for neuropathic pain, bracing that does not chafe the skin, care of diabetic foot ulcers, selective strengthening of affected muscles, and conditioning and tilt-table exercises for dysautonomia that produces fatigue and postural hypotension.

CRITICAL ILLNESS POLYNEUROPATHY

Critical illness polyneuropathy and myopathy (CIP) have become a frequent cause of diffuse weakness, deconditioning, and disabilty that requires inpatient rehabilitation.[59–61] The self-limited disorder is associated closely with sepsis, organ failure, ventilator dependence, and use of neuromuscular blocking agents and steroids. In prospective studies, CIP may affect 80% of adults and children with these risk factors. At university hospital rehabilitation centers, CIP is common in patients who have a stormy course after organ transplantation and in trauma patients. The patients have profound muscle atrophy without fasciculations, muscles feel pasty to palpation, and deep tendon reflexes may be preserved. A systemic inflammatory response evoked by sepsis appears to cause the axonal polyneuropathy, predominantly of motor axons, and myopathy.[62] The pathology of the myopathy includes nonnecrotizing and acute necrotizing involvement of fibers, or selective loss of thick myosin filaments. Most patients regain strength and mobility within a few weeks to 3 months of physical therapy, but QOL often does not recover in the first year or more after hospital discharge.[63]

We prefer to admit patients with CIP as soon as they are stable enough to begin to participate in inpatient rehabilitation, even if they do not yet have the endurance to spend 3 hours a day in active therapy. The sooner these patients get away from the stress and medical focus of the acute care setting and enter a milieu that encourages them to assist themselves, stay out of bed, and do light resistance exercises throughout the day, the quicker their progress increases. Patients are encouraged to work their arms and legs against the resistance of a stretchable rubber *Theraband* for 10 repetitions in various planes every hour, even when resting in bed. Nearly all patients who are not still encephalopathic from ongoing toxic-metabolic complications will improve their strength from movement only against gravity at admission to the ability to offer resistance in proximal muscles within 3 weeks of the inpatient stay. This gain in strength leads to the ability to move from sitting to standing and to ambulate with a walker. A prolonged foot-drop suggests a motor neuropathy from the CIP or a peroneal nerve palsy from compression of the nerve at the head of the fibula during the ICU stay, leading to the need for an AFO.

Myopathies

Although the level of resistance may have to be modified by patients with a disease of muscle, especially with an inflammatory myositis, strengthening is feasible. Eccentric exercise may cause muscle damage not brought about by isometric exercise.

The most common hereditary myopathy is DMD with its dystrophin deficiency. Dystrophin reinforces the sarcolemmal membrane of muscle fibers, so mechanical stress from an eccentric contraction could injure fibers. Strengthening is feasible, however, without inducing much of a rise in creatine kinase muscle enzyme. In DMD, weakness evolves in the hip flexors and gluteal muscles and leads to a lordotic stance, The plantar flexors are stronger than the tibialis anterior, so children walk on their toes. Tendon shortening gradually increases across all joints. Gait becomes unsafe. Some patients choose to use a wheelchair, whereas others choose to use a polypropylene knee-ankle-foot orthosis (KAFO) to prolong ambulation for 1 or 2 years. Contractures may require tendon lengthening or casting before fitting the braces, however. A spinal fusion for scoliosis is less likely to be used for DMD than for patients with spinal muscular atrophy, a congenital myopathy, or poliomyelitis, because of the inexorable course of DMD. A few other procedures have a place in long-lasting myopathies. For example, people with facioscapulohumeral (FSH) dystrophy may benefit from a thoracoscapular fusion that allows the deltoid muscle to assist abduction, elevation, and flexion of the arm.

Patients with polymyositis or with inclusion-body myositis, the most common cause of a myopathy in older adults, may have a transient rise in the creatine kinase after strength training. The elevation does not persist, whereas strength and endurance for repetitive contractions do improve.[64] In treating the inflammatory myopathies or when using steroids to manage other immune-mediated diseases, a steroid myopathy can confound the determination of whether the drug or the disease is producing proximal weakness. Disuse also augments paresis from a neuromuscular disease. Modest resistive exercise[65] and a reduction to low dose or alternate day steroids can allow strength to recover.

Muscle may respond to various drugs such as human growth hormone, insulin-like growth factor, and albuterol, a beta-2 agonist (see Chapter 2). Trials to date have not revealed efficacy of drug alone. For example, a randomized 1-year trial of albuterol and placebo in patients with FSH dystrophy revealed no overall gain in strength, although muscle mass increased by imaging and other evidence of an anabolic effect was found.[66] The subjects in this trial did not exercise in conjunction with the drug, which may have limited its effect on strengthening.

MYASTHENIA GRAVIS

Myasthenia gravis is an antibody-mediated autoimmune disease, but 15% of patients with generalized myasthenia have no detectable antibodies to nicotinic acetylcholine receptors. Over the age of 50 years, and especially over age 70 years, myasthenia gravis may affect many more patients who decline functionally than is appreciated. Up to 25% of elderly patients do not have antibodies to the receptors and others show no decrement in the evoked responses to repetitive nerve simulation. The proper diagnosis may not be considered unless physicians check for fatigability of strength with repetitive limb movements followed by rapid improvement with brief rest or after injection of edrophonium chloride. Figure 12–2

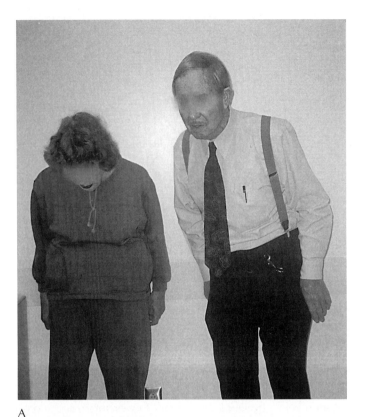

A

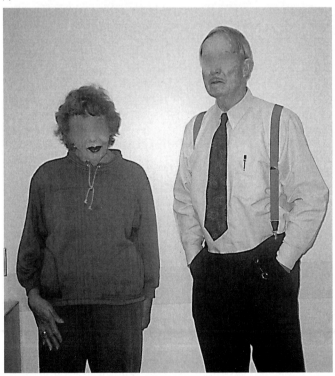

B

Figure 12–2. (A) Two patients presented with the complaint of leaning forward as they walked. No evidence for a dystonia was found. (B) Both discovered that by placing a hand across the groin on the thigh, they could right themselves and walk. The patient on the left has an ill-defined neuromuscular disease and the patient on the right has seropositive myasthenia gravis. Both have weakness of the trunk, abdominal, and pelvic muscles, which causes the forward stoop from the fulcrum of the low back. Both demonstrate fatigability with 10 repetitive movements against gravity of most arm and leg muscle groups. This weakness recedes within a minute of resting. Segmental sensory inputs across the hip appeared to activate a focused contraction for extension of some of the affected muscles, allowing erect stance. We have also seen this postural stoop sign in a patient with seronegative myasthenia gravis and in a patient with postpolio syndrome.

shows a patient with a neuromuscular disease with fatigability lessened by pyridostigmine who had no antibodies and a patient with symptoms of undiagnosed myasthenia gravis of at least 5 years duration. The patients presented with proximal weakness and profound truncal muscle paresis that caused them to lean forward after walking modest distances. Light resistance exercises and use of a rolling walker improved their mobility. Strength training will improve maximal muscle force and endurance in patients with myasthenia gravis.[67] Patients who are treated with steroids must routinely perform isometric exercises to avoid a steroid-induced myopathy.

PARKINSON'S DISEASE

Parkinson's disease is the second most common neurodegenerative disease and affects 1% to 2% of people over 65 years of age. Risk factors for the rigidity, bradykinesia, resting tremor, and postural instability include advancing age and family history. Defective genes for protein clearance through the ubiquitin-proteasome pathway, including genes for Parkin, α-synuclein, and a ubiquitin C hydrolase, cause genetically transmitted Parkinson's.[68] Genetic and environmental stressors probably cause idiopathic Parkinson's disease as proteins deposit in dopaminergic cells of the substantia nigra.

An increasing number of dopaminergic receptor agonists and drugs that prolong the effects of dopamine have joined levodopa/carbidopa and anticholinergic agents for the medical therapy of the symptoms of the disease.[69] Transplantation of cells that produce glial-derived neurotrophic factor[70] and implants of dopaminergic cells may benefit patients, if the new supply of dopamine does not induce movement disorders.[71] Unilateral pallidotomy and thalamotomy are used occasionally. Chronic high-frequency electrical stimulation by implanted electrodes in the ventral thalamus, subthalamic nucleus, or putamen can alleviate tremor and hypokinesia, but intracerebral hemorrhages and infections may complicate the implantation. Cognition may also be affected by deep brain stimulators. Bilateral stimulation of the subthalamic nucleus produced motor benefits in one trial, but induced frontostriatal circuit dysfunction (see Chapter 1) especially in older patients, causing

a decline in working memory, speech fluency, speed of mental processing, and consolidation of long-term memory.[72] Many of these interventions, however, seem to improve aspects of QOL.[73]

Interventions

Although drug therapy, deep brain stimulation, and the near-term hope of dopaminergic cell implantation dominate the approach to Parkinsons's, modest rehabilitative interventions can lessen impairments and disabilities. Indeed, physical and occupational therapy approaches may augment the benefit of the newer, more invasive therapies. Physical therapy was the only treatment for Parkinson's patients prior to the discovery of L-DOPA, although one of the first controlled trials revealed no benefit on global outcome measures.[74] The interventions, however, were based upon neurodevelopmental approaches rather than on task-oriented therapies. When training strategies take into account some of the pathophysiologic impairments of patients, outcomes can improve, at least during the intervention. Of interest, in an animal model of Parkinson's disease, forced physical activity after a lesion of the nigra helped prevent further neuronal degeneration.[75]

Bradykinesia, or slow ongoing movements, and akinesia, or the inability to make willed movements, compromise the activities of many patients. The problem partly arises from within the subcortical processes that precede and support motor cortex activation, the pattern of muscle firing, and the production of simultaneous and sequential movements.[76] Patients can, however, be trained to increase the speed of a skilled movement such as buttoning a shirt, although with more practice than healthy control subjects require.[77] Moreover, the practice of whole body movements twice a week for 3 months, along with problem-solving to best carry out these sitting, kneeling, standing up, and throwing activities, improves the speed of mobility in moderately disabled people with Parkinson's disease.[78] Range of motion activities are an important component of exercise, given that up to 12% of patients have a frozen shoulder[79] and many have limited hip flexion associated with reduced leg strength that can slow gait speed.[80]

Although large amplitude limb and truncal movements and general fitness and flexibility exercises may improve function, few studies have offered proof or insight into how best to accomplish this. A randomized, crossover study compared regular activity to 1 hour of repetitive stretching and endurance training, along with balance, gait, and fine motor exercises. The sessions were performed 3 times a week with a progressive number of repetitions for 4 weeks.[81] The Parkinson's disease patients had moderate disability ratings on the United Parkinson's Disease Rating Scale (UPDRS). The total UPDRS score and the ADL and motor subscores, particularly the bradykinesia and rigidity components, improved significantly with exercise. Depression scores and anti-Parkinson's medication dosages did not change. Without an ongoing formal exercise program, patients lost their gains 6 months later. Another study found that the combination of drug treatment and physical therapy improved some measures of motor performance.[82] Associated with passive, active, and walking exercises, the walking speed of the treated patients improved.

Approaches that employ cued movements are especially interesting. For example, visual, auditory, and somatosensory stimuli of an appropriate intensity, frequency, and timing during gait may trigger muscle activation to improve locomotion. Patients with Parkinson's disease often have reduced range of motion at the hip, knee, and ankle joints along with greater flexion in the trunk, which results in a short stride length, suggesting that patients have a motor set deficit in regulating movement amplitude. In one study, visual cues such as stepping to reach targets improved several measures of gait.[83] Visual feedback during walking may reduce a patient's reliance on kinesthetic feedback. In a well-designed trial, patients increased their stride length and walking velocity by 30%, into the range for healthy controls, by using taped step length markers and by a subject-mounted, laser light device that also cued the patients to take longer steps.[84]

The cerebral circuit activated by visually cued walking in patients with Parkinson's disease is the lateral premotor cortex, which especially responds to external cues needed for axial and proximal limb movements, along with the posterior parietal cortex and the cerebellum.[85] Failure of the basal ganglia-supplementary motor cortex circuit to elaborate an internally driven motor sequence may make patients more likely to respond to external triggers for walking. The auditory stimulus of rhythmic music, for example, entrains faster stepping and increases stride length.[86] A randomized trial compared 4 weeks of inpatient rehabilitation to no treatment of patients with moderate parkinsonian disability. The therapy emphasized rhythmic movements with visual and auditory cues, movement speed, gait, ADLs, and speech intelligibility.[87] The treated group improved significantly on the FIM, the UPDRS, and walking speed at the end of the intervention, but much of this gain reversed itself by 6 months after treatment stopped.

The mechanical and multisensory effects of practice in walking on a moving treadmill belt may enhance the rhythmicity of locomotion or at least allow step training for balance, strengthening, and fitness. For patients at risk for falls, an overhead support device is attached to a harness worn by the patient. Greater stepping speed and postural control was entrained using BWSTT for 4 weeks with 20% weight support, compared to conventional gait training.[88] The benefit may arise from inducing practice with greater hip extension caused by the moving belt and by training at speeds that exceed the patient's usual overground walking velocity. A solidly balanced rolling walker with large wheels can improve the automaticity of stepping, but it may encourage unsafe festination in some patients.

Fatigue is one of the most common symptoms in parkinsonian patients, affecting approximately 60%. Studies suggest that fatigue and poor exercise tolerance especially affect the most rigid and hypokinetic side of the body.[89] The fatigue lessens with levodopa treatment, suggesting that the effortfulness of movement or the central dopamine deficiency itself causes fatigue. Orthostatic hypotension and depression may add to fatigue and to cognitive dysfunction. The prevalence of depression is approximately 40% and is associated with neuronal loss in the locus coeruleus at autopsy and with reduction of postsynaptic 5-hydroxytryptamine binding in the cortex.[90] Thus, serotonergic and noradrenergic antidepressants ought to be most effective.

Short-term trials, then, show that parkinsonian patients can reduce their symptoms and improve their function with focused phyiscal and occupational rehabilitation therapies. Speech therapy improves prosody, breath support for speaking, and intelligibility. Delayed auditory feedback provided by an electronic device may aid self-control of volume and speed of articulation (see Chapter 5). Tremor during reaching may lessen with weighting the upper extremity, but drug therapies that include beta-blockers are more likely to help. Assistive devices such as a 4-wheel rolling walker for balance, using partial resistors on the back wheels for patients who rapidly festinate, may improve safety. Removing environmental hazards to walking such as plush carpets and raised floor thresholds also enhances safety.

Unfortunately, most health insurers make it difficult to provide formal rehabilitation for patients with a chronic disease. We have found that a 3-day inpatient rehabilitation stay immediately following implantation of a deep brain stimulator serves the patient well. Various stimulation frequencies can be tried and their value assessed during ADLs and gait. For other patients, a pulse of outpatient PT and OT to establish a home exercise program may serve them well if repeated every 6–12 months.

MULTIPLE SCLEROSIS

Multiple sclerosis carries a lifetime of prognostic uncertainty in regard to subsequent impairments, disabilities, and difficulties in participation. Opportunities for rehabilitative interventions over the short and long term depend upon the frequency and severity of attacks, the duration of remissions, the rate of progression, the secondary medical complications, symptomatic fatigue and spasticity, and the side-effects of pharmacologic treatments.

Epidemiology of Disability

Multiple sclerosis is the most common chronic disabling CNS disease of young adults, affecting 1 per 1000 people in Western countries. Although prevalence rates vary considerably among populations and studies, the sex and age-adjusted prevalence of probable and definite MS was 167 per 100,000 in Olmsted County, Minnesota.[91] Approximately 50% of patients with MS have a progressive disease by 10–15

years after onset and 50% of all patients have reached a Kurtzke Expanded Disability Status Scale (EDSS) score of 6.[92] By 15 years, approximately 20% of patients are confined to wheelchairs. By 25 years after onset, only 10%–20% walk well. Thus, approximately 50% of women with MS must use a wheelchair by 50 years of age. More favorable prognostic characteristics include onset at age less than 40 years old in females, optic neuritis or sensory symptoms at onset, a relapsing-remitting course, and a low frequency of attacks over the first 5 years.

A study from France of 1560 patients with relapsing-remitting MS at onset found that the median time to reach a score of 4, 6, and 7 on the Kurtzke Disability Status Scale was 11, 23, and 33 years, respectively.[93] The scores represent a change from limited walking up to 500 meters (EDSS 4) to walking with unilateral support no more than 100 meters without rest (EDSS 5) to walking no more than 10 meters while holding objects for support (EDSS 6). Patients with progressive disease from onset declined to those scores at 0, 7, and 13 years, respectively.

In the Olmstead County population, one-third of MS subjects had a marked paraparesis or quadriparesis, 25% required intermittent or continuous bladder catheterization, 4% required supervision for cognitive dysfunction, 53% worked fulltime, and 28% needed outside financial support. Fatigue was a significant problem for 43%. Table 12–1 shows the level of disability in these subjects based upon the Incapacity Status Scale of the Minimal Record of Disability for Multiple Sclerosis. Symptoms reported by clinic pa-

Table 12–1. **Percentage of Population with Multiple Sclerosis Needing Assistance for Activities of Daily Living**

Activity	Assistive Device	Human Assistance
Ambulation	13	28
Stair climbing	31	26
Bathing	18	23
Dressing	10	20
Transfers	14	18
Feeding	12	9

Source: Data adapted from Rodriguez et al., 1994.[91]

Table 12–2. **Symptoms in 656 Patients with Multiple Sclerosis**

Symptom	No Difficulty in ADLs (%)	Interferes With ADLs (%)
Fatigue	21	56
Imbalance	24	50
Paresis	18	45
Sensory	39	24
Bladder	25	34
Spasticity	23	26
Bowel	19	20
Memory	21	16
Depression	18	18
Pain	15	21
Lability	24	8
Visual	14	16
Tremor	14	13
Speech	12	11

ADL, activities of daily living.
Source: Adapted from Kraft G et al., 1986.[199]

tients with MS often interfere with ADLs (Table 12–2). An MS-Related Symptom Checklist of 22 items correlates with the location of the burden of plaques in patients.[94]

A comparison of scales for impairment, disability, and QOL is presented in Chapter 7. The FIM has found increasing use as a reliable and valid measure of the physical care needs of patients with MS,[95] but no single measurement tool is likely to reflect the complex interactions of a rehabilitative intervention. The Multiple Sclerosis Functional Composite Measure, which includes a timed 25-foot walk, the 9-Hole Peg Test, and the Paced Auditory Serial Addition Test (PASAT), has become the standard scale for impairment. Quality of life correlates negatively with signs of pyramidal tract, brain stem, and visual impairment.[96] Significant associations are reported between scores on tools such as the Multiple Sclerosis Quality of Life-54 (MSQOL-54) and severity of symptoms, level of independence for ambulation, employment limitations, hospital admissions, and symptoms of depression.[97] Other promising disease-specific tools include the Leeds Quality of Life Scale,[97a] the 29-item Multiple Sclerosis Impact Scale, which seems more sensitive to changes than the EDSS, and the six-item Multiple Sclerosis Walking Scale.[97b]

The morbidity and disability caused by MS may decline or be delayed as more patients come to benefit from interferon beta, interferon beta-1a, glatiramer acetate, mitoxantrone, and other agents that reduce the rate of relapses, of progression, and of the evolution of MRI lesions.[98]

Pathophysiology

Acute relapses are primarily a function of inflammatory demyelination with destruction of oligodendrocytes, invasion of T-cells and monocytes, and reactive astrogliosis. Axon cylinders are mostly spared. Clinical improvement is associated with resolution of edema and inflammation, sodium channel reorganization for conduction along demyelinated axons, and some remyelination. Axonal injury may lead to functional adaptations in the cortical representations for movements (see Color Fig. 3–7 in separate color insert), such as increased activation in cortex around a U-fiber lesion, in the supplementary motor area, and the ipsilateral primary sensorimotor cortex, and a shift posteriorly of this activation during a finger tapping task.[99,100] Thus, task-oriented practice may lead to substitution of function when restitution is incomplete (see Chapter 2). Progression of disease and disability often involves axonal transection and degeneration.[101] Most patients have a relapsing-remitting course for the first 8–15 years that transforms into a secondary progressive course. By that time, mechanisms of partial network sparing and representational plasticity may be unable to serve a substitute function.

Rehabilitative Interventions

Problems such as spasticity, paresis, sensory loss, dysarthria, dysphagia, a neurogenic bladder that affects up to 75% of patients with detrusor hyperreflexic or detrusor–sphincter dyssynergia, sexual dysfunction, cognitive impairment, paroxysmal pain, and functional disabilities are managed much as they would be for patients with stroke or SCI. Frontal lobe demyelination often results in euphoria or emotional lability.

Treatments for spasticity are reviewed in Chapter 8. A Cochrane review of the use of antispasticity agents in patients with MS concludes that of the 23 placebo-controlled trials and 13 comparative trials that met selection criteria, only 3 showed a statistically significant difference between test drugs.[102] As is the case for most trials of such agents, the absolute and comparative efficacy and tolerability make guidelines for the use of these drugs difficult. Clinicians and patients must set a goal for the continued administration of agents, try drug holidays, and experiment with different agents to make certain the substances truly reduce spasms or clonus that interferes with ADLs, have some positive affect on movement, lessen pain from spasms or severe hypertonicity, or improve perineal accessibility and care for the immobile patient. Tizanidine has the most consistent effect on the Ashworth score for measuring clinical hypertonicity,[103,104] but functional changes are rarely documented beyond this passive range of motion test. Transcutaneous nerve stimulation sometimes decreases painful spasms when placed over the affected muscles.[105]

As in SCI, the advent of intermittent bladder catheterization by a clean technique has probably reduced morbidity and mortality more than any other recent intervention. Drugs that increase bladder capacity are especially valuable adjuncts (see Chapter 8). Although cognitive and especially frontal executive dysfunction accompany the disconnections by white matter plaques in up to 50% of people with MS, global intellectual impairment is unusual.[106] The PASAT evaluates concentration and working memory and the Mini–Mental Status Examination is a useful serial measure.[107] Compensatory memory strategies (see Table 11–16) can aid patients who develop mild subcortical dementia-like impairments.

The Beck Depression Inventory or other simple tools reveal that 30%–40% of patients are depressed during the time of the illness.[108] Depression may relate to both physiologic and psychologic factors. Counseling and education may help patients lessen their sense of loss of self-image and feelings of vulnerability as physical impairments and disabilities alter their lives. Support groups that share feelings and problem-solving strategies are invaluable to many patients and their families. Persons with MS often improve their mood with selective serotonin-reuptake inhibitors. These drugs occasionally increase spasms and hypertonicity.

Some problems are more nearly unique to patients with MS. Heat sensitivity is especially prominent, although muscle fatigue and lassitude can follow heat exposure in any patient with a neurologic disease, especially with stroke, myelopathies, or myasthenia gravis. Visual impairment from an optic neuritis may require magnifying lenses or braille materials. Diplopia sometimes responds to a prism, but patients more often prefer to cover one of their eyes, unless the resulting loss of depth perception is disabling. Pendular nystagmus causing oscillopsia often interferes with ADLs, vision, and balance. It has been successfuly reduced with isoniazid in some cases.[109] An action tremor may also respond to up to 1200 mg of isoniazid or to propanolol, acetazolamide, glutethemide, benzodiazepines, or mysoline, although functional gains are generally modest. Deep brain electrical stimulation lessens tremor in some instances. Limb ataxia can be dampened by slightly weighting the distal limb or the utensils used by the patient. Paroxysmal pain can be treated with carbamazepine and other interventions for central pain and dysesthesia (see Chapter 8). Motorized scooters enable community mobility for persons with MS who find walking to be too effortful or unsafe.

FATIGUE

Fatigability is the most serious symptom for 40% of patients with MS. Its possible origins include impaired central conduction that increases paresis with activity, slowed neural processing, increases in body temperature that affect conduction velocity, and exhausting efforts related to impairments. Patients with MS demonstrate more fatigue than healthy contol subjects during sustained muscle contractions, repetitive contractions, and ambulation; this fatigability does not necessarily involve muscle groups that are most affected by the disease.[110] The fatigue is not limited to physical activities. In a single session of cognitive testing, greater self-reported fatigue and a decline in scores on neuropsychologic tests of visual and verbal memory and of verbal fluency were found for patients with MS compared to healthy controls.[111] The healthy subjects tended to improve with a sustained effort. Patients often complain of fatigue during continuous concentration.

The symptoms and signs of fatigue are not readily measured. Fatigue in MS is not an all-

or-none phenomenon; it varies in severity and with differing circumstances, and it is largely subjective. Thus, tight correlations between pathology, physiology, and clinical measures are unlikely. Some important relationships have been found, however.

Miller and colleagues[112] related biochemical changes in the muscles of patients with spastic paraparesis to their greater than normal fatigability. With repetitive electrical stimulation of the peroneal nerve, the tetanic decline in tension of the tibialis anterior muscle and the decline in phosphocreatine and intracellular pH was greater than in normal controls. Also, the half-relaxation time was prolonged; this is the number of milliseconds from the time of the last stimulus to the time at which the peak tension had decayed by half. The investigators believe this prolongation reflects a reduced rate of ATP production and slowed calcium ATPase activity in the membrane of the sarcoplasmic reticulum. At least some aspects of fatigability with central lesions, then, may arise from secondary changes in muscle fibers associated with altered metabolism. Secondary changes in muscle may also contribute to stretch-related hypertonicity (see Chapters 2 and 8).

An electrophysiologic study by Sheean and colleagues[113] found an abnormal 45% decline in strength during maximum muscle contractions compared to a 20% decline in healthy controls. Using transcranial magnetic stimulation and EMG responses, the mechanism of fatigability did not appear related to a frequency-dependent conduction block or to a decline in maximum speed of voluntary movements. Of course, TMS only tests the pyramidal tract from BA 4, so other descending pathways or ascending modulating pathways from sensory or cerebellar inputs to motor cortex may yet be implicated in activity-dependent conduction block. The degree of exercise-induced fatigue did not correlate with the usual level of symptomatic fatigue of patients, so other factors must be at play. Lack of motivation was not an important cause of fatigue in this study. Symptoms of fatigue also do not correlate with the MRI measure of regional and global numbers of plaque.[114] Sheean and colleagues suggest that central fatigue in MS is most likely caused by impaired drive to the primary motor cortex. These investigators also found that 3,4-diaminopyridine lessened reports of fatigue in patients with MS and a mod-

est but significant decrease in a fatigue index derived during an exercise test with the adductor pollicus muscle.[115]

The notion of impaired cortical drive as a mechanism of fatigue is compatible with the fMRI findings shown in Figure 3–7 for a patient with demonstrable fatigability with exercise. Demyelination of the U-fibers under the primary motor cortex representation for the back and hip presumably limited sensory drive and output from this region. Functional MRI may reveal other correlates with fatigue, such as hypoactivity in corticocortical and cortico-subcortical networks for motor planning and the execution of movements. Other investigators found an association between symptoms of fatigue and a reduction in glucose metabolism by ^{18}F-fluorodeoxyglucose PET in the frontal cortex and the basal ganglia caused by subcortical demyelination.[116] Impaired motor planning or other cognitive functions associated with diminished prefrontal drive may also contribute to fatigue. An abnormal balance between cortical excitation and inhibition, based on changes in EEG frequencies during simple motor tasks, also fits with impaired function of motor-related cortices as a cause of physical fatigue.[117]

Fatigue of a different sort may arise from malaise associated with depression, from poor sleep, and from medical causes such as a bladder infection or side effect of medications. Evidence-based practices and a Fatigue Questionnaire are provided in a booklet from the Multiple Sclerosis Council.[118] Cooling, energy-conservation techniques during activities, and assistive devices can reduce fatigue for some patients. During resistive and aerobic exercises, persons with MS should drink cold fluids, exercise under a fan or in an air-conditioned environment, and, if very sensitive to overheating, try wearing a cooling jacket device.

Medications may reduce fatigability and lassitude, and improve impairments caused by a conduction block. Amantadine,[119] 100–200 mg daily, and pemoline,[120] 75 mg daily, have lessened fatigue in short-term controlled trials. Methylphenidate, d-amphetamine, modafinil, and other drugs have also been reported anecdotally to benefit occasional patients.

Long-term oral treatment with 4-aminopyridine (4-AP) at 0.5 mg/kg has also reduced fatigue.[121,122] Both 4-AP and 3,4-diaminopyridine (3,4-DAP), from 40 to 100 mg per day, block potassium channels in demyelinated axons to potentially improve conduction (see Chapter 2). The aminopyridines have improved some neurologic impairments, particularly those that are sensitive to heat.[123] In controlled trials using different methodologies, 4-AP has improved ADLs and neurophysiologic parameters in some patients,[124] but it has not clearly decreased disability in other trials.[125] It has not benefitted neuropsychologic performance either, at least in small group cross-over trials.[126] Fampridine, a sustained release form, improved walking speed compared to a placebo, but not strength or scores on the EDSS in another trial with only 10 subjects.[127] Potential adverse reactions include paresthesias, imbalance, and dizziness. Seizures have occurred at a high serum concentration. Gastrointestinal pain is more frequent with 3,4-DAP. Digitalis also restores high-frequency impulse transmission in demyelinated central and peripheral fibers and may reverse a conduction block in patients with MS.[128]

Clinical Trials

Rehabilitation-related trials include studies of exercise and of inpatient and outpatient therapy.

Disease severity and disability complicate strategies to train patients to improve muscle strength and cardiopulmonary fitness, but an individualized exercise prescription can often overcome these limitations. Muscle weakness tends to be greater with concentric than with eccentric muscle contractions, with alternating flexion-extension compared with isolated flexion movements, and with high-speed compared with low-speed contractions. This pattern is typical of upper motoneuron dysfunction. Many patients prefer pool exercise at cool temperatures, which takes advantage of the patient's buoyancy for support while allowing work against the resistance of the water.

Aerobic training by arm–leg bicycle ergometry significantly decreased fatigue, depression, and anxiety and improved fitness in a controlled trial of ambulatory MS patients.[129] Patients exercised for 30 minutes at 60% of their maximal aerobic capacity 4 times a week for 15 weeks. A fan helped cool them during exertion. Some neurologic symptoms worsened during and shortly after exercise, but no exacerbations

of MS were related to the program. Quality of life was rated as improved after the intervention, but symptoms of fatigue were unchanged. Another small trial compared a Bobath approach and a more task-oriented approach to physical therapy for approximately 15 sessions.[130] Both groups improved their mobility, but no between-group gains in walking velocity were found. The intensity of locomotor training probably did not differ much, so walking speed would not be expected to increase. Other potential flaws in this study include not having a blinded observer carry out the outcome measures and having the same therapist treat both groups. We have employed BWSTT to allow patients with MS who walk with assistive devices to practice walking at speeds that exceed their overground velocity, resulting in 15%–25% increases in velocity. This approach must be carried out with frequent periods of rest and cooling measures.

At least eight prospective and four retrospective studies of inpatient rehabilitation show the benefit of this approach to reduce disability.[131] Several well-designed trials are especially important. A randomized, wait-list controlled study of 66 patients with mild to severe secondary progressive MS used a multidisciplinary team to train the 32 inpatients to meet patient-centered goals.[132] Disability and handicap improved significantly in the treated group 6 weeks after onset of the program. On the FIM, 72% of the treated patients improved and 25% deteriorated, compared to 29% and 62%, respectively, of people in the control group. The same investigators followed 50 patients who had mostly secondary progressive MS for a mean of 15 years at 3-month intervals following inpatient rehabilitation.[133] Although neurologic status deteriorated over time, inpatient gains for disability measured by the FIM and handicap measured by the London Handicap Scale were maintained for 6 months. The physical component of QOL using the Short Form-36 (see Chapter 7) was maintained for 10 months. Thus, outpatient services may be needed within 6 months of an inpatient pulse of rehabilitation.

DAY CARE

Day care programs offer another approach to the long-term outpatient management of disabled patients with MS. Di Fabio and colleagues at the Minneapolis Multiple Sclerosis Achievement Center reported on 46 subjects with chronic progressive MS, 20 given a weekly day treatment program for 1 year and 26 who were wait-listed.[134] Their program integrated physical and occupational therapy with supportive services. The Minneapolis center has previously shown that program costs are lower than the cost of nursing home placement and such programs can extend the time until nursing home placement is necessary. In this trial, at 1 year, the treated group had significantly fewer MS-related symptoms and less fatigue with a fairly high effect size, and a trend toward less loss of functional status, again with a good effect size despite no change in level of impairment.

Although encouraging, the Minneapolis study had some potentially confounding problems that the authors recognized. The wait-listed control and treated groups were not randomized. Their subjects, who had EDSS scores of 5–8, were selected because the screening process suggested that the subjects would continue to decline without regular intervention. Although the two groups appeared similar at the time of the initial data collection, sampling bias could have confounded the results. In addition, the attrition rate for the year was approximately 30%, mostly caused by illness or moving from the area. Thus, they ended up with a rather small number of subjects compared to the 12 independent variables measured at the initial assessment. The largest number of dropouts occurred in the control group for "unknown reasons" and the dropouts were significantly more impaired than those who remained in the study. The control group did not receive any specific attention during the year of wait-listing. Along with lack of randomization, these design flaws may have biased the results and their generalizability. Finally, the clinical meaning of the outcome measures used by the investigators is unclear. No composite or dimensional scores from a QOL tool were employed. The National MS Society has made recommendations for the development of adult day services, but has not studied the efficacy of a system of care that ascribes to those recommendations.

A day program may include general physical fitness exercises, group recreation, gardening, and local travel that help maintain or build self-care and community skills, along with psychosocial supports for clients and caregivers. Interactive lectures from experts can improve education regarding disability. Supervision in a program can stabilize medical conditions and prevent secondary complications to minimize hospitalizations. The major emphasis, however, is to improve self-care and home and community ADLs, maintain or improve mobility, optimize cognitive functioning, improve emotional status and self-esteem, prevent social isolation, and give participants a chance to regain greater control of their environments. Some of the specific learning tasks may include the correct use of medications, recognizing and dealing with symptoms, optimizing nutrition and exercise, reducing stress and conflicts, using community resources, and managing emergencies, new symptoms, and psychological responses to illness. Participants share and explore ways to cope with symptoms and disabilities. Day programs also provide supports and respite for caregivers and families. Programs also ought to foster research for clinical interventions and outcomes. A program can include pilot studies of therapeutic modules to be tested for their efficacy in enhancing cognitive, emotional, and functional abilities. One potentially valuable type of trial, for example, could test the efficacy of a self-management program such as that developed by Lorig and colleagues to increase self-efficacy.[135] In their trial of people with a variety of chronic diseases, the treated group improved in important variables of health behavior—number of minutes of exercise per week, increased practice of cognitive symptom management, less health distress, and fewer hospitalizations.

Across these inpatient and outpatient trials, physical and occupational therapy interventions carried out within the milieu of other organized supports can lead to gains in fitness, physical functioning, aspects of QOL, and the need for fewer home care services. Immune suppression, immunomodulating therapies, biologic interventions such as remyelination by transplantation of oligodendrocytes or Schwann cells, and other neuroprotection and neural repair approaches will have to be combined with rehabilitation-related problem solving and interventions to try to lessen impairments and disabilities. Activity-dependent reorganizational plasticity appears to be at work throughout much of the course of the disease, so task-related motor and cognitive training should be offered if functional independence starts to wane.

PEDIATRIC DISEASES

The rehabilitation of infants and children requires clinicians to establish goals based partly upon needs at a particular chronologic and developmental stage. Realistic motor, psychosocial, educational, lifestyle, and vocational objectives must be considered throughout the disabled person's life.

Ethical issues regarding disabled children are especially vexing. Children are dependent upon the values and beliefs of parents, clergy, physicians, and the world around them. From the moment of diagnosis of cerebral palsy or of meningomyelocele, decisions must be made in the best interest of the infant or child amid clinical and moral uncetainty about treatments and their alternatives.[136] Psychologic and financial burdens and familial stress also affect decision making. Family counseling and support groups can help the child's caregivers to work through their obligations, beliefs, and courses of action. One of the dilemmas is that families, patients, and therapists often demand more physical therapy when, in the absence of good clinical trials and outcome measures, the potential benefit is uncertain.

Cerebral Palsy

Cerebral palsy (CP) is a perinatal, nonprogressive disorder that occurs in approximately 2.5 per 1000 births in developed countries. Over 100,000 Americans under the age of 18 have the symptom complex of cerebral palsy, which can include arrested or delayed motor development, cognitive impairments, and epilepsy in approximately one-third of patients.[137] In some surveys, up to one-half of victims have mental retardation. The direct and indirect costs for the 275,000 Americans with serious disability from CP is approximately $5 billion per year. The WeeFIM and FIM (see Chapter 7) appear to capture much of the disability of youngsters with spastic diplegia and quadriplegia.[138]

For rehabilitation, the most practical classification is based on which limbs are affected, the presence of hypotonia or spasticity, and the presence of a movement disorder such as athetosis. These differences among individuals increase the difficulty of studying a particular intervention. For example, in hemiplegic cerebral palsy, studies suggest abnormal spinal branching of corticospinal axons from the undamaged motor cortex to ipsilateral motoneurons.[139,140] This novel path may account for mirror movements. More importantly, this developmental neuroplasticity may offer therapy approaches that are not relevant to the patient with spastic diplegia from bicerebral periventricular leukomalacia.

Although many styles of intervention have had allure for parents and therapists, their benefits have generally not been evaluated. Most formal studies of rehabilitative interventions have been undertaken in infants and children with spastic diplegia. One controlled trial compared a program of motor, sensory, language, and cognitve stimulation to physical therapy with a neurodevelopmental (NDT) approach.[141] The infants were 12–19 months old and received either 12 months of physical therapy or 6 months of physical therapy followed by the stimulation. Over this short term, young patients in the stimulation program were more likely to walk and had a higher mental quotient. The small sample size, the uncertain longer-term implications, and the possibility that physical therapy may delay the onset of walking if primarily aimed at altering tone and pushing the child toward more normal patterns of movement, rather than practicing walking, leave rehabilitationists with intriguing questions about the best therapeutic approach. In another small study, weekly NDT for infants improved scores on tests of motor development more than monthly therapy for 6 months.[142] Although greater intensity of treatment may be a critical component of therapy, this modest intervention with uncertain between-treatment care cannot be considered a clear-cut efficacy study.

In older children and adults, EMG biofeedback,[143] fitness training,[144] and a short pulse of therapy for specific limb and trunk impairments and singular disabilities can benefit persons with well-defined problems. Few trials have applied motor learning principles or a task-oriented approach. A pilot study of BWSTT (see Chapter 6) found modest, but statistically significant gains in the ability to walk or to perform transfers in most of the 6 nonambulators and for 4 who walked with help who had had 3 sessions weekly for 3 months.[145] Subjects trained at treadmill speeds of less than 1 mph.

Muscle strengthening programs may be underutilized. Most children and adults show weakness on testing across many muscle groups. Studies with fewer than a dozen patients suggest that even a 5-year-old child can selectively increase the strength of a muscle group with 3 sessions of resistance exercises a week for 6 weeks, leading to an increase in stride length, less of a crouching gait, and higher walking velocity as cadence increases.[146] Fast walking speed rose 10% on average in youngsters who walked at 80 cm/second before treatment. The combination of strengthening the hip and knee flexors and extensors and BWSTT at speeds that reach 2 mph needs to be compared to another form of task-oriented physical therapy for walking. Adults with CP do seem very likely to benefit from a lifelong program of selective muscle strengthening and fitness exercise.

SPASTICITY

Much of the rehabilitation work in CP concerns the management of spasticity and ambulation in youngsters with spastic diplegia. One study showed that contractures of the soleus could be prevented if dorsiflexion of the ankles was maintained with a slight force for at least 6 hours within every 24 hours.[147] Such splinting can be done during sleep. Inhibitive casting and AFOs and KAFOs are often used to limit tone or to compensate for paresis.

Drug and surgical interventions for spasticity-associated complications ought to proceed from treatments with the fewest side effects that are least invasive to more risky approaches. Hypertonicity in children can be lessened with anti-spasticity medications (see Chapter 8), but their side effects and potential to excessively reduce the extensor tone needed for stance limits their use. Oral baclofen is almost always tried. Levodopa/carbidopa may lessen stiffness, muscle cocontractions, and involuntary movements in patients with extensive periventricular lesions.[148] Intrathecal baclofen has reduced tone and improved ADLs for both the upper and lower extremities and can be titrated to allow enough tone to stand and walk.[149] Nerve and motor point blocks, especially at the hip adductors, hamstrings, and triceps surae allow a more localized approach. Focal injections of botulinum toxin, combined with serial casting, splint-

ing, and physiotherapy, may improve skin care, gait, and upper extremity function and ought to be tried before more invasive procedures.[150]

Muscle-tendon recession and release surgeries for the lower extremities in children with spastic diplegia aim to improve dynamic joint alignment. Using standardized techniques at the hip (gracilis and adductor longus release), knee (semitendinosis tenotomy, semimembranosis and biceps femoris recession), and ankle (gastocnemius-soleus recession), surgery followed by physical therapy and splinting was associated with a 25% increase in walking velocity and 18% increase in stride length within 9 months and maintained 2 years later.[151] This study did not include a control group. Tendon releases must not overcorrect the shortening. Electromyography and formal gait analysis studies should precede these approaches so that the optimal muscle–tendon can be chosen to try to correct the deviations that affect ambulation. Rhizotomy of selected dorsal lumbar roots in carefully chosen spastic diplegic youngsters, followed by extensive physical therapy, can decrease tone and improve functional mobility,[152,153] although the ultimate role of the procedure is equivocal. A meta-analysis of three randomized controlled trials revealed less hypertonicity and a very modest functional improvement with rhizotomy plus PT versus PT alone.[153a] A key aspect for the design of trials of the muscle-tendon or rhizotomy interventions will require investigators to grapple with the issue of what constitutes the one or two important outcomes that lessen disability enough to make the interventions efficacious and cost-effective.

Other efforts by the rehabilitation team include improving oromotor function, speech, and swallowing disorders associated with a pseudobulbar palsy, managing cognitive and behavioral problems, and monitoring for potential orthopedic issues such as scoliosis and hip dislocation. Pain of at least moderate severity, lasting at least 3 months, is reported by two-thirds of adults with CP.[154] Most pain is experienced in the back and legs. Exercise and stretching exercises help relieve the pain in 90%.

Myelomeningocele

This neural tube defect occurs in approximately 1 per 1000 births. Approximately 75% of infants also have progressive hydrocephalus and all have an Arnold Chiari Type II malformation with caudal displacement of the cerebellar vermis and aqueductal stenosis.

A defect within the thoracic spine or at the L-1 to L-2 level generally prevents assisted ambulation in older children. At the L-3 level, approimately 50% of youngsters may walk, at L-4, approximately 67% walk, and at the L-5 and sacral levels, 80% ambulate.[155] A syrinx, symptomatic Chiari malformation, scoliosis, advancing age, and hip flexion contractures interfere with ambulation, especially in children with lesions below L-2. Overall, only approximately 30% of children become functionally independent. Early bracing can allow a child with a high lesion to walk, perhaps through adolescence, which may result in fewer bone fractures, pressure sores, and more independent ADLs. Bracing may also increase the need for orthopedic interventions and physical therapy.[156] Assistive devices may extend the age for walking despite high lesions by reducing energy requirements. Scoliosis, clubfoot, hip dislocation, shunt failure, a tethered cord, and bladder dysfunction are among the complications that may require surgical intervention. This entity is ripe for a neural repair strategy that restores innervation to the bladder or proximal muscles, perhaps by implanting peripheral nerve into the cord above the lesion and extending it out to the end organ (see Chapter 2).

BALANCE DISORDERS

Frailty and Falls in the Elderly

By the year 2020, approximately 17% of Americans will be over the age of 65 years and 45% of this group will be over the age of 75 years. The relationship between greater impairments producing greater disabilities is less linear for elderly persons who do not have a specific neurologic disease than, say, for patients with stroke. The precise pathology is often more obscure or multifactorial in people who decline physically and cognitively with aging.

Much clinical research has gone into the issues of geriatric rehabilitation, particularly related to the prevention of falls and the management of the functional disabilities that can accompany aging. The yearly incidence of falls increases from 25% among 70-year-olds living in the community to 35% after the age of 75

years; half of these elderly persons fall repeatedly.[157] Approximately 5% of falls cause a fracture and another 10% result in serious injury. Falls are a strong risk factor for placement in nursing homes.[158] For many geriatric patients, the intrinsic and external causes of falls interact (Table 12–3); a drug causes mild delirium, arthritis makes weight bearing on the knees painful, and residual impairments from an old mild hemiparesis combine to make the person stumble over a raised crack on a sidewalk. Risks for a serious injury from falls in disabled elderly persons differ from independent persons. A Finnish study associated single status, low body mass index, impaired visual acuity, use of long-acting benzodiazepines, and impaired gait with injuries in the disabled group compared to insomnia and diminished sensation in the feet from a peripheral neuropathy in the able group.[159] Weakness of the iliopsoas was another common finding in disabled subjects.

Although tests of postural instability using force plates have become a growth industry for trying to predict who is at risk for a fall, the simplest physical tests are the manual examination of leg muscle strength, balance, and

Table 12–3. **Risks Identified by Studies of Nonsyncopal Falls in Elderly Persons**

Environmental hazards
Use of sedatives and antidepressants
Cognitive impairment
Postural hypotension, often related to medication
Impaired vision
Decreased hip or knee strength
Difficulty standing up or tandem walking
Foot, knee, and hip pain or limited range of motion
Neurologic disease
  Parkinsonism
  Cervical myelopathy
  B_{12} deficiency
  Polyneuropathy
  Vestibular disorder
  Stroke with hemiparesis
  Multiple subcortical infarcts
  Normal pressure hydrocephalus
  Toxic-metabolic encephalopathy
  Seizures
  Vasovagal syncope

speed on standing up from a chair, and observation of a short walk and turning. A prospective study of persons over age 70 found that timed tests of standing in semitandem and tandem stance, walking 8 feet, and rising from a chair and sitting down five times predicted subsequent risk for disability in mobility and ADLs by 4 years later.[160]

Of interest, poor hand grip strength, which correlates with general strength, predicts a risk for falls in older persons and, if present in midlife, predicts slow walking, difficulty arising from a chair, and limitations in ADLs 25 years later.[161] Muscle weakness before age 65 years presumably lessens a person's reserve as aging-related disabilities increase. Impaired walking velocity and single-leg stance time are also associated with decreased white matter volume and a greater volume of abnormal white matter signals by MRI.[162] These lesions may predispose to dysequilibrium and falls. Indeed, a prospective study of elderly patients with dysequilibrium complaints of uncertain cause found strong associations between falls, concerns about falling, cerebral atrophy, and white matter lesions.[163]

INTERVENTIONS

Preventing falls is feasible. Most rehabilitation interventions are straight forward. Environmental hazards such as steps, loose rugs, slick floors, loose slippers, pets, poor lighting, low beds and toilets, and raised floor thresholds can be corrected. Drugs that sedate, confuse, or cause postural hypotension should be reconsidered (Table 12–4). Older persons who report symptoms of depression are at higher risk for a decline in physical performance related to mobility.[164] Counseling and antidepressant agents may improve the drive for better physical functioning, although few clinical trials show this. On the other hand, antidepressant medications, including tricyclics, SSRIs, and trazadone increase the risk for falls, especially in residents of nursing homes.[165]

Some studies find no particular characteristics during formal gait analysis that separate fallers from nonfallers,[166] but others suggest features that a visual inspection of ambulation may detect, such as reduced angular velocity of hip extension.[167]

Resistance exercises can improve leg strength and mobility even in the frail elderly.[19] A spe-

Table 12–4. Medications Most Associated with Falls in Elderly Persons

Propoxyphene

Benzodiazepines

Chlorpropamide

Anticholinergics (e.g., diphenhydramine, amitriptyline, chlorpheniramine)

Antidepressants

Barbiturates

Meperidine

cial effort should be made to assess the hip, knee, and ankle muscle groups and to strengthen weak muscles. Falls prevention also ought to include strengthening muscles that help a person arise from the floor. Supplements of human growth hormone may also increase muscle mass, but side effects, so far, outweigh physical benefits and costs.[168] Older patients may experience carpal tunnel syndrome, fluid retention, and arthralgias from growth hormone. Stretching for hip and ankle flexibility and practicing balance exercises can also help to defray some of the risks for a fall. Pain management for arthritis and other sources of discomfort during walking and assistive devices, such as canes and walkers, can also reduce risk.

The intensity of an intervention depends on the patient's setting. During the acute hospital stay of elderly patients, a geriatric rehabilitation unit was shown to improve function, decrease nursing home placements, and potentially reduce mortality.[169] After hip and knee surgery, inpatient rehabilitation benefits patients and should make them less likely to fall.[170] On the other hand, a 4-month trial of physical therapy for frail nursing home residents, which included range of motion, strengthening and endurance exercises, balance and coordination training, and work on mobility, revealed modest improvements, but not fewer falls.[171]

A physical therapy evaluation should be part of a falls assessment for the elderly person who lives at home. A controlled community trial of 301 people who had risk factors for falling and were over the age of 70 years showed a significant reduction for falls during a 1-year intervention.[172] The risk dropped from 47% in the controls to 35% in the group managed for targeted risk factors by a nurse and physical therapist. Targeted findings included postural hypotension (see Chapter 8), use of sedatives, use of more than four medications, inability to do a safe toilet or tub transfer, home environmental hazards, and impaired gait, balance, and strength.

Thus, exercise, particularly a selective program of strengthening, conditioning, stretching, and balance for physical impairments, along with practice in ADLs and community activities, should reduce the number of falls. In turn, confidence in physical skills can ease the fear of falling that puts self-limitations on the lives of the frail elderly. By designing interventions for specific physical disabilities, as well as for depressive symptoms, the rehabilitation team can prevent a downward spiral in the quality of life of elderly persons.

Rehabilitation interventions have been employed to mitigate the risk of disability in older community dwellers who live in subsidized apartments. A randomized trial compared a 9-month program for 2 hours a week of occupational therapy to a social activity control group and to an untreated control group.[173] The treated group received instruction in ADLs, instrumental ADLs, exercise, nutrition, energy conservation, adaptive equipment, and experienced a range of physical and social activities. All domains of QOL on the SF-36 significantly improved for the treated group, including physical functioning, role functioning, vitality, and mental health. Thus, health-promoting activities that are individualized and increase personal control may be a valuable addition to the prophylactic care of an aging population.

Vestibular Dysfunction

Dizziness is a common and disabling symptom. Vertigo from acute peripheral vestibular dysfunction generally improves over time, but some patients have residual unsteadiness, symptoms that can be related to mismatches in vestibulo-ocular gain, and episodic positional vertigo. During the rehabilitation of patients after traumatic brain injury or brainstem stroke, dizziness and vertigo from central vestibular dysfunction may interfere with mobility training. The neurochemistry and neuropharmacology of the central and peripheral vestibular systems are complex and far from well understood.[174] With central dysfunction, judicious trials of antihistamines, anticholinergics, and anticonvulsants may lessen symptoms that do not respond to a phenothiazine or benzodiazepine.

Debilitating psychiatric symptoms that include anxiety are associated with vestibular dysfunction.[175] A community study found that 11% of respondents reported both dizziness and anxiety.[176] Psychologic factors may exacerbate vestibular symptoms and vestibular symptoms often induce anxiety. Symptoms especially interface in patients with panic disorders. Rehabilitative movement therapies can reduce or eliminate symptoms related to unilateral vestibular hypofunction and benign positional vertigo (BPV). Pharmacologic management of an anxiety disorder along with counseling about triggers for vestibular dysfunction are needed for patients in whom panic attacks and dizziness interact.[177] Sertraline, for example, may help such patients.

Specific vestibular exercises soon after acute peripheral vestibular dysfunction may accelerate the rate of central vestibular compensation.[178] Patients with ongoing vestibular dysfunction tend to self-limit their head and eye movements. The rehabilitation approach encourages activity and specific exercises such as walking on uneven surfaces, moving in different directions with eyes open or closed, making repetitive head and body rotations and tilts, and practicing saccadic and smooth pursuit eye movements to stimuli. Vestibular Habituation Training offers a detailed method of evaluation and exercise aimed at encouraging adaptation within the connections of the vestibular pathways.[179] No controlled trials of exercises for central or peripheral vestibular symptoms have been published, however.

The incidence of BPV is 141 per 100,000 at age 50 and approximately 190 per 100,000 by age 85.[180] The attacks are triggered by debris from the otolith that gravitates through the endolymph during head positional changes.[181] When the floating material reaches the most dependent part of the canal, it settles on the cupula and produces forces that initiate short duration vertigo. A single or a series of rapid head and trunk tilting maneuvers can loosen the debris and disperse it into the cavity of the utricle.[182] In the single Semont liberatory maneuver for BPV arising from the posterior canal, patients start out seated with the head turned 45° toward the unaffected ear. They are taken from the sitting to a side-lying position with the head tilted back approximately 105° toward the affected ear, a movement that induces vertigo. They hold this position for 3 to 5 minutes. Then, they roll quickly to the opposite side with the nose down. If this induces the typical nystagmus of BPV, they hold this position for 5 minutes and then sit up very slowly. Some clinicians recommend that patients then hold the head upright for 48 hours.

ALZHEIMER'S DISEASE

This all-too-common degenerative disease affects approximately 8% of people over the age of 65 and nearly 30% of people over the age of 85 years. Direct and indirect (family caregiver) costs approach $100 billion each year.[183] Over the 8 to 10 years of progressing dementia, victims become increasingly disabled in ADLs. The centrally acting acetylcholinesterase inhibitors provide modest cognitive and behavioral benefits. Much of the focus of treatment is still on educating the family.

Physical therapy can improve mobility despite the dementia.[184] The approach to ADLs and social activities must take advantage of the ability of many patients with Alzheimer's disease to learn skills through procedural memory.[185] This motor learning depends upon corticocerebellar and striatal structures, rather than upon the mesial temporal networks that bear the brunt of the degeneration. A controlled trial showed that motor learning and the transfer of motor skills requires constant practice, rather than random, blocked, or no practice for patients with Alzheimer's disease.[186] Thus, training to help patients maintain ADLs requires consistent repetition without interference to optimize learning. Approximately 10% of nursing homes certified by Medicare and Medicaid have special care units for these patients. A study of special units, of conventional care in facilities that include special units, and of nursing homes without such units revealed no differences in the percentage of patients who declined during a 1-year follow-up.[187] Without specific practice, 30% deteriorated in ADLs such as walking, eating, dressing, and continence. Exercise and skills practice can be carried out by trained caregivers.[188]

EPILEPSY

Children with refractory epilepsy are increasing coming to surgery for a partial lobectomy or hemispherectomy.[189] Children with perinatal lesions that cause their seizures may have reorganized the brain prior to hemispherectomy and can be quite resilient, showing only modest new impairments in hand and foot function or language. Figure 12–3 (in separate color insert) reveals the network for motor control of the left and right leg during ankle dorsiflexion following a right partial hemispherectomy in a youngster who suffered a perinatal left hemispheric stroke and frequent seizures. The ipsilesional SMA and anterior cingulate cortex that were spared are highly activated along with contralesional parietal cortex and lateral BA 6. No new impairment in walking was apparent by a few months after surgery. These regions had likely reorganized during the child's development to carry out leg movements, when walking could not recruit M1 and S1 due to the stroke. Primary sensorimotor cortex of the unaffected hemisphere activates rather normally during ankle movement of the unaffected leg.

Psychosocial rehabilitation can help patients reintegrate into the community and find employment.[190] Vocational rehabilitation is especially helpful. Cognitive and behavioral rehabilitation may also be needed after a temporal lobectomy more often than remediation is offered.[190a] Both left and right temporal lobectomy patients have difficulty remembering the content of past actions, as well as whether they had performed the action, someone else had, or they imagined having carried it out. Also, emotional learning after a right lobectomy and verbal learning after a left lobectomy may be impaired. Disease-specific quality of life tools can help monitor outcomes for surgery and for new medications.[191]

CONVERSION DISORDERS WITH NEUROLOGIC SYMPTOMS

Hemiparesis, paraparesis, or monoparesis that has no neuropathologic basis can arise from a conversion disorder and from malingering. The suspicion of hysterical paralysis evolves from a history of injury that would not be expected to produce profound impairments. Sometimes, the astute clinician can discern the special psychologic meaning that the symptoms and signs hold for the patient. For example, the patient's father may have had numbness that was ignored by his physician and later the father died with a stroke. In some instances, symptoms of CNS dysfunction may have been present at the onset of, say, a transient cervical spinal cord injury with dysesthesias. Persistent disability subsequently arises from the inconsistent explanations by physicians regarding the cause of those symptoms, from repeated radiologic testing that leaves the patient suspecting that the doctors have not nailed down a definitive diagnosis and prognosis, or perhaps from an unrecognized posttraumatic stress disorder.

The examination may reveal odd patterns of sensory loss and paresis, changing examination findings, give-way weakness, unilateral loss of sensation to pin or vibration that splits the midline of the sternum or forehead, remarkably better use of the limb in a functional setting than on specific testing, and an indifferent affect. Although malingerers may behave in a similar fashion, they tend to try to convince the clinician about how disabled they are and how much they depend on a financial settlement or other secondary gain. For nonmalingerers, psychotherapy and physical and occupational therapies merged with behavioral conditioning approaches can lead to motor recovery. The physician and therapist should set definite goals with the patient, provide positive feedback and support for each small accomplishment, and not reinforce symptoms and signs of disability. Education often helps a patient better understand the original source of the symptoms.

CHRONIC FATIGUE SYNDROME

Patients with the chronic fatigue syndrome (CFS) often come to the attention of specialists in rehabilitation. A lot of sociopolitical baggage accompanies this diagnosis. Consumer groups and clinicians who believe in specific causes may villify those who do not. The prevalence of at least 6 months of new-onset fatigue unexplained by a medical diagnosis is 0.5% in American women and 0.3% in men.[192] These persons report a lower functional status than matched patients with congestive heart failure.[193] The syndrome may include fibromyalgia, depression, and an irritable bowel. Al-

though some reports have suggested abnormalities on MRI scans and by single photon emission tomography, these data have not held up in better-designed comparison studies.

General conditioning exercises and energy conservation techniques may improve daily functioning in sedentary patients. The syndrome has been associated with neurally mediated hypotension in some instances, which can respond to sodium loading,[194] but a randomized trial of fludrocortisone did not alter the course of the disease.[195] Comorbid psychiatric conditions may relieve these symptoms, but may not alter the somatic complaints. Cognitive-behavioral therapy has helped some patients and antidepressant medications may lessen the cost of care within 6 months.[193] Impaired working memory and attention on effortful tasks is common[196] and may respond to cognitive remediation strategies. A systematic review of the literature concluded that graded exercise and cognitive behavioral therapy are the most promising interventions.[197]

ACQUIRED IMMUNODEFICIENCY SYNDROME

The myriad neurologic complications of infection by the human immunodeficiency virus (HIV) require ongoing assessment and management. Rehabilitative efforts can optimize strength, mobility, fitness, ADLs, and cognition for the neurobehavioral problems, dementia, myelopathy, mononeuritis or polyneuropathy, and myopathy that can compromise patients. Fortunately, medical treatment over the past 5 years has greatly reduced the neurologic complications of the disease.[198]

SUMMARY

Rehabilitationists can find opportunities to diminish disabilities associated with every neurologic disease and any neurologic complication of a medical illness. The physician with skills in rehabilitation can serve patients well by acting as the general practitioner or "quarterback" for the person's long-term care as it relates to the disease. With a chronic or progressive central or peripheral neurologic disease, proactive interventions can sometimes delay or prevent deterioration in the quality of a patient's life. New treatments for these diseases may be more effective in reducing disability if accompanied by a rehabilitation program that emphasizes strengthening, conditioning, and task-oriented practice of motor and cognitive skills, along with psychosocial supports and assistive devices.

REFERENCES

1. Berger A, Schaumburg H. Rehabilitation of focal nerve injuries. J Neurol Rehabil 1988; 2:65–91.
2. Ringel S, Neville H. The rehabilitation of muscular disorders. J Neurol Rehabil 1990; 4:203–215.
3. Cohn R, Campbell K. Molecular basis of muscular dystrophies. Muscle Nerve 2000; 23:1456–1471.
4. Fletcher S, Wilton S, Howell J. Gene therapy and molecular approaches to the treatment of hereditary muscular disorders. Curr Opin Neurol 2000; 13:553–560.
5. Chakravarthy M, Davis B, Booth F. IGF-I restores satellite cell proliferative potential in immobilized old skeletal muscle. Appl Physiol 2000; 89:1365–1379.
6. Singleton J, Feldman E. Insulin-like growth factor-1 in muscle metabolism and myotherapies. Neurobiol Dis 2001; 8:541–554.
7. Grounds M. Muscle regeneration: molecular aspects and therapeutic implications. Curr Opin Neurol 1999; 12:535–543.
8. Dobkin B. Exercise fitness and sports for individuals with neurologic disability. In: Gordon S, Gonzalez-Mestre X, Garrett W, eds. Sports and Exercise in Midlife. Rosemont, IL: American Academy of Orthopedic Surgeons, 1993:235–252.
9. Phillips B, Mastaglia F. Exercise therapy in patients with myopathy. Curr Opin Neurol 2000; 13:547–552.
10. Bohannon R. Exercise training variables influencing the enhancement of voluntary muscle strength. Clin Rehabil 1990; 4:325–331.
11. Aitkens S, McCrory M, Kilmer D, Bernauer E. Moderate resistance exercise program: Its effect in slowly progressive neuromuscular disease. Arch Phys Med Rehabil 1993; 74:711–715.
12. Kilmer D, McCrory M, Wright N, Aitkens S, Bernauer E. The effect of a high resistance exercise program in slowly progressive neuromuscular disease. Arch Phys Med Rehabil 1994; 75:560–563.
13. Kobashigawa J, Leaf D, Lee N, Gleeson M, Liu H, Hamilton M, Moriguchi J, Kawata N, Einhorn K, Herlihy E, Laks H. A controlled trial of exercise rehabilitation after heart transplantation. N Engl J Med 1999; 340:272–277.
14. Brinkmann J, Ringel S. Effectiveness of exercise in progressive neuromuscular disease. J Neurol Rehabil 1991; 5:195–199.
15. Taivassalo T, Shoubridge E, Chen J, Kennaway N, DiMauro S, Arnold D, Haller R. Aerobic conditioning in patients with mitochondrial myopathies: Physiological, biochemical, and genetic effects. Ann Neurol 2001; 50:133–141.
16. Milner-Brown H, Miller R. Muscle strengthening through high-resistance weight training in patients with neuromuscular disorders. Arch Phys Med Rehabil 1988; 69:14–19.
17. Miller R. The effects of aging upon nerve and muscle function and their importance for neurorehabilitation. J Neurol Rehabil 1995; 9:175–181.
18. Cooper R, Quatrano L, Axelson P. Research on physical activity and health among people with disabilities: a consensus statement. J Rehabil Res Dev 1999; 36:142–154.
19. Fiatarone M, O'Neill E, Ryan N, Clements KM, Solares G, Nelson M, Roberts S, Kehayias J, Lipsitz L, Evans W. Exercise training and nutritional supplementation for physical frailty in very elderly people. N Engl J Med 1994; 330:1769–1775.
20. Annoni J-M, Chevrolet J, Kesselring J. Respiratory problems in chronic neurological disorders. Crit Rev Phys Rehabil Med 1993; 5:155–192.
21. Heckmatt J, Dubowitz V. Night-time nasal ventilation in neuromuscular disease. Lancet 1990; 1:579–581.
22. Bach J. Pulmonary rehabilitation considerations for Duchenne muscular dystrophy. Crit Rev Phys Rehabil Med 1992; 3:239–269.
23. Bach J. Intubation and tracheostomy paradigm paralysis. Neurology 2000; 55:613–614.
24. Bach J. Amyotrophic lateral sclerosis: Predictors for prolongation of life by noninvasive respiratory aids. Arch Phys Med Rehabil 1995; 76:828–832.
25. Annane D, Chevrolet J, Chevret S, Raphael J. Nocturnal mechanical ventilation for chronic hypoventilation in patients with neuromuscular and chest wall disorders. In: Review C, ed. The Cochrane Library: Oxford: Update Software, 2000.
26. Nomori H, Ishihara T. Pressure-controlled ventilation via a mini-tracheostomy tube for patients with neuromuscular disease. Neurology 2000; 55:698–702.
27. Reynolds J, Mendell J. Another approach to ventilatory failure in neuromuscular disease. Neurology 2000; 55:611–612.
28. Bach J, Barnett V. Ethical considerations in the management of individuals with severe neuromuscular disorders. Am J Phys Med Rehabil 1994; 73:134–140.
29. Moss A, Casey P, Stocking C, Roos R, Brooks B, Siegler M. Home ventilation for ALS patients. Neurology 1993; 43:438–443.
30. Munsat T, Andres P, Finison L, Conlon T, Thibodeau L. The natural history of motoneuron loss in amyotrophic lateral sclerosis. Neurology 1988; 38:409–413.
31. Andres P, Finison L, Conlon T, Munsat T. Use of composite scores (megascores) to measure deficit in ALS. Neurology 1988; 38:405–408.
32. Slavin M, Jette D, Andres P, Munsat T. Lower extremity muscle force measures and functional ambulation in patients with amyotrophic lateral sclerosis. Arch Phys Med Rehabil 1998; 79:950–954.
33. Maselli R, Wollman R, Leung C, Distad B, Palombi S, Richman D, Salazar-Grueso E, Roos R. Neuromuscular transmission in amyotrophic lateral sclerosis. Muscle Nerve 1993; 16:1193–1203.
34. Kubler A, Neumann N, Kaiser J, Kotchoubey B, Hinterberger T, Birbaumer N. Brain-computer communication: Self-regulation of slow cortical potentials for verbal communication. Arch Phys Med Rehabil 2001; 82:1533–1539.
35. Gregory S, Siderowf A, Golaszewski A, McCluskey

L. Gastrostomy insertion in ALS patients with low vital capacity: Respiratory support and survival. Neurology 2002; 58:485–488.

36. Windebank A, Litchy W, Daube J, Kurland L. Late effects of paralytic poliomyelitis in Olmsted County, Minnesota. Neurology 1991; 41:501–507.

37. Sonies B, Dalakas M. Dysphagia in patients with the post-polio syndrome. N Eng J Med 1991; 324:1162–1167.

38. Goerss J, Atkinson E, Winderbank A, O'Fallon W, Melton LJ 3rd. Fractures in an aging population of poliomyelitis survivors: A community based study in Olmstead County. Mayo Clin Proc 1994; 69:333–339.

39. Windebank A, Litchy W, Daube J, Iverson R. Lack of progression of neurologic deficit in survivors of paralytic polio: A 5-year prospective population-based study. Neurology 1996; 46:80–84.

40. Ivanyi B, Nollet F, Redekop W. Late onset polio sequelae: disabilities and handicaps in a population-based cohort of the 1956 poliomyelitis outbreak in the Netherlands. Arch Phys Med Rehabil 1999; 80:687–690.

41. Kemp B, Krause J. Depression and life satisfaction among people ageing with post-polio and spinal cord injury. Disabil Rehabil 1999; 21:241–249.

42. Trojan D, Cashman N. Pathophysiology and diagnosis of post-polio syndrome. NeuroRehabil 1997; 8:83–92.

43. Sharma K, Kent-Braun J, Miller R, Mynhier M, Weiner M. Excessive muscular fatigue in the postpoliomyelitis syndrome. Neurology 1994; 44:642–646.

44. Sunnerhagen K, Carlsson U, Sandberg A, Stalberg E, Hedberg M, Grimby G. Electrophysiologic evaluation of muscle fatigue development and recovery in late polio. Arch Phys Med Rehabil 2000; 81:770–776.

45. Nollet F, Beelen A, Sargeant A, de Visser M, Lankhorst G, de Jong B. Submaximal exercise capacity and maximal power output in polio subjects. Arch Phys Med Rehabil 2001; 82:1678–1685.

46. Jones D, Speier J, Canine K, Owen R, Stull G. Cardiorespiratory responses to aerobic training by patients with postpoliomyelitis sequelae. JAMA 1989; 261:3255–3258.

47. Einarsson G. Muscle conditioning in late poliomyelitis. Arch Phys Med Rehabil 1991; 72:11–14.

48. Agre J, Rodriquez A, Franke T. Strength, endurance, and work capacity after muscle strengthening exercise in postpolio subjects. Arch Phys Med Rehabil 1997; 78:681–686.

49. Perry J, Mulroy S, Renwick S. The relationship of lower extremity strength and gait parameters in patients with post-polio syndrome. Arch Phys Med Rehabil 1993; 74:165–169.

50. Dalakas M. Why drugs fail in postpolio syndrome: lessons from another clinical trial. Neurology 1999; 53:1166–1167.

51. Trojan D, Collet J, Shapiro S, Tandan R, Granger C, Robinson A, Finch L, Ducruet T, Jubelt B, Miller R, Agre J, Munsat T, Hollander D, Cashman N. A multicenter, randomized, double-blinded trial of pyridostigmine in postpolio syndrome. Neurology 1999; 53:1225–1233.

52. Gupta K, Shetty K, Agre J, Cuisinier M, Rudman I, Rudman D. Human growth hormone effect on serum IGF-I and muscle function in poliomyelitis survivors. Arch Phys Med Rehabil 1994; 75:889–894.

53. Vickrey B, Hays R, Beckstrand M. Development of a health-related quality of life measure for peripheral neuropathy. Neurorehabil Neural Repair 2000; 14:93–104.

54. Fletcher D, Lawn N, Wolter T, Wijdicks E. Long-term outcome in patients with Guillain-Barre syndrome requiring mechanical ventilation. Neurology 2000; 54:2311–2315.

55. Lennon S, Koblar S, Hughes R. Reasons for persistent disability in Guillain-Barre syndrome. Clin Rehabil 1993; 7:1–8.

56. Bergin P, Miller D, Hirsch N, Murray N. Failure of 3,4-diaminopyridine to reverse conduction block in inflammatory demyelinating neuropathies. Ann Neurol 1993; 34:406–409.

57. Mackinnon S, Dellon A. Surgery of the Peripheral Nerve. New York: Thieme, 1988:521–533.

58. Feldman E, Russell J, Sullivan K, Golovoy D. New insights into the pathogenesis of diabetic neuropathy. Curr Opin Neurol 1999; 12:553–563.

59. Ruff R. Acute illness myopathy. Neurology 1996; 46:600–601.

60. Bolton C, Young G, Zochodne D. The neurological complications of sepsis. Ann Neurol 1993; 33:94–100.

61. Wheeler, A, Bernard G. Treating patients with severe sepsis. New Engl J Med 1999; 340:207–214.

62. Guttridge D, Mayo M, Madrid L, Wang C, Baldwin A. NF-kappaB-induced loss of myoD messenger RNA: possible role in muscle decay and cachexia. Science 2000; 289:2363–2365.

63. Zifko U. Long-term outcome of critical care illness polyneuropathy. Muscle Nerve 2000; 23(suppl 9):S49–S52.

64. Spector S, Lemmer J, Koffman B, Fleisher T, Feuerstein IM, Hurley B, Dalakas M. Safety and efficacy of strength training in patients with sporadic inclusion body myositis. Muscle Nerve 1997; 20:1242–1248.

65. Czerwinski S, Kurowski T, O'Neill T, Hickson R. Initiating regular exercise protects against muscle atrophy from glucocorticoids. J Appl Physiol 1987; 63:1504–1510.

66. Kissel J, McDermott M, Mendell J, King W, Pandya S, Griggs R, Tawil R. Randomized, double-blinded, placebo-controlled trial of albuterol in facioscapulohumeral dystrophy. Neurology 2001; 57:1434–1440.

67. Lohi E-L, Lindberg C, Andersen O. Physical training effects in myasthenia gravis. Arch Phys Med Rehabil 1993; 74:1178–1180.

68. Mouradian M. Recent advances in the genetics and pathogenesis of Parkinson's disease. Neurology 2002; 58:179–185.

69. Jankovic J. New and emerging therapies for Parkinson disease. Arch Neurol 1999; 56:785–790.

70. Zurn A, Widmer H, Aebischer P. Sustained delivery of GDNF: towards a treatment for Parkinson's disease. Brain Res Rev 2001; 36:222–229.

71. Freed C, Greene P, Breeze R, Tsai W, DuMouchel W, Kao R, Dillon S, Winfield H, Culver S, Trojanowski J, Eidelberg D, Fahn S. Transplantation of embryonic dopamine neurons for severe Parkinson's disease. N Engl J Med 2001; 344:710–719.

72. Saint-Cyr J, Trepanier L, Kumar R, Lozano A, Lang A. Neuropsychological consequences of chronic bilateral stimulation of the subthalamic nucleus in parkinson's disease. Brain 2000; 123:2091–2108.

73. Straits-Troster K, Fields J, Wilkinson S, Pahwa R, Lyons K, Koller W, Troster A. Health-related quality of life in Parkinson's disease after pallidotomy and deep brain stimulation. Brain Cognit 2000; 42:399–416.

74. Gibberd F, Page N, Spencer K, Kinnear E, Hawksworth J. Controlled trial of physiotherapy and occupational therapy for Parkinson's disease. Br Med J 1981; 282:1196.

75. Tillerson JL, Cohen AD, Philhower J, Miller GW, Zigmond MJ, Schallert T. Forced limb-use effects on the behavioral and neurochemical effects of 6-hydroxydopamine. J Neurosci 2001; 21:4427–4435.

76. Benecke R, Rothwell J, Dick J, Marsden C. Disturbance of sequential movements in patients with Parkinson's disease. Brain 1987; 110:361–379.

77. Soliveri P, Brown R, Jahanshahi M, Marsden C. Effect of performance of a skilled motor task in patients with Parkinson's disease. J Neurol Neurosurg Psychiatry 1992; 55:454–460.

78. Yekutiel M, Pinhasov A, Shahar G, Sroka H. A clinical trial of the re-education of movement in patients with Parkinson's disease. Clin Rehabil 1991; 5:207–214.

79. Riley D, Lang A, Blair R, Birnbaum A, Reid B. Frozen shoulder and other shoulder disturbances in parkinson's disease. J Neurol Neurosurg Psychiatry 1989; 52:63–66.

80. Bowes S, Charlett A, Dobbs R, Lubel D, Mehta R, O'Neill C, Weller C, Hughes J, Dobbs S. Gait in relation to ageing and idiopathic Parkinsonism. Scand J Rehabil Med 1992; 24:157–160.

81. Comella C, Stebbins G, Brown-Toms N, Goetz C. Physical therapy and Parkinson's disease: A controlled clinical trial. Neurology 1994; 44:376–378.

82. Formisano R, Pratesi I, Modarelli F, Bonifati V, Meco G. Rehabilitation and Parkinson's disease. Scand J Rehabil Med 1992; 24:157–160.

83. Bagley S, Kelly B, Tunnicliffe N. The effect of visual cues on the gait of independently mobile Parkinson's disease patients. Physiotherapy 1991; 77:415–420.

84. Lewis G, Byblow W, Walt S. Stride length regulation in Parkinson's disease: The use of extrinsic, visual cues. Brain 2000; 123:2077–90.

85. Hanakawa T, Fukuyama H, Katsumi Y, Honda M, Shibasaki H. Enhanced lateral premotor activity during paradoxical gait in Parkinson's disease. Ann Neurol 1999; 45:329–336.

86. Thaut M, McIntosh G, Rice R, Miller R, Rathbun J, Brault J. Rhythmic auditory stimulation in gait training for Parkinson's disease patients. Mov Disord 1996; 11:193–200.

87. Patti F, Reggio A, Nicoletti F, Sellaroli T. Effects of rehabilitation therapy on Parkinson's disability and functional independence. J Neurol Rehabil 1996; 10:223–231.

88. Miyai I, Fujimoto Y, Ueda Y, Yamamoto H, Nozaki S, Saito T, Kang J. Treadmill training with body weight support: Its effect on Parkinson's disease. Arch Phys Med Rehabil 2000; 81:849–52.

89. Ziv I, Avraham M, Michaelov Y. Enhanced fatigue during motor performance in patients with Parkinson's disease. Neurology 1998; 51:1583–1586.

90. Brooks D, Doder M. Depression in Parkinson's disease. Curr Opin Neurol 2001; 14:465–470.

91. Rodriguez M, Siva A, Ward J, Kurland L, Stolp-Smith K, O'Brien P. Impairment, disability, and handicap in multiple sclerosis. Neurology 1994; 44:28–33.

92. Weinshenker B, Bass B, Rice G, Noseworthy J, Carriere W, Baskerville J, Ebers G. The natural history of multiple sclerosis: A geographically-based study. Brain 1989; 112:133–146.

93. Confavreux C, Vukusic S, Moreau T, Adeleine P. Relapses and progression of disability in multiple sclerosis. N Engl J Med 2000; 343:1430–1438.

94. Gulick E. Model confirmation of the MS-Related Symptom Checklist. Nurs Res 1989; 38:147–153.

95. Granger C, Cotter A, Hamilton B, Fiedler R, Hens M. Functional assessment scales: A study of persons with multiple sclerosis. Arch Phys Med Rehabil 1990; 71:870–875.

96. Rudick R, Miller D, Clough J, Gragg L, Farmer R. Quality of life in multiple sclerosis. Arch Neurol 1992; 49:1237–1242.

97. Vickrey B, Hays R, Harooni R, Myers L, Ellison G. A health-related quality of life measure for multiple sclerosis. Qual Life Res 1995; 4:187–206.

97a. Ford HL, Tennant G, Whalley A. Developing a disease-specific quality of life measure for people with MS. Clin Rehabil 2001; 15:247–258.

97b. Hobart JC, Lamping D, Fitzpatrick R. The Multiple Sclerosis Impact Scale: A new patient-based outcome measure. Brain 2001; 124:962–973.

98. Goodin D, Frohman E, Garmany G, Halper J, Likosky W, Lublin F, Silberberg D, Stuart W, van den Noort S. Disease modifying therapies in multiple sclerosis. Neurology 2002; 58:169–178.

99. Reddy H, Narayanan S, Arnoutelis R, Jenkinson M, Antel J, Matthews P, Arnold D. Evidence for adaptive functional changes in the cerebral cortex with axonal injury from multiple sclerosis. Brain 2000; 123:2314–2320.

100. Lee M, Reddy H, Johansen-Berg H, Pendlebury S, Jenkinson M, Smith S, Palace J, Matthews P. The motor cortex shows adaptive functional changes to brain injury from multiple sclerosis. Ann Neurol 2000; 47:606–613.

101. Trapp B, Peterson J, Ransohoff R, Rubick R, Mork S, Bo L. Axonal transection in the lesions of multiple sclerosis. N Engl J Med 1998; 338:278–285.

102. Shakespeare D, Boffild M, Young C. Anti-spasticity agents for multiple sclerosis (Cochrane Review). The Cochrane Library, Issue 4: Oxford: Update Software, 2001.

103. Smith C, Birnbaum G, Carter J, Greenstein J, Lublin F. Tizanidine treatment of spasticity caused by multiple sclerosis. Neurology 1994; 44(Suppl 9):S34–S43.

104. Nance P, Sheremata W, Lynch S, Vollmer T, Hudson S, Francis G, O'Connor P, Cohen J, Schapiro R, Whitham R, Mass M, Lindsey J, Shellenberger K. Relationship of the antispasticity effect of tizanidine to plasma concentration in patients with multiple sclerosis. Arch Neurol 1997; 54:731–736.

105. Mattison P. Transcutaneous electrical nerve stimulation in the management of painful muscle spasm in multiple sclerosis. Clin Rehabil 1993; 7:45–48.

106. DeLuca J, Johnson S. Cognitive impairments in multiple sclerosis. NeuroRehabil 1993; 3(4):9–16.

107. Beatty W, Goodkin D. Screening for cognitive impairment in multiple sclerosis. Arch Neurol 1990; 47:297–301.

108. Sullivan M, Weinshenker B, Mikail S, Bishop S.

Screening for major depression in the early stages of MS. Can J Neurol Sci 1995; 22:228–231.

109. Traccis S, Rosati C, Monaco M. Successful treatment of acquired pendular elliptical nystagmus in multiple sclerosis with isoniazid and base-out prisms. Neurology 1990; 40:492–494.

110. Schwid S, Thornton C, Pandya S. Quantitative assessment of motor fatigue and strength in MS. Neurology 1999; 53:743–750.

111. Krupp L, Elkins L. Fatigue and declines in cognitive functioning in multiple sclerosis. Neurology 2000; 55:934–939.

112. Miller R, Green A, Moussavi R, Carson P, Weiner M. Excessive muscular fatigue in patients with spastic paraparesis. Neurology 1990; 40:1271–1274.

113. Sheean G, Murray N, Rothwell J, Miller D, Thompson A. An electrophysiological study of the mechanism of fatigue in multiple sclerosis. Brain 1997; 120:299–315.

114. Bakshi R, Miletich R, Henschel K. Fatigue in multiple sclerosis: Cross-sectional correlation with brain MRI findings in 71 patients. Neurology 1999; 53:1151–1153.

115. Sheean G, Murray N, Rothwell J, Miller D, Thompson A. An open-labelled clinical and electrophysiological study of 3,4 diaminopyridine in the treatment of fatigue in multiple sclerosis. Brain 1998; 121:967–975.

116. Roelcke U, Kappos L, Lechner-Scott J, Brunnschweiler H, Leenders K, Huber S, Ammann W, Plohmann A, Dellas S, Maguire R, Missimer JI, Radu E, Steck A. Reduced glucose metabolism in the frontal cortex and basal ganglia of multiple sclerosis patients with fatigue. Neurology 1997; 48:1566–1571.

117. Leocani L, Colombo B, Magnani G, et al. Fatigue in multiple sclerosis is associated with abnormal cortical activation to voluntary movement-EEG evidence. NeuroImage 2001; 13:1186–1192.

118. Kinkel R, Conway K, Copperman L, Forwell S, Hugos C. Fatigue and multiple sclerosis. Multiple Sclerosis Council for Clinical Practice Guidelines. Washington, D.C.: Paralysed Veterans of America, 1998.

119. Canadian MS Research Group. A randomized controlled trial of amantadine in fatigue associated with multiple sclerosis. Can J Neurol Sci 1987; 14:273–278.

120. Weinshenker B, Penman M, Bass R, Ebers G, Rice G. A double-blind, randomized crossover trial of pemoline in fatigue associated with multiple sclerosis. Neurology 1992; 42:1468–1471.

121. Polman C, Bertelsmann F, van Loenen A, Koetsier J. 4-aminopyridine in the treatment of patients with MS. Arch Neurol 1994; 51:292–296.

122. Polman C, Bertelsmann F, de Waal R, van Dieman, Uitdehaag B, van Loenen A, Koetsier J. 4-aminopyridine is superior to 3,4-diaminopyridine in the treatment of patients with multiple sclerosis. Arch Neurol 1994; 51:1136–1139.

123. Bever C. The current status of studies of aminopyridines in patients with multiple sclerosis. Ann Neurol 1994; 36:S118–S121.

124. van Dieman H, Polman C, van Dongen T, van Loenen A, Nauta J, Taphoorn M, van Walbeek H, Koetsier J. The effect of 4-aminopyridine on clinical signs in multiple sclerosis. Ann Neurol 1992; 32:123–130.

125. Bever C, Young D, Anderson P, Krumholz A, Conway K, Leslie J, Eddington N, Plaisance K, Panitch H, Dhib-Jalbut S. The effects of 4-aminopyridine in multiple sclerosis patients. Neurology 1994; 44:1054–1059.

126. Smits R, Emmen H, Bertelsmann F, Kulig B, van Loenen A, Polman C. The effects of 4-aminopyridine on cognitive function in patients with multiple sclerosis. Neurology 1994; 44:1701–1705.

127. Schwid S, Petrie M, McDermott M, Tierney D, Mason D, Goodman A. Quantitative assessment of sustained-release 4-aminopyridine for symptomatic treatment of multiple sclerosis. Neurology 1997; 48:817–21.

128. Kaji R, Happel L, Sumner A. Effect of digitalis on clinical symptoms and conduction variables in patients with multiple sclerosis. Ann Neurol 1990; 28:582–584.

129. Petajan J, Gappmaier E, White A, Spencer M, Mino L, Hicks R. Impact of aerobic training on fitness and quality of life in multiple sclerosis. Ann Neurol 1996; 39:432–441.

130. Lord S, Wade D, Halligan P. A comparison of two physiotherapy treatment approaches to improve walking in multiple sclerosis: A pilot randomized controlled study. Clin Rehabil 1998; 12:477–486.

131. Thompson A. The effectiveness of neurological rehabilitation in multiple sclerosis. J Rehabil Res Dev 2000; 37:455–461.

132. Freeman J, Langdon D, Hobart J, Thompson A. The impact of inpatient rehabilitation on progressive multiple sclerosis. Ann Neurol 1997; 42:236–44.

133. Freeman J, Langdon D, Hobart J, Thompson A. Inpatient rehabilitation in multiple sclerosis: Do the benefits carry over into the community? Neurology 1999; 52:50–56.

134. Di Fabio R, Soderberg J, Choi T, Hansen C, Shapiro R. Extended outpatient rehabilitation: Its influence on symptom frequency, fatigue and functional status for persons with progressive multiple sclerosis. Arch Phys Med Rehabil 1998; 79:141–146.

135. Lorig K, Sobel D, Stewart A, Brown B, Bandura A, Ritter P, Gonzalez V, Laurent D, Holman H. Evidence suggesting that a chronic disease self-management program can improve health status while reducing hospitalization. Med Care 1999; 37:5–14.

136. Banja J, Jann B. Ethical issues in treating pediatric rehabilitation patients. NeuroRehabil 1993; 3(3):44–52.

137. Kuban K, Leviton A. Cerebral palsy. N Eng J Med 1994; 330:188–195.

138. Azaula M, Msall M, Buck G, Tremont M, Wilczenski F, Rogers B. Measuring functional status and family support in older school-aged children with cerebral palsy: Comparison of three instruments. Arch Phys Med Rehabil 2000; 81:307–311.

139. Farmer S, Harrison L, Ingram D, Stephens J. Plasticity of central motor pathways in children with hemiplegic cerebral palsy. Neurology 1991; 41:1505–1510.

140. Eyre J, Tayulor J, Villagra F, Smith M, Miller S. Evidence of activity-dependent withdrawal of corticospinal projections during human development. Neurology 2001; 57:1543–1554.

141. Palmer F, Shapiro B, Wachtel R, Allen M, Hiller J, Harryman S, Mosher B, Meinert C, Capute A. The

effects of physical therapy on cerebral palsy. N Eng J Med 1991; 318:803–808.

142. Mayo N. The effect of physical therapy for children with motor delay and cerebral palsy. Am J Phys Med Rehabil 1991; 70:258–267.

143. Colborne G, Wright V, Naumann S. Feedback of triceps surae EMG in gait of children with cerebral palsy: A controlled study. Arch Phys Med Rehabil 1994; 75:40–45.

144. Fernandez J, Pitetti K. Training of ambulatory individuals with cerebral palsy. Arch Phys Med Rehabil 1993; 74:468–472.

145. Schindl M, Forstner C, Kern H, Hesse S. Treadmill training with partial body weight support in non-ambulatory patients with cerebral palsy. Arch Phys Med Rehabil 2000; 81:301–306.

146. Damiano D, Abel M. Functional outcomes of strength training in spastic cerebral palsy. Arch Phys Med Rehabil 1998; 79:119–125.

147. Tardeu C, Lespargot A, Tabary C, Bret M. For how long must the soleus muscle be stretched each day to prevent contracture? Dev Med Child Neurol 1988; 30:3–10.

148. Brunstrom J, Bastian A, Wong M, Mink J. Motor benefit from levodopa in spastic quadriplegic cerebral palsy. Ann Neurol 2000; 47:662–665.

149. Albright A, Barron W, Fasick M, Barry M, Shultz B. Continuous intrathecal baclofen infusion for spasticity of cerebral origin. JAMA 1993; 270:2475–2477.

150. Molenaers G, Desloovere K, Eyssen M, Decat J, Jonkers I, De Cock P. Botulinum toxin type A treatment of cerebral palsy: An integrated approach. Europ J Neurol 1999; 6:S51–S57.

151. Abel M, Damiano D, Pannunzio M, Bush J. Muscle-tendon surgery in diplegic cerebral palsy: Functional and mechanical changes. J Pediatr Orthopaed 1999; 19:366–375.

152. Peacock W, Staudt L. Functional outcomes following selective posterior rhizotomy in children with cerebral palsy. J Neurosurg 1991; 74:380–385.

153. Buckon C, Thomas S, Pierce R, Piatt J Jr, Aiona M. Developmental skills of children with spastic diplegia: Functional and qualitative changes after selective dorsal rhizotomy. Arch Phys Med Rehabil 1997; 78:946–951.

154. Schwartz L, Engel J, Jensen M. Pain in persons with cerebral palsy. Arch Phys Med Rehabil 1999; 80: 1243–1246.

155. Beaty J, Canale S. Orthopedic aspects of myelomeningocele. J Bone Joint Surg 1990; 72A:626–630.

156. Mazur J, Shurtleff D, Menelaus M, Colliver J. Orthopedic management of high-level spinal bifida. J Bone Joint Surg 1989; 71A:56–61.

157. Tinetti M, Speechley M. Prevention of falls among the elderly. N Engl J Med 1989; 320:1055–1059.

158. Tinetti M, Williams C. Falls, injuries due to falls, and the risk of admission to a nursing home. N Engl J Med 1997; 337:1279–1284.

159. Koski K, Luukinen H, Laippala P, Kivela S. Risk factors for major injurious falls among the home-dwelling elderly by functional abilities. Gerontology 1998; 44:232–238.

160. Guralnik J, Ferrucci L, Simonsick E, Salive M, Wallace R. Lower-extremity function in persons over the age of 70 years as a predictor of subsequent disability. N Engl J Med 1995; 332:556–561.

161. Rantanen T, Guralnik J, Foley D, Masaki K, Leveille S, Curb J, White L. Midlife hand grip strength as a predictor of old age disability. JAMA 1999; 281: 558–560.

162. Guttmann C, Benson R, Warfield S, Wei X, Anderson M, Hall C. White matter abnormalities in mobility-impaired older persons. Neurology 2000; 54: 1277–1283.

163. Kerber K, Enrietto J, Jacobson K, Baloh R. Disequilibrium in older people. Neurology 1998; 51:574–580.

164. Penninx B, Guralnik J, Ferucci L, Simonsick E, Deeg D, Wallace R. Depressive symptoms and physical decline in community-dwelling older persons. JAMA 1998; 279:1720–1726.

165. Thapa P, Gideon P, Cost T, Milam A, Ray W. Antidepressants and the risk of falls among nursing home residents. N Engl J Med 1998; 339:875–881.

166. Gehlsen G, Whaley M. Falls in the elderly: Part 1, Gait. Arch Phys Med Rehabil 1990; 71:735–738.

167. Kerrigan D, Lee L, Nieto T, Markman J, Collins J, Riley P. Kinetic alterations independent of walking speed in elderly fallers. Arch Phys Med Rehabil 2000; 81:730–735.

168. Rudman D, Feller A, Nagraj H, Gergans G, Lalitha P, Goldberg A, Schlenker R, Cohn L, Rudman I, Mattson D. Effects of human growth hormone in men over 60 years old. N Eng J Med 1990; 323:1–6.

169. Applegate W, Miller S, Graney M, Elam J, Burns R, Akins D. A randomized, controlled trial of a geriatric assessment unit in a community rehabilitation hospital. N Engl J Med 1990; 322:1572–1578.

170. Munin M, Rudy T, Glynn N, Crossett L, Rubash H. Early inpatient rehabilitation after elective hip and knee arthroplasty. JAMA 1998; 279:847–852.

171. Mulrow C, Gerety M, Kanten D, Cornell J, DeNino L, Chiodo L, Aguilar C, O'Neil M, Rosenberg J, Solis R. A randomized trial of physical rehabilitation for very frail nursing home residents. JAMA 1994; 271: 513–524.

172. Tinetti M, Baker D, McAvay G, Claus E, Garrett P, Gottschalk M, Koch M, Trainor K, Horwitz R. A multifactorial intervention to reduce the risk of falling among elderly people living in the community. N Eng J Med 1994; 331:821–827.

173. Clark F, Azen S, Zemke R, Jackson J, Carlson M, Mandel D, Hay J, Josephson K, Cherry B, Hessel C, Palmer J, Lipson L. Occupational therapy for independent-living older adult. JAMA 1997; 278:1321–1326.

174. Smith P. Pharmacology of the vestibular system. Curr Opin Neurol 2000; 13:31–37.

175. Eagger S, Luxon L, Davies R, Coelho A, Ron M. Psychiatric morbidity in patients with peripheral vestibular disorder. J Neurol Neurosurg Psychiatry 1992; 55:383–387.

176. Yardley L, Owen N, Nazareth I, Luxon L. Prevalence and presentation of dizziness in a general practice community sample of working age people. Br J Gen Pract 1998; 48:1131–1136.

177. Staab J. Diagnosis and treatment of psychologic symptoms and psychiatric disorders in patients with dizziness and imbalance. Otolaryngol Clin North Am 2000; 33:617–635.

178. Strupp M, Arbusow V, Maag K, Gall C, Brandt T. Vestibular exercises improve central vestibulospinal compensation after vestibular neuritis. Neurology 1998; 51:838–844.

179. Norre M. Rehabilitation treatments for vertigo and related syndromes. Crit Rev Phys Rehabil Med 1990; 2:101–120.
180. Froehling D, Silverstein M, Mohr D, Beatty C, Offord K, Ballard D. Benign positional vertigo: Incidence and prognosis in Olmsted County, Minnesota. Mayo Clin Proc 1991; 66:596–601.
181. Troost B, Patton J. Exercise therapy for positional vertigo. Neurology 1992; 42:1441–1444.
182. Brandt T, Steddin S, Daroff R. Therapy for benign paroxysmal positioning vertigo, revisited. Neurology 1994; 44:796–800.
183. Small G, Rabins P, Barry P, Buckholtz N, Dekosky S, Ferris S, Finkel S, Gwyther L, Khachaturian Z, Lebowitz B, McRae T, Morris J, Oakley F, Schneider L, Stremin J, Sunderland T, Teri L, Tune L. Diagnosis and treatment of Alzheimer disease and related disorders. JAMA 1997; 278:1363–1371.
184. Pomeroy V. The effect of physiotherapy input on mobility skills of elderly people with severe dementing illness. Clin Rehabil 1993; 7:163–170.
185. Eslinger P, Damasio A. Preserved motor learning in Alzheimer's disease: Implications for anatomy and behavior. J Neurosci 1986; 6:3006–3009.
186. Dick M, Hsieh S, Dick-Muehlke C, Davis D, Cotman C. The variability of practice hypothesis in motor learning: Does it apply to Alzheimer's disease? Brain Cogn 2000; 44:470–489.
187. Phillips C, Sloane P, Hawes C, Koch G, Han J, Spry K, Dunteman G, Williams R. Effects of residence in Alzheimer disease special care units on functional outcomes. JAMA 1997; 278:1340–1344.
188. Teri L, McCurry S, Buchner D, Logsdon R, LaCroix A, Kukull W, Barlow W, Larson E. Exercise and activity level in Alzheimer's disease: A potential treatment focus. J Rehabil Res Dev 1998; 35:411–419.
189. Engel J. Etiology as a risk factor for medically refractory epilepsy: A case for early surgical intervention. Neurology 1998; 51:1243–1244.
190. Fraser R, Gumnit R, Dobkin B, Thorbecke R. Psychosocial rehabilitation: A pre- and post-operative perspective. In: Engel J, ed. Surgical Treatment of the Epilepsies. New York: Raven Press, 1993.
190a. Rausch R. Epilepsy surgery within the temporal lobe and its short-term and long-term effects on memory. Curr Opin Neurol 2002; 15:185–189.
191. Birbeck G, Kim S, Hays R, Vickrey B. Quality of life measures in epilepsy: How well can they detect change over time? Neurology 2000; 54:1822–1827.
192. Jason L, Richman J, Rademaker A, Jordan K, Plioplys A, Taylor R, McCredy W, Huang C, Plioplys S. A community-based study of chronic fatigue syndrome. Arch Inten Med 1999; 159:2129–2137.
193. Natelson B. Chronic fatigue syndrome. JAMA 2001; 285:2557–2559.
194. Bou-Holaigah I, Rowe P, Kan J, Calkins H. The relationship between neurally mediated hypotension and the chronic fatigue syndrome. JAMA 1995; 274:961–967.
195. Rowe P, Calkins H, DeBusk K, McKensie R, Anand R, Sharma G, Cuccherini B, Soto N, Hohman P, Snader S, Lucas K, Wolff M, Straus S. Fludrocortisone acetate to treat neurally mediated hypotension in chronic fatigue syndrome: A randomized controlled trial. JAMA 2001; 285:52–59.
196. Joyce E, Blumenthal S, Wessely S. Memory, attention, and executive function in chronic fatigue syndrome. J Neurol Neurosurg Psychiatry 1996; 60:495–503.
197. Whiting P, Bagnall A-M, Sowden A, Cornell J, Mulrow C, Ramirez G. Interventions for the treatment and management of chronic fatigue syndrome. JAMA 2001; 286:1360–1368.
198. d'Arminio Monforte A, Duca P, Vago L, Grassi M, Moroni M. Decreasing incidence of CNS AIDS-defining events associated with antiretroviral therapy. Neurology 2000; 54:1856–1859.
199. Kraft G, Freal J, Coryll J. Disability, disease duration and rehabilitation service needs in multiple sclerosis: Patient perspectives. Arch Phys Med Rehabil 1986; 67:164–178.

Index

Page numbers followed by f and t indicate figures and tables, respectively.